BIOPHARMACEUTICALS
BIOCHEMISTRY AND BIOTECHNOLOGY

Second Edition

BIOPHARMACEUTICALS
BIOCHEMISTRY AND BIOTECHNOLOGY

Second Edition

Gary Walsh

Industrial Biochemistry Programme
CES Department
University of Limerick, Ireland

WILEY

First Edition 1998 © John Wiley & Sons, Ltd

Copyright © 2003 John Wiley & Sons Ltd, The Atrium, Southern Gate, Chichester, West Sussex PO19 8SQ, England

Telephone (+44) 1243 779777

E-mail (for orders and customer service enquiries): cs-books@wiley.co.uk
Visit our Home Page on www.wileyeurope.com or www.wiley.com

Reprinted January 2004

Other Wiley Editorial Offices

John Wiley & Sons Inc., 111 River Street, Hoboken, NJ 07030, USA

Jossey-Bass, 989 Market Street, San Francisco, CA 94103-1741, USA

Wiley-VCH Verlag GmbH, Boschstr. 12, D-69469 Weinheim, Germany

John Wiley & Sons Australia Ltd, 33 Park Road, Milton, Queensland 4064, Australia

John Wiley & Sons (Asia) Pte Ltd, 2 Clementi Loop #02-01, Jin Xing Distripark, Singapore 129809

John Wiley & Sons Canada Ltd, 22 Worcester Road, Etobicoke, Ontario, Canada M9W 1L1

Wiley also publishes its books in a variety of electronic formats. Some content that appears in print may not be available in electronic books.

British Library Cataloguing in Publication Data

A catalogue record for this book is available from the British Library

ISBN 0 470 84326 8 (ppc)
ISBN 0 470 84327 6 (pbk)

Typeset by Dobbie Typesetting Ltd, Tavistock, Devon
Printed and bound in Great Britain by Antony Rowe Ltd, Chippenham, Wilts
This book is printed on acid-free paper responsibly manufactured from sustainable forestry in which at least two trees are planted for each one used for paper production.

I dedicate this book to my beautiful son Shane, born during the revision of Chapter 6. I include his photograph in the hope that a Hollywood producer, looking for a child film star, will spot it and immediately offer to make us suitably rich. In the future, I also hope to use it to embarrass him during his teenage years, by showing it to all his cool, sophisticated friends.

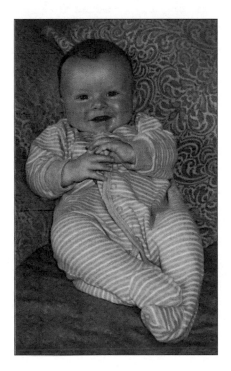

Contents

Preface

Advances in our understanding of the molecular principles underlining both health and disease has revealed the existence of many regulatory polypeptides of significant medical potential. The fact that such polypeptides are produced naturally within the body only in minute quantities initially precluded their large-scale medical application. The development in the 1970s of the twin techniques of genetic engineering and hybridoma technology marked the birth of the modern biotech era. These techniques facilitate the large-scale production of virtually any protein, and proteins of medical interest produced by these methodologies have been coined 'biopharmaceuticals'. More recent developments in biomedical research highlights the clinical potential of nucleic acid-based therapeutic agents. Gene therapy and anti-sense technology are likely to become a medical reality within a decade. The term 'biopharmaceutical' now also incorporates the polynucleotide sequences utilized for such purposes.

This book attempts to provide a balanced overview of the biopharmaceutical industry, not only in terms of categorizing the products currently available, but also illustrating how these drugs are produced and brought to market. Chapter 1 serves as an introduction to the topic, and also focuses upon several 'traditional' pharmaceutical substances isolated (initially at least) from biological sources. This serves as a backdrop for the remaining chapters, which focus almost exclusively upon recently developed biopharmaceutical products. The major emphasis is placed upon polypeptide-based therapeutic agents, while the potential of nucleic acid-based drugs is discussed in the final chapter.

In preparing the latest edition of this textbook, I highlight the latest developments within the sector, provide a greater focus upon actual commercial products thus far approved and how they are manufactured, and I include substantial new sections detailing biopharmaceutical drug delivery and how advances in genomics and proteomics will likely impact upon (bio)pharmaceutical drug development.

The major target audience is that of advanced undergraduates or postgraduate students pursuing courses in relevant aspects of the biological sciences. The book should prove particularly interesting to students undertaking programmes in biotechnology, biochemistry, the pharmaceutical sciences, medicine or any related biomedical subject. A significant additional target audience are those already employed in the (bio)pharmaceutical sector, who wish to gain a better overview of the industry in which they work.

The successful completion of this text has been made possible by the assistance of several people to whom I owe a depth of gratitude. Chief amongst these is Sandy Lawson, who appears to be able to read my mind as well as my handwriting. Thank you to Nancy, my beautiful wife, who suffered most from my becoming a social recluse during the preparation of this text. Thank you, Nancy, for not carrying out your threat to burn the manuscript on various occasions, and for helping with the proof-reading. I am also very grateful to the staff of John Wiley and Sons Ltd for the professionalism and efficiency they exhibited while bringing this book through the publication process. The assistance of companies who provided information and photographs for inclusion in the text is also gratefully acknowledged, as is the cooperation of those publishers who granted me permission to include certain copyrighted material. Finally, a word of appreciation to all my colleagues at Limerick, who continue to make our university such a great place to work.

Gary Walsh
Limerick, November 2002

Chapter 1

Pharmaceuticals, biologics and biopharmaceuticals

INTRODUCTION TO PHARMACEUTICAL PRODUCTS

Pharmaceutical substances form the backbone of modern medicinal therapy. Most traditional pharmaceuticals are low molecular mass organic chemicals (Table 1.1). Although some (e.g. aspirin) were originally isolated from biological sources, most are now manufactured by direct chemical synthesis. Two types of manufacturing companies thus comprise the 'traditional' pharmaceutical sector; the chemical synthesis plants, which manufacture the raw chemical ingredients in bulk quantities, and the finished product pharmaceutical facilities, which purchase these raw bulk ingredients, formulate them into final pharmaceutical products, and supply these products to the end-user.

In addition to chemical-based drugs, a range of pharmaceutical substances (e.g. hormones and blood products) are produced by or extracted from biological sources. Such products, some major examples of which are listed in Table 1.2, may thus be described as products of biotechnology. In some instances, categorizing pharmaceuticals as products of biotechnology or chemical synthesis becomes somewhat artificial, e.g. certain semi-synthetic antibiotics are produced by chemical modification of natural antibiotics produced by fermentation technology.

BIOPHARMACEUTICALS AND PHARMACEUTICAL BIOTECHNOLOGY

Terms such as 'biologic', 'biopharmaceutical' and 'products of pharmaceutical biotechnology' or 'biotechnology medicines' have now become an accepted part of the pharmaceutical literature. However, these terms are sometimes used interchangeably and can mean different things to different people.

While it might be assumed that 'biologic' refers to any pharmaceutical product produced by biotechnological endeavour, its definition is more limited. In pharmaceutical circles, 'biologic'

Biopharmaceuticals: Biochemistry and Biotechnology, Second Edition. Gary Walsh
John Wiley & Sons Ltd: ISBN 0 470 84326 8 (ppc), ISBN 0 470 84327 6 (pbk)

Table 1.1. Some traditional pharmaceutical substances which are generally produced by direct chemical synthesis

Drug	Molecular formula	Molecular mass	Therapeutic indication
Acetaminophen (paracetamol)	$C_8H_9NO_2$	151.16	Analgesic
Ketamine	$C_{13}H_{16}ClNO$	237.74	Anaesthetic
Levamisole	$C_{11}H_{12}N_2S$	204.31	Anthelmintic
Diazoxide	$C_8H_7ClN_2O_2S$	230.7	Anti-hypertensive
Acyclovir	$C_8H_{11}N_5O_3$	225.2	Anti-viral agent
Zidovudine	$C_{10}H_{13}N_5O_4$	267.2	Anti-viral agent
Dexamethasone	$C_{22}H_{29}FO_5$	392.5	Anti-inflammatory and immunosuppressive agent
Misoprostol	$C_{22}H_{38}O_5$	382.5	Anti-ulcer agent
Cimetidine	$C_{10}H_{16}N_6$	252.3	Anti-ulcer agent

Table 1.2. Some pharmaceuticals which were traditionally obtained by direct extraction from biological source material. Many of the protein-based pharmaceuticals mentioned below are now also produced by genetic engineering

Substance	Medical application
Blood products (e.g. coagulation factors)	Treatment of blood disorders such as haemophilia A or B
Vaccines	Vaccination against various diseases
Antibodies	Passive immunization against various diseases
Insulin	Treatment of diabetes mellitus
Enzymes	Thrombolytic agents, digestive aids, debriding agents (i.e. cleansing of wounds)
Antibiotics	Treatment against various infectious agents
Plant extracts (e.g. alkaloids)	Various, including pain relief

generally refers to medicinal products derived from blood, as well as vaccines, toxins and allergen products. Thus, some traditional biotechnology-derived pharmaceutical products (e.g. hormones, antibiotics and plant metabolites) fall outside the strict definition.

The term 'biopharmaceutical' was first used in the 1980s and came to describe a class of therapeutic protein produced by modern biotechnological techniques, specifically via genetic engineering or (in the case of monoclonal antibodies) by hybridoma technology. This usage equated the term 'biopharmaceutical' with 'therapeutic protein synthesized in engineered (non-naturally occurring) biological systems'. More recently, however, nucleic acids used for purposes of gene therapy and antisense technology (Chapter 11) have come to the fore and they too are generally referred to as 'biopharmaceuticals'. Moreover, several recently approved proteins are used for *in vivo* diagnostic as opposed to therapeutic purposes. Throughout this book therefore, the term 'biopharmaceutical' refers to protein or nucleic acid based pharmaceutical substances used for therapeutic or *in vivo* diagnostic purposes, which are produced by means other than direct extraction from natural (non-engineered) biological sources (Tables 1.3 and 1.4).

As used herein, 'biotechnology medicines' or 'products of pharmaceutical biotechnology' are afforded a much broader definition. Unlike the term 'biopharmaceutical', the term

Table 1.3. A summary of the definition of the terms 'biologic', 'biopharmaceutical' and 'biotechnology medicine' as used throughout this book. Reprinted from European Journal of Pharmaceutical Sciences, vol 15, Walsh, Biopharmaceuticals and Biotechnology, p 135–138, ©2002, with permission from Elsevier Science

Biopharmaceutical	A protein or nucleic acid based pharmaceutical substance used for therapeutic or *in vivo* diagnostic purposes, which is produced by means other than direct extraction from a native (non-engineered) biological source
Biotechnology medicine/ product of pharmaceutical biotechnology	Any pharmaceutical product used for therapeutic or *in vivo* diagnostic purposes, which is produced in full or in part by biotechnological means
Biologic	A virus, therapeutic serum, toxin, antitoxin, vaccine, blood, blood component or derivative, allergenic product or analogous product, or arsphenamine or its derivatives or any other trivalent organic arsenic compound applicable to the prevention, cure or treatment of disease or conditions of human beings

'biotechnology' has a much broader and long-established meaning. Essentially, it refers to the use of biological systems (e.g. cells or tissues) or biological molecules (e.g. enzymes or antibodies) for or in the manufacture of commercial products. Therefore, the term is equally applicable to long-established biological processes, such as brewing, and more modern processes, such as genetic engineering. As such, the term 'biotechnology medicine' is defined here as 'any pharmaceutical product used for a therapeutic or *in vivo* diagnostic purpose, which is produced in full or in part by either traditional or modern biotechnological means'. Such products encompass, for example, antibiotics extracted from fungi, therapeutic proteins extracted from native source material (e.g. insulin from pig pancreas) and products produced by genetic engineering (e.g. recombinant insulin) (Tables 1.3 and 1.4).

HISTORY OF THE PHARMACEUTICAL INDUSTRY

The pharmaceutical industry, as we now know it, is barely 60 years old. From very modest beginnings it has grown rapidly, reaching an estimated value of $100 billion by the mid-1980s. Its current value is likely double this figure or more. There are well in excess of 10 000 pharmaceutical companies in existence, although only about 100 of these can claim to be of true international significance. These companies manufacture in excess of 5000 individual pharmaceutical substances used routinely in medicine.

The first stages of development of the modern pharmaceutical industry can be traced back to the turn of the twentieth century. At that time (apart from folk cures), the medical community had at their disposal only four drugs that were effective in treating specific diseases:

- Digitalis, extracted from foxglove, was known to stimulate heart muscle and hence was used to treat various heart conditions.
- Quinine, obtained from the barks/roots of a plant (*Cinchona* sp.), was used to treat malaria.
- Pecacuanha (active ingredient is a mixture of alkaloids), used for treating dysentery, was obtained from the bark/roots of the plant species *Cephaelis*.
- Mercury, for the treatment of syphilis.

Table 1.4. The categorization of pharmaceutically significant biological molecules using the indicated definitions as listed in Table 1.3. Reproduced in modified form from European Journal of Pharmaceutical Sciences, vol 15, Walsh, Biopharmaceuticals and Biotechnology, p 135–138, ©2002, with permission from Elsevier Science

Pharmaceutical product	Biopharmaceutical?	Biotechnology medicine?	Biologic?
Recombinant protein	Yes	Yes	No
Monoclonal antibody	Yes	Yes	No
Proteins obtained by direct extraction from native source (e.g. blood derived clotting factors)	No	Yes	Some (e.g. blood factors and polyclonal antibodies)
Gene therapy products	Yes	Yes	No
Antisense oligonucleotides manufactured by direct chemical synthesis	Yes	No	No
Antisense oligonucleotides produced by enzymatic synthesis	Yes	Yes	No
Peptides manufactured by direct chemical synthesis	No	No	No
Peptides, if obtained by direct extraction from native producer source	No	Yes	No
Antibiotics obtained by direct extraction from native producer, or by semi-synthesis	No	Yes	No
Plant-based products obtained by direct extraction from a native producer, or by semi-synthesis (e.g. taxol)	No	Yes	No
Cell/tissue-based therapeutic agents	No	Yes	No

The lack of appropriate safe and effective medicines contributed in no small way to the low life expectancy characteristic of those times.

Developments in biology (particularly the growing realization of the microbiological basis of many diseases), as well as a developing appreciation of the principles of organic chemistry, helped underpin future innovation in the fledgling pharmaceutical industry. The successful synthesis of various artificial dyes, which proved to be therapeutically useful, led to the formation of pharmaceutical/chemical companies such as Bayer and Hoechst in the late 1800s, e.g. scientists at Bayer succeeded in synthesizing aspirin in 1895.

Despite these early advances, it was not until the 1930s that the pharmaceutical industry began to develop in earnest. The initial landmark discovery of this era was probably the discovery and chemical synthesis of the sulpha drugs. These are a group of related molecules derived from the red dye, *Prontosil rubrum*. These drugs proved effective in the treatment of a wide variety of bacterial infections (Figure 1.1). Although it was first used therapeutically in the early 1920s, large-scale industrial production of insulin also commenced in the 1930s.

The medical success of these drugs gave new emphasis to the pharmaceutical industry, which was boosted further by the commencement of industrial-scale penicillin manufacture in the early 1940s. Around this time, many of the current leading pharmaceutical companies (or their forerunners) were founded. Examples include Ciba Geigy, Eli Lilly, Wellcome, Glaxo and Roche. Over the next two to three decades, these companies developed drugs such as tetracyclines, corticosteroids, oral contraceptives, antidepressants and many more. Most of these pharmaceutical substances are manufactured by direct chemical synthesis.

THE AGE OF BIOPHARMACEUTICALS

Biomedical research continues to broaden our understanding of the molecular mechanisms underlining both health and disease. Research undertaken since the 1950s has pinpointed a host of proteins produced naturally in the body which have obvious therapeutic applications. Examples include the interferons, and interleukins, which regulate the immune response; growth factors such as erythropoietin, which stimulates red blood cell production; and neurotrophic factors, which regulate the development and maintenance of neural tissue.

While the pharmaceutical potential of these regulatory molecules was generally appreciated, their widespread medical application was in most cases rendered impractical due to the tiny quantities in which they were naturally produced. The advent of recombinant DNA technology (genetic engineering) and monoclonal antibody technology (hybridoma technology) overcame many such difficulties, and marked the beginning of a new era of the pharmaceutical sciences.

Recombinant DNA technology has had a four-fold positive impact upon the production of pharmaceutically important proteins:

- *It overcomes the problem of source availability.* Many proteins of therapeutic potential are produced naturally in the body in minute quantities. Examples include interferons (Chapter 4), interleukins (Chapter 5) and colony stimulating factors (Chapter 6). This rendered impractical their direct extraction from native source material in quantities sufficient to meet likely clinical demand. Recombinant production (Chapter 3) allows the manufacture of any protein in whatever quantity it is required.
- *It overcomes problems of product safety.* Direct extraction of product from some native biological sources has, in the past, led to the unwitting transmission of disease. Examples include the transmission of blood-borne pathogens such as hepatitis B, C and HIV via infected blood products and the transmission of Creutzfeldt–Jakob disease to persons receiving human growth hormone preparations derived from human pituitaries.
- *It provides an alternative to direct extraction from inappropriate/dangerous source material.* A number of therapeutic proteins have traditionally been extracted from human urine. The fertility hormone FSH, for example, is obtained from the urine of post-menopausal women, while a related hormone, hCG, is extracted from the urine of pregnant women (Chapter 8). Urine is not considered a particularly desirable source of pharmaceutical products. While several products obtained from this source remain on the market, recombinant forms have now also been approved. Other potential biopharmaceuticals are produced naturally in downright dangerous sources. Ancrod, for example, is a protein displaying anti-coagulant activity (Chapter 9) and, hence, is of potential clinical use; however, it is produced naturally by the Malaysian pit viper. While retrieval by milking snake venom is possible, and indeed may be quite an exciting procedure, recombinant production in less dangerous organisms, such as *Escherichia coli* or *Saccharomyces cerevisiae*, would be considered preferable by most.
- *It facilitates the generation of engineered therapeutic proteins displaying some clinical*

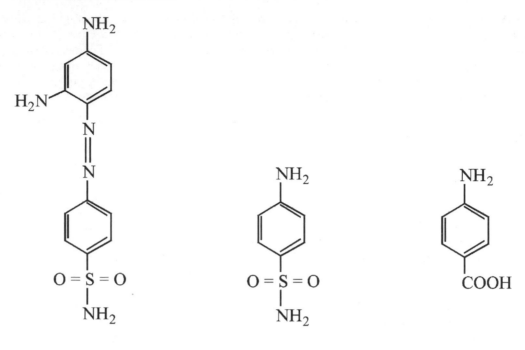

Prontosil rubrum
(a)

Sulphanilamide
(b)

PABA
(c)

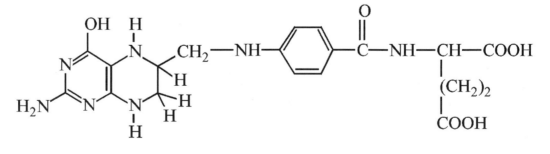

Tetrahydrofolic acid
(d)

Table 1.5. Selected engineered biopharmaceutical types/products, which have now gained marketing approval. These and additional such products will be discussed in detail in subsequent chapters

Product description/type	Alteration introduced	Rationale
Faster-acting insulins (Chapter 8)	Modified amino acid sequence	Generation of faster-acting insulin
Slow-acting insulins (Chapter 8)	Modified amino acid sequence	Generation of slow-acting insulin
Modified tissue plasminogen activator (tPA: Chapter 9)	Removal of three of the five native domains of tPA	Generation of a faster-acting thrombolytic (clot degrading) agent
Modified blood factor VIII (Chapter 9)	Deletion of one domain of native factor VIII	Production of a lower molecular mass product
Chimaeric/humanized antibodies (Chapter 10)	Replacement of most/virtually all of the murine amino acid sequences with sequences found in human antibodies	Greatly reduced/eliminated immonogenicity. Ability to activate human effector functions
'Ontak', a fusion protein (Chapter 5)	Fusion protein consisting of the diphtheria toxin linked to interleukin-2	Targets toxin selectively to cells expressing an IL-2 receptor

advantage over the native protein product. Techniques such as site-directed mutagenesis facilitate the logical introduction of pre-defined changes in a protein's amino acid sequence. Such changes can be minimal, such as the insertion, deletion or alteration of a single amino acid residue, or can be more substantial, e.g. the alteration or deletion of an entire domain, or the generation of a novel hybrid protein. Such changes can be made for a number of reasons and several engineered products have now gained marketing approval. An overview summary of some engineered product types now on the market is provided in Table 1.5. These and other examples will be discussed in subsequent chapters.

Despite the undoubted advantages of recombinant production, it remains the case that many protein-based products extracted directly from native source material remain on the market. These products have proved safe and effective and selected examples are provided in Table 1.2. In certain circumstances, direct extraction of native source material can prove equally/more attractive than recombinant production. This may be for an economic reason, e.g. if the protein is produced in very large quantities by the native source and is easy to extract/purify, as is the case for human serum albumin (Chapter 9). Also, some blood factor preparations purified from

---

Figure 1.1. (*Opposite*) Sulpha drugs and their mode of action. The first sulpha drug to be used medically was the red dye prontosil rubrum (a). In the early 1930s, experiments illustrated that the administration of this dye to mice infected with haemolytic streptococci prevented the death of the mice. This drug, while effective *in vivo*, was devoid of *in vitro* antibacterial activity. It was first used clinically in 1935 under the name Streptozon. It was subsequently shown that prontosil rubrum was enzymatically reduced by the liver, forming sulphanilamide, the actual active antimicrobial agent (b). Sulphanilamide induces its effect by acting as an anti-metabolite with respect to *para*-aminobenzoic acid (PABA) (c). PABA is an essential component of tetrahydrofolic acid (THF) (d). THF serves as an essential co-factor for several cellular enzymes. Sulphanilamide (at sufficiently high concentrations) inhibits manufacture of THF by competing with PABA. This effectively inhibits essential THF-dependent enzyme reactions within the cell. Unlike humans, who can derive folates from their diets, most bacteria must synthesize it *de novo*, as they cannot absorb it intact from their surroundings

donor blood actually contain several different blood factors and hence can be used to treat several haemophilia patient types. Recombinant blood factor preparations, on the other hand, contain but a single blood factor and hence can be used to treat only one haemophilia type (Chapter 9).

The advent of genetic engineering and monoclonal antibody technology underpinned the establishment of literally hundreds of start-up biopharmaceutical (biotechnology) companies in the late 1970s and early 1980s. The bulk of these companies were founded in the USA, with smaller numbers of start-ups emanating from Europe and other world regions.

Many of these fledgling companies were founded by academics/technical experts who sought to take commercial advantage of developments in the biotechnological arena. These companies were largely financed by speculative monies attracted by the hype associated with the establishment of the modern biotech era. While most of these early companies displayed significant technical expertise, the vast majority lacked experience in the practicalities of the drug development process (Chapter 2). Most of the well-established large pharmaceutical companies, on the other hand, were slow to invest heavily in biotech research and development. However, as the actual and potential therapeutic significance of biopharmaceuticals became evident, many of these companies did diversify into this area. Most either purchased small established biopharmaceutical concerns or formed strategic alliances with them. An example was the long-term alliance formed by Genentech (see later) and the well-established pharmaceutical company, Eli Lilly. Genentech developed recombinant human insulin, which was then marketed by Eli Lilly under the trade name, Humulin. The merger of biotech capability with pharmaceutical experience helped accelerate development of the biopharmaceutical sector.

Many of the earlier biopharmaceutical companies no longer exist. The overall level of speculative finance available was not sufficient to sustain them all long-term (it can take 6–10 years and $200–500 million to develop a single drug; Chapter 2). Furthermore, the promise and hype of biotechnology sometimes exceeded its ability to actually deliver a final product. Some biopharmaceutical substances showed little efficacy in treating their target condition, and/or exhibited unacceptable side effects. Mergers and acquisitions also led to the disappearance of several biopharmaceutical concerns. Table 1.6 lists the major pharmaceutical concerns which now manufacture/market biopharmaceuticals approved for general medical use. Box 1.1 provides a profile of three well-established dedicated biopharmaceutical companies.

BIOPHARMACEUTICALS: CURRENT STATUS AND FUTURE PROSPECTS

By mid-2002, some 120 biopharmaceutical products had gained marketing approval in the USA and/or EU. Collectively, these represent a global biopharmaceutical market in the region of $15 billion (Table 1.7). A detailed list of the approved products is provided in Appendix 1. The products include a range of hormones, blood factors and thrombolytic agents, as well as vaccines and monoclonal antibodies (Table 1.8). All but one are protein-based therapeutic agents. The exception is Vitravene, an antisense oligonucleotide (Chapter 11), first approved in the USA in 1998. Many additional nucleic acid-based products for use in gene therapy or antisense technology (Chapter 11) are currently in clinical trials.

Many of the initial biopharmaceuticals approved were simple replacement proteins (e.g. blood factors and human insulin). The ability to logically alter the amino acid sequence of a protein, coupled to an increased understanding of the relationship between protein structure and function has facilitated the more recent introduction of several engineered therapeutic

Table 1.6. Pharmaceutical companies who manufacture and/or market biopharmaceutical products approved for general medical use in the USA and EU

Genetics Institute	Hoechst AG
Bayer	Aventis Pharmaceuticals
Novo Nordisk	Genzyme
Centeon	Schwartz Pharma
Genentech	Pharmacia and Upjohn
Centocor	Biotechnology General
Boehringer Mannheim	Serono
Galenus Mannheim	Organon
Eli Lilly	Amgen
Ortho Biotech	Dompe Biotec
Schering Plough	Immunex
Hoffman-la-Roche	Bedex Laboratories
Chiron	Merck
Biogen	SmithKline Beecham
Pasteur Mérieux MSD	Medeva Pharma
Immunomedics	Cytogen
Novartis	Med Immune
Abbott	Roche
Wyeth	Isis pharmaceuticals
Unigene	Sanofi-Synthelabo

proteins (Table 1.5). Thus far, the vast majority of approved recombinant proteins have been produced in *E. coli*, *S. cerevisiae* or in animal cell lines (most notably Chinese hamster ovary (CHO) cells or baby hamster kidney (BHK) cells). The rationale for choosing these production systems is discussed in Chapter 3.

While most biopharmaceuticals approved to date are intended for human use, a number of products destined for veterinary application have also come on the market. One early example of this is recombinant bovine growth hormone (somatotrophin), approved in the USA in the early 1990s and used to increase milk yields from dairy cattle. Additional examples of approved veterinary biopharmaceuticals include a range of recombinant vaccines and an interferon-based product (Table 1.9).

At least 500 potential biopharmaceuticals are currently being evaluated in clinical trials. Vaccines and monoclonal antibody-based products represent the two biggest product categories. Regulatory factors (e.g. hormones and cytokines), as well as gene therapy and antisense-based products, also represent significant groupings. While most protein-based products likely to gain marketing approval over the next 2–3 years will be produced in engineered *E. coli*, *S. cerevisiae* or animal cell lines, some products now in clinical trials are being produced in the milk of transgenic animals (Chapter 3). Additionally, plant-based transgenic expression systems may potentially come to the fore, particularly for the production of oral vaccines (Chapter 3).

Interestingly, the first generic biopharmaceuticals are already entering the market. Patent protection for many first-generation biopharmaceuticals (including recombinant human growth hormone, insulin, erythropoietin, α-interferon and granulocyte colony stimulating factor) has now come/is now coming to an end. Most of these drugs command an overall annual market value in excess of US$ 1 billion, rendering them attractive potential products for many biotechnology/pharmaceutical companies. Companies already producing, or about to produce,

Box 1.1.   Amgen, Biogen and Genentech

Amgen, Biogen and Genentech represent three pioneering biopharmaceutical companies that remain in business. Founded in the 1980s as AMGen (Applied Molecular Genetics), Amgen now employs over 9000 people worldwide, making it one of the largest dedicated biotechnology companies in existence. Its headquarters are situated in Thousand Oaks, California, although it has research, manufacturing, distribution and sales facilities worldwide. Company activities focus upon developing novel (mainly protein) therapeutics for application in oncology, inflammation, bone disease, neurology, metabolism and nephrology. By mid-2002, six of its recombinant products had been approved for general medical use (the erythropoietin-based products, 'Aranesp' and 'Epogen' (Chapter 6), the colony stimulating factor-based products, 'Neupogen' and 'Neulasta' (Chapter 6) as well as the interleukin-1 receptor antagonist, 'Kineret' and the anti-rheumatoid arthritis fusion protein, Enbrel (Chapter 5)). Total product sales for 2001 reached US$ 3.5 billion and the company reinvested 25% of this in R&D. In July 2002, Amgen acquired Immunex Corporation, another dedicated biopharmaceutical company founded in Seattle in the early 1980s.

Biogen was founded in Geneva, Switzerland in 1978 by a group of leading molecular biologists. Currently, its international headquarters are located in Paris and it employs in excess of 2000 people worldwide. The company developed and directly markets the interferon-based product, 'Avonex' (Chapter 4), but also generates revenues from sales of other Biogen-discovered products which are licensed to various other pharmaceutical companies. These include Schering Plough's 'Intron A' (Chapter 4) as well as a number of hepatitis B-based vaccines sold by SmithKline Beecham (SKB) and Merck (Chapter 10). By 2001, worldwide sales of Biogen-discovered products had reached US$ 3 billion. Biogen reinvests ca. 33% of its revenues back into R&D and has ongoing collaborations with several other pharmaceutical and biotechnology companies.

Genentech was founded in 1976 by scientist Herbert Boyer and the venture capitalist, Robert Swanson. Headquartered in San Francisco, it employs almost 5000 staff worldwide and has 10 protein-based products on the market. These include human growth hormones ('Nutropin', Chapter 8), the antibody-based products 'Herceptin' and 'Rituxan' (Chapter 10) and the thrombolytic agents 'Activase' and 'TNKase' (Chapter 9). The company also has 20 or so products in clinical trials. In 2001, it generated some US$ 2.2 billion in revenues, 24% of which it reinvested in R&D.

generic biopharmaceuticals include Genemedix (UK), Sicor and Ivax (USA), Congene and Microbix (Canada) and BioGenerix (Germany); e.g. Genemedix secured approval for sale of a recombinant colony-stimulating factor in China in 2001 and is also commencing the manufacture of recombinant erythropoietin; Sicor currently markets human growth hormone and interferon-α in Eastern Europe and various developing nations. The widespread approval and marketing of generic biopharmaceuticals in regions such as the EU and USA is, however, unlikely to occur in the near future, mainly due to regulatory issues.

To date (mid-2002) no gene therapy based product has thus far been approved for general medical use (Chapter 11). Although gene therapy trials were initiated as far back as 1990, the

Table 1.7. Approximate annual market values of some leading approved biopharmaceutical products. Data gathered from various sources, including company home pages, annual reports and industry reports

Product and (Company)	Product description and (use)	Annual sales value (US$, billions)
Procrit (Amgen/Johnson & Johnson)	Erythropoietin (treatment of anaemia)	2.7
Epogen (Amgen)	Erythropoietin (treatment of anaemia)	2.0
Intron A (Schering Plough)	Interferon-α (treatment of leukaemia)	1.4
Neupogen (Amgen)	Colony stimulating factor (treatment of neutropenia)	1.2
Avonex (Biogen)	Interferon-β (treatment of multiple sclerosis)	0.8
Embrel (Immunex)	Monoclonal antibody (treatment of rheumatoid arthritis)	0.7
Betasteron (Chiron/Schering Plough)	Interferon-β (treatment of multiple sclerosis)	0.6
Cerezyme (Genzyme)	Glucocerebrosidase (treatment of Gaucher's disease)	0.5

Table 1.8. Summary categorization of biopharmaceuticals approved for general medical use in the EU and/or USA by August 2002. Refer to Appendix 1 for further details

Product type	Examples	Number approved	Refer to Chapter
Blood factors	Factors VIII and IX	7	9
Thrombolytic agents	Tissue plasminogen activator (tPA)	6	9
Hormones	Insulin, growth hormone, gonadotrophins	28	8
Haemapoietic growth factors	Erythropoietin, colony stimulating factors	7	6
Interferons	Interferons-α, -β, -γ	15	4
Interleukin-based products	Interleukin-2	3	5
Vaccines	Hepatitis B surface antigen	20	10
Monoclonal antibodies	Various	20	10
Additional products	Tumour necrosis factor, therapeutic enzymes	14	Various

results have been disappointing. Many technical difficulties remain, e.g. in relation to gene delivery and regulation of expression. Product effectiveness was not apparent in the majority of trials undertaken and safety concerns have been raised in several trials.

Only one antisense-based product has been approved to date (in 1998) and, although several such antisense agents continue to be clinically evaluated, it is unlikely that a large number of

Table 1.9. Some recombinant (r) biopharmaceuticals recently approved for veterinary application in the EU

Product	Company	Indication
Vibragen Omega (r feline interferon omega)	Virbac	Reduction of mortality/clinical symptoms associated with canine parvovirus
Fevaxyl Pentafel (combination vaccine containing r feline leukaemia viral antigen as one component)	Fort Dodge Laboratories	Immunization of cats against various feline pathogens
Porcilis porcoli (combination vaccine containing r E. coli adhesins)	Intervet	Active immunization of sows
Porcilis AR-T DF (combination vaccine containing a recombinant modified toxin from *Pasteurella multocida*)	Intervet	Reduction in clinical signs of progressive atrophic rhinitis in piglets
Porcilis pesti (combination vaccine containing r classical swine fever virus E_2 subunit antigen)	Intervet	Immunization of pigs against classical swine fever
Bayovac CSF E2 (combination vaccine containing r classical swine fever virus E_2 subunit antigen)	Intervet	Immunization of pigs against classical swine fever

such products will be approved over the next 3–4 years. Despite the disappointing results thus far generated by nucleic acid-based products, future technical advances will almost certainly ensure the approval of gene therapy- and antisense-based products in the intermediate future.

Technological developments in areas such as genomics, proteomics and high-throughput screening are also beginning to impact significantly upon the early stages of drug development (Chapter 2). For example, by linking changes in gene/protein expression to various disease states, these technologies will identify new drug targets for such diseases. Many/most such targets will themselves be proteins, and drugs will be designed/developed specifically to interact with them. They may be protein-based or (more often) low molecular mass ligands.

TRADITIONAL PHARMACEUTICALS OF BIOLOGICAL ORIGIN

The remaining chapters of this book are largely dedicated to describing the major biopharmaceuticals currently in use and those likely to gain approval for use in the not-too-distant future. Before undertaking this task, however, it would be useful to overview briefly some of the now-traditional pharmaceutical substances originally obtained from biological sources. This will provide a more comprehensive foundation for the study of biopharmaceuticals and facilitate a better overall appreciation of how biotechnology, in whatever guise, impacts upon the pharmaceutical industry.

As previously indicated, some of these biological substances are now synthesized chemically, although many continue to be extracted from their native biological source material. Animals, plants and microorganisms have all yielded therapeutically important compounds, as described below.

Table 1.10. Some pharmaceutical substances originally isolated from animal sources. While some are still produced by direct extraction from the native source, others are now also produced by direct chemical synthesis (e.g. peptides and some steroids), or by recombinant DNA technology (most of the polypeptide products). Abbreviations: hGH=human growth hormone; FSH=follicle stimulating hormone; hCG=human chorionic gonadotrophin; HSA=human serum albumin; HBsAg=hepatitis B surface antigen

Product	Indication	Original source
Insulin	Diabetes mellitus	Porcine/bovine pancreatic tissue
Glucagon	Used to reverse insulin-induced hypoglycaemia	Porcine/bovine pancreatic tissue
hGH	Treatment of short stature	Originally human pituitaries
FSH	Subfertility/infertility	Urine of post-menopausal women
hCG	Subfertility/infertility	Urine of pregnant women
Blood coagulation factors	Haemophilia and other related blood disorders	Human blood
HSA	Plasma volume expander	Human plasma/placenta
Polyclonal antibodies	Passive immunization	Serum of immunized animals/ humans
H Bs Ag	Vaccination against hepatitis B	Plasma of hepatitis B carriers
Urokinase	Thrombolytic agent	Human urine
Peptide hormones (e.g. gonadorelin, oxytocin, vasopressin)	Various	Mostly from pituitary gland
Trypsin	Debriding agent	Pancreas
Pancrelipase	Digestive enzymes	Pancreas
Glucocerebrosidase	Gaucher's disease	Placenta
Steroid (sex) hormones	Various, including subfertility	Gonads
Corticosteroids	Adrenal insufficiency, anti-inflammatory agents, immunosuppressants	Adrenal cortex
Prostaglandins	Various, including uterine stimulants, vasodilators and inhibition of gastric acid secretion	Manufactured in most tissues
Adrenaline	Management of anaphylaxis	Adrenal gland

Pharmaceuticals of animal origin

A wide range of pharmaceutical substances are derived from animal sources (Table 1.10). Many are protein-based and detailed description of products such as insulin and other polypeptide hormones, antibody preparations, vaccines, enzymes, etc., have been deferred to subsequent chapters. (Many of the therapeutic proteins are now also produced by recombinant DNA technology. Considerable overlap would have been generated had a product obtained by direct extraction from native sources been discussed here, with further discussion of a version of the same product produced by recombinant DNA technology at a later stage.) Non-proteinaceous pharmaceuticals originally derived from animal sources include steroid (sex) hormones, corticosteroids and prostaglandins. A limited discussion of these substances is presented below, as they will not be discussed in subsequent chapters. Most of these substances are now prepared synthetically.

The sex hormones

The male and female gonads, as well as the placenta of pregnant females and, to a lesser extent, the adrenal cortex, produce a range of steroid hormones which regulate the development and maintenance of reproductive and related functions. As such, these steroid sex hormones have found medical application in the treatment of various reproductive dysfunctions.

While these steroids directly regulate sexual function, their synthesis and release are, in turn, controlled by gonadotropins — polypeptide hormones produced by the pituitary gland. The biology and medical applications of the gonadotropins are outlined in Chapter 8. Sex hormones produced naturally may be classified into one of three groups:

- the androgens;
- the oestrogens;
- progesterone.

While these steroids can be extracted directly from human tissue, in most instances they can also be synthesized chemically. Direct chemical synthesis methodology has also facilitated the development of synthetic steroid analogues. Many such analogues exhibit therapeutic advantages over the native hormone, e.g. they may be more potent, be absorbed intact from the digestive tract, or exhibit a longer duration of action in the body. The majority of sex steroid hormones now used clinically are chemically synthesized.

The androgens   The androgens are the main male sex hormones. They are produced by the Leydig cells of the testes, as well as in the adrenals. They are also produced by the female ovary. As in the case of all other steroid hormones, the androgens are synthesized in the body, using cholesterol as their ultimate biosynthetic precursor. The major androgen produced by the testes is testosterone, of which 4–10 mg is secreted daily into the bloodstream by healthy young men. Testosterone synthesis is stimulated by the gonadotrophin, luteinizing hormone.

Testosterone is transported in the blood bound to transport proteins, the most important of which are albumin (a non-specific carrier) and testosterone–oestradiol binding globulin (TEBG), a 40 kDa polypeptide which binds testosterone and oestrogens with high affinity.

Testosterone and other androgens induce their characteristic biological effects via binding to a specific intracellular receptor. These hormones promote:

- induction of sperm production;
- development/maintenance of male secondary sexual characteristics;
- general anabolic (growth-promoting) effects;
- regulation of gonadotrophin secretion.

The actions of androgens are often antagonized by oestrogens, and vice versa. This forms the basis of androgen administration in some forms of breast cancer, and oestrogen administration in the treatment of prostate cancer. Anti-androgenic compounds have also been synthesized. These antagonize androgen action due to their ability to compete with androgens for binding to the receptor.

Androgens are used medically as replacement therapy in male hypogonadal disorders (i.e. impaired functioning of the testes). They are administered to adolescent males displaying delayed puberty to promote an increase in the size of the scrotum and other sexual organs. Androgens are also sometimes administered to females, particularly in the management of some

Table 1.11.   Major androgens/anabolic steroids used medically

Hormone	Description	Use
Danazol	Synthetic androgen. Suppresses gonadotrophin production. Exhibits some weak androgenic activity	Oral administration in the treatment of endometriosis, benign breast disorders, menorrhagia, premenstrual syndrome and hereditary angioedema
Methyltestosterone	Synthetic androgen, longer circulatory half-life than testosterone	Replacement therapy for male hypogonadal disorders. Breast cancer in females
Oxymetholone	Synthetic androgen	Treatment of anaemia
Stanozolol	Synthetic androgen	Treatment of some clinical presentations of Behçet's syndrome and management of hereditary angioedema
Testosterone	Main androgen produced by testes. Esterified forms display longer circulatory half lives	Treatment of male hypogonadism. Also sometimes used in treatment of post-menopausal breast carcinoma and osteoporosis

forms of breast cancer. The major androgens used clinically are listed in Table 1.11, and their chemical structures are outlined in Figure 1.2.

Oestrogens   Oestrogens are produced mainly by the ovary in (non-pregnant) females. These molecules, which represent the major female sex steroid hormones, are also produced by the placenta of pregnant females. Testosterone represents the immediate biosynthetic precursor of oestrogens. Three main oestrogens have been extracted from ovarian tissue (oestrone, β-oestradiol and oestriol). β-oestradiol is the principal oestrogen produced by the ovary. It is 10 times more potent than oestrone and 25 times more potent than oestriol, and these latter two oestrogens are largely by-products of β-oestradiol metabolism.

Oestrogens induce their various biological effects by interacting with intracellular receptors. Their major biological activities include:

- stimulation of the growth and maintenance of the female reproductive system (their principal effect);
- influencing bone metabolism; as is evidenced from the high degree of bone decalcification (osteoporosis) occurring in post-menopausal women;
- influencing lipid metabolism.

Natural oestrogens generally only retain a significant proportion of their activity if administered intravenously. Several synthetic analogues have been developed which can be administered orally. Most of these substances also display more potent activity than native oestrogen. The most important synthetic oestrogen analogues include ethinyloestradiol and diethylstilboestrol (often simply termed stilboestrol). These are orally active and are approximately 10 and 5 times (respectively) more potent than oestrone.

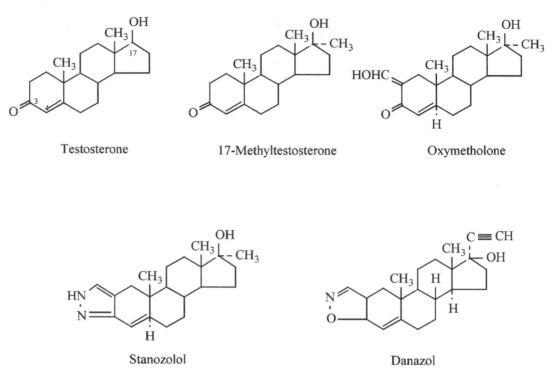

Figure 1.2.   Chemical structure of the major synthetic and native androgens used clinically

Oestrogens are used to treat a number of medical conditions, including:

- replacement therapy for medical conditions underlined by insufficient endogenous oestrogen production;
- for alleviation of menopausal/post-menopausal disorders/symptoms;
- combating post-menopausal osteoporosis;
- treatment of some cancer forms, notably prostate and breast cancer;
- as an active ingredient in several oral contraceptive preparations.

The major oestrogen preparations used medically are outlined in Table 1.12, and their chemical structure is illustrated in Figure 1.3. The widest clinical application of oestrogens relate to their use as oral contraceptives. Most such contraceptive pills contain an oestrogen in combination with a progestin (discussed later).

Several synthetic anti-oestrogens have also been developed. These non-steroidal agents, including clomiphene and tamoxifen (Figure 1.4) inhibit oestrogen activity by binding their intracellular receptors, but fail to elicit a subsequent cellular response. Such anti-oestrogens have also found clinical application. Many female patients with breast cancer improve when either endogenous oestrogen levels are reduced (e.g. by removal of the ovaries) or anti-oestrogenic compounds are administered. However, not all patients respond. Predictably, tumours exhibiting high levels of oestrogen receptors are the most responsive.

Table 1.12. Major oestrogens used medically

Hormone	Description	Use
Ethinyloestradiol	Synthetic oestrogen	Used for oestrogen replacement therapy in deficient states, both pre- and post-menopausal. Treatment of prostate cancer (male), breast cancer (post-menopausal women). Component of many oral contraceptives
Mestranol	Synthetic oestrogen	Treatment of menopausal, post-menopausal or menstrual disorders. Component of many oral contraceptives
Oestradiol	Natural oestrogen	Oestrogen replacement therapy in menopausal, post-menopausal or menstrual disorders. Management of breast cancer in post-menopausal women and prostate cancer in man
Oestrone	Natural oestrogen	Uses similar to oestradiol
Quinestrol	Synthetic oestrogen, with prolonged duration of action	Oestrogen deficiency
Stilboestrol	Synthetic oestrogen (non-steroidal)	Treatment of breast/prostate cancer. Management of menopausal/post-menopausal disorders

Progesterone and progestogens Progesterone is the main hormone produced by the corpus luteum during the second half of the female menstrual cycle (Chapter 8). It acts upon the endometrial tissue (lining of the womb). Under its influence, the endometrium begins to produce and secrete mucus, which is an essential prerequisite for subsequent implantation of a fertilized egg. In pregnant females, progesterone is also synthesized by the placenta, and its continued production is essential for maintenance of the pregnant state. Administration of progesterone to a non-pregnant female prevents ovulation and, as such, the progestogens (discussed below) are used as contraceptive agents. Progesterone also stimulates breast growth, and is immunosuppressive at high doses.

Only minor quantities of intact biologically active progesterone are absorbed if the hormone is given orally. Progestogens are synthetic compounds which display actions similar to that of progesterone. Many progestogens are more potent than progesterone itself and can be absorbed intact when administered orally.

Progesterone, and particularly progestogens, are used for a number of therapeutic purposes, including:

- treatment of menstrual disorders;
- treatment of endometriosis (the presence of tissue similar to the endometrium at other sites in the pelvis);
- management of some breast and endometrial cancers;
- hormone replacement therapy, where they are used in combination with oestrogens;
- contraceptive agents, usually in combination with oestrogens.

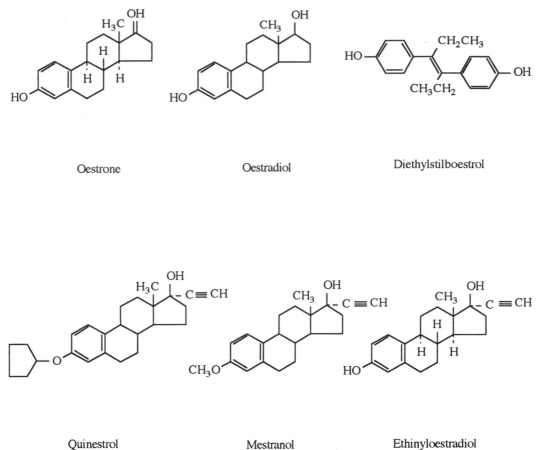

Oestrone   Oestradiol   Diethylstilboestrol

Quinestrol   Mestranol   Ethinyloestradiol

Figure 1.3. Chemical structure of the major synthetic and native oestrogens used clinically

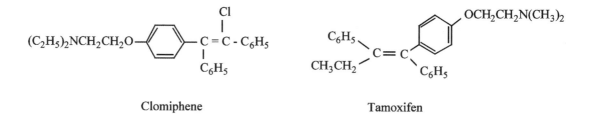

Clomiphene   Tamoxifen

Figure 1.4.   Structure of clomiphene and tamoxifen, two non-steroidal synthetic anti-oestrogens that have found medical application

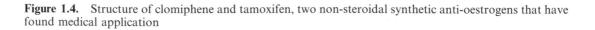

Table 1.13. Progesterone and major progestogens used clinically

Hormone	Description	Use
Progesterone	Hormone produced naturally by corpus luteum, adrenals and placenta. Serum half-life is only a few minutes	Dysfunctional uterine bleeding. Sustaining pregnancy in threatening abortion
Chlormadinone	Synthetic progestogen	Menstrual disorders. Oral contraceptive
Ethynodiol diacetate	Synthetic progestogen	Component of many combined oral contraceptives. Progesterone replacement therapy
Medroxyprogesterone acetate	Synthetic progestogen	Treatment of menstrual disorders, endometriosis and hormone responsive cancer. Also used as long-acting contraceptive
Megestrol acetate	Synthetic progestogen	Treatment of endometrial carcinoma and some forms of breast cancer
Norethisterone	Synthetic progestogen	Abnormal uterine bleeding. Endometriosis, component of some oral contraceptives and in hormone replacement therapy

Table 1.13 lists some progestogens which are in common medical use, and their structures are presented in Figure 1.5.

A wide range of oestrogens and progesterone are used in the formulation of oral contraceptives. These contraceptive pills generally contain a combination of a single oestrogen and a single progestogen. They may also be administered in the form of long-acting injections.

These combined contraceptives seem to function by inducing feedback inhibition of gonadotrophin secretion which, in turn, inhibits the process of ovulation (Chapter 8). They also induce alterations in the endometrial tissue that may prevent implantation. Furthermore, the progestogen promotes thickening of the cervical mucus, which renders it less hospitable to sperm cells. This combination of effects is quite effective in preventing pregnancy.

Corticosteroids

The adrenal cortex produces in excess of 50 steroid hormones, which can be divided into 3 classes:

- glucocorticoids (principally cortisone and hydrocortisone, also known as cortisol);
- mineralocorticoids (principally deoxycorticosterone and aldosterone);
- sex corticoids (mainly androgens, as previously discussed).

Glucocorticoids and mineralocorticoids are uniquely produced by the adrenal cortex, and are collectively termed corticosteroids. Apart from aldosterone, glucocorticoid secretion is regulated by the pituitary hormone, corticotrophin. The principal corticosteroids synthesized in the body are illustrated in Figure 1.6. Glucocorticoids generally exhibit weak mineralocorticoid actions and vice versa.

The glucocorticoids induce a number of biological effects (Table 1.14), but their principal actions relate to modulation of glucose metabolism. The mineralocorticoids regulate water and

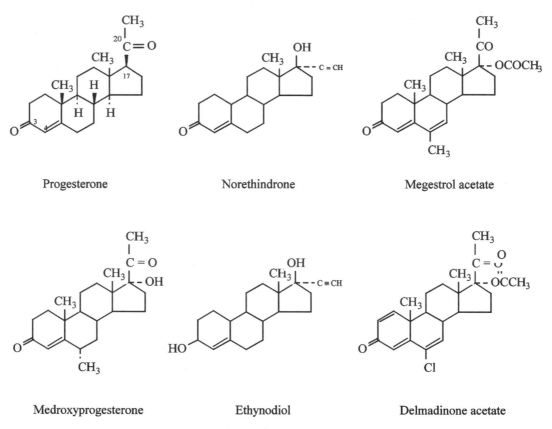

Progesterone   Norethindrone   Megestrol acetate

Medroxyprogesterone   Ethynodiol   Delmadinone acetate

Figure 1.5. Chemical structure of progesterone and the major progestogens used clinically

electrolyte metabolism. They generally increase renal reabsorption of Na^+, and promote Na^+–K^+–H^+ exchange. This typically results in increased serum Na^+ concentrations and decreased serum K^+ concentrations. Elevated blood pressure is also usually induced.

Various synthetic corticosteroids have also been developed. Some display greater potency than the native steroids, while others exhibit glucocorticoid activity with little associated mineralocorticoid effects, or vice versa. The major glucocorticoids used clinically are synthetic. They are usually employed as:

- replacement therapy in cases of adrenal insufficiency;
- anti-inflammatory agents;
- immunosuppressive agents.

Examples of the corticosteroids used most commonly in the clinic are presented in Table 1.15 and Figure 1.7.

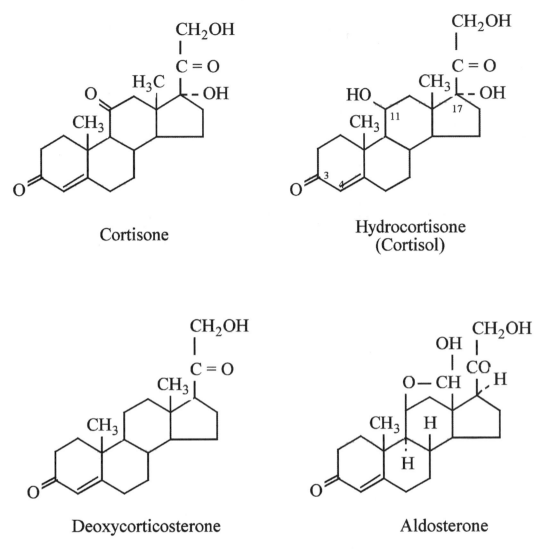

Figure 1.6. Corticosteroids produced naturally in the adrenal cortex

Catecholamines

The adrenal medulla synthesizes two catecholamine hormones, adrenaline (epinephrine) and noradrenaline (norepinephrine) (Figure 1.8). The ultimate biosynthetic precursor of both is the amino acid tyrosine. Subsequent to their synthesis, these hormones are stored in intracellular vesicles, and are released via exocytosis upon stimulation of the producer cells by neurons of the sympathetic nervous system. The catecholamine hormones induce their characteristic biological effects by binding to one of two classes of receptors, the α- and β-adrenergic receptors. These receptors respond differently (often oppositely) to the catecholamines.

Table 1.14. Some biological effects of glucocorticoids. Reproduced from Smith *et al.* (1983), *Principles of Biochemistry* (mammalian biochemistry), by kind permission of the publisher, McGraw Hill International, New York

System	Effect	Basis for change
General	Increase survival and resistance to stress	Composite of many effects (see below)
Intermediary metabolism		
Carbohydrate	Increase fasting levels of liver glycogen	Increase gluconeogenesis and glycogenesis
	Decrease insulin sensitivity	Inhibition of glucose uptake, increase gluconeogenesis
Lipid	Increase lipid mobilization from depots	Facilitate actions of lipolytic hormones
Proteins and nucleic acid	Increase urinary nitrogen during fasting	Anti-anabolic (catabolic) effect
Inflammatory and allergic phenomena and effects on leukocyte function	Anti-inflammatory and immunosuppressive	Impair cellular immunity
	Lymphocytopenia, eosinopenia, granulocytosis	Decrease influx of inflammatory cells into areas of inflammation
		Impair formation of prostaglandins
		Lymphoid sequestration in spleen, lymph node and other tissues
		Lymphocytolytic effect (not prominent in humans)
Haematologic system	Mild polycythaemia	Stimulation of erythropoiesis
Fluid and electrolytes	Promote water excretion	Increase glomerular filtration rate; inhibit vasopressin release
Cardiovascular	Increase cardiac output and blood pressure	
	Increase vascular reactivity	Not known
Bone and calcium	Lower serum Ca^{2+}	Inhibition of vitamin D function on intestinal Ca^{2+} absorption
	Osteoporosis	Inhibition of osteoblast function
Growth	Inhibit growth (pharmacologic doses)	Inhibition of cell division and DNA synthesis
Secretory actions	Tendency to increased peptic ulceration	Stimulate secretion of gastric acid and pepsinogen
Central nervous system	Changes in mood and behaviour	Unknown
Fibroblasts and connective tissue	Poor wound healing and thinning of bone (osteoporosis)	Impair fibroblast proliferation and collagen formation

Adrenaline and noradrenaline induce a wide variety of biological responses, including:

- stimulation of glycogenolysis and gluconeogenesis in the liver and skeletal muscle;
- lipolysis in adipose tissue;
- smooth muscle relaxation in the bronchi and skeletal blood vessels;
- increased speed and force of heart rate.

Table 1.15. Corticosteroids which find clinical use

Hormone	Description	Use
Betamethasone	Synthetic corticosteroid, displays glucocorticoid activity, lacks mineralocorticoid activity	Use mainly as anti-inflammatory and immunosuppressive effect
Deoxycortone acetate	Modified form of natural corticosteroid (deoxycortone). Is a mineralocorticoid, displays no significant glucocorticoid action	Used to treat Addison's disease and other adrenocortical deficiency states
Dexamethasone	Synthetic glucocorticoid, lacks mineralocorticoid activity	Used to treat range of inflammatory diseases. Used to treat some forms of asthma, also cerebral oedema and congenital adrenal hyperplasia
Fludrocortisone acetate	Synthetic corticosteroid with some glucocorticoid and potent mineralocorticoid activity	Administered orally to treat primary adrenal insufficiency
Hydrocortisone (cortisol)	Natural glucocorticoid	Used to treat all conditions for which corticosteroid therapy is indicated
Methylprednisolone	Synthetic glucocorticoid	Used as an anti-inflammatory agent and as an immunosuppressant

In general, the diverse effects induced by catecholamines serve to mobilize energy resources and prepare the body for immediate action—the 'fight or flight' response.

Catecholamines, as well as various catecholamine agonists and antagonists, can be synthesized chemically and many of these have found medical application.

The major clinical applications of adrenaline include:

- emergency management of anaphylaxis;
- emergency cardiopulmonary resuscitation;
- addition to some local anaesthetics (its vasoconstrictor properties help to prolong local action of the anaesthetic).

Noradrenaline is also sometimes added to local anaesthetics, again because of its vasoconstrictive properties. A prominent activity of this catecholamine is its ability to raise blood pressure. It is therefore used to restore blood pressure in acute hypotensive states.

Prostaglandins

The prostaglandins (PGs) are yet another group of biomolecules that have found clinical application. These molecules were named 'prostaglandins', as it was initially believed that their sole site of synthesis was the prostate gland. Subsequently, it has been shown that prostaglandins are but a sub-family of biologically active molecules, all of which are derived from arachidonic acid, a 20-carbon polyunsaturated fatty acid (Figure 1.9). These families of molecules, collectively known as ecosanoids, include the prostaglandins, thromboxanes and leukotrienes.

The principal naturally-occurring prostaglandins include prostaglandin E_1 (PGE_1), as well as PGE_2, PGE_3, $PGF_{1\alpha}$, $PGF_{2\alpha}$ and $PGF_{3\alpha}$ (Figure 1.10). All body tissues are capable of

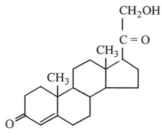

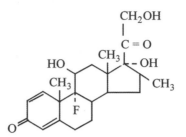

Deoxycorticosterone
acetate

Betamethasone

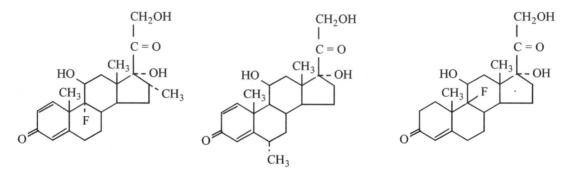

Dexamethasone   Methylprednisolone   Fludrocortisone

Figure 1.7. Structure of some of the major corticosteroids that have found routine therapeutic application

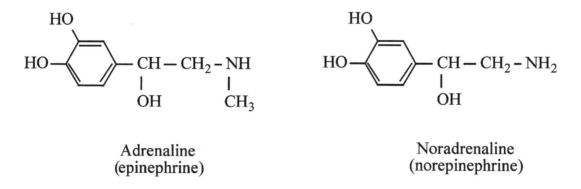

Adrenaline
(epinephrine)

Noradrenaline
(norepinephrine)

Figure 1.8. Structure of adrenaline and noradrenaline. Both are catecholamines (amide-containing derivatives of catechol, i.e. 1,2-dihydroxybenzene)

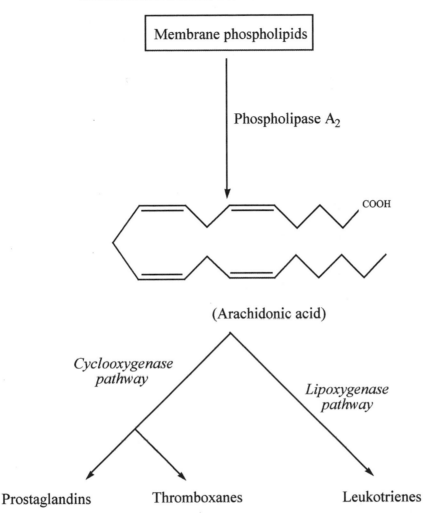

Figure 1.9. Overview of the biosynthesis of ecosanoids. The 20 carbon fatty acid arachidonic acid is released from cell membrane phospholipids by the actions of phospholipase A_2. Free arachidonic acid forms the precursor of prostaglandins and thromboxanes via the multi-enzyme cyclooxygenase pathway, while leukotrienes are formed via the lipoxygenase pathway

synthesizing endogenous prostaglandins and these molecules display an extremely wide array of biological effects, including:

- effects upon smooth muscle;
- the induction of platelet aggregation (PGEs mostly);
- alteration of metabolism and function of various tissues/organs (e.g. adipose tissue, bone, kidney, neurons);
- mediation of inflammation;
- modulation of the immune response.

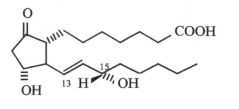

PGE$_1$

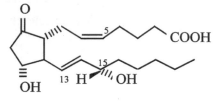

PGE$_2$

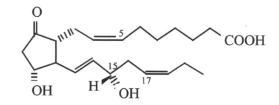

PGE$_3$

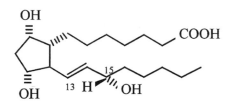

PGF$_{1\alpha}$

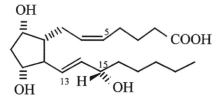

PGF$_{2\alpha}$

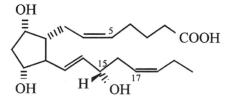

PGF$_{3\alpha}$

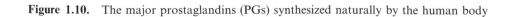

Figure 1.10.   The major prostaglandins (PGs) synthesized naturally by the human body

Their actions on smooth muscle, in particular, can be complex. For example, both PGEs and PGFs induce contraction of uterine and gastrointestinal smooth muscle. On the other hand, PGEs stimulate dilation of vascular and bronchial smooth muscle, whereas PGFs induce constriction of these muscle types.

Although prostaglandins in some ways resemble hormones, they fail to fit the classical definition of a hormone in several respects, e.g. their synthesis is not localized to a specialized gland and they act primarily in a paracrine rather than true endocrine fashion. The diverse biological actions of the prostaglandins underpin their diverse clinical applications. Synthetic analogues have also been developed which display some clinical advantage over native PGs (e.g. greater stability, longer duration of action, more specific biological effects). The major clinical uses of native or synthetic prostaglandins can be grouped as follows:

- *Obstetrics and gynaecology*: several prostaglandin preparations (mainly E_2, $F_{2\alpha}$ and their analogues) are used to induce uterine contraction. The purpose can be either to induce labour as part of the normal childbirth procedure, or to terminate a pregnancy;
- *Induction of vasodilation and inhibition of platelet aggregation*: prostaglandin E_1 and its analogues are most commonly employed and are used to treat infants with congenital heart disease;
- *Inhibition of gastric acid secretion*: an effect promoted in particular by PGE_1 and its analogues.

In some circumstances, inhibition of endogenous prostaglandin synthesis can represent a desirable medical goal. This is often achieved by administration of drugs capable of inhibiting the cyclooxygenase system. Aspirin is a well known example of such a drug, and it is by this mechanism that it induces its analgesic and anti-inflammatory effects.

Pharmaceutical substances of plant origin

The vast bulk of early medicinal substances were plant-derived. An estimated 3 billion people worldwide continue to use traditional plant medicines as their primary form of healthcare. At least 25% of all prescription drugs sold in North America contain active substances which were originally isolated from plants (or are modified forms of chemicals originally isolated from plants). Many of these were discovered by a targeted knowledge-based ethnobotanical approach. Researchers simply recorded plant-based medical cures for specific diseases and then analysed the plants for their active ingredients. Plants produce a wide array of bioactive molecules via secondary metabolic pathways. Most of these probably evolved as chemical defence agents against infections or predators.

While some medicinal substances continue to be directly extracted from plant material, in many instances plant-derived drugs can now be manufactured, at least in part, by direct chemical synthesis. In addition, chemical modification of many of these plant 'lead' drugs have yielded a range of additional therapeutic substances.

The bulk of plant-derived medicines can be categorized into a number of chemical families, including alkaloids, flavonoids, terpenes and terpenoids, steroids (e.g. cardiac glycosides), as well as coumarins, quinines, salicylates and xanthines. A list of some better-known plant-derived drugs is presented in Table 1.16.

Table 1.16. Some drugs of plant origin

Drug	Chemical type	Indication	Plant producer
Aspirin	Salicylate	Analgesic, anti-inflammatory	*Salix alba* (white willow tree) and *Filipendula ulmaria* (meadowsweet)
Atropine	Alkaloid	Pupil dilator	*Atropa belladonna* (deadly nightshade)
Caffeine	Xanthine	Increases mental alertness	*Camellia sinensis*
Cocaine	Alkaloid	Ophthalmic anaesthetic	*Erythoxylum coca* (coca leaves)
Codeine	Alkaloid	Analgesic, cough suppressor	*Papaver somniferum* (opium poppy)
Dicoumarol	Coumarin	Anti-coagulant	*Melilotus officinalis*
Digoxin	Steroid	Increases heart muscle contraction	*Digitalis purpurea* (purple foxglove)
Digitoxin	Steroid	Increases heart muscle contraction	*Digitalis purpurea*
Ipecac	Alkaloid	Induces vomiting	*Psychotria ipecacuanha*
Morphine	Alkaloid	Analgesic	*Papaver somniferum* (opium poppy)
Pseudoephedrine	Alkaloid	Clears nasal congestion	*Ephedra sinica*
Quinine	Alkaloid	Malaria	*Cinchona pubescens* (fever tree)
Reserpine	Alkaloid	Antihypertensive (reduces blood pressure)	*Rauvolfia serpentina* (Indian snakeroot)
Scopalamine	Alkaloid	Motion sickness	*Datura stramonium* (Jimson weed)
Taxol	Terpenoid	Ovarian, breast cancer	*Taxus brevifolia* (western yew tree)
Theophylline	Xanthine	Anti-asthmatic, diuretic	*Camellia sinensis*
Vinblastine	Alkaloid	Hodgkin's disease	*Catharanthus roseus* (rosy periwinkle)
Vincristine	Alkaloid	Leukaemia	*Catharanthus roseus*

Alkaloids

Alkaloids may be classified as relatively low molecular mass bases containing one or more nitrogen atoms, often present in a ring system. They are found mainly in plants (from which over 6000 different alkaloids have been extracted). They are especially abundant in flowering plants, particularly lupins, poppies, tobacco and potatoes. They also are synthesized by some animals, insects, marine organisms and microorganisms. Most producers simultaneously synthesize several distinct alkaloids.

The solubility of these substances in organic solvents facilitates their initial extraction and purification from plant material using, for example, petroleum ether. Subsequent chromatographic fractionation facilitates separation of individual alkaloid components. Many alkaloids are poisonous (and have been used for this purpose), although at lower concentrations they may be useful therapeutic agents. Several of the best known alkaloid-based drugs are discussed below. The chemical structure of most of these is presented in Figure 1.11.

Atropine and scopalamine   Atropine is found in the berries of the weeds deadly nightshade and black nightshade. It is also synthesized in the leaves and roots of *Hyoscyamus muticusi*. At high

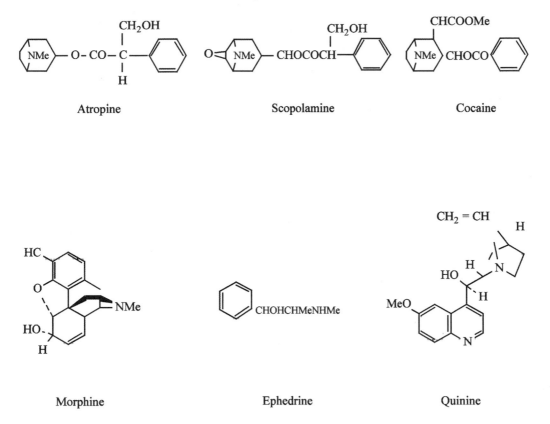

Figure 1.11. Chemical structure of some better-known alkaloids that have found medical application

concentrations it is poisonous but, when more dilute, displays a number of beneficial medical applications. Atropine sulphate solutions (1%, w/v) are used in ophthalmic procedures to dilate the pupil. It is also sometimes used as a pre-anaesthetic, as it inhibits secretion of saliva and mucus in the respiratory tract, which protects the patient from bronchoconstriction. Its ability to inhibit gastric secretion underlines its occasional use in the treatment of some stomach ulcers. Scopalamine, found in the leaves of the plant *Hyoscyamus niger*, shares some properties with atropine. Its major medical use is to treat motion sickness.

Morphine and cocaine   Morphine is medically the most important alkaloid present in opium. Opium itself consists of the dried milky exudate extracted from unripe capsules of the opium poppy (*Papaver somniferum*), which is grown mainly in Asia, but also in some parts of India and China. Morphine is a powerful analgesic and has been used to treat severe pain. However, its addictive properties complicate its long-term medical use and it is also a drug of abuse. In addition to morphine, opium also contains codeine, which has similar, but weaker, actions.

Cocaine is extracted from coca leaves (*Erythoxylum coca*), which grows predominantly in South America and the Far East. Indigenous populations used coca leaves for medicinal and recreational purposes (chewing them could numb the mouth, give a sense of vitality and reduce the sensation of hunger). Cocaine was first isolated in 1859 and (until its own addictive nature was discovered) was used to treat morphine addiction and as an ingredient in soft drinks. It also proved a powerful topical anaesthetic and coca leaf extract (and, subsequently, pure cocaine) was first introduced as an eye anaesthetic in Europe by Dr Carl Koller (who subsequently became known as Coca Koller). This represented its major medical application. While it is now rarely used medically, several derivatives (e.g. procaine, lignocaine, etc.) find widespread use as local anaesthetics.

Additional plant alkaloids   Additional plant alkaloids of medical note include ephedrine, papaverine, quinine, vinblastine and vincristine.

Ephedrine is the main alkaloid produced in the roots of *Ephedra sinica*, preparations of which have found medical application in China for at least 5000 years. It was first purified from its natural source in 1887, and its chemical synthesis was achieved in 1927. It was initially used in cardiovascular medicine, but subsequently found wider application in the treatment of mild hayfever and asthma. It is also used as a nasal decongestant and cough suppressant.

Papaverine is an opium alkaloid initially isolated in the mid-1800s. It relaxes smooth muscle and is a potent vasodilator. As such it is used to dilate pulmonary and other arteries. It is therefore sometimes of use in the treatment of angina pectoris (usually caused by partial blockage of the coronary artery), heart attacks and bronchial spasms.

Quinine is an alkaloid produced by various *Cinchona* species (e.g. *Cinchona pubescens* or fever tree), which are mainly native to South America. The bark of these trees were initially used to treat malaria. Quinine itself was subsequently isolated in 1820 and found to be toxic not only to the protozoan *Plasmodium* (which causes malaria) but also to several other protozoan species.

The Madagascar periwinkle plant (*Vinca rosea*) produces in the region of 60 alkaloids, including vinblastine and vincristine. These two closely related alkaloids (which are obtained in yields of 3 and 2 g/tonne of leaves, respectively) are important anti-tumour agents. They are used mainly to treat Hodgkin's disease and certain forms of leukaemia. They exert their effect by binding to tubulin, thus inhibiting microtubule formation during cell division.

Ergot alkaloids   Ergot is a parasitic fungus which grows upon a variety of grains. It synthesizes over 30 distinct alkaloids, of which ergometrine is the most medically significant. This alkaloid stimulates contractions of the uterus when administered intravenously. It is sometimes used to assist labour and to minimize bleeding following delivery.

Another ergot derivative is the well known hallucinogenic drug, D-lysergic diethylamide (LSD). Other fungi also produce hallucinogenic/toxic alkaloids. These include the hallucinogenic psilocybin (produced by a number of fungi, including *Psilocybe mexicana*). These are often consumed by Mexican Indians during religious ceremonies.

Flavonoids, xanthines and terpenoids

Flavonoids are 15-carbon polyphenols produced by all vascular plants. Well over 4000 distinct flavonoids have now been identified, a limited number of which display therapeutic activity. These substances are generally degraded if taken orally, and are administered medically via the intravenous route. This is probably just as well (the average Western daily diet contains approximately 1 g of flavonoids). A number of flavonoids appear to display anti-viral activity and, hence, are of pharmaceutical interest (Figure 1.12).

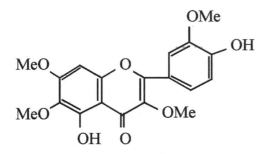

Chrysosplenol B

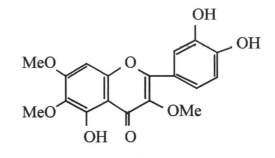

Axillarin

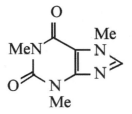

Caffeine

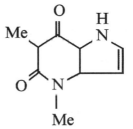

Theophylline

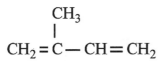

Isoprene

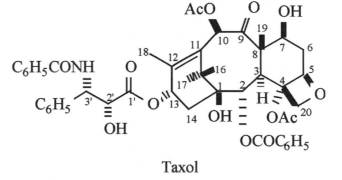

Taxol

Figure 1.12. Some flavonoids, xanthines and terpenoids. Chrysoplenol B and axillarin are two flavonoids exhibiting anti-viral activity against Rhinovirus (causative agent of the common cold). Examples of xanthines include caffeine and theophylline. Terpenes are polymers of the 5-carbon compound isoprene. Perhaps the best-known such substance discovered in recent years is the diterpenoid taxol, which is used as an anti-tumour agent

The principal xanthines of medical interest include caffeine, theophylline and aminophylline. Caffeine is synthesized by several plants and was originally isolated from tea in 1838. It is a methylxanthine (Figure 1.12) which stimulates the central nervous system, increasing mental alertness. It also acts as a diuretic and stimulates gastric acid secretion. It is absorbed upon oral administration and is frequently included in drugs containing an analgesic, such as aspirin or paracetamol.

Theophilline is also a minor constituent of tea, but is prepared by direct chemical synthesis for medical use. It functions to relax smooth muscle and, therefore, can be used as a bronchodilator in the treatment of asthma and bronchitis. Aminophylline is a derivative of theophilline (theophylline ethylenediamine), which is often used in place of theophilline due to its greater aqueous solubility.

Terpenes are polymers of the 5-carbon compound isoprene (Figure 1.12) and, as such, generally display properties similar to those of hydrocarbons. Terpenoids are substituted terpenes (i.e. contain additional chemical groups, such as an alcohol, phenols, aldehydes, ketones, etc.). Only a few such substances could be regarded as true drugs. Terpenes, such as limonene, menthol and camphor, form components of various essential oils with pseudo-pharmaceutical uses. A number of these molecules, however, exhibit anti-tumour activity, of which taxol is by far the most important.

The diterpenoid taxol (Figure 1.12) was first isolated from the pacific yew tree (*Taxus brevifolia*) in the late 1960s. Its complete structure was elucidated by 1971. Difficulties associated with the subsequent development of taxol as a useful drug mirror those encountered during the development of many plant-derived metabolites as drug products. Its low solubility made taxol difficult to formulate into a stable product, and its low natural abundance required large-scale extraction from its native source.

Despite such difficulties, encouraging *in vitro* bioassay results against transformed cell lines fuelled pre-clinical studies aimed at assessing taxol as an anti-cancer agent. Initial clinical trials in humans commenced in 1983 using a product formulated as an emulsion in a modified castor oil. Initial difficulties associated with allergic reactions against the oil were largely overcome by modifying the treatment regimen used. Large-scale clinical trials proved the efficacy of taxol as an anti-cancer agent, and it was approved for use in the treatment of ovarian cancer by the US Food and Drug Administration (FDA) in 1992.

Direct extraction from the bark of *T. brevifolia* yielded virtually all of the taxol used clinically up to almost the mid-1990s. The yield of active principle was in the range 0.007–0.014%. Huge quantities of bark were thus required to sustain taxol production (almost 30 000 kg bark were extracted in 1989 to meet requirements during large-scale clinical trials). A major (late) intermediate in the biosynthesis of taxol is 10-decacetylbaccatin (10-DAB). This can be obtained from the leaves (needles) of many species of yew, and at concentrations in excess of 0.1%. Chemical methods have been developed allowing synthesis of taxol from 10-DAB, and much of the taxol now used therapeutically is produced in this way. Semi-synthesis of taxol also facilitates generation of taxol analogues, some of which have also generated clinical interest. Although semi-synthesis of taxol is relatively straightforward, its total *de novo* synthesis is extremely complex. The cost of achieving *de novo* synthesis ensures that this approach will not be adopted for commercial production of this drug.

An alternative route of taxol production under investigation entails the use of plant cell culture techniques. Plant cell culture is considered to be an economically viable production route for plant-derived drugs, if the drug commands a market value in excess of $1000–2000/kg. While many commonly used plant-derived metabolites fall into this category, plant cell culture has not generally been adopted for their industrial production. In many cases, this is because the plant cell lines fail to produce the desired drug, or produce it in minute quantities. Several cultures of *T. brevifolia*, however, have been shown to produce taxol. Interestingly, a fungus, *Taxomyces andreanae* (isolated growing on *T. brevifolia*) also produces taxol, although at very low levels. Genetic manipulation of this fungus may, however, yet yield mutants capable of synthesizing taxol in quantities rendering production by this means economically viable.

Betulinic acid is a five-ringed triterpene which has recently generated interest as an anti-cancer agent. It is produced in relatively substantial quantities in the bark of the white birch tree, from which it can easily be isolated. Initial studies indicate that betulinic acid is capable of selectively destroying melanoma cells by inducing apoptosis. Over the past number of years, the incidence of melanoma has increased at a faster rate than any other cancer. In the region of 7000 patients die annually from this condition in the USA alone. Although early surgery produces a 10-year survival rate of greater than 90%, treatment of late (metastatic) melanoma is more problematic. The current most effective drug (dacarbazine) is only effective in 25% of cases. A more effective drug would be a valuable therapeutic tool in combating advanced cases of this cancer.

Cardiac glycosides and coumarins

Cardiac glycosides are steroids to which a carbohydrate component is attached. Although produced by a variety of plants, the major cardiac glycosides that have found medical use have been isolated from species of *Digitalis* (foxgloves). 'Digitalis' in pharmaceutical circles has also come to mean a crude extract of dried foxglove leaves. This contains two glycoside components — digoxin and digitoxin — which increase heart muscle contraction. These drugs are in widespread use in the treatment of heart failure; both can be administered either orally or by injection. Digoxin induces an immediate but short-lived effect, whereas digitoxin is slower-acting but its effects are prolonged.

Coumarins are also synthesized by a variety of plant species. Medically, the most significant coumarins are dicoumarol and its derivative, warfarin. Dicoumarol was initially discovered as the active substance in mouldy sweet clover hay, which could induce haemorrhagic disease in cattle. Dicoumarol and warfarin are now used clinically as anticoagulants, as discussed in Chapter 9.

Aspirin

Few drugs have gained such widespread use as aspirin. The story of aspirin begins in the annals of folk medicine, where willow bark and certain flowers (e.g. *Filipendula ulmaria*) were used to relieve rheumatic and other pain. The bark of the white and black willow was subsequently found to contain salicin (Figure 1.13), which is metabolized to salicylic acid when ingested by humans. The flowers of *F. ulmaria* (meadowsweet) were also found to contain salicylic acid, which possesses anti-pyretic, anti-inflammatory and analgesic properties. Although it was an effective pain reliever, it irritates the stomach lining, and it was not until its modification to acetylsalicylate by Bayer chemists that it found widespread medical application (Figure 1.13). Bayer patented its acetylsalicylate drug under the trade name 'Aspirin' in 1900.

Pharmaceutical substances of microbial origin

Microorganisms produce a wide variety of secondary metabolites, many of which display actual or potential therapeutic application. Antibiotics are by far the most numerous such substances

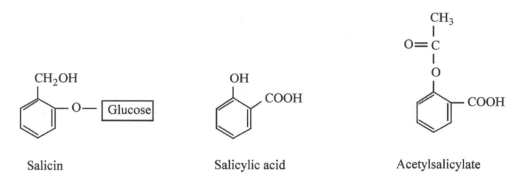

Figure 1.13. Chemical structure of salicin, salicylic acid and acetylsalicylate

and this family of pharmaceuticals arguably has had the greatest single positive impact upon human healthcare in history. A detailed discussion of antibiotics goes far beyond the scope of this text and, as such, only a brief overview is presented here. The interested reader is referred to the further reading section at the end of this chapter.

Antibiotics are generally defined as low molecular mass microbial secondary metabolites which, at low concentrations, inhibit the growth of other microorganisms. To date, well in excess of 10 000 antibiotic substances have been isolated and characterized. Overall, antibiotics are a chemically heterogeneous group of molecules, although (as described later) many can be classified into different families based upon similarity of chemical structure.

While chemically heterogeneous, it is interesting to note that in excess of half the antibiotic substances described to date are produced by a single bacterial order, the Actinomycetales. Within this order, the genus *Streptomyces* are particularly prolific producers of antibiotic substances. Although several fungal genera are known to produce antibiotics, only two (*Aspergillus* and *Penicillium*) do so to a significant extent. Indeed, the first antibiotic to be used medically — penicillin — was extracted from *Penicillium notatum*.

Sir Alexander Fleming first noted the ability of the mould *P. notatum* to produce an antibiotic substance (which he called penicillin) in 1928. However, he also noted that when penicillin was added to blood *in vitro*, it lost most of its antibiotic action, and Fleming consequently lost interest in his discovery. In the late 1930s, Howard Florey, Ernst Chain and Norman Heatley began to work on penicillin. They purified it and, unlike Fleming, studied its effect on live animals. They found that administration of penicillin to mice after their injection with lethal doses of streptococci protected the mice from an otherwise certain death.

The Second World War conferred urgency to their research and they began large-scale culture of *Penicillium* in their laboratory (mostly in bedpans). However, low levels of antibiotic production rendered large-scale medical trials difficult. The first human to be treated was Albert Alexander, a policeman. Although dying from a severe bacterial infection, he responded immediately to penicillin treatment. Supplies were so scarce that medical staff collected his urine to extract traces of excreted penicillin. He was almost cured 4 days after commencement of treatment, but supplies ran out. He relapsed and died. The first serious clinical trials in 1940–1941 proved so encouraging that massive effort was expended (particularly in the USA) to develop large-scale penicillin production systems. This succeeded and, before the end of the war,

Table 1.17. Major families of antibiotics

β-Lactams
Tetracyclines
Aminoglycoside antibiotics
Macrolides
Ansamycins
Peptide/glycopeptide antibiotics
Miscellaneous antibiotics

it was in plentiful supply. At this stage, scientists also initiated screening programmes to identify additional antibiotics. Streptomycin was an early success in this regard. It was first isolated in 1944 from a strain of *Streptomyces griseus*.

Today there are in excess of 100 antibiotics available on the market. Due to the availability of such a wide range, many pharmaceutical companies cut back or abandoned ongoing antibiotic screening programmes during the 1980s. However, the emergence of microbial strains resistant to most antibiotics threatens medical reversion effectively to a pre-antibiotic era. These developments have rejuvenated interest in discovering new antibiotics and many pharmaceutical companies have recommenced antibiotic screening programmes.

When grouped on the basis of similarities in their chemical structure, most antibiotics fall into the categories listed in Table 1.17. β-Lactams, which include penicillins and cephalosporins, exhibit a characteristic β-lactam core ring structure (a four-atom cyclic amide) (Figure 1.14). They induce their bacteriocidal activity by inhibiting the synthesis of peptidoglycan, an essential component of the bacterial cell wall.

Penicillins refer to a family of both natural and semi-synthetic antibiotics. Although all exhibit a 6-aminopenicillanic acid core ring structure (Figure 1.15), they differ in the structure of their side-chains. Naturally produced penicillins include penicillins G and V. Semi-synthetic penicillins can be manufactured by enzymatic removal of a natural penicillin side-chain (using

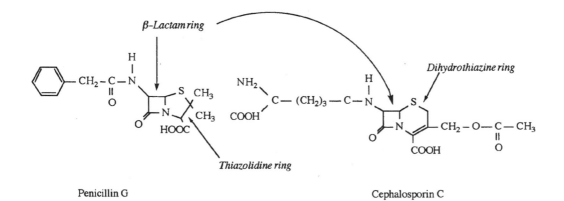

Penicillin G   Cephalosporin C

Figure 1.14.   Structure of penicillin G and cephalosporin C, two of the best-known β-lactam antibiotics. Both exhibit the 4-atom β-lactam ring

(a)

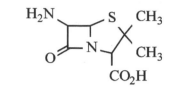

(b)

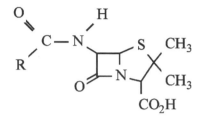

(c)   <u>NAME</u>   <u>SUBSTITUENT (R)</u>

PENICILLIN G (NATURAL)

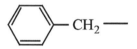

PENICILLIN V (NATURAL)

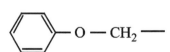

METHICILLIN (SEMISYNTHETIC)

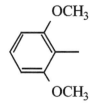

AMPICILLIN (SEMISYNTHETIC)

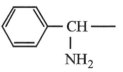

Figure 1.15. Structure of 6-aminopenicillanic acid (a); generalized penicillin structure (b) and side-groups present in two natural penicillins and two semisynthetic penicillins (c)

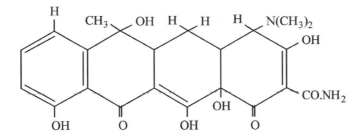

Figure 1.16. Chemical structure of the antibiotic tetracycline. Other members of the tetracycline family (see also Table 1.18) also display this characteristic 4-ring structure

penicillin acylase). Downward adjustment of the reaction pH to 4.3 results in precipitation of the resultant 6-aminopenicillanic acid ring, which can then be easily harvested. Novel side-chains can subsequently be attached, yielding semi-synthetic penicillins. Examples of the latter include phenethicillin, propicillin and oxacillin. Some semi-synthetic penicillins are effective against bacterial pathogens that have become resistant to natural penicillins. Others are acid-stable, allowing their oral administration.

Cephalosporins display an antibiotic mechanism of action identical to that of the penicillins. Cephalosporin C (Figure 1.14) is the prototypic natural cephalosporin and is produced by the fungus *Cephalosporium acremonium*. Most other members of this family are semi-synthetic derivatives of cephalosporin C. Chemical modification normally targets side-chains at position 3 (the acetoxymethyl group) or 7 (derived from D-α-aminoadipic acid).

Tetracyclines are a family of antibiotics which display a characteristic 4-fused-core ring structure (Figure 1.16). They exhibit broad antimicrobial activity and induce their effect by inhibiting protein synthesis in sensitive microorganisms. Chlortetracycline was the first member of this family to be discovered (in 1948). Penicillin G and streptomycin were the only antibiotics in use at that time, and chlortetracycline was the first antibiotic employed therapeutically that retained its antimicrobial properties upon oral administration. Since then, a number of additional tetracyclines have been discovered (all produced by various strains of *Streptomyces*), and a variety of semi-synthetic derivatives have also been prepared (Table 1.18).

Tetracyclines gained widespread medical use due to their broad spectrum of activity, which includes not only Gram-negative and Gram-positive bacteria, but also mycoplasmas, rickettsias, chlamydias and spirochaetes. However, adverse effects (e.g. staining of teeth and gastro-intestinal disturbances), along with the emergence of resistant strains, now somewhat limits their therapeutic applications.

Table 1.18. Natural and semi-synthetic tetracyclines which have gained medical application

Natural	Semi-synthetic
Chlortetracycline	Methacycline
Oxytetracycline	Doxycycline
Tetracycline	Minocycline
Demeclocycline	

Table 1.19. Some aminoglycoside antibiotics which have gained significant therapeutic application. Producer microorganisms are listed in brackets. In addition to naturally produced aminoglycosides, a number of semi-synthetic derivatives have also found medical application. Examples include amikacin, a semi-synthetic derivative of kanamycin and netilmicin, an N-ethyl derivative of sissomicin

---

Streptomycin (*Streptomyces griseus*)
Tobramycin (*Streptomyces tenebrarius*)
Framycetin (*Streptomyces* spp.)
Neomycin (*Streptomyces* spp.)
Kanamycin (*Streptomyces* spp.)
Paromycin (*Streptomyces* spp.)
Gentamicin (*Micromonospora purpurea*)
Sissomicin (*Micromonospora* spp.)

The aminoglycosides are a closely related family of antibiotics produced almost exclusively by members of the genus *Streptomyces* and *Micromonospora* (Table 1.19). Most are polycationic compounds, composed of a cyclic amino alcohol to which amino sugars are attached. They all induce their bacteriocidal effect by inhibiting protein synthesis (apparently by binding to the 30 S and, to some extent, the 50 S, ribosomal subunits). Most are orally inactive, generally necessitating their parenteral administration.

The aminoglycosides are most active against Gram-negative rods. Streptomycin was the first aminoglycoside to be used clinically. Another notable member of this family, gentamicin, was first purified from a culture of *Micromonospora purpurea* in 1963. Its activity against *Pseudomonas aeruginosa* and *Serratia marcescens* renders it useful in the treatment of these (often life-threatening) infections.

The macrolides and ansamycins

The macrolides are a large group of antibiotics. They are characterized by a core ring structure containing 12 or more carbon atoms (closed by a lactone group), to which one or more sugars are attached. The core ring of most anti-bacterial macrolides consists of 14 or 16 carbon atoms, while that of the larger anti-fungal and anti-protozoal macrolides contain up to 30 carbons. This family of antibiotics are produced predominantly by various species of *Streptomyces*. Antibacterial macrolides induce their effects by inhibiting bacterial synthesis (anti-fungal/ protozoal macrolides appear to function by interfering with sterols, thus compromising membrane structure). The only member of this family that enjoys widespread therapeutic use is erythromycin, which was discovered in 1952.

Ansamycins, like the macrolides, are synthesized by condensation of a number of acetate and propionate units. These antibiotics, which are produced by several genera of the Actinomycetales, display a characteristic core aromatic ring structure. Amongst the best-known family members are the rifamycins, which are particularly active against Gram-positive bacteria and mycobacteria. They have been used, for example, in the treatment of *Mycobacterium tuberculosis*.

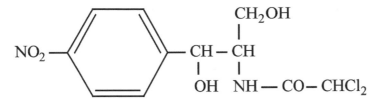

Figure 1.17. Chemical structure of chloramphenicol, the first broad-spectrum antibiotic to gain clinical use

Peptide and other antibiotics

Peptide antibiotics consist of a chain of amino acids which often have cyclized, forming a ring-like structure. The first such antibiotics isolated were bacitracin and gramicidin, although neither are used clinically due to their toxicity. While a number of microbes produce peptide antibiotics, relatively few such antibiotics are applied therapeutically. Polymyxins are the most common exception. Vancomycin, a glycopeptide, has also gained therapeutic application. It functions by interfering with bacterial cell wall synthesis, and is particularly active against Gram-positive cocci.

A variety of additional antibiotics are known that, based on their chemical structure, do not fit into any specific antibiotic family. Perhaps the most prominent such antibiotic is chloramphenicol (Figure 1.17). Chloramphenicol was first isolated from a culture of *Streptomyces venezuelae* in 1947, but it is now obtained by direct chemical synthesis. It was the first truly broad-spectrum antibiotic to be discovered, and was found effective against Gram-negative and Gram-positive bacteria, rickettsias and chlamydias. It retains activity when administered orally and functions by inhibiting protein synthesis. However, due to its adverse effects upon bone marrow function, clinical application of chloramphenicol is undertaken with caution. Its main use has been to combat *Salmonella typhi*, *Haemophilus influenzae* (especially in cases of meningitis) and *Bacteroides fragilis* (an anaerobe which can cause cerebral abscess formation). Some semi-synthetic derivatives of chloramphenicol (e.g. thiamphenicol) have also been developed for clinical use.

CONCLUSION

Most major life form families (microorganisms, plants and animals) have each yielded a host of valuable therapeutic substances. Many pharmaceutical companies and other institutions continue to screen plants and microbes in the hope of discovering yet more such therapeutic agents. However, in recent years, more and more emphasis is being placed upon developing the 'body's own drugs' as commercially produced pharmaceutical substances. Most such drugs are protein-based, and these biopharmaceuticals represent an exciting new family of pharmaceutical products. The number of such drugs gaining approval for general medical use continues to grow, as does their range of therapeutic applications. A fuller discussion of these biopharmaceuticals forms the basis of the remaining chapters of this text. In addition, the reader's attention is drawn to Appendix 2 of this book, which contains a list of Internet sites of relevance to the biopharmaceutical sector. Much additional valuable information may be downloaded from these sites.

FURTHER READING

Books

Buckingham, J. (1996). *Dictionary of Natural Products*. Chapman & Hall, London.

Crommelin, D. & Sindelar, R. (2002) *Pharmaceutical Biotechnology*, 2nd Edn. Taylor & Francis, London.

Goldberg, R. (2001). *Pharmaceutical Medicine, Biotechnology and European Law*. Cambridge University Press, Cambridge.

Grindley, J. & Ogden, J. (2000). *Understanding Biopharmaceuticals. Manufacturing and Regulatory Issues*. Interpharm Press, Denver, CO.

Kucers, A. (1997). *Use of Antibiotics: A Clinical Review of Antibacterial, Antifungal and Antiviral Drugs*, 5th edn. Butterworth–Heinemann, Oxford.

Lincini, G. (1994). *Biotechnology of Antibiotics and Other Bioactive Microbial Metabolites*. Plenum, New York.

Lubiniecki, A. (1994). *Regulatory Practice for Biopharmaceutical Production*. Wiley, Chichester.

Mann, J. (1998). *Bacteria and Antibacterial Agents*. Oxford University Press, Oxford.

Manske, R. (1999). *Alkaloids*. Academic Press, London.

Oxender, D. & Post, L. (1999). *Novel Therapeutics from Modern Biotechnology*. Springer-Verlag, Berlin.

Pezzuto, J. (1993). *Biotechnology and Pharmacy*. Chapman & Hall, London.

Reese, R. (2000). *Handbook of Antibiotics*. Lippincott, Williams & Wilkins, Philadelphia, PA.

Roberts, M. (1998). *Alkaloids*. Plenum, New York.

Smith, E. *et al.* (1983). Mammalian biochemistry. In *Principles of Biochemistry*. McGraw Hill, New York.

Strohl, W. (1997). *Biotechnology of Antibiotics*. Marcel Dekker, New York.

Walsh, G. & Murphy, B. (Eds) (1998). *Biopharmaceuticals: An Industrial Perspective*. Kluwer Academic, Dordrecht.

Articles

General biopharmaceutical

Drews, J. (1993). Into the twenty-first century. Biotechnology and the pharmaceutical industry in the next 10 years. *Bio/ Technology* **11**, 516–520.

Olson, E. & Ratzkin, B. (1999). Pharmaceutical biotechnology. *Curr. Opin. Biotechnol.* **10**, 525–527.

Walsh, G. (2000). Biopharmaceutical benchmarks. *Nature Biotechnol.* **18**, 831–833.

Walsh, G. (2002). Biopharmaceuticals and biotechnology medicines: an issue of nomenclature. *Eur. J. Pharmaceut. Sci.* **15**, 135–138.

Weng, Z. & DeLisi, C. (2000). Protein therapeutics: promises and challenges of the twenty-first century. *Trends Biotechnol.* **20**(1), 29–36.

Natural products

Attaurrahman-Choudhary, M. (1997). Diterpenoid and steroidal alkaloids. *Nat. Prod. Rep.* **14**(2), 191–203.

Billstein, S. (1994). How the pharmaceutical industry brings an antibiotic drug to the market in the United States. *Antimicrob. Agents Chemother.* **38**(12), 2679–2682.

Bruce, N. *et al.* (1995). Engineering pathways for transformations of morphine alkaloids. *Trends Biotechnol.* **13**, 200–205.

Chopra, I. *et al.* (1997). The search for anti-microbial agents effective against bacteria resistant to multiple antibiotics. *Antimicrob. Agents Chemother.* **41**(3), 497–503.

Cordell, G. *et al.* (2001). The potential of alkaloids in drug discovery. *Phytother. Res.* **15**(3), 183–205.

Dougherty, T. *et al.* (2002). Microbial genomics and novel antibiotic discovery. *New Technol. New Drugs Curr. Pharmaceut. Design* **8**(13), 1119–1135.

Facchini, P. (2001). Alkaloid biosynthesis in plants: biochemistry, cell biology, molecular regulation and metabolic engineering applications. *Ann. Rev. Plant Physiol. Plant Mol. Biol.* **52**, 29–66.

Flieger, M. *et al.* (1997). Ergot alkaloids — sources, structures and analytical methods. *Folia Microbiol.* **42**(1), 3–29.

Glass, J. *et al.* (2002). *Streptococcus pneumoniae* as a genomics platform for broad spectrum antibiotic discovery. *Curr. Opin. Microbiol.* **5**(3), 338–342.

Gournelis, D. *et al.* (1997). Cyclopeptide alkaloids. *Nat. Prod. Rep.* **14**(1), 75–82.

Hancock, R. (1997). Peptide antibiotics. *Lancet* **349**(9049), 418–422.

Kalant, H. (1997). Opium revisited — a brief review of its nature, composition, non-medical use and relative risks. *Addiction* **92**(3), 267–277.

Kaufmann, C. & Carver, P. (1997). Antifungal agents in the 1990s — current status and future developments. *Drugs* **53**(4), 539–549.

Krohn, K. & Rohr, J. (1997). Angucyclines — total synthesis, new structures and biosynthetic studies of an emerging new class of antibiotics. *Topics Curr. Chem.* **188**, 127–195.

McManus, M. (1997). Mechanisms of bacterial resistance to anti-microbial agents. *Am. J. Health Syst. Pharm.* **54**(12), 1420–1433.

Marston, A. *et al.* (1993). Search for antifungal, molluscicidal and larvicidal compounds from African medicinal plants. *J. Ethnopharmacol.* **38**, 215–233.

Michael, J.P. (1997). Quinoline, quinazoline and acridone alkaloids. *Nat. Prod. Rep.* **14**(1), 11–20.

Nicolas, P. & Mor, A. (1995). Peptides as weapons against microorganisms in the chemical defence system of vertebrates. *Ann. Rev. Microbiol.* **49**, 277–304.

Normark, B. & Normark, S. (2002). Evolution and spread of antibiotic resistance. *J. Intern. Med.* **252**(2), 91–106.

Tudzynski, P. *et al.* (2001). Biotechnology and genetics of ergot alkaloids. *Appl. Microbiol. Biotechnol.* **57**(5–6), 593–605.

Walsh, C. (2002). Combinatorial biosynthesis of antibiotics, challenges and opportunities. *Chembiochem.* **3**(2–3), 125–134.

Chapter 2

The drug development process

In this chapter, the life history of a successful drug will be outlined (summarized in Figure 2.1). A number of different strategies are adopted by the pharmaceutical industry in their efforts to identify new drug products. These approaches range from random screening of a wide range of biological materials to knowledge-based drug identification. Once a potential new drug has been identified, it is then subjected to a range of tests (both *in vitro* and in animals) in order to characterize it in terms of its likely safety and effectiveness in treating its target disease.

After completing such pre-clinical trials, the developing company apply to the appropriate government-appointed agency (e.g. the FDA in the USA) for approval to commence clinical trials (i.e. to test the drug in humans). Clinical trials are required to prove that the drug is safe and effective when administered to human patients, and these trials may take 5 years or more to complete. Once the drug has been characterized, and perhaps early clinical work is under way, the drug is normally patented by the developing company, in order to ensure that it receives maximal commercial benefit from the discovery.

Upon completion of clinical trials, the developing company collates all the pre-clinical and clinical data they have generated, as well as additional pertinent information, e.g. details of the exact production process used to make the drug. They submit this information as a dossier (a multi-volume work) to the regulatory authorities. Regulatory scientific officers then assess the information provided and decide (largely on criteria of drug safety and efficacy) whether the drug should be approved for general medical use.

If marketing approval is granted, the company can sell the product from then on. As the drug has been patented, they will have no competition for a number of years at least. However, in order to sell the product, a manufacturing facility is required, and the company will also have to gain manufacturing approval from the regulatory authorities. In order to gain a manufacturing licence, a regulatory inspector will review the proposed manufacturing facility. The regulatory authority will only grant the company a manufacturing licence if they are satisfied that every aspect of the manufacturing process is conducive to consistently producing a safe and effective product.

Regulatory involvement does not end even at this point. Post-marketing surveillance is generally undertaken, with the company being obliged to report any subsequent drug-induced side effects/adverse reactions. The regulatory authority will also inspect the manufacturing facility from time to time in order to ensure that satisfactory manufacturing standards are maintained.

Biopharmaceuticals: Biochemistry and Biotechnology, Second Edition by Gary Walsh
John Wiley & Sons Ltd: ISBN 0 470 84326 8 (ppc), ISBN 0 470 84327 6 (pbk)

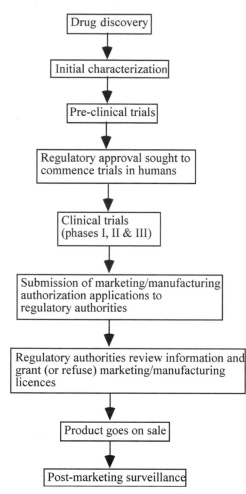

Figure 2.1. An overview of the life history of a successful drug. Patenting of the product is usually also undertaken, often during the initial stages of clinical trial work

DRUG DISCOVERY

The discovery of virtually all the biopharmaceuticals discussed in this text was a knowledge-based one. Continuing advances in the molecular sciences have deepened our understanding of the molecular mechanisms which underline health and disease. An understanding at the molecular level of how the body functions in health, and the deviations that characterize the development of a disease, often renders obvious potential strategies likely to cure/control that disease. Simple examples illustrating this include the use of insulin to treat diabetes, or the use of growth hormone to treat certain forms of dwarfism (Chapter 8). The underlining causes of these types of disease are relatively straightforward, in that they are essentially promoted by the deficiency/absence of a single regulatory molecule. Other diseases, however, may be multifactorial and, hence, more complex. Examples here include cancer and inflammation. Nevertheless, cytokines such as interferons and interleukins, known to stimulate the immune response/regulate inflammation, have proved to be therapeutically useful in treating several such complex diseases (Chapters 4 and 5).

An understanding, at the molecular level, of the actions of various regulatory proteins, or the progression of a specific disease does not, however, automatically translate into pinpointing an effective treatment strategy. The physiological responses induced by the potential biopharmaceutical *in vitro* (or in animal models) may not accurately predict the physiological responses seen when the product is administered to a diseased human. For example, many of the most promising biopharmaceutical therapeutic agents (e.g. virtually all the cytokines; Chapter 4), display multiple activities on different cell populations. This makes it difficult, if not impossible, to predict what the overall effect administration of any biopharmaceutical will have on the whole body, hence the requirement for clinical trials.

In other cases, the widespread application of a biopharmaceutical may be hindered by the occurrence of relatively toxic side effects (as is the case with tumour necrosis factor α (TNF-α), Chapter 5). Finally, some biomolecules have been discovered and purified because of a characteristic biological activity which, subsequently, was found not to be the molecule's primary biological activity. TNF-α again serves as an example. It was first noted because of its cytotoxic effects on some cancer cell types *in vitro*. Subsequently, trials assessing its therapeutic application in cancer proved disappointing, due not only to its toxic side effects but also to its moderate, at best, cytotoxic effect on many cancer cell types *in vivo*. TNF's major biological activity *in vivo* is now known to be as a regulator of the inflammatory response.

In summary, the 'discovery' of biopharmaceuticals, in most cases, merely relates to the logical application of our rapidly increasing knowledge of the biochemical basis of how the body functions. These substances could be accurately described as being the body's own pharmaceuticals. Moreover, rapidly expanding areas of research, such as genomics and proteomics, will likely hasten the discovery of many more such products, as discussed below.

While biopharmaceuticals are typically proteins derived from the human body, most conventional drugs have been obtained from sources outside the body (e.g. plant and microbial metabolites, synthetic chemicals, etc.). Although they do not form the focus of this text, a brief overview of strategies adopted in the discovery of such 'non-biopharmaceutical' drugs is appropriate, and is summarized later in this chapter.

The impact of genomics and related technologies upon drug discovery

The term 'genomics' refers to the systematic study of the entire genome of an organism. Its core aim is to sequence the entire DNA complement of the cell and to physically map the genome arrangement (assign exact positions in the genome to the various genes/non-coding regions). Prior to the 1990s, the sequencing and study of a single gene represented a significant task. However, improvements in sequencing technologies and the development of more highly automated hardware systems now render DNA sequencing considerably faster, cheaper and more accurate. Modern sequencing systems can sequence in excess of 1000 bases/h. Such innovations underpin the 'high-throughput' sequencing necessary to evaluate an entire genome sequence within a reasonable time frame. As a result, the genomes of almost 70 microorganisms have thus far been completely or almost completely sequenced (Table 2.1). In addition, various public and private bodies are currently sequencing the genomes of various plants and animals, including those of wheat, barley, chicken, dog, cow, pig, sheep, mouse and rat. The human genome project commenced in 1990, with an initial target completion date set at 2005. A 'rough draft' was published in February 2001, with the final completed draft expected in 2003. The total human

Table 2.1. Genome size (expressed as the number of nucleotide base pairs present in the entire genome of various microorganisms whose genome sequencing is complete/near complete). MB (megabase) = million bases

Microbe	Genome size (MB)	Microbe	Genome size (MB)
Agrobacterium tumefaciens	5.3	*Neisseria meningitidis*	2.27
Aquifex aeolicus	1.5	*Salmonella typhi*	4.8
Bacillus subtilis	4.2	*Streptococcus pneumoniae*	2.2
Campylobacter jejuni	1.64	*Sulfolobus solfataricus*	2.99
Clostridium acetobutylicum	4.1	*Thermoplasma acidophilum*	1.56
Escherichia coli	4.6	*Vibrio cholerae*	4.0
Haemophilus influenzae	1.83	*Yersinia pestis*	4.65
Helicobacter pylori	1.66	*Saccharomyces cerevisiae*	13.0
Mycobacterium leprae	3.26	*Candida albicans*	15.0
Mycobacterium tuberculosis	4.4		

genome size is in the region of 3.2 gigabases (Gb), approximately 1000 times larger than a typical bacterial genome (Table 2.1). Less than one-third of the genome is transcribed into RNA. Only 5% of that RNA is believed to encode polypeptides and the number of polypeptide-encoding genes is estimated to be of the order of 30 000 — well below the initial 100 000–120 000 estimates.

From a drug discovery/development perspective, the significance of genome data is that it provides full sequence information of every protein the organism can produce. This should result in the identification of previously undiscovered proteins which will have potential therapeutic application, i.e. the process should help identify new potential biopharmaceuticals. The greatest pharmaceutical impact of sequence data, however, will almost certainly be the identification of numerous additional drug targets. It has been estimated that all drugs currently on the market target one (or more) of a maximum of 500 targets. The majority of such targets are proteins (mainly enzymes, hormones, ion channels and nuclear receptors). Hidden in the human genome sequence data is believed to be anywhere between 3000 and 10 000 new protein-based drug targets. Additionally, present in the sequence data of many human pathogens (e.g. *Helicobacter pylori*, *Mycobacterium tuberculosis* and *Vibrio cholerae*; Table 2.1) is sequence data of hundreds, perhaps thousands, of pathogen proteins that could serve as drug targets against those pathogens (e.g. gene products essential for pathogen viability or infectivity).

While genome sequence data undoubtedly harbours new drug leads/drug targets, the problem now has become one of specifically identifying such genes. Impeding this process is the fact that (at the time of writing) the biological function of between one-third and half of sequenced gene products remains unknown. The focus of genome research is therefore now shifting towards elucidating the biological function of these gene products, i.e. shifting towards 'functional genomics'.

Assessment of function is critical to understanding the relationship between genotype and phenotype and, of course, for the direct identification of drug leads/targets. The term 'function' traditionally has been interpreted in the narrow sense of what isolated biological role/activity the gene product displays (e.g. is it an enzyme and, if so, what specific reaction does it catalyse?). In the context of genomics, gene function is assigned a broader meaning, incorporating not only the isolated biological function/activity of the gene product, but also relating to:

- where in the cell that product acts and, in particular, what other cellular elements it influences/interacts with;
- how such influences/interactions contribute to the overall physiology of the organism.

The assignment of function to the products of sequenced genes can be pursued via various approaches, including:

- sequence homology studies;
- phylogenetic profiling;
- Rosetta Stone method;
- gene neighbourhood method;
- knock-out animal studies;
- DNA array technology (gene chips);
- proteomics approach;
- structural genomics approach.

With the exception of knock-out animals, these approaches employ, in part at least, sequence structure/data interrogation/comparison. The availability of appropriate highly powerful computer programs renders these approaches 'high-throughput'. However, even by applying these methodologies, it will not prove possible to immediately identify the function of all gene products sequenced.

Sequence homology studies depend upon computer-based (bioinformatic) sequence comparison between a gene of unknown function (or, more accurately, of unknown gene product function) and genes whose product has previously been assigned a function. High homology suggests likely related functional attributes. Sequence homology studies can assist in assigning a putative function to 40–60% of all new gene sequences.

Phylogenetic profiling entails establishing a pattern of the presence or absence of the particular gene coding for a protein of unknown function across a range of different organisms whose genomes have been sequenced. If it displays an identical presence/absence pattern to an already characterized gene, then in many instances it can be inferred that both gene products have a related function.

The Rosetta Stone approach is dependent upon the observation that sometimes two separate polypeptides (i.e. gene products X and Y) found in one organism occur in a different organism as a single fused protein, XY. In such circumstances, the two protein parts (domains), X and Y, often display linked functions. Therefore, if gene X is recently discovered in a newly sequenced genome and is of unknown function, but gene XY of known function has been previously discovered in a different genome, the function of the unknown X can be deduced.

The gene neighbourhood method is yet another computation-based method. It depends upon the observation that if two genes are consistently found side by side in the genome of several different organisms, they are likely to be functionally linked.

Knock-out animal studies, in contrast to the above methods, are dependent upon phenotype observation. The approach entails the generation and study of mice in which a specific gene has been deleted. Phenotypic studies can sometimes yield clues as to the function of the gene knocked out.

Gene chips

Although sequence data provides a profile of all the genes present in a genome, it gives no information as to which genes are switched on (transcribed) and, hence, which are functionally active at any given time/under any given circumstances. Gene transcription results in the production of RNA, either messenger RNA (mRNA; usually subsequently translated into a polypeptide) or ribosomal or transfer RNA (rRNA or tRNA, which have catalytic or structural functions). The study of under which circumstances an RNA species is expressed/not expressed in the cell/organism can provide clues as to the biological function of the RNA (or, in the case of mRNA, the function of the final polypeptide product). Furthermore, in the context of drug lead/target discovery, the conditions under which a specific mRNA is produced can also point to putative biopharmaceuticals/drug targets. For example, if a particular mRNA is only produced by a cancer cell, that mRNA (or, more commonly, its polypeptide product) may represent a good target for a novel anti-cancer drug.

Levels of RNA (usually specific mRNAs) in a cell can be measured by well-established techniques such as Northern blot analysis or by polymerase chain reaction (PCR) analysis. However, the recent advent of DNA microarray technology has converted the identification and measurement of specific mRNAs (or other RNAs if required) into a 'high-throughput' process. DNA arrays are also termed 'oligonucleotide arrays', 'gene chip arrays' or simply, 'chips'.

The technique is based upon the ability to anchor nucleic acid sequences (usually DNA-based) on plastic/glass surfaces at very high density. Standard griding robots can put on up to 250 000 different short oligonucleotide probes or 10 000 full-length complementary DNA (cDNA) sequences per cm^2 of surface. Probe sequences are generally produced/designed from genome sequence data and hence chip production is often referred to as 'downloading the genome on a chip'. RNA can be extracted from a cell and probed with the chip. Any complementary RNA sequences present will hybridize with the appropriate immobilized chip sequence (Figure 2.2). Hybridization is detectable as the RNA species are first labelled. Hybridization patterns obviously yield critical information regarding gene expression.

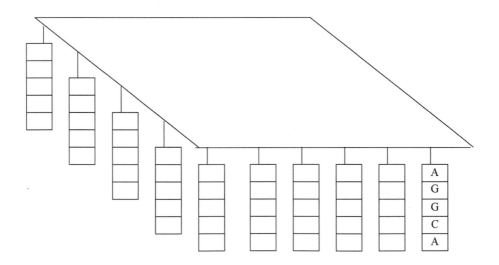

Figure 2.2. Generalized outline of a gene chip. In this example, short oligonucleotide sequences are attached to the anchoring surface (only the outer rows are shown). Each probe displays a different nucleotide sequence, and the sequences used are usually based upon genome sequence information. The sequence of one such probe is shown as AGGCA. By incubating the chip, e.g. with total cellular mRNA, under appropriate conditions, any mRNA with a complementary sequence (UCCGU in the case of the probe sequence shown) will hybridize with the probes. In reality, probes will have longer sequences than the one shown above

Proteomics

While virtually all drug targets are protein-based, the inference that protein expression levels can be accurately (if indirectly) detected/measured via DNA array technology is a false one, because:

- mRNA concentrations do not always directly correlate with the concentration of the mRNA-encoded polypeptide.
- a significant proportion of eukaryote mRNAs undergo differential splicing and, therefore, can yield more than one polypeptide product (Figure 2.3).

Additionally, the cellular location at which the resultant polypeptide will function often cannot be predicted from RNA detection/sequences nor can detailed information regarding how the polypeptide product's functional activity will be regulated (e.g. via post-translational mechanisms such as phosphorylation, partial proteolysis, etc.). Therefore, protein-based drug leads/targets are often more successfully identified by direct examination of the expressed protein complement of the cell, i.e. its proteome. Like the transcriptome (total cellular RNA content) and in contrast to the genome, the proteome is not static with changes in cellular

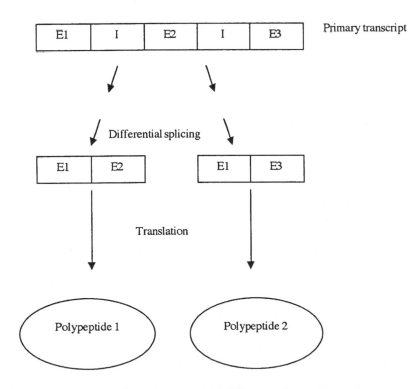

Figure 2.3. Differential splicing of mRNA can yield different polypeptide products. Transcription of a gene sequence yields a 'primary transcript' RNA. This contains coding regions (exons) and non-coding regions (introns). A major feature of the subsequent processing of the primary transcript is 'splicing', the process by which introns are removed, leaving the exons in a contiguous sequence. Although most eukaryotic primary transcripts produce only one mature mRNA (and hence code for a single polypeptide) some can be differentially spliced, yielding two or more mature mRNAs. The latter can therefore code for two or more polypeptides. E = exon; I = intron

conditions triggering changes in cellular protein profiles/concentrations. This field of study is termed 'proteomics'.

Proteomics is, therefore, closely aligned to functional genomics and entails the systematic and comprehensive analysis of the proteins expressed in the cell and their function. Classical proteomic studies generally entailed initial extraction of the total protein content from the target cell/tissue, followed by separation of the proteins therein using two-dimensional (2-D) electrophoresis (Chapter 3). Isolated protein 'spots' could then be eluted from the electrophoretic gel and subjected to further analysis; mainly to Edman degradation, in order to generate partial amino acid sequence data. The sequence data could then be used to interrogate protein sequence databanks, e.g. in order to assign putative function by sequence homology searches (Figure 2.4). 2-D electrophoresis, however, is generally capable of resolving no more than 2000 different proteins, and proteins expressed at low levels may not be detected at all if their gel concentration is below the (protein) staining threshold. The latter point can be particularly significant in the context of drug/target identification, as most such targets are likely to be kinases and other regulatory proteins which are generally expressed within cells at very low levels.

More recently, high-resolution chromatographic techniques (particularly reverse-phase and ion exchanged-based HPLC) have been applied in the separation of proteome proteins and high-resolution mass spectrometry is being employed to aid high-throughput sequence determination.

Structural genomics

Related to the discipline of proteomics is that of structural genomics. The latter focuses upon the large-scale, systematic study of gene product structure. While this embraces rRNA and tRNA, in practice the field focuses upon protein structure. The basic approach to structural genomics entails the cloning and recombinant expression of cellular proteins, followed by their purification and three-dimensional (3-D) structural analysis. High-resolution determination of a protein's structure is amongst the most challenging of molecular investigations. By the year 2000, protein structure databanks housed in the region of 12 000 entries. However, such databanks are highly redundant, often containing multiple entries describing variants of the same molecule. For example, in excess of 50 different structures of 'insulin' have been deposited (e.g. both native and mutated/engineered forms from various species, as well as insulins in various polymeric forms and in the presence of various stabilizers and other chemicals). In reality, by the year 2000, the 3-D structure of approximately 2000 truly different proteins had been resolved.

Until quite recently, X-ray crystallography was the technique used almost exclusively to resolve the 3-D structure of proteins. As well as itself being technically challenging, a major limitation of X-ray crystallography is the requirement for the target protein in crystalline form. It has thus far proved difficult or impossible to induce the majority of proteins to crystallize. Nuclear magnetic resonance (NMR) is an analytical technique which can also be used to determine the three-dimensional structure of a molecule without the necessity for crystallization. For many years, even the most powerful NMR machines could resolve the 3-D structure of only relatively small proteins (less than 20–25 kDa). However, recent analytical advances now render it possible to successfully analyse much larger proteins by this technique.

The ultimate goal of structural genomics is to provide a complete 3-D description of any gene product. Also, as the structures of more and more proteins of known function are elucidated, it should become increasingly possible to link specific functional attributes to specific structural attributes. As such, it may prove ultimately feasible to predict protein function if its structure is known, and vice versa.

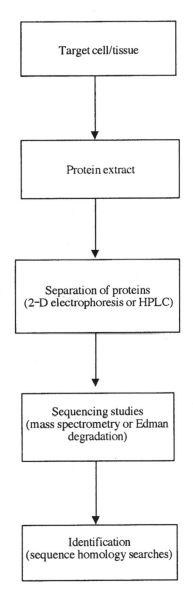

Figure 2.4. The proteomics approach. Refer to text for details

Pharmacogenetics

'Pharmacogenetics' relates to the emerging discipline of correlating specific gene DNA sequence information (specifically sequence variations) to drug response. As such, the pursuit will ultimately impinge directly upon the drug development process and should allow doctors to make better-informed decisions regarding what exact drug to prescribe to individual patients.

Different people respond differently to any given drug, even if they present with essentially identical disease symptoms, e.g. optimum dose requirements can vary significantly.

Furthermore, not all patients respond positively to a specific drug (e.g. interferon-β is of clinical benefit to only one in three multiple sclerosis patients; see Chapter 4). The range and severity of adverse effects induced by a drug can also vary significantly within a patient population base.

While the basis of such differential responses can sometimes be non-genetic (e.g. general state of health, etc), genetic variation amongst individuals remains the predominant factor. While all humans display almost identical genome sequences, some differences are evident. The most prominent widespread-type variations amongst individuals are known as single nucleotide polymorphisms (SNPs, sometimes pronounced 'snips'). SNPs occur in the general population at an average incidence of one in every 1000 nucleotide bases and hence the entire human genome harbours 3 million or so. SNPs are not mutations; the latter arise more infrequently, are more diverse and are generally caused by spontaneous/mutagen-induced mistakes in DNA repair/ replication. SNPs occurring in structural genes/gene regulatory sequences can alter amino acid sequence/expression levels of a protein and hence affect its functional attributes. SNPs largely account for natural physical variations evident in the human population (e.g. height, colour of eyes, etc.).

The presence of a SNP within the regulatory or structural regions of a gene coding for a protein which interacts with a drug could obviously influence the effect of the drug on the body. In this context, the protein product could, for example, be the drug target or perhaps an enzyme involved in metabolizing the drug.

The identification and characterization of SNPs within human genomes is, therefore, of both academic and applied interest. Several research groups continue to map human SNPs and over 1.5 million have thus far been identified.

By identifying and comparing SNP patterns from a group of patients responsive to a particular drug with patterns displayed by a group of unresponsive patients, it may be possible to identify specific SNP characteristics linked to drug efficacy. In the same way, SNP patterns or characteristics associated with adverse reactions (or even a predisposition to a disease) may be uncovered. This could usher in a new era of drug therapy, where drug treatment could be tailored to the individual patient. Furthermore, different drugs could be developed with the foreknowledge that each would be efficacious when administered to specific (SNP-determined) patient sub-types. A (distant) futuristic scenario could be visualized where all individuals could carry chips encoded with SNP details relating to their specific genome, allowing medical staff to choose the most appropriate drugs to prescribe in any given circumstance.

Linking specific genetic determinants to many diseases, however, is unlikely to be as straightforward as implied thus far. The progress of most diseases, and the relative effectiveness of allied drug treatment, is dependent upon many factors, including the interplay of multiple gene products. 'Environmental' factors, such as patient age, sex and general health, also play a prominent role.

The term 'pharmacogenomics' is one which has entered the 'genomic' vocabulary. Although sometimes used almost interchangeably with pharmacogenetics, it more specifically refers to studying the pattern of expression of gene products involved in a drug response.

Plants as a source of drugs

Traditionally, drug discovery programmes within the pharmaceutical industry relied heavily upon screening various biological specimens for potential drugs. Prior to the 1950s, the vast bulk of drug substances discovered were initially extracted from vascular plants (see also

Chapter 1). Examples include digoxin and digitoxin, originally isolated from the foxglove (a member of the genus *Digitalis*), as well as aspirin, codeine and taxol.

Today, well over 100 drugs (accounting for 25% of all prescriptions issued in the USA), were initially isolated from vascular plants. While some are still extracted from their native source, most are now obtained more cheaply and easily by direct chemical synthesis or semi-synthesis.

Plants are a rich potential source of drugs as they produce a vast array of novel bioactive molecules, many of which probably serve as chemical defences against infection or predation. In addition, the variety of different plant species present on the earth is staggering. There exist well over 265 000 flowering species alone, of which less that 1% have, thus far, been screened for the presence of any bioactive molecules of potential therapeutic use.

Two screening approaches may be adopted with respect to plants. The most straightforward entails random collection of vegetation in areas supporting a diversity of plant growth. Although there have been a few notable successes recorded (e.g. taxol) by pursuing this approach, the success rate of identifying a new useful drug is quite low.

Targeted screening approaches specifically zone in upon plants more likely to contain bioactive molecules in the first place. For example, plants which seem to be immune from predation may well be producing substances toxic to, for example, insects. These in turn are also likely to have some effect on human cells.

A more commonly employed targeted search strategy is that of the ethnobotanical approach (ethnobotany is the study of the relationships between plants and people). This entails interaction of the drug discoverer with indigenous communities in areas where herbal or plant-based medicines form the basis of therapeutic intervention. Researchers simply collect plant specimens used as local cures. Furthermore if, for example, interest is focused upon discovering an antiviral agent, plants used in the treatment of diseases known to be caused by viruses are given special attention (in some instances, scientists have even used non-human guides in targeting certain plants, e.g. some have studied the plant types fed to sick monkeys by other members of the monkey troop).

The collection procedure itself is straightforward. After cataloguing and identification, 1–2 kg of the plant material is dried, or stored in alcohol and brought back to the lab. The plant material is crushed and extracted with various solvents (most plant-derived bioactive molecules are low molecular mass substances, soluble in organic solvents of varying polarity). After removal of the solvent, the extracts are screened for desirable biological activities (e.g. inhibition of microbial growth, selective toxicity towards various human cancer cell lines, etc.).

If an interesting activity is described, larger quantities (10–100 kg) of the plant material are collected, from which chemists purify and characterize the active principle. The active principle is known as a 'lead compound'. Chemists will then usually attempt to modify the lead compound in order to render it more therapeutically useful (e.g. make it more potent, or perhaps increase its hydrophobicity so that it can pass through biological membranes). This is then subjected to further pre-clinical trials, and chemists determine whether an economically feasible method, allowing the drug's chemical synthesis, can be developed.

Microbial drugs

Microorganisms, particularly bacteria and fungi, have also proved to be a rich source of bioactive molecules such as antibiotics and anticancer agents (Chapter 1). Again, as in the case of plants, an incredibly rich array of microbial species inhabit the earth and their characteristic metabolic flexibility generates an enormous bank of potential pharmaceutical products. Most are also easy to culture, and large-scale fermentation technology, which allows bulk-scale production of products, is well established. Soil microorganisms in particular have proved to be an incredibly rich source of bioactive molecules, especially antibiotics.

Rational drug design

While large-scale systematic screening of natural (or synthetic) substances have yielded the bulk of modern pharmaceuticals, the use of more sophisticated knowledge-based approaches to drug discovery are now becoming increasingly routine.

Structure-based drug design relies heavily upon computer modelling to modify an existing drug or design a new drug which will interact specifically with a selected molecular target important in disease progression. A prerequisite to this approach is that the 3-D structure of the drug's target be known. Targets are normally proteins (e.g. specific enzymes or perhaps receptors for hormones or other regulatory molecules). Predictive computer modelling software is available that allows generation of a likely 3-D structure from amino acid (i.e. primary sequence) data. However, this approach will not yield a sufficiently accurate representation to be of significant use to the drug designer. The exact 3-D structure must be determined by X-ray crystallography. The generation of protein crystals, of sufficiently high quality to facilitate X-ray analysis is far from straightforward, and has somewhat limited progress in this area to date. The ability to determine 3-D structure of at least small proteins by NMR analysis may add impetus to this field.

If the 3-D structure of the target protein has been resolved, molecular modelling software facilitates rational design of a small ligand capable of fitting precisely into a region of the target (e.g. an enzyme's active site). The hope is that such a ligand would modify the target activity in a therapeutically beneficial manner. For example, a ligand capable of blocking the activity of retroviral reverse transcriptase would show promise as an effective AIDS therapeutic agent. Also, because the putative therapeutic agent has been custom-designed to fit its target ligand, its potency and specificity should be high.

This rational approach to drug design has been adopted in developing a specific inhibitor of the human cellular enzyme, purine nucleoside phosphorylase (PNP). PNP functions in the purine salvage pathway, catalysing the reversible reaction shown below:

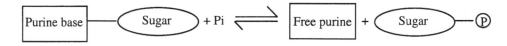

The free purine released can then be used in the biosynthesis of new nucleic acids within the cell.

Synthetic analogues of purine nucleosides are used medically as anti-cancer or anti-viral agents (they interfere with normal synthesis of nucleic acids and, hence, retard cell growth/viral infection; an example is 2'-3'-dideoxynosine, used to treat AIDS). PNP, however, can cleave these drugs, thus negating their therapeutic effect. PNP also appears to play a more prominent role in the metabolism of T lymphocytes when compared to other cells of the immune system. Thus, an effective inhibitor of this enzyme might prove useful in combating autoimmune diseases such as diabetes, rheumatoid arthritis, psoriasis and multiple sclerosis—all of which are characterized by excessive T cell activity.

X-ray crystallographic analysis illustrated that three amino acids in the purine-binding pocket of PNP form H-bonds with the purine rings, while the sugar residue interacts with additional active-site amino acids via hydrophobic bonds (Figure 2.5). Design of an effective inhibitor

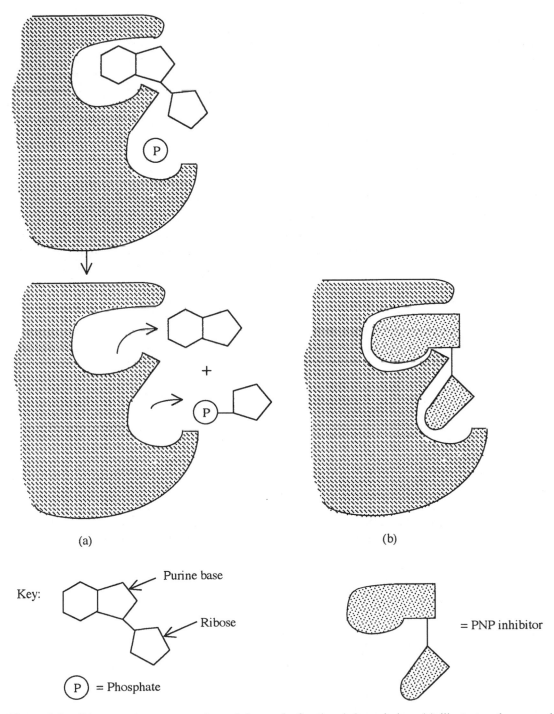

Figure 2.5. Diagramatic representation of the goal of rational drug design: (a) illustrates the normal catalytic activity exhibited by purine nucleoside phosphorylase (PNP); (b) represents an effective inhibitor of PNP, which fits well into the active site thereby blocking its normal enzymatic activity

centred around developing a molecule that fitted into the active site, and engaged in stronger H-bonding or additional hydrophobic interactions with the active site residues.

Without using computer modelling, identification of a potent inhibitor would, on average, require screening of hundreds of thousands of candidates, take up to 10 years and cost several million dollars. With computer modelling, the time and cost are cut to a fraction of this and, in this case, less than 60 compounds were prepared/modified to yield a highly effective inhibitor, BCX-34. This inhibitor molecule contains a 9-deazaguanine group (to fill the sugar binding site) and an acetate group (to fill the phosphate binding site). It is 100 times more potent than the best inhibitor previously identified by classical techniques, and it has performed well in initial clinical trials in treating psoriasis and cutaneous T cell lymphoma.

Combinatorial approaches to drug discovery

The concept of rational drug design drew emphasis away from the traditional random screening approach to drug discovery. However, the evelopment of techniques capable of generating large numbers of novel synthetic chemicals (combinatorial libraries), coupled with high-throughput screening methods, has generated fresh interest in the random screening approach.

Libraries can be generated relatively inexpensively and in a short time period. While many larger pharmaceutical companies maintain libraries of several hundred thousand natural and synthetic compounds, combinatorial chemistry can generate millions of compounds with relative ease. Peptides, for example, play various regulatory roles in the body, and several enjoy therapeutic application (e.g. GnRH; Chapter 8). Synthetic peptide libraries, containing peptides displaying millions of amino acid sequence combinations, can now be generated by combinatorial chemistry with minimal requirement for expensive equipment. Two approaches can be followed to generate a combinatorial peptide library: 'split synthesis' and 'T-bag synthesis'.

The split level approach, for example, results in the creation of a large peptide library in which the peptides are grown on small synthetic beads. Peptides grown on any single bead will all be of identical amino acid sequences. Individual amino acids can be coupled to the growing chain by straightforward solid phase peptide synthesis techniques (Box 2.1). In the split-level approach, a pool of beads are equally distributed into separate reaction vessels, each containing a single amino acid in solution. After chemical coupling to the beads, the beads are recovered, pooled and randomly distributed into the reaction vessels once more. This cycle can be repeated several times to extend the peptide chain. A simplified example is provided in Figure 2.6. While the example presented in Figure 2.6 is straightforward, a hexapeptide library containing every possible combination of all 20 commonly occurring amino acids would contain 64 million (20^6) different peptide species. Such a library, although more cumbersome, would be generated using exactly the same strategy.

The combinatorial approach is characterized not only by rapid synthesis of vast peptide libraries but also by rapid screening of these libraries (i.e. screening of the library to locate any peptides capable of binding to a ligand of interest — perhaps an enzyme or a hormone receptor). The soluble ligand is first labelled with an easily visible tag, often a fluorescent tag. This is then added to the beads. Binding of the ligand to a particular peptide will effectively result in staining of the bead to which the peptide is attached. This bead can then be physically separated from the other beads, e.g. using a microforceps. The isolated bead is then washed in 8 M guanidine hydrochloride (to remove the screening ligand) and the sequence of the attached peptide is then elucidated using a microsequencer. Typically, a bead will have 50–200 pmol of peptide attached, while the lower limit of sensitivity of most microsequencers is of the order of 5 pmol. Once its amino acid sequence is elucidated, it can be synthesized in large quantities for further study.

A library containing several million beads can be screened in a single afternoon. Furthermore, the library is reusable, as it may be washed in 8 M guanidine hydrochloride and then re-screened using a different probe. This split synthesis approach displays the ability to generate peptide libraries of incredible variety, variety that can be further expanded by incorporation of, for example, D-amino acids or rarely occurring amino acids.

Overall, therefore, various approaches may be adopted in the quest to discover new drugs. The approach generally adopted in biopharmacentical discovery differs from most other approaches in that biopharmaceuticals are produced naturally in the body. Discovery of a biopharmaceutical product, therefore, becomes a function of an increased knowledge of how the body itself functions. After its initial discovery, the physicochemical and biological characteristics of the potential drug can then be studied.

Initial product characterization

The physicochemical and other properties of any newly identified drug must be extensively characterized prior to its entry into clinical trials. As the vast bulk of biopharmaceuticals are proteins, a summary overview of the approach taken to initial characterization of these biomolecules is presented. A prerequisite to such characterization is initial purification of the protein. Purification to homogeneity usually requires a combination of three or more high-resolution chromatographic steps. The purification protocol is designed carefully, as it usually forms the basis of subsequent pilot and process-scale purification systems. The purified product is then subjected to a battery of tests, which aim to characterize it fully. Moreover, once these characteristics have been defined, they form the basis of many of the quality control (QC) identity tests routinely performed on the product during its subsequent commercial manufacture. As these identity tests are discussed in detail in Chapter 3, only an abbreviated overview is presented here, in the form of Figure 2.7.

In addition to the studies listed in Figure 2.7, stability characteristics of the protein, e.g. with regard to temperature, pH and incubation with various potential excipients, are undertaken. Such information is required in order to identify a suitable final product formulation, and to give an early indication of the likely useful shelf-life of the product.

PATENTING

The discovery and initial characterization of any substance of potential pharmaceutical application is followed by its patenting. The more detail given relevant to the drug's physicochemical characteristics, a method of synthesis and its biological effects, the better the chances of successfully securing a patent. Thus patenting may not take place until pre-clinical trials and phase I clinical trials are completed. Patenting, once successfully completed, does not grant the patent holder an automatic right to utilize/sell the patented product — it must first be proved safe and effective in subsequent clinical trials and then be approved for general medical use by the relevant regulatory authorities.

What is a patent and what is patentable?

A patent may be described as a monopoly granted by a government to an inventor, such that only the inventor may exploit the invention/innovation for a fixed period of time (up to 20

Box 2.1.   The chemical synthesis of peptides

A number of approaches may be adopted to achieve chemical synthesis of a peptide. The Merrifield solid phase synthesis method is perhaps the most widely used. This entails sequential addition of amino acids to a growing peptide chain anchored to the surface of modified polystyrene beads. The modified beads contain reactive chloromethyl ($-CH_2Cl$) groups.

The individual amino acid building blocks are first incubated with di-*tert*-butyl dicarbonate, thus forming a *tert*-butoxycarbonyl amide (BOC) amino acid derivative.

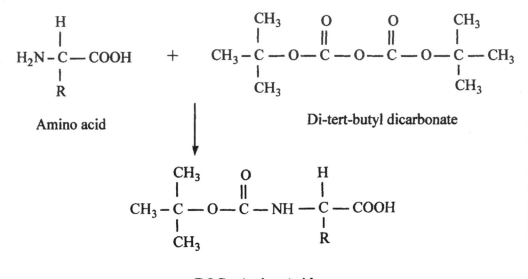

The BOC group protects the amino acid amino group, thus ensuring that addition of each new amino acid to the growing peptide chain occurs via the amino acid's carboxyl group (Step 1 below). Coupling of the first amino acid to the bead is achieved under alkaline conditions. Subsequent treatment with trifluoroacetic acid removes the BOC group (Step 2 below). Next, a second BOC-protected amino acid is added, along with a coupling reagent (DCC, Step 3). This promotes peptide bond formation. Additional amino acids are coupled by repeating this cycle of events. Note that the peptide is grown from its carboxy-terminal end. After the required peptide is synthesized (a dipeptide in the example below), it is released from the bead by treatment with anhydrous hydrogen fluoride. Automated computer-controlled peptide synthesizers are available commercially, rendering routine peptide manufacture for pharmaceutical or other purposes.

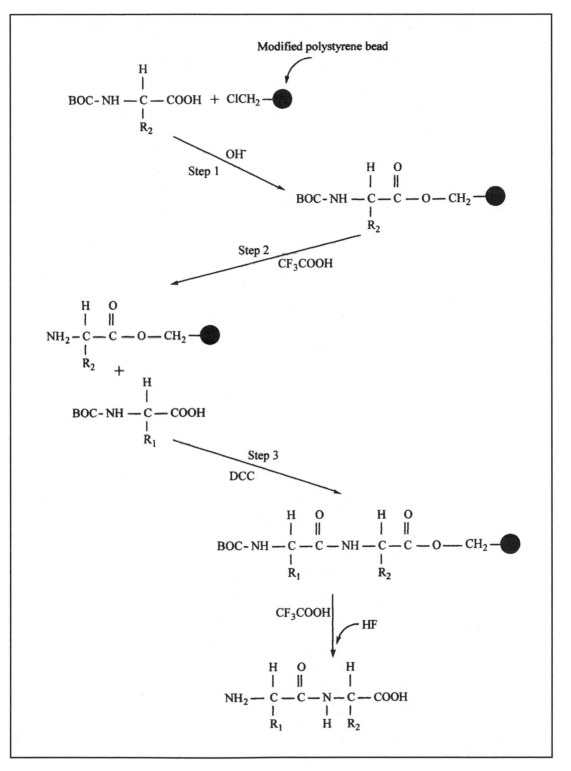

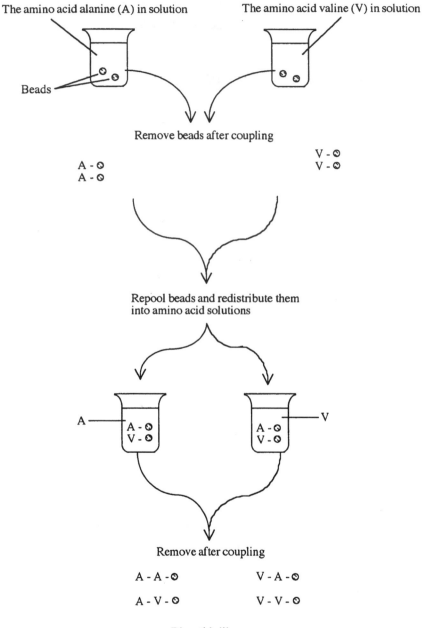

Figure 2.6. The use of the split synthesis technique to generate a dipeptide library. After the two coupling steps shown are completed, the four possible (2^2) dipeptide sequence combinations are found. Note that any single bead will have multiple copies of the (identical) dipeptide attached and not just a single copy as shown above. This synthesis technique is economical and straightforward to undertake and requires no sophisticated equipment. The coupling steps, etc. utilized are based upon standard peptide synthesizing techniques, such as the Merrifield method (Box 2.1)

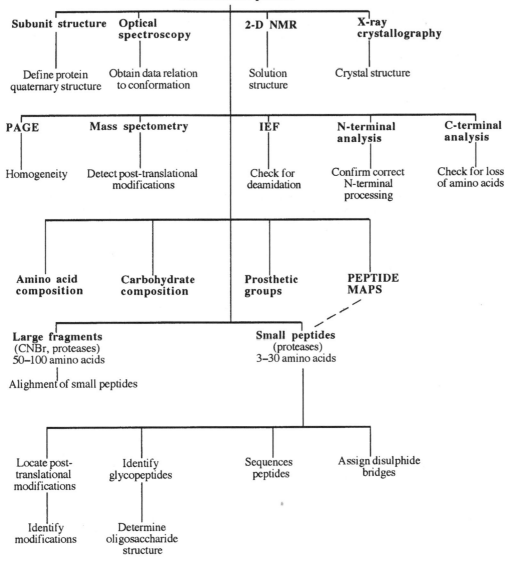

Figure 2.7. Task tree for the full structural characterization of a therapeutic protein. Reprinted by permission from *Bio/Technology* **9** (1991), p. 922

years). In return, the inventor makes available a detailed technical description of the invention/ innovation so that, when the monopoly period has expired, it may be exploited by others without the inventor's permission.

A patent, therefore, encourages innovation by promoting research and development. It can also be regarded as a physical asset, which can be sold or licensed to third parties for cash. Patents also represent a unique source of technical information regarding the patented product.

The philosophy underlining patent law is fairly similar throughout the world. Thus, although there is no worldwide patenting office, patent practice in different world regions is often quite similar. This is fortuitous, as there is a growing tendency towards world harmonization of patent law, fuelled by multinational trade agreements.

In order to be considered patentable, an invention/innovation must satisfy several criteria, the most important four of which are:

- novelty;
- non-obviousness;
- sufficiency of disclosure;
- utility.

To be novel, the invention/innovation should not be what is described as 'prior art', i.e. it should not be something already known or described previously. Prior disclosure of the invention/innovation, e.g. by publishing its details in a scientific (or other) journal, or a verbal description given, e.g. at a scientific meeting, puts this innovation in the public arena. This can effectively make it 'prior art'. While this can hinder a subsequent patent application, it may not be entirely fatal. To preclude a successful subsequent patent application, prior publication usually must be 'enabling', i.e. the detail given must be sufficient to allow an average person, familiar with the discipline relating to the patent (i.e. 'a person with ordinary skill and knowledge in the art'), to repeat the experiment or process described. A bare prior disclosure, which describes the innovation but not to an enabling level, will not normally prevent its subsequent patenting. Patenting law in relation to this point is more flexible in the USA. Here, even in the case of an existing enabling publication, patenting is usually possible as long as the patent is filed in under 1 year after the date of that publication.

The USA, unlike many other world regions, also adopts the 'first to invent' principle. Put simply (although patent disputes are rarely simple), if two inventors file similar patents, the patent will be granted to the one who proves that he/she was the first to 'invent' the 'product', even if he/she was not the first to file for a patent. Proving you were the first to invent can be complex and usually hinges around the availability of full and detailed laboratory notebooks or other records as to how and when the invention was made.

Non-obviousness (inventiveness) means that the invention/innovation process must not be something that would be immediately obvious to somebody skilled in the art. Non-obviousness, although it sounds straightforward, is often a difficult concept to apply in practice. Obviousness could be described as a simple and logical progression of prior art, thus non-obviousness requires an additional ingredient of inspiration or often chanced good luck.

Sufficiency of disclosure is a more straightforward requirement. Sufficient technical detail must be provided in the patent application such that somebody of ordinary technical skill in the area could reproduce/repeat the innovation. Utility or industrial applicability is the last major prerequisite to patenting. This simply means that the innovation must have some applied use.

Patent types

Patent types can be subdivided into 'Product', 'Process' and 'Use' patents. In the first case, a specific substance is patented (e.g. a revolutionary new car engine, a new cytokine with applicability in cancer treatment, a novel microorganism capable of degrading oil, etc.). In the case of process patents, a specific novel process, rather than an end product, is patented (e.g. a new combination of chromatographic methods capable of purifying a therapeutic protein with very high yield). Use patents are appropriate when a novel application for a specific substance is discovered, particularly if the substance itself is not patentable. An example might be the inclusion of a specific chemical that boosts yields of end product in a microbial industrial fermentation process. To be successfully filed, all of these patent types must satisfy the four major criteria already discussed.

The patent application

The patent application process can be both lengthy and costly. Generally, it takes 2–5 years from the initial filing date to get a patent approved, and the anticipated cost would be in the region of $10 000 per country. Any patent is a national right, granted by the government of the country in question. In the USA, the government patenting organization is known as the Patent and Trademark Office (PTO). While there are national patenting agencies within Europe, most European countries are members of the European Patent Organization (EuPO, based in Munich, Germany). These member countries have adapted national patent law such that, in most instances, any patent application approved by the EuPO can be enforced automatically in the constituent countries.

Many of the most significant patenting regions (e.g. Japan, the USA and Europe) are also signatories of the International Patent Cooperation Treaty (PCT). This allows for an initial review of the patent application to be undertaken by a single patent office. The office then provides a summary assessment of this application, which provides an indication of the likely response that would be obtained from individual PCT countries. For many, this initial assessment plays a major role in deciding whether to proceed with the patent application in individual countries.

The patent application document may be considered under a number of headings (Table 2.2). After the title comes the abstract, which identifies the innovation and the innovation area. Relevant prior art is then overviewed in detail in the 'background' section. This is drawn mainly from published research articles and pre-existing patents. An adequate preparation of this section relies on prior completion of a comprehensive literature and patent search. Next, a short paragraph that details the problem the innovation will solve is presented. This should emphasize why the innovation should be considered novel and non-obvious. This in turn is followed by a detailed technical description of the innovation, such that an ordinary person skilled in the art could reproduce it. If, for example, microbial cultures or animal cells form part of the innovation, these must be deposited in an approved depository (e.g. the American Type Culture

Table 2.2. Headings of the most important sections found in a generalized patent application

Patent title
Abstract
Background to patent application
Outline of problems the innovation will solve
Detailed technical description of innovation
The specific patent claims

Collection, ATCC). The last section of the patent outlines exactly what claims are being made for the innovation.

While the inventor often prepares the first draft of the patent application, a patent specialist is normally employed to prepare a final draft and guide the application through the patenting process.

After its submission to a patent office, the patent application is briefly reviewed and, if all the required information is provided, a formal filing date is issued. A detailed examination of the patent will then be undertaken by patent office experts, whose assessment will be based upon the four main criteria previously outlined. A report is subsequently issued accepting or rejecting the patent claim. The applicant is given the opportunity to reply, or modify the patent and resubmit it for further evaluation. In some cases, two or three such cycles may be undertaken before the patent is granted (or perhaps finally rejected).

The normal duration of a patent is 20 years. In most world jurisdictions, patent protection on pharmaceutical substances is extended, often by up to 5 years. This is to offset the time lost between the patenting date and final approval of the drug for general medical use.

Patenting in biotechnology

Many products of nature (e.g. specific antibiotics, microorganisms, proteins, etc.) have been successfully patented. It might be argued that simply to find any substance naturally occurring on the earth is categorized as a discovery, and would be unpatentable because it lacks true novelty or any inventive step. However, if you enrich, purify or modify a product of nature such that you make available the substance for the first time in an industrially useful format, that product/process is generally patentable. In other words, patenting is possible if the 'hand of man' has played an obvious part in developing the product.

In the USA, purity alone often facilitates patenting of a product of nature (Table 2.3). The PTO recognizes purity as a change in form of the natural material. For example, although vitamin B_{12} was a known product of nature for many years, it was only available in the form of a crude liver extract, which was of no use therapeutically; development of a suitable production (fermentation) and purification protocol allowed production of pure, crystalline vitamin B_{12} which could be used clinically. On this basis, a product patent was granted in the USA.

Using the same logic, the US PTO has, for example, granted patents for pure cultures of specific microorganisms, as well as medically important proteins [e.g. factor VIII, purified from blood (Chapter 9) and erythropoietin, purified from urine (Chapter 6)].

Table 2.3 Some products of nature which are generally patentable under US patent law. Additional patenting criteria (e.g. utility) must also be met. For many products, the patent will include details of the process used to purify the product. However, process patents can be filed, as can use patents. Refer to text for further details

A pure microbial culture
Isolated viruses
Specific purified proteins (e.g. erythropoietin)
Purified nucleic acid sequences (including isolated genes, plasmids, etc.)
Other purified biomolecules (e.g. antibiotics, vitamins, etc.)

Rapid technological advances in the biological sciences raises complex patenting issues, and patenting law as applied to modern biotechnology is still evolving.

In the late 1980s, the PTO confirmed that they would consider issuing patents for non-human multicellular organisms, including animals. The first transgenic animal was patented in 1988 by Harvard University. The 'Harvard mouse' carried a gene which made it more susceptible to cancer and, hence, more sensitive in detecting possible carcinogens.

Another area of biotechnology patent law relates to the patenting of genes and DNA sequences. Thus far, patents have been issued for some human genes, largely on the basis of the use of their cloned products (e.g. erythropoietin and tissue plasminogen activator). The human genome project continues to make available vast quantities of DNA sequence information — of both genes and non-coding regions. Moreover, the function of the bulk of the putative genes sequences at the moment remain unknown.

Most of the groups working on this project are funded by public bodies. Some sequencing groups, however, are funded by private companies. These wish to see a payback on their investment. Gaining a patent for a nucleotide sequence that is of medical or diagnostic use would provide very significant payback potential.

Patenting DNA sequences came under heavy legal and public scrutiny in 1992, when the US National Institutes of Health (NIH) filed a patent application on partial human cDNA sequences of unknown function. This patent was rejected, and the consensus has emerged that patent protection should only be considered for nucleotide sequences that can be used for specific purposes, e.g. for a sequence which can serve as a diagnostic marker or codes for a protein product of medical value. This appears to be a reasonable approach, as it balances issues of public interest with encouraging innovation in the area.

The issue of patenting genetic material or transgenic plants or animals remains a contentious one. The debate is not confined to technical and legal argument — ethical and political issues, including public opinion, also impinge on the decision-making process. The increasing technical complexity and sophistication of the biological principles and processes upon which biotechnological innovations are based also render resolution of legal patenting issues more difficult.

A major step in clarifying EU-wide law with regard to patenting in biotechnology stems from the introduction of the 1998 European patent directive. This directive (EU law) confirms that biological materials (e.g. specific cells, proteins, genes, nucleotide sequences, antibiotics, etc.) which previously existed in nature, are potentially patentable. However, in order to actually be patentable, they must (a) be isolated/purified from their natural environment and/or be produced via a technical process (e.g. recombinant DNA technology in the case of recombinant proteins), and (b) they must conform to the general patentability principles regarding novelty, non-obviousness, utility and sufficiency of disclosure. The 'utility' condition, therefore, in effect prevents patenting of gene/genome sequences of unknown function. The directive also prohibits the possibility of patenting inventions if their exploitation would be contrary to public order or morality. Thus, it is not possible to patent:

- the human body;
- the cloning of humans;
- the use of human embryos for commercial purposes;
- modifying germ line identity in humans;
- modifying the genetic complement of an animal if the modifications cause suffering without resultant substantial medical benefits to the animal or to humans.

DELIVERY OF BIOPHARMACEUTICALS

An important issue, which must be addressed during the pre-clinical phase of the drug development process, relates to the route by which the drug will be delivered or administered. To date, the vast majority of biopharmaceuticals approved for general medical use are administered by direct injection (i.e. parenterally), usually either intravenously (i.v.), subcutaneously (s.c.—directly under the skin) or intramuscularly (i.m.—into muscle tissue); s.c. or i.m. administration is generally followed by slow release of the drug from its depot site into the bloodstream. Amongst the few exceptions to this parenteral route are the enzyme DNase, used to treat cystic fibrosis (Chapter 9), and platelet-derived growth factor (PDGF), used to treat certain skin ulcers (Chapter 7). However, neither of these products is required to reach the bloodstream in order to achieve its therapeutic effect. In fact, in each case, the delivery system delivers the biopharmaceutical directly to its site of action (DNase is delivered directly to the lungs via aerosol inhalation, while PDGF is applied topically—directly on the ulcer surface—as a gel).

Parenteral administration is not perceived as a problem in the context of drugs that are administered infrequently, or as a once-off dose to a patient. However, in the case of products administered frequently or daily (e.g. insulin to diabetics), non-parenteral delivery routes would be preferred. Such routes would be more convenient, less invasive, less painful and generally would achieve better patient compliance. Alternative potential delivery routes include oral, nasal, transmucosal, transdermal or pulmonary routes. While such routes have proved possible in the context of many drugs, routine administration of biopharmaceuticals by such means has proved to be technically challenging. Obstacles encountered include their high molecular mass, their susceptibility to enzymatic inactivation and their potential to aggregate.

Oral delivery systems

Oral delivery is usually the preferred system for drug delivery, due to its convenience and the high level of associated patient compliance generally attained. Biopharmaceutical delivery via this route has proved problematic for a number of reasons:

- inactivation due to stomach acid. Prior to consumption of a meal, stomach pH is usually below 2.0. Although the buffering action of food can increase the pH to neutrality, the associated stimulation of stomach acid secretion subsequently reduces the ambient pH back down to 3.0–3.5. Virtually all biopharmaceuticals are acid-labile and are inactivated at low pH values;
- inactivation due to digestive proteases. Therapeutic proteins would represent potential targets for digestive proteases such as pepsin, trypsin and chymotrypsin;
- their (relatively) large size and hydrophilic nature renders difficult the passage of intact biopharmaceuticals across the intestinal mucosa;
- orally absorbed drugs are subjected to first-pass metabolism. Upon entry into the bloodstream, the first organ encountered is the liver, which usually removes a significant proportion of absorbed drugs from circulation.

Given such difficulties, it is not unsurprising that bioavailabilities below 1% are often recorded in the context of oral biopharmaceutical drug delivery. Strategies pursued to improve bioavailability include physically protecting the drug via encapsulation, formulation as microemulsions/microparticulates, as well as inclusion of protease inhibitors and permeability enhancers.

Encapsulation within an enteric coat (resistant to low pH values) protects the product during stomach transit. Microcapsules/spheres utilized have been made from various polymeric substances, including cellulose, polyvinyl alcohol, polymethylacrylates and polystyrene. Delivery systems based upon the use of liposomes and cyclodextrin-protective coats have also been developed. Included in some such systems also are protease inhibitors, such as aprotinin and ovomucoids. Permeation enhancers employed are usually detergent-based substances, which can enhance absorption through the gastrointestinal lining.

More recently, increasing research attention has focused upon the use of 'mucoadhesive delivery systems' in which the biopharmaceutical is formulated with/encapsulated in molecules which interact with the intestinal mucosa membranes. The strategy is obviously to retain the drug at the absorbing surface for a prolonged period. Non-specific (charge-based) interactions can be achieved by the use of polyacrylic acid, while more biospecific interactions are achieved by using selected lectins or bacterial adhesion proteins. Despite intensive efforts, however, the successful delivery of biopharmaceuticals via the oral route remains some way off.

Pulmonary delivery

Pulmonary delivery currently represents the most promising alternative to parenteral delivery systems for biopharmaceuticals. While the lung is not particularly permeable to solutes of low molecular mass (e.g. sucrose or urea), macromolecules can be absorbed into the blood via the lungs surprisingly well. In fact, pulmonary macromolecular absorption generally appears to be inversely related to molecular mass, up to a mass of about 500 kDa. Many peptides/proteins delivered to the deep lung are detected in the blood within minutes and bioavailabilities approaching or exceeding 50% (relative to subcutaneous injection) have been reported for therapeutic proteins such as colony-stimulating factors and some interferons. Although not completely understood, such high pulmonary bioavailability may stem from:

- the lungs' very large surface area;
- their low surface fluid volume;
- thin diffusional layer;
- relatively slow cell surface clearance;
- the presence of proteolytic inhibitors.

Additional advantages associated with the pulmonary route include:

- the avoidance of first-pass metabolism;
- the availability of reliable, metered nebulizer-based delivery systems capable of accurate dosage delivery, in either powder or liquid form;
- levels of absorption achieved without the need to include penetration enhancers, which are generally too irritating for long-term use.

Although obviously occurring in practice, macromolecules absorbed via the pulmonary route must cross a number of biological barriers to get into the blood. These are:

- a protective monolayer of insoluble phospholipid, termed 'lung surfactant', and its underlying surface lining fluid, which lies immediately above the lung epithelial cells;
- the epithelial cells lining the lung;
- the interstitium (an extracellular space) and the basement membrane, composed of a layer of interstitial fibrous material;

- the vascular endothelium—the monolayer of cells which constitute the walls of the blood vessels.

Passage through the epithelium and endothelial cellular barriers likely represents the greatest challenge to absorption. Although the molecular details remain unclear, this absorption process appears to occur via one of two possible means—transcytosis or paracellular transport (Figure 2.8).

Although no biopharmaceutical product delivered to the bloodstream via the pulmonary route has been approved to date, several companies continue to pursue active research and development programmes in the area. Amongst the leading product candidates is 'Exubera', an inhalable dry powder insulin formulation currently being evaluated by Pfizer and Aventis Pharma in Phase III clinical studies. The inhaled insulin is actually more rapidly absorbed than if administered subcutaneously and appears to achieve equivalent glycaemic control. While promising, final approval or otherwise of this product also depends upon additional safety studies which are currently under way.

Nasal, transmucosal and transdermal delivery systems

A nasal-based biopharmaceutical delivery route is considered potentially attractive as:

- it is easily accessible;
- nasal cavities are serviced by a high density of blood vessels;

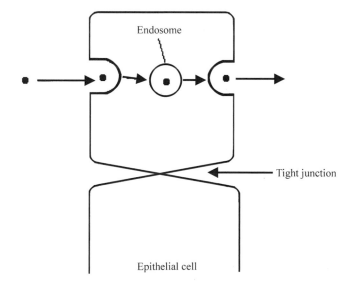

Figure 2.8. Likely mechanisms by which macromolecules cross cellular barriers in order to reach the bloodstream from (in this case) the lung. Transcytosis entails direct uptake of the macromolecule at one surface via endocytosis, travel of the endosome vesicle across the cell, with subsequent release on the opposite cell face via exocytosis. Paracellular transport entails the passage of the macromolecules through 'leaky' tight junctions found between some cells

- nasal microvilli generate a large potential absorption surface area;
- nasal delivery ensures the drug by-passes first-pass metabolism.

However, the route does display some disadvantages, including:

- clearance of a proportion of administered drug occurs due to its deposition upon the nasal mucous blanket, which is constantly cleared by ciliary action;
- the existence of extracellular nasal proteases/peptidases;
- low uptake rates for larger peptides/polypeptides.

Peptide/protein uptake rates across the nasal epithelia are dependent upon molecular mass. Relatively small peptides, such as oxytocin, desmopressin and LHRH analogues, cross relatively easily and several such products used medically are routinely delivered nasally. Larger molecules (of molecular mass greater than 10 kDa) generally do not cross the epithelial barrier without the concurrent administration of detergent-like uptake enhancers. Long-term use of enhancers is prohibited due to their damaging cellular effects.

Research efforts also continue to explore mucosal delivery of peptides/proteins via the buccal, vaginal and rectal routes. Again, bioavailabilities recorded are low with modest increases observed upon inclusion of permeation enhancers. Additional barriers also exist, e.g. relating to low surface areas, relatively rapid clearance from the mouth (buccal) cavity and the cyclic changes characteristic of vaginal tissue. Various strategies have been adopted in an attempt to achieve biopharmaceutical delivery across the skin (transdermal systems). Most have met with, at best, modest success thus far. Strategies employed include the use of a jet of helium or the application of a low voltage to accelerate proteins through the skin.

PRE-CLINICAL TRIALS

In order to gain approval for general medical use, the quality, safety and efficacy of any product must be demonstrated. Demonstration of conformance to these requirements, particularly safety and efficacy, is largely attained by undertaking clinical trials. However, preliminary data, especially safety data, must be obtained prior to the drug's administration to human volunteers. Regulatory authority approval to commence clinical trials is based largely upon pre-clinical pharmacological and toxicological assessment of the potential new drug in animals. Such pre-clinical studies can take up to 3 years to complete, and at a cost of anywhere between $10 million and $30 million. On average, approximately 10% of potential new drugs survive pre-clinical trials.

In many instances, there is no strict set of rules governing the range of tests that must be undertaken during pre-clinical studies. However, guidelines are usually provided by regulatory authorities. The range of studies generally undertaken with regard to traditional chemical-based pharmaceuticals are discussed below (see also Table 2.4). Most of these tests are equally applicable to biopharmaceutical products.

Pharmacokinetics and pharmacodynamics

Pharmacology may be described as the study of the properties of drugs and how they interact with/affect the body. Within this broad discipline exist (somewhat artificial) sub-disciplines, including pharmacokinetics and pharmacodynamics.

Table 2.4.   The range of major tests undertaken on a potential new drug during pre-clinical trials. The emphasis at this stage of the drug development process is upon assessing safety. Satisfactory pharmacological, and particularly toxicological, results must be obtained before any regulatory authority will permit commencement of human trials

---

Pharmacokinetic profile
Pharmacodynamic profile
Bioequivalence and bioavailability
Acute toxicity
Chronic toxicity
Reproductive toxicity and teratogenicity
Mutagenicity
Carcinogenicity
Immunotoxicity
Local tolerance

Pharmacokinetics relates to the fate of a drug in the body, particularly its ADME, i.e.:

- absorption into the body;
- distribution within the body;
- metabolism by the body;
- excretion from the body;

The results of such studies not only help to identify any toxic effects but also point to the most appropriate method of drug administration, as well as the most likely effective dosage regime to employ. Generally, ADME studies are undertaken in two species, usually rats and dogs, and studies are repeated at various different dosage levels. All studies are undertaken in both males and females.

If initial clinical trials reveal differences in human versus animal model pharmacokinetic profiles, additional pharmacokinetic studies may be necessary using primates.

Pharmacodynamic studies deal more specifically with how the drug brings about its characteristic effects. Emphasis in such studies is often placed upon how a drug interacts with a cell/organ type, the effects and side effects it induces, and observed dose–response curves.

Bioavailability and bioequivalence are also usually assessed in animals. Such studies are undertaken as part of pharmacokinetic and/or pharmacodynamic studies. Bioavailability relates to the proportion of a drug that actually reaches its site of action after administration. As most biopharmaceuticals are delivered parenterally (e.g. by injection), their bioavailability is virtually 100%. On the other hand, administration of biopharmaceuticals by mouth would, in most instances, yield a bioavailability at or near 0%. Bioavailability studies would be rendered more complex if, for example, a therapeutic peptide was being administered intranasally.

Bioequivalence studies come into play if any change in product production/delivery systems is being contemplated. These studies would seek to identify if such modifications still yield a product equivalent to the original one in terms of safety and efficacy. Modifications could include an altered formulation or method of administration, dosage regimes, etc.

Toxicity studies

Comprehensive toxicity studies are carried out by animal testing in order to ascertain whether the product exhibits any short-term or long-term toxicity. Acute toxicity is usually assessed by administration of a single high dose of the test drug to rodents. Both rats and mice (male and female) are usually employed. The test material is administered by two means, one of which should represent the proposed therapeutic method of administration. The animals are then monitored for 7–14 days, with all fatalities undergoing extensive post-mortem analysis.

Earlier studies demanded calculation of an LD_{50} value (i.e. the quantity of the drug required to cause death of 50% of the test animals). Such studies required large quantities of animals, were expensive, and attracted much attention from animal welfare groups. Their physiological relevance to humans was often also questioned. Nowadays, in most world regions, calculation of the approximate lethal dose is sufficient.

Chronic toxicity studies also require large numbers of animals and, in some instances, can last for up to 2 years. Most chronic toxicity studies demand daily administration of the test drug (parenterally for most biopharmaceuticals). Studies lasting 1–4 weeks are initially carried out in order to, for example, assess drug levels required to induce an observable toxic effect. The main studies are then initiated and generally involve administration of the drug at three different dosage levels. The highest level should ideally induce a mild but observable toxic effect, while the lowest level should not induce any ill effects. The studies are normally carried out in two different species — usually rats and dogs, and using both males and females. All animals are subjected to routine clinical examination and periodic analyses, e.g. of blood and urine, are undertaken. Extensive pathological examination of all animals is undertaken at the end of the study.

The duration of such toxicity tests varies. In the USA, the FDA usually recommends a period of up to 2 years, while in Europe the recommended duration is usually much shorter. Chronic toxicity studies of biopharmaceuticals can also be complicated by their likely stimulation of an immune response in the recipient animals.

Reproductive toxicity and teratogenicity

All reproductive studies entail ongoing administration of the proposed drug at three different dosage levels (ranging from non-toxic to slightly toxic) to different groups of the chosen target species (usually rodents). Fertility studies aim to assess the nature of any effect of the substance on male or female reproductive function. The drug is administered to males for at least 60 days (one full spermatogenesis cycle). Females are dosed for at least 14 days before they are mated. Specific tests carried out include assessment of male spermatogenesis, female follicular development, as well as fertilization, implantation and early fetal development.

These reproductive toxicity studies complement teratogenicity studies, which aim to assess whether the drug promotes any developmental abnormalities in the fetus (a teratogen is any substance/agent which can induce fetal developmental abnormalities; examples include alcohol, radiation and some viruses). Daily doses of the drug are administered to pregnant females of at least two species (usually rats and rabbits). The animals are sacrificed close to term and a full autopsy on the mother and fetus ensues. Post-natal toxicity evaluation often forms an extension of such studies. This entails administration of the drug to females both during and after pregnancy, with assessment of mother and progeny not only during pregnancy, but also during the lactation period.

Mutagenicity, carcinogenicity and other tests

Mutagenicity tests aim to determine whether the proposed drug is capable of inducing DNA damage, either by inducing alterations in chromosomal structure or by promoting changes in nucleotide base sequence. While mutagenicity tests are prudent and necessary in the case of chemical-based drugs, they are less so for most biopharmaceutical substances. In many cases, biopharmaceutical mutagenicity testing is likely to focus more so on any novel excipients added to the final product, rather than the biopharmaceutical itself ('excipient' refers to any substances other than the active ingredient, present in the final drug formulation).

Mutagenicity tests are usually carried out *in vitro* and *in vivo*, often using both prokaryotic and eukaryotic organisms. A well-known example is the Ames test, which assesses the ability of a drug to induce mutation reversions in *E. coli* and *Salmonella typhimurium*.

Longer-term carcinogenicity tests are undertaken, particularly if (a) the product's likely therapeutic indication will necessitate its administration over prolonged periods (a few weeks or more) or (b) if there is any reason to suspect that the active ingredient or other constituents could be carcinogenic. These tests normally entail ongoing administration of the product to rodents at various dosage levels for periods of up to (or above) 2 years.

Some additional animal investigations are also undertaken during pre-clinical trials. These include immunotoxicity and local toxicity tests. Again, for many biopharmaceuticals, immunotoxicity tests (i.e. the product's ability to induce an allergic or hypersensitive response) are often inappropriate or impractical. The regulatory guidelines suggest that further studies should be carried out if a biotechnology drug is found capable of inducing an immune response. However, many of the most prominent biopharmaceuticals (e.g. cytokines) actually function to modulate immunological activities in the first place.

Many drugs are administered to localized areas within the body by, for example, subcutaneous (s.c.) or intramuscular (i.m.) injection. Local toxicity tests appraise whether there is any associated toxicity at/surrounding the site of injection. Predictably, these are generally carried out by s.c. or i.m. injection of product to test animals, followed by observation of the site of injection. The exact cause of any adverse response noted (i.e. active ingredient or excipient) is usually determined by their separate subsequent administration.

Pre-clinical pharmacological and toxicological assessment entails the use of thousands of animals. This is both costly and, in many cases, politically contentious. Attempts have been made to develop alternatives to using animals for toxicity tests, and these have mainly centred around animal cell culture systems. A whole range of animal and human cell types may be cultured, at least transiently, *in vitro*. Large-scale and fairly rapid screening can be undertaken by, for example, microculture of the target animal cells in microtitre plates, followed by addition of the drug and an indicator molecule.

The indicator molecule serves to assess the state of health of the cultured cells. The dye, neutral red, is often used (healthy cells assimilate the dye, dead cells do not). The major drawback to such systems is that they do not reflect the complexities of living animals and, hence, may not accurately reflect likely results of whole-body toxicity studies. Regulatory authorities are (rightly) slow to allow replacement of animal-based test protocols until the replacement system has been shown to be reliable and is fully validated.

The exact range of pre-clinical tests that regulatory authorities suggest be undertaken for biopharmaceutical substances remains flexible. Generally, only a sub-group of the standard tests for chemical-based drugs are appropriate. Biopharmaceuticals pose several particular difficulties, especially in relation to pre-clinical toxicological assessment. These difficulties stem from several factors (some of which have already been mentioned), including:

- the species specificity exhibited by some biopharmaceuticals, e.g. growth hormone as well as several cytokines, means that the biological activity they induce in man is not mirrored in test animals;
- for biopharmaceuticals, greater batch-to-batch variability exists compared to equivalent chemical-based products;
- induction of an immunological response is likely during long-term toxicological studies;
- lack of appropriate analytical methodologies in some cases.

In addition, tests for mutagenicity and carcinogenicity are probably not required for most biopharmaceutical substances. The regulatory guidelines and industrial practices relating to biopharmaceutical pre-clinical trials thus remain in an evolutionary mode.

CLINICAL TRIALS

Clinical trials serve to assess the safety and efficacy of any potential new therapeutic 'intervention' in its intended target species. In our context, an intervention represents the use of a new biopharmaceutical. Examples of other interventions could be, for example, a new surgical procedure, or a novel medical device. While veterinary clinical trials are based upon the same principles, this discussion is restricted to investigations in humans. Clinical trials are also prospective rather than retrospective in nature, i.e. participants receiving the intervention are followed forward with time.

Clinical trials may be divided into three consecutive phases (Table 2.5). During phase I trials, the drug is normally administered to a small group of healthy volunteers. The aims of these studies are largely to establish:

- the pharmacological properties of the drug in humans (including pharmacokinetic and pharmacodynamic considerations);
- the toxicological properties of the drug in humans (with establishment of the maximally tolerated dose, MTD);
- the appropriate route and frequency of administration of the drug to humans.

Thus, the emphasis of phase I trials largely remains upon assessing drug safety. If satisfactory results are obtained during phase I studies, the drug then enters phase II trials. These studies aim to assess both the safety and effectiveness of the drug when administered to volunteer patients (i.e. persons suffering from the condition the drug claims to cure or alleviate).

Table 2.5. The clinical trial process. A drug must satisfactorily complete each phase before it enters the next phase. Note that the average duration listed here relates mainly to traditional chemical-based drugs. For biopharmaceuticals, the cumulative duration of all clinical trials is, on average, under 4 years

Trial phase	Evaluation undertaken (and usual number of patients)	Average duration (years)
I	Safety testing in healthy human volunteers (20–80)	1
II	Efficacy and safety testing in small number of patients (100–300)	2
III	Large scale efficacy and safety testing in substantial numbers of patients (1000–3000)	3
IV	Post-marketing safety surveillance undertaken for some drugs that are administered over particularly long periods of time (number of patients varies)	Several

The design of phase II trials is influenced by the phase I results. Phase II studies typically last for anything up to 2 years, with anywhere between a few dozen and 100 or more patients participating, depending upon the trial size.

If the drug proves safe and effective, phase III trials are initiated. In the context of clinical trials, 'safe' and 'effective' are rarely used in the absolute sense. 'Safe' generally refers to a favourable risk:benefit ratio, i.e. the benefits should outweigh any associated risk. A drug is rarely 100% effective in all patients. Thus, an acceptable level of efficacy must be defined, ideally prior to trial commencement. Depending upon the trial context, 'efficacy' could be defined as prevention of death or prolonging of life by a specific time frame. It could also be defined as alleviation of disease symptoms or enhancement of the quality of life of sufferers (often difficult parameters to measure objectively). An acceptable incidence of efficacy should also be defined (particularly for phase II and III trials), e.g. the drug should be efficacious in, say, 25% of all patients. If the observed incidence is below the minimal acceptable level, clinical trials are normally terminated.

Phase III clinical trials are designed to assess the safety and efficacy characteristics of a drug in greater detail. Depending upon the trial size, hundreds if not thousands of patients are recruited, and the trial may last for up to 3 years. These trials serve to assess the potential role of the new drug in routine clinical practice — the phase III results will largely dictate whether or not the prospective drug subsequently gains approval for general medical use.

Even if a product gains marketing approval (on average 10–20% of prospective drugs that enter clinical trials are eventually commercialized), the regulatory authorities may demand further post-marketing surveillance studies. These are often termed 'phase IV clinical trials'. They aim to assess the long-term safety of a drug, particularly if the drug is administered to patients for periods of time longer than the phase III clinical trials. The discovery of more long-term unexpected side effects can result in subsequent withdrawal of the product from the market.

Both pre-clinical and clinical trials are underpinned by a necessity to produce sufficient quantities of the prospective drug for its evaluation. Depending on the biopharmaceutical product, this could require from several hundred grams to over a kilo of active ingredient. Typical production protocols for biopharmaceutical products are outlined in detail in Chapter 3. It is important that a suitable production process be designed prior to commencement of pre-clinical trials, that the process be amenable to scale-up and, as far as is practicable, that it is optimized (Figure 2.9). The material used for pre-clinical and clinical trials should be produced using the same process by which it is intended to undertake final commercial-scale manufacture.

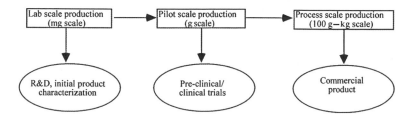

Figure 2.9.   Scale-up of proposed biopharmaceutical production process to generate clinical trial material, and eventually commercial product. No substantive changes should be introduced to the production protocol during scale-up

Extensive early development work is thus essential. Any significant deviation from the production protocol, used to generate the trial material, could invalidate all the clinical trial results with respect to the proposed commercialized product (changes in the production process could potentially change the final product characteristics — both the active ingredient and contaminant profile).

Clinical trial design

Proper and comprehensive planning of a clinical trial is essential to the successful development of any drug. Clinical trial design is a subject whose scope is too broad to be undertaken in this text, and only a brief overview of the subject is presented below. The interested reader is referred to the Further Reading section at the end of this chapter. The general principles presented below are relevant to phase II, and particularly phase III, clinical trials. As the bulk of the estimated $300–500 million required to develop a drug is spent on clinical trials, a poorly planned and/or executed clinical trial can be very costly to the drug developer.

The first issue to be considered when developing a trial protocol is to define precisely what questions the trial results should be capable of answering. As previously discussed, the terms 'safety' and 'efficacy' are difficult to define in a therapeutic context. An acceptable meaning of these concepts, however, should be committed to paper prior to planning of the trial.

Trial size and study population

A clinical trial must obviously have a control group against which the test (intervention) group can be compared. The control group may receive (a) no intervention at all; (b) a placebo (i.e. a substance such as saline, which will have no pharmacological or other effect); (c) the therapy most commonly used at that time to combat the target disease/condition.

The size of the trial will be limited by a number of factors, including:

- economic considerations (level of supporting financial resources);
- size of population with target condition;
- size of population with target condition after additional trial criteria have been imposed (e.g. specific age bracket, lack of complicating medical conditions, etc.);
- size of eligible population willing to participate in the trial.

While a comprehensive phase III trial would require at least several hundred patients, smaller trials would suffice if, for example:

- the target disease is very serious/fatal;
- there are no existing acceptable alternative treatments;
- the target disease population is quite small;
- the new drug is clearly effective and exhibits little toxicity.

Choosing the study population is obviously critical to adequate trial design. The specific criteria of patient eligibility should be clearly pre-defined as part of the primary question the trial strives to answer.

A number of trial design types may be used (Table 2.6), each having its own unique advantages and disadvantages. The most scientifically pure is a randomized, double-blind trial (see later). However, in many instances, alternative trial designs are chosen based on ethical or other grounds. In most cases, two groups are considered: control and test. However, these designs can be adapted to facilitate more complex sub-grouping.

Table 2.6.   Some clinical trial design types. Refer to text for full details

Randomized control studies (blinded or unblinded)
Historical control studies (unblinded)
Non-randomized concurrent studies (unblinded)
Cross over trial design
Factorial design
Hybrid design
Large simple clinical trials

Randomized control studies

This trial design, which is the most scientifically desirable, involves randomly assigning participants into either control or test groups, with concurrent testing of both groups. Randomness means that each participant has an equal chance of being assigned to one or other group. This can be achieved by, for example, flipping a coin or drawing names from a hat. Randomness is important as it:

- removes the potential for bias (conscious or subconscious) and thus will produce comparable groups in most cases;
- guarantees the validity of subsequent statistical analysis of trial results.

The trial may also be unblinded or blinded. In an unblinded ('open') trial, both the investigators and participants know to which group any individual has been assigned. In a single-blind trial, only the investigator is privy to this information, while in double-blind trials, neither the investigator nor the participants know to which group any individual is assigned. Obviously, the more blind the trial, the less scope for systematic error introduced by bias.

The most significant objection to the randomized control design is an ethical one. If a new drug is believed to be beneficial, many feel it is ethically unsound to effectively deprive up to half the trial participants from receiving the drug. One modification that overcomes the ethical difficulties is the use of historical control trials. In this instance, all the trial participants are administered the new drug and the results are compared to previously run trials in which a comparable group of participants were used. The control data are thus obtained from previously published or unpublished trial results. This trial design is non-randomized and non-concurrent. While it bypasses ethical difficulties associated with withholding the new drug from any participant, it is vulnerable to bias. The trial designers have no influence over the criteria set for their control group. Furthermore, historical data can distort the result, as beneficial responses in the test subjects may be due not only to the therapeutic intervention but to generally improved patient management practices. This can be particularly serious if the control data are old (in some trials it was obtained 10–20 years previously).

Additional trial designs

Non-randomized concurrent clinical trials initially assign participants to a control or test group in a non-random fashion. These trials are run concurrently, but are unblinded. This introduces a danger that the control and intervention groups are not strictly comparable.

Cross-over design trials represent an adaptation of randomized control trials in which each participant acts as his/her own control. In the simplest scenario, each participant will receive either a placebo or the test drug for the first half of the trial and will receive the alternative treatment for the second half. The order of placebo versus test drug for any individual is randomized. Hence, at any time point, approximately half the test participants will be receiving the placebo and the other half the test substance.

The major benefit of this design is the associated reduction in variability. This allows investigators to use smaller participant numbers to detect a specific response. This trial type, however, may only be used if there is sufficient evidence to show there is no carry-over effect from the first half to the second half of the trial. An extreme example of non-conformance to this requirement would be if the patient received the test drug during the first phase and was completely cured by it.

Factorial design represents yet another trial design of interest. This may be used to evaluate the effect of two or more interventions upon participants in a single trial (Table 2.7) and, hence, can be economically attractive.

Hybrid trial designs also have been used under certain circumstances. These generally combine elements of both historical and randomized control studies. They may be of particular interest if a substantial amount of control data are already available in the literature. Under such circumstances, a smaller proportion of the trial participants serve as control, whereas the majority of participants form the test group.

In some cases, the concept of a large, simple clinical trial has gained favour. This trial type would only be considered in cases where the intervention is easily administered and the outcome is easily measured. In such instances, simplified trial criteria are enforced, with the major prerequisites being recruitment of relatively large numbers of participants and randomization.

Table 2.7. Illustration of factorial design. In this example, any one of three potential interventions (placebo, drug 1, drug 2) are possible. Each participant will receive two of the possible three interventions

Participant group	Treatment received
A	Drug 1 and drug 2
B	Drug 1 and placebo
C	Drug 2 and placebo
D	Placebo and placebo

Table 2.8. Typical issues addressed when designing a clinical trial protocol. The trial objectives should clearly define what questions the trial should answer. The study design section should contain comprehensive information detailing trial size, criteria used to choose the study population, and enrolment procedures. Description of intervention section should give the background to the intervention itself, its therapeutic rationale and how it is to be administered. Measurement of response should detail the data to be collected, how it will be collected and analysed. The organization and administration section should give full details of all the investigators, where the trial is being run, and its project management details

Trial objectives
Study design
Description of intervention
Measurement of response
Study organization and administration

No matter what its design, a well-planned clinical trial requires development of a suitable trial protocol prior to its commencement. The protocol documents outline all pertinent aspects of the trial (Table 2.8) and should be made available to trial participants and other interested parties. A core prerequisite of any trial is that participants be fully informed regarding the intervention and any likely associated effects.

THE ROLE AND REMIT OF REGULATORY AUTHORITIES

The pharmaceutical industry is one of the most highly regulated industries known. Governments in virtually all world regions continue to pass tough laws to ensure that every aspect of pharmaceutical activity is tightly controlled. All regulations pertaining to the pharmaceutical industry are enforced by (government-established) regulatory agencies. The role and remit of some of the major world regulatory authorities is outlined below. In the context of this chapter, particular emphasis is placed upon their role with regard to the drug development process.

The Food and Drug Administration

The Food and Drug Administration (FDA) is the American regulatory authority. Its mission statement defines its goal simply as being 'to protect public health'. In fulfilling this role, it regulates many products/consumer items (Table 2.9), the total annual value of which is estimated to be $1 trillion. A more detailed list of the type of products regulated by the FDA is presented in Table 2.10. Its work entails inspecting/regulating almost 100 000 establishments in the USA (or those abroad who export regulated products for American consumption). The agency employs over 9000 people, of whom in the region of 4000 are concerned with enforcing drug law. The FDA's total annual budget is in the region of $1 billion.

The FDA was founded in 1927. An act of Congress officially established it as a governmental agency in 1988, and it now forms a part of the USA Department of Health and Human Services. The FDA Commissioner is appointed directly by the President (with the consent of the US Senate).

Table 2.9. The main product categories (along with their annual sales value), which the FDA regulate

$500 billion-worth of food
$350 billion-worth of medical devices
$100 billion-worth of drugs
$50 billion-worth of cosmetics and toiletries

Table 2.10. A more detailed outline of the substances regulated by the FDA

Foods, nutritional supplements
Drugs: chemical-based, biologics and biopharmaceuticals
Blood supply and blood products
Cosmetics/toiletries
Medical devices
All radioactivity-emitting substances
Microwave ovens
Advertising and promotional claims relating to the above product types

The FDA derives most of its statutory powers from the Federal Food, Drug and Cosmetic (FD & C) Act, legislation originally signed into law in 1930, but which has been amended several times since. The agency interprets and enforces these laws. In order to achieve this, it draws up regulations based upon the legislation. Most of the regulations themselves are worded in general terms, and are supported by various FDA publications that explain/interpret these regulations in far greater detail. The publications include: *Written Guidelines*, *Letters to Industry* and the *Points to Consider* series of documents. As technological and other advances are made, the FDA further supplements their support publication list.

A partial organizational structure of the FDA is presented in Figure 2.10. The core activities of biopharmaceutical drug approval/regulation is undertaken mainly by the Center for Drug Evaluation and Research (CDER) and the Center for Biologics Evaluation and Research (CBER).

The major FDA responsibilities with regard to drugs include:
- to assess pre-clinical data, and decide whether a potential drug is safe enough to allow commencement of clinical trials;
- to protect the interests and rights of patients participating in clinical trials;
- to assess pre-clinical and clinical trial data generated by a drug and decide whether that drug should be made available for general medical use (i.e. whether it should be granted a marketing licence);

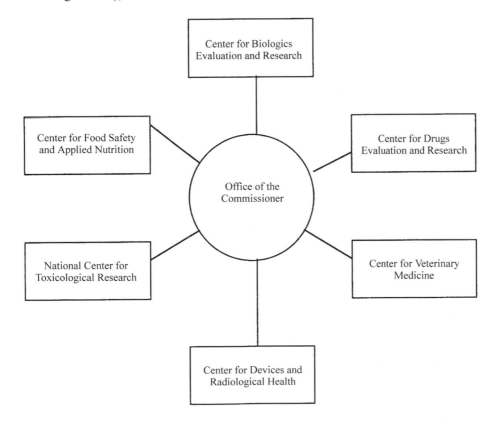

Figure 2.10. Partial organizational structure of the FDA, displaying the various centres primarily responsible for regulating drugs, devices and food

- to oversee the manufacture of safe effective drugs (inspect and approve drug manufacturing facilities on the basis of compliance to the principles of good manufacturing practice as applied to pharmaceuticals);
- to ensure the safety of the US blood supply.

In relation to the drug development process, CDER oversees and regulates the development and marketing approval of mainly chemical-based drugs. CBER is more concerned with biologics. 'Biologic' has traditionally been defined in a narrow sense and has been taken to refer to vaccines and viruses, blood and blood products, as well as antiserum, toxins and antitoxins used for therapeutic purposes. Because of this, many established pharmaceutical products (e.g. microbial metabolites and hormones) have come under appraisal by CDER, even though one might initially assume they would come under the biologics umbrella (Table 2.11).

Biopharmaceutical products have not fallen neatly into either category and the decision to refer any biotech-derived drug to CBER or CDER is taken on a case-by-case basis. Tissue plasminogen activator (tPA; Chapter 9), for example, is licensed as a biologic, whereas erythropoietin (EPO; Chapter 6) comes under the auspices of CDER. The majority of biopharmaceuticals, however, are assessed by CBER.

The criteria used by CBER and CDER regulators in assessing product performance during the drug development process are similar, i.e. safety, quality and efficacy. However, the administrative details can vary in both name and content. Upon concluding pre-clinical trials, all the data generated regarding any potential new drug are compiled in a dossier and submitted to CDER or CBER in the form of an investigational new drug application (IND application). The FDA assesses the application, and if it does not object within a specific time frame (usually 30 days), clinical trials can begin. The FDA usually meet with the drug developers at various stages, to be updated and often to give informal guidance/advice. Once clinical trials have been completed, all the data generated during the entire development process are compiled in a multi-volume dossier.

The dossier submitted to CDER is known as a new drug application (NDA) which, if approved, allows the drug to be marketed. If the drug is a CBER-regulated one, a biologics licence application (BLA) is submitted.

The investigational new drug application

An investigational new drug (IND) is a new chemical-based, biologic or biopharmaceutical substance for which the FDA has given approval to undergo clinical trials. An IND application

Table 2.11 Some traditional pharmaceutical products produced by/extracted from biological sources, which come under the auspices of CDER for regulatory purposes. The specific reviewing divisions within CDER which deal with these products are also listed

Product	Reviewing division
Most antibiotics	Division of anti-infective drug products
Anticoagulants, fibrinolytics, prostaglandins	Division of gastrointestinal and coagulation drug products
Enzymes	Division of medical imaging, surgical and dental drug products
Insulin, somatostatin, growth hormone, gonadotrophins, vasopressin, oxytocin	Division of metabolic and endocrine drug products

Table 2.12. The major itemized points which must be included/addressed in an IND application to CDER or CBER

FDA Form 1571
Table of (IND) contents
Introduction
Proposed trial detail and protocol (general investigational plan)
Investigator's brochure
Chemistry (or biology, as appropriate), manufacturing, and control detail
Pharmacology and toxicology data
Any previous human experience regarding the drug substance
Any additional information

should contain information detailing pre-clinical findings, method of product manufacture and proposed protocol for initial clinical trials (Table 2.12).

In some instances, the FDA and drug sponsor (company/institution submitting the IND) will agree to hold a pre-IND meeting. This aims to acquaint the FDA officials with the background to/content of the IND application, and to get a feel for whether the IND application will be regarded as adequate (see below) by the FDA. An IND application can consist of up to 15 volumes of approximately 400 pages each. Once received by the FDA, it is studied to ensure that:

- it contains sufficient/complete information required;
- the information supplied supports the conclusion that clinical trial subjects would not be exposed to an unreasonable risk of illness/injury (the primary FDA role being to protect public health);
- the clinical investigator named is qualified to conduct the clinical trials;
- the sponsor's product brochures are not misleading or incomplete.

Based on their findings, the FDA may grant the application immediately or may require additional information, which the sponsor then submits as IND amendments (Figure 2.11). Once clinical trials begin, the sponsor must provide the FDA with periodic updates, usually in the form of annual reports. Unscheduled reports must also be submitted under a variety of circumstances, including:

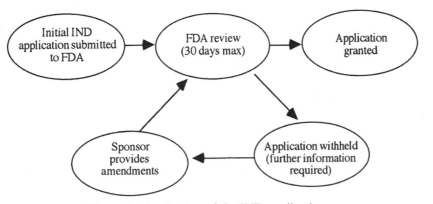

Figure 2.11. Outline of the IND application process

- if any amendments to the trial protocol are being considered;
- if any new scientific information regarding the product is obtained;
- if any unexpected safety observations are made.

During the clinical trial phase, the sponsor and FDA will meet on one or more occasions. A particularly important meeting is often the end of phase II meeting. This aims primarily to evaluate and agree upon phase III plans and protocols. This is particularly important, as phase III trials are the most costly and generate the greatest quantity of data used later to support the drug approval application.

The new drug application

Upon completion of clinical trials, the sponsor will collate all the pre-clinical, clinical and other pertinent data (Table 2.13) and submit this to FDA in support of an application to allow the new drug to be placed upon the market. For CDER-related drugs, this submission document is termed a new drug application (NDA).

The NDA must be an integrated document. It often consists of 200–300 volumes, which can represent a total of over 120 000 pages. Several copies of the entire document, and sections thereof, are provided to CDER. The FDA then classify the NDA based upon the chemical type of the drug and its therapeutic potential. Generally, drugs of high therapeutic potential (e.g. new drugs capable of curing/alleviating serious/terminal medical conditions) are appraised by CDER in the shortest time.

After initial submission of the NDA, the FDA has 45 days in which to preliminarily inspect the document — to ensure that everything is in order. They then 'file' the NDA, or if more information/better information management is needed, they refuse to file until such changes are implemented by the sponsor.

Once filed, an NDA undergoes several layers of review (Figure 2.12). A primary review panel generally consists of a chemist, a microbiologist, a pharmacologist, a biostatistician, a medical officer and a biopharmaceutics scientist. Most hold PhDs in their relevant discipline. The team is organized by a project manager or consumer safety officer (CSO). The CSO initially forwards relevant portions of the NDA to the primary review panel member with the appropriate expertise.

Table 2.13. An overview of the contents of a typical new NDA. The multi-volume document is often organized into 15 different sections, the titles of which are provided below

1	Index
2	Overall summary
3	Chemistry, manufacturing and control section
4	Sampling, methods of validation, package and labelling
5	Non-clinical pharmacology and toxicology data
6	Human pharmacokinetics and bioavailability data
7	Microbiology data
8	Clinical data
9	Safety update reports
10	Statistical section
11	Case report tabulations
12	Case report forms
13 and 14	Patent information and certification
15	Additional pertinent information

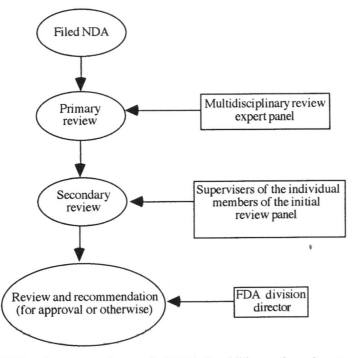

Figure 2.12. The CDER review process for a typical NDA. In addition to the review stages described, the FDA also may consult with a technical advisory committee. The members of the advisory committee are not routinely involved in IND or NDA assessment. The FDA is not obliged to follow any advice given by the advisory committee, but it generally does so

Each reviewer then prepares a review report. This is forwarded to their supervisory officers, who undertake a second review. All of the reports are then sent to the division director who, in turn, recommends rejection or approval, or asks the sponsor to provide more information. On average, this entire process takes 12 months.

Even when the NDA is approved and the product goes on sale, the sponsor must provide the FDA with further occasional reports. These can be in the form of scheduled annual reports, but unscheduled reports are also required in instances such as the occurrence of an unexpected adverse response to the drug.

A similar general approach is taken by CBER with regard to drugs being developed under their auspices. The CBER 'licensing process' for a new drug consists of three phases: the IND phase (already discussed), the pre-marketing approval phase (licensure phase) and the post-marketing surveillance phase. The pre-marketing approval phase (i.e. clinical trial phase) aims to generate data which proves the potency, purity and safety of the product. Upon completion of clinical trials, the sponsor collates the data generated and submits it to the FDA in the form of a biologics licence application, which must provide a comprehensive description of both the product and product manufacture (including methods of QC analysis, product stability data, labelling data and, of course, safety and efficacy data).

A small number of biotechnology products are classified as medical devices and hence are regulated by the Center for Devices and Radiological Health. The first approved biotech product to come under the auspices of the CDRH was OP-1 implant. Marketed by Stryker

Biotech, OP-1 implant is a sterile powder composed of recombinant human osteogenic protein-1 (OP-1) along with bovine collagen. It is used to treat fractured bones that fail to heal. The product is mixed with sterile saline immediately before application, which entails surgical insertion of the paste into the fracture.

European regulations

The overall philosophy behind granting a marketing authorization for a new drug is broadly similar in the USA and Europe. There are, however, major differences in the systems by which these philosophies are implemented in the two regions.

The European Union (EU) is currently composed of 15 member states and a total population of 371 million (compared with 249 million in the USA and 124 million in Japan — the other two world pharmaceutical markets). The total European pharmaceutical market value stands at €70 billion, representing almost 33% of world sales (the US and Japanese figures are 31% and 21%, respectively). Annual expenditure on European pharmaceutical R&D stands at about €17 billion.

Prominent within the EU organizational structure is the European Commission. The Commission is composed of 20 commissioners (with at least one being from each member state) and several thousand civil servants. The major function of the European Commission is to propose new EU legislation and to ensure enforcement of existing legislation (European drug law, therefore, comes under the auspices of the Commission).

Two forms of legal instrument can be issued from the centralized European authorities: a 'regulation' and a 'directive'. A regulation is a strong legal instruction which, once passed, must be implemented immediately, and without modification, by national governments. A directive is a looser legal term, and provides an individual member state with 18 months to translate the flavour of that law into national law. Pharmaceutical law within the EU has been shaped by both directives and regulations, as discussed later.

National regulatory authorities

In all European countries, there exist national regulatory authorities. These authorities are appointed by the government of the country in question and are usually located in the national Ministry of Health. They serve to apply national and European law with regard to the drug development process. In many countries, different arms of the regulatory authorities are responsible for authorizing and assessing clinical trials, assessing the resultant drug dossier and deciding on that basis whether or not to grant a (national) marketing authorization/product licence. They are also often responsible for issuing manufacturing licences to companies (Chapter 3).

In the past, a company wishing to gain a marketing licence within Europe usually applied for separate marketing authorizations on a country-by-country basis. This entailed significant duplication of effort, because:

- the drug dossiers needed to be translated into various European languages;
- national laws often differed and, hence, different expectations/dossier requirements were associated with different countries;
- the time scale taken for dossier assessment varied from country to country.

Attempts to harmonize European pharmaceutical laws were accelerated in the 1980s. From 1985 onwards, a substantial number of European pharmaceutical directives have been adopted.

Table 2.14. The nine-volume series that comprises *The Rules Governing Medicinal Products in the European Union*

1, *Pharmaceutical Legislation*	Medicinal products for human use
2, *Notice to Applicants*	Medicinal products for human use
3, *Guidelines*	Medicinal products for human use
4, *Good Manufacturing Practices*	Medicinal products for human and veterinary use
5, *Pharmaceutical Legislation*	Veterinary medicinal products
6, *Notice to Applicants*	Veterinary medicinal products
7, *Guidelines*	Veterinary medicinal products
8, *Maximum residue limits*	Veterinary medicinal products
9, *Pharmacovigilance*	Medicinal products for human and veterinary use

This entire legislation has been published in the form of a nine-volume series entitled *The Rules Governing Medicinal Products in the European Union* (Table 2.14). These volumes form the basis of EU-wide regulation of virtually every aspect of pharmaceutical activity.

The EMEA and the new EU drug approval systems

In 1993, a significant advance was made in simplifying the procedures relating to drug marketing authorization applications in the EU. At that time, the legal basis of a new drug approval system was formed by an EU regulation and three directives. Central to this was the establishment of the European Medicines Evaluation Agency (EMEA), which is based in London and began work in January 1995. Two new marketing authorization (drug registration) procedures for human or veterinary drugs are now in place within the EU:

- a centralized procedure in which applications for a marketing licence are forwarded directly to the EMEA;
- a decentralized procedure based upon mutual acceptance or recognition of national authority decisions. Disputes arising from this system are arbitrated by the EMEA.

The EMEA comprises:

- a management board, consisting of representatives of each EU member state as well as representatives of the European Commission and European Parliament. This group functions mainly to coordinate EMEA activities and manage its budget;
- pre-authorization evaluation of medicines for human use unit. This unit provides scientific advice relating to quality, safety and efficacy issues, as well as relating to orphan drugs;
- post-authorization evaluation of medicines for human use. This regulatory affairs unit is responsible for issues such as post-marketing surveillance of drugs;
- veterinary medicines and inspections. This unit is responsible for veterinary marketing authorization procedures as well as inspections.

Central to the functioning of the EMEA are three committees:

- the Committee for Proprietary Medicinal Products (CPMP). This committee is composed of 35 technical experts drawn from the various EU member countries. It is primarily responsible for formulating the EMEA's opinion on any medicinal product being considered for marketing approval under the centralized procedure;

- the Committee for Veterinary Medicinal Products (CVMP), whose structure and role is similar to the CPMP except that it is concerned with animal medicines;
- the Committee for Orphan Medicinal Products (COMP), composed of a representative from each EU member state, as well as EMEA and patient representatives. The COMP assesses applications relating to experimental medicines being granted 'orphan' status. Orphan medicines are those intended to treat rare diseases, and orphan designation results in a reduction of the fees charged by the EMEA when assessing marketing authorization applications.

Unlike the FDA, the EMEA itself does not directly undertake appraisals of drug dossiers submitted to support marketing authorization applications under the centralized procedure. Instead (as discussed in detail below), they forward the dossier to selected national EU regulatory bodies, who undertake the appraisal, and the EMEA makes a recommendation to approve (or not) the application, based upon the national body's report. The overall role of the EMEA is thus to coordinate and manage the new system. The EMEA's annual budget is of the order of €70 million. The key objectives of the EMEA may be summarized as:

- protection of public and animal health by ensuring the quality, safety and efficacy of medicinal products for human and veterinary use;
- to strengthen the ideal of a single European market for human and veterinary pharmaceuticals;
- to support the European pharmaceutical industry as part of the EU industrial policy.

The centralized procedure

Under the centralized procedure, applications are accepted with regard to (a) products of biotechnology; (b) new chemical entities (NCEs: drugs in which the active ingredient is new). Biotech products are grouped as 'list A', NCEs as 'list B'. Marketing approval application for biotech products must be considered under the centralized procedure, whereas NCEs can be considered under centralized or decentralized mechanisms.

Upon receipt of a marketing authorization application under centralized procedures, the EMEA staff carry out an initial appraisal to ensure that it is complete and has been compiled in accordance with the appropriate EU guidelines (Box 2.2). This appraisal must be completed within 10 days, at which time (if the application is in order), it is given a filing date. The sponsor also pays an appropriate fee. The EMEA then has 210 days to consider the application. In the case of human drugs, the application immediately comes before the CPMP (which convenes 2–3 days a month).

Two rapporteurs are then appointed (committee members who are responsible for getting the application assessed). The rapporteurs generally arrange to have the application assessed by their respective home national regulatory authority. Once assessment is complete, the reports are presented via the rapporteur to the CPMP. After discussion, the CPMP issue an 'opinion' (i.e. a recommendation that the application be accepted, or not). This opinion is then forwarded to the European Commission, who have another 90 days to consider it. They usually accept the opinion and 'convert' it into a decision (they—and not the EMEA directly—have the authority to issue a marketing authorization). The single marketing authorization covers the entire EU. Once granted it is valid for 5 years after which it must be renewed. The total time in which a decision must be taken is 300 days (210 + 90), which is

Box 2.2.   The marketing authorization application in the EU

The dossier submitted to EU authorities, when seeking a manufacturing authorization, must be compiled according to specific EU guidelines. It generally consists of four parts, as follows:

Part I   (A)   Administrative data
         (B)   Summary of product characteristics
         (C)   Expert reports

Part II (A)   Composition of the product
         (B)   Method of product preparation
         (C)   Control of starting materials
         (D)   Control tests on intermediate products
         (E)   Control tests on finished product
         (F)   Stability tests
         (Q)   Bioavailability/bioequivalence and other information

Part III (A)   Single dose toxicity
         (B)   Repeated dose toxicity
         (C)   Reproductive studies
         (D)   Mutagenicity studies
         (E)   Carcinogenicity studies
         (F)   Pharmacodynamics
         (G)   Pharmacokinetics
         (H)   Local tolerance
         (Q)   Additional information

Part IV (A)   Clinical pharmacology
         (B)   Clinical trial results
         (Q)   Additional information

Part I (A) contains information which identifies the product, its pharmaceutical form and strength, route of administration and details of the manufacturer. The summary of product characteristics summarizes the qualitative and quantitative composition of the product, its pharmaceutical form, details of pre-clinical and clinical observations, as well as product particulars, such as a list of added excipients, storage conditions, shelf-life, etc. The expert reports contain written summaries of pharmaceutical, pre-clinical and clinical data.

Parts II, III and IV then make up the bulk of technical detail. They contain detailed breakdown of all aspects of product manufacture and control (Part II), pre-clinical data (Part III) and clinical results (Part IV).

considerably shorter than the average approval times in many other world regions. The 300 day deadline only applies in situations where the CPMP do not require any additional information from the sponsor. In many cases, additional information is required and when this occurs, the 300 day 'clock' stops until the additional information is received.

Mutual recognition

The mutual recognition procedure is an alternative means by which a marketing authorization may be sought. It is open to all drug types except products of biotechnology. Briefly, if this procedure is adopted by a sponsor, the sponsor applies for a marketing licence, not to the EMEA but to a specific national regulatory authority (chosen by the sponsor). The national authority then has 210 days to assess the application.

If adopted by the national authority in question, the sponsor can seek marketing licences in other countries on that basis. For this bilateral phase, other states in which marketing authorization are sought have 60 days in which to review the application. The theory, of course, is that no substantive difficulty should arise at this stage, as all countries are working to the same set of standards as laid down in *The Rules Governing Medicinal Products in the European Union*.

A further 30 days is set aside in which any difficulties that arise may be resolved. The total application duration is 300 days. If one or more states refuse to grant the marketing authorization (i.e. mutual recognition breaks down), the difficulties are referred back to the EMEA. The CPMP will then make a decision ('opinion'), which is sent to the European Commission. The Commission, taking into account the CPMP opinion, will make a final decision, which is a binding one.

Drug registration in Japan

The Japanese are the greatest consumers of pharmaceutical products per capita in the world. The Ministry of Health and Welfare in Japan has overall responsibility to implement Japanese pharmaceutical law. Within the department is the Pharmaceutical Affairs Bureau (PAB), which exercises this authority.

There are three basic steps in the Japanese regulatory process:

- approval ('shonin') must be obtained to manufacture or import a drug;
- a licence ('kyoka') must also be obtained;
- an official price for the drug must be set.

The PAB undertakes drug dossier evaluations, a process which normally takes 18 months. The approval requirements/process for pharmaceuticals (including biopharmaceuticals) are, in broad terms, quite similar to those in the USA. PAB have issued specific requirements (Notification 243) for submission of recombinant protein drugs.

Applications are initially carefully checked by a single regulatory examiner to ensure conformance to guidelines. Subsequently, the application is reviewed in detail by a sub-committee of specialists. Clear evidence of safety, quality and efficacy are required prior to approval.

In addition, the Japanese normally insist that at least some clinical trials be carried out in Japan itself. This position is adopted due, for example, to differences in the body size and metabolism of the Japanese compared to US or European citizens. Also, the quantity of active ingredient present in Japanese drugs is lower than in many other world regions. Hence, trials must be undertaken to prove product efficacy under intended Japanese usage conditions.

World harmonization of drug approvals

There is a growing trend in the global pharmaceutical industry towards internationalization. Increasingly, mergers and other strategic alliances are a feature of world pharmaceutical activity. Many companies are developing drugs which they aim to register in several world regions. Differences in regulatory practices and requirements in these different regions considerably complicates this process.

Development of harmonized requirements for world drug registrations would be of considerable benefit to pharmaceutical companies and to patients for whom many drugs would be available much more quickly.

The ICH process (International Conference on Harmonization of technical requirements for registration of pharmaceuticals for human use) brings together experts from both the regulatory authorities and pharmaceutical industries based in the EU, USA and Japan. The aim is to achieve greater harmonization of technical/guidelines relating to product registration in these world regions, and considerable progress has been made in this regard over the last decade. The 'members' comprising ICH are experts from the European Commission, the European Federation of Pharmaceutical Industries Association (EFPIA), the Japanese Ministry of Health and Welfare, the Japanese Pharmaceutical Manufacturers Assocaition (JPMA), the FDA and the Pharmaceutical Research and Manufacturers of America (PhRMA). The ICH process is supported by an ICH secretariat, based in Geneva, Switzerland.

CONCLUSION

The drug discovery and development process is a long and expensive one. A wide range of strategies may be adopted in the quest for identifying new therapeutic substances. Most biopharmaceuticals, however, have been discovered directly as a consequence of an increased understanding of the molecular mechanisms underlining how the body functions, in both health and disease.

Before any newly discovered drug is placed on the market, it must undergo extensive testing in order to assure that it is both safe and effective in achieving its claimed therapeutic effect. The data generated by these tests (i.e. pre-clinical and clinical trials), are then appraised by independent, government-appointed regulatory agencies, who ultimately decide whether a drug should gain a marketing license. While the drug development process may seem cumbersome and protracted, the cautious attitude adopted by regulatory authorities has served the public well in ensuring that only drugs of the highest quality finally come onto the market.

FURTHER READING

Books

Adjei, H. (1997). *Inhalation Delivery of Therapeutic Peptides and Proteins*. J.A. Majors Co., Atlanta, GA.

Ansel, H. (1999). *Pharmaceutical Dosage Forms and Drug Delivery Systems*. Lippincott Williams & Wilkins, Philadelphia, PA.

Askari, F. (2003). *Beyond the Genome — The Proteomics Revolution*. Prometheus, Frome, UK.

Crommelin, D. (2002). *Pharmaceutical Biotechnology*. Routledge, London.

De Jong, M. (1998). *FAQs on EU Pharmaceutical Regulatory Affairs*. Brookwood Medical, Richmond, UK.

Desalli, R. (2002). *The Genomics Revolution*. Joseph Henry Press.

Ferraiolo, B. (1992). *Protein Pharmacokinetics and Metabolism*. Plenum, New York.

Giffels, J. (1996). *Clinical Trials*. Demos Medical, London.

Goldberg, R. (2001). *Pharmaceutical Medicine, Biotechnology and European Patent Law*. Cambridge University Press, Cambridge.

Grindley, J. & Ogden, J. (2000). *Understanding Biopharmaceuticals. Manufacturing and Regulatory Issues*. Interpharm, Denver, CO.

Hunt, S. (2000). *Functional Genomics*. Oxford University Press, Oxford.

Knight, H. (2001). *Patent Strategy*. Wiley, Chichester.

Krogsgaard, L. (2002). *Textbook of Drug Design and Discovery*. Taylor and Francis, London.

McNally, E. (Ed), (2000). *Protein Formulation and Delivery*. Marcel Dekker, New York.

Oxender, D. & Post, L. (1999). *Novel Therapeutics from Modern Biotechnology*. Springer-Verlag, Berlin.

Pennington, S. (2000). *Proteomics*. BIOS Scientific, Oxford.

Poste, G. (1999). *The Impact of Genomics on Healthcare*. Royal Society of Medicine Press, London.

Scolnick, E. (2001). *Drug Discovery and Design*. Academic Press, London.

Venter, J. (2000). *From Genome to Therapy*. Wiley, Chichester.

Articles

Clinical trials and regulatory authorities

Beatrice, M. (1997). FDA regulatory reform. *Curr. Opin. Biotechnol.* **18**(3), 370–378.

Crooke, S. (1995). Comprehensive reform of the new drug regulatory process. *Bio/Technology* **13**, 25–29.

Graffeo, A. (1994). The do's and don'ts of preclinical development. *Bio/Technology* **12**, 865.

Helms, P. (2002). Real world pragmatic clinical trials: what are they and what do they tell us? *Pediat. Allergy Immunol.* **13**(1), 4–9.

Jefferys, D. & Jones, K. (1995). EMEA and the new pharmaceutical procedures for Europe. *Eur. J. Clin. Pharmacol.* **47**, 471–476.

Kaitin, K. (1997). FDA reform: setting the stage for efforts to reform the agency. *Drug Inf. J.* **31**, 27–33.

Kessler, D. & Feiden, K. (1995). Faster evaluation of vital drugs. *Sci. Am.* **March**, 26–32.

Lubiniecki, A. (1997). Potential influence of international harmonization of pharmaceutical regulations on biopharmaceutical development. *Curr. Opin. Biotechnol.* **8**(3), 350–356.

Pignatti, F *et al.* (2002). Clinical trials for registration in the European Union: the EMEA 5-year experience in oncology. *Crit. Rev. Oncol. Haematol.* **42**(2), 123–135.

Sauer, F. (1997). A new and fast drug approval system in Europe. *Drug Inf. J.* **31**, 1–6.

Walsh, G. (1999). Drug approval in Europe. *Nature Biotechnol.* **17**, 237–240

Patenting

Allison, J. & Lemley, M. (2002). The growing complexity of the United States patenting system. *Boston Univ. Law Rev.* **82**(1), 77–144.

Barton, J. (1991). Patenting life. *Sci. Am.* **March**, 18–24.

Berks, A. (1994). Patent information in biotechnology. *Trends Biotechnol.* **12**, 352–364.

Crespi, R. (1993). Biotechnological inventions and the patent law: outstanding issues. *Biotechnol. Genet. Eng. Rev.* **11**, 229–261.

Crespi, R. (1994). Protecting biotechnological inventions. *Trends Biotechnol.* **12**, 395–397.

Johnson, E. (1996). A benchside guide to patents and patenting. *Nature Biotechnol.* **14**, 288–291.

Orr, R. & O'Neill, C. (2000). Patent review: therapeutic applications of antisense oligonucleotides, 1999–2000. *Curr. Opin. Mol. Therapeut.* **2**(3), 325–331.

Drug development

Bugg, C. *et al.* (1993). Drugs by design. *Sci. Am.* **December**, 92–98.

Cox, P. & Balick, M. (1994). The ethanobotanical approach to drug discovery. *Sci. Am.* **June**, 60–65.

Drews, J. (2000). Drug discovery: a historical perspective. *Science* **287**(5460), 1960–1964.

Dykes, C. (1996). Genes, disease and medicine. *Br. J. Clin. Pharmacol.* **42**(6), 683–695.

Ecker, D. & Crooke, S. (1995). Combinatorial drug discovery: which methods will produce greatest value? *Bio/Technology* **13**, 351–359.

Geisow, M. J. (1991) Characterizing recombinant proteins. *Bio/Technology*, **9**(10), 921–922.

Hodgson, J. (1993). Pharmaceutical screening: from off the wall to off the shelf. *Bio/Technol.* **11**, 683–688.

Lowman, H. (1997). Bacteriophage display and discovery of peptide leads for drug development. *Ann. Rev. Biophys. Biomol. Struct.* **26**, 401–424.

Medynski, D. (1994). Synthetic peptide combinatorial libraries. *Bio/Technology* **12**, 709–710.
Saragovi, H. *et al.* (1992). Loops and secondary structure mimetics: development and applications in basic science and rational drug discovery. *Bio/Technology* **10**, 773–777.
Scicinski, J. (1995). Chemical libraries in drug discovery. *Trends Biotechnol* **13**, 246–247.

Genomics, proteomics and related technologies

Baba, Y. (2001). Development of novel biomedicine based on genome science. *Eur. J. Pharmaceut. Sci.* **13**(1), 3–4.
Brenner, S. (2001). A tour of structural genomics. *Nature Rev. Genet.* **2**(10), 801–809.
Cunningham, M. (2000) Genomics and proteomics, the new millennium of drug discovery and development. *J. Pharmacol. Toxicol. Methods* **44**(1), 291–300.
Debouck, C. & Goodfellow, P. (1999). DNA microarrays in drug discovery and development. *Nature Genet.* **21**, 48–50.
Gabig, M. & Wegrzyn, G. (2001). An introduction to DNA chips: principles, technology, applications and analysis. *Acta Biochim. Polon.* **48**(3), 615–622.
Jain, K. (2001). Proteomics: new technologies and their applications. *Drug Discovery Today* **6**(9), 457–459.
Jain, K. (2001). Proteomics: delivering new routes to drug discovery, part 2. *Drug Discovery Today* **6**(16), 829–832.
Kassel, D. (2001). Combinatorial chemistry and mass spectrometry in the twenty-first century drug development laboratory. *Chem. Rev.* **101**(2), 255–267.
Lesley, S. (2001). High-throughput proteomics: protein expression and purification in the post-genomic world. *Protein Expr. Purif.* **22**(2), 159–164.
McLeod, H. & Evans, W. (2001). Pharmacogenomics: unlocking the human genome for better drug therapy. *Ann. Rev. Pharmacol. Toxicol.* **41**, 101–121.
Page, M. *et al.* (1999). Proteomics: a major new technology for the drug discovery process. *Drug Discovery Today* **4**(2), 55–62.
Ramsay, G. (1998) DNA chips: state of the art. *Nature Biotechnol.* **16**(1), 40–44.
Roses, A. (2000). Pharmacogenetics and the practice of medicine. *Nature* **405**(6788), 857–865.
Schmitz, G. *et al.* (2001). Pharmacogenomics: implications for laboratory medicine. *Clin. Chim. Acta* **308**(1–2), 43–53.
Searls, D. (2000). Using bioinformatics in gene and drug discovery. *Drug Discovery Today* **5**(4), 135–143.
Terstappen, G. & Reggiani, A. (2001). *In silico* research in drug discovery. *Trends Pharmacol. Sci.* **22**(1), 23–26.
Wamg, J. & Hewick, R. (1999). Proteomics in drug discovery. *Drug Discovery Today* **4**(3), 129–133.
Wieczorek, S. & Tsongalis, G. (2001). Pharmacogenomics: will it change the field of medicine? *Clin. Chim. Acta* **308**(1–2), 1–8.
Wilgenbus, K. & Lichter, P. (1999). DNA chip technology ante portas. *J. Mol. Med.* **77**(11), 761–768.
Wolf, C. *et al.* (2000). Science, medicine and the future — pharmacogenetics. *Br. Med. J.* **320**(7240), 987–990.

Drug delivery

Davis, S. (2001). Nasal vaccines. *Adv. Drug Delivery Rev.* **51**, 21–42.
Kompella, U. *et al.* (2001). Delivery systems for penetration enhancement of peptide and protein drugs: design considerations. *Adv. Drug Delivery Rev.* **46**, 211–245.
Patton, J. *et. al.* (1999). Inhaled insulin. *Adv. Drug Delivery Rev.* **35**, 235–247.
Patton, J. (1996). Mechanism of macromolecule absorption by the lungs. *Adv. Drug Delivery Rev.* **19**(1), 3–36.

Chapter 3

The drug manufacturing process

The manufacture of pharmaceutical substances is one of the most highly regulated and rigorously controlled manufacturing processes known. In order to gain a manufacturing licence, the producer must prove to the regulatory authorities that not only is the product itself safe and effective, but that all aspects of the proposed manufacturing process comply to the highest safety and quality standards. Various elements contribute to the safe manufacture of quality pharmaceutical products. These include:

- the design and layout of the manufacturing facility;
- raw materials utilized in the manufacturing process;
- the manufacturing process itself;
- the training and commitment of personnel involved in all aspects of the manufacturing operation;
- the existence of a regulatory framework which assures the establishment and maintenance of the highest quality standards with regard to all aspects of manufacturing.

This chapter aims to overview the manufacturing process. It concerns itself with four major themes: (a) a description of the infrastructure of a typical manufacturing facility, and some relevant operational issues — much of the detail presented in this section is equally applicable to facilities manufacturing non-biological-based pharmaceutical products; (b) sources of biopharmaceuticals; (c) upstream and downstream processing of biopharmaceutical products; and (d) analysis of the final biopharmaceutical product. Before delving into specific aspects of pharmaceutical manufacturing, various publications, such as international pharmacopoeias and guides to good manufacturing practice for medicinal products, will be discussed. These publications play a central role in establishing criteria which guarantee the consistent production of safe and effective drugs.

INTERNATIONAL PHARMACOPOEIA

Many thousands of pharmaceutical substances are routinely manufactured by the pharmaceutical industry. Two of the most important determinants of final product safety and efficacy are: (a) the standard of raw materials used in the manufacturing process; and (b) the standard (i.e. specification) to which the final product is manufactured. Most pharmaceutical substances are

Biopharmaceuticals: Biochemistry and Biotechnology, Second Edition by Gary Walsh
John Wiley & Sons Ltd: ISBN 0 470 84326 8 (ppc), ISBN 0 470 84327 6 (pbk)

manufactured to exacting specifications laid down in publications termed 'pharmacopoeias'. There are more than two dozen pharmacopoeias published world-wide, most notably the *United States Pharmacopoeia* (USP), the *European Pharmacopoeia* (Eur. Ph.) and the *Japanese Pharmacopoeia*. The products listed in these international pharmacopoeias are invariably generic drugs (i.e. drugs no longer patent-protected, which can be manufactured in any pharmaceutical facility holding the appropriate manufacturing licence). The vast bulk of such substances are traditional chemical-based drugs, and biological substances such as insulin and various blood products. Two sample monographs from the *European Pharmacopoeia* are reproduced in Appendix 3. Future editions of such pharmacopoeias are likely to include a growing number of biopharmaceuticals, particularly as many of these begin to lose their patent protection.

Martindale, The Extra Pharmacopoeia

Martindale, The Extra Pharmacopoeia (often simply referred to as 'Martindale') represents an additional publication of relevance to the pharmaceutical industry. Unlike the pharmacopoeias discussed above, Martindale is not a book of standards. The aim of this encyclopaedic publication is to provide concise, unbiased information (largely summarized from the peer-reviewed literature) regarding drugs of clinical interest.

The first edition of Martindale was published in 1883 by William Martindale and the 30th edition was published in 1993. It contains information in monograph format on over 5000 drugs in clinical use. The vast bulk of substances described are chemical-based pharmaceuticals, as well as traditional biological substances such as antibiotics, certain hormones and blood products. Recent editions, however, carry increasing numbers of monographs detailing biopharmaceuticals—a reflection of their growing importance in the pharmaceutical industry.

Martindale is largely organized into chapters that detail groups of drugs having similar clinical uses or actions (Table 3.1). The information presented in a monograph detailing any particular drug will usually include:

- its physiochemical characteristics;
- absorption and fate;
- uses and appropriate mode of administration;
- adverse/side effects;
- suitable dosage levels.

In addition, summaries of published papers/reviews of the substance in question are included. Because of its clinical emphasis, Martindale represents a valuable drug information source to pharmacists and clinicians, but also provides much relevant drug information to personnel engaged in pharmaceutical manufacturing.

GUIDES TO GOOD MANUFACTURING PRACTICE

All aspects of pharmaceutical manufacture must comply with the most rigorous standards to ensure consistent production of a safe, effective product. The principles underlining such standards are summarized in publications which detail good manufacturing practice (GMP). Pharmaceutical manufacturers must be familiar with the principles laid down in these publications and they are legally obliged to ensure adoption of these principles to their specific manufacturing process. Regulatory authority personnel will assess compliance of the manufacturer with these principles by undertaking regular inspections of the facility. The

Table 3.1. List of the major headings under which various drugs are described in *Martindale, The Extra Pharmacopoeia*

Analgesics and anti-inflammatory agents	Cardiac inotropic agents	Non-ionic surfactants
Anthelmintics	Chelating agents, antidotes and antagonists	Nutritional agents and vitamins
Anti-arrhythmic agents	Colouring agents	Opioid analgesics
Anti-bacterial agents	Contrast media	Organic solvents
Anti-coagulants	Corticosteroids	Paraffins and similar bases
Anti-depressants	Cough suppressants, expectorants and mucolytics	Parasympathomimetics
Anti-diabetic agents	Dermatological agents	Pesticides and repellants
Anti-epileptics	Diagnostic agents	Preservatives
Anti-fungal agents	Disinfectants	Prophylactic anti-asthma agents
Anti-gout agents	Diuretics	Prostaglandins
Anti-hypertensive agents	Dopaminergic anti-parkinsonian agents	Radiopharmaceuticals
Anti-malarials	Electrolytes	Sex hormones
Anti-migraine agents	Gases	Skeletal muscle relaxants
Anti-muscarinic agents	Gastrointestinal agents	Soaps and other anionic surfactants
Anti-neoplastic agents and immunosuppressants	General anaesthetics	Stabilizing and suspending agents
Anti-protozoal agents	Haemostatics	Stimulants and anorectics
Anti-thyroid agents	Histamine H_1-receptor antagonists	Sunscreen agents
Anti-viral agents	Hypothalamic and pituitary hormones	Sympathomimetics
Anxiolytic sedatives, hypnotics and neuroleptics	Iodine and iodides	Thrombolytic agents
	β-Adrenoceptor blocking agents	Iron and iron components
	Thyroid agents	Blood and blood products
Lipid-regulating agents	Vaccines, immunoglobulins and antisera	Blood substitutes and plasma expanders
Local anaesthetics	Vasodilators	Calcium-regulating agents
Nitrates and other anti-angina agents	Xanthines	

subsequent granting/renewing (or refusing/revoking) of a manufacturing licence depends largely upon the level of compliance found during the inspection.

Although separate guides to pharmaceutical GMP are published in different world regions the principles outlined in them all are largely similar. In Europe, for example, the European Union (EU) publishes the *EU Guide to Good Manufacturing Practice for Medicinal Products.* This guide consists of a number of chapters, each of which is concerned with a specific aspect of pharmaceutical manufacture (Table 3.2). The principles therein often appear little more than common-sense guidelines, e.g. the principles outlined in the chapter detailing GMP in relation to personnel could be summarized as:

- an adequate number of sufficiently qualified, experienced personnel must be employed by the manufacturer;
- key personnel, such as the heads of production and quality control, must be independent of each other;

Table 3.2. List of chapter titles present in the *Guide to Good Manufacturing Practice in the European Community* (i.e. Vol. IV of the *Rules Governing Medicinal Products in the European Union*)

1	Quality management
2	Personnel
3	Premises and equipment
4	Documentation
5	Production
6	Quality control
7	Contract manufacture and analysis
8	Complaints and product recall
9	Self-inspection

- personnel should have well-defined job descriptions, and should receive training such that they can adequately perform all their duties;
- issues of personal hygiene should be emphasized, so as to prevent product contamination as a result of poor hygiene practices.

The chapter detailing premises and equipment describes similar obvious principles, such as:

- all premises and equipment should be designed, operated and serviced such that it is capable of carrying out its intended function effectively;
- facility design and equipment use should be such as to avoid cross-contamination or mix-up between different products;
- sufficient storage area must be provided, and a clear demarcation must exist between storage zones for materials at different levels of processing (i.e. raw materials, partially processed product, finished product, rejected product, etc.);
- quality control labs must be separated from production and must be designed and equipped to a standard allowing them to fulfil their intended function.

Some of the principles outlined in the guide are sufficiently general to render them applicable to most manufacturing industries. However, many of the guidelines are far more specific in nature (e.g. guidelines relating to the requirement for dedicated facilities when manufacturing specific products, including some antibiotics and hormones). In addition to the main chapters, the EU guide also contains a series of 14 annexes (Table 3.3). These lay down guidelines relating mainly to the manufacture of specific pharmaceutical substances, such as radioactive pharmaceuticals or products derived from human blood or human plasma. One such annex (manufacture of biological medicinal products for human use) is included as appendix 4 of this textbook.

Most of the principles outlined in such guides to GMP are equally as applicable to the manufacture of traditional pharmaceuticals as to the newer biopharmaceutical preparations. However, the regulatory authorities have found it necessary to publish additional guidelines relating to many of the newer biotechnology-based biopharmaceuticals. Examples include the 'Points to Consider' series, which contain guidelines relating to safe production, e.g. of therapeutic monoclonal antibodies by hybridoma technology, and recombinant biopharmaceuticals produced by genetic engineering (Table 3.4).

Guides to GMP and ancillary publications are among the most significant publications governing the practical aspects of drug manufacture in the pharmaceutical industry. The

Table 3.3. List of the specific annexes now associated with good manufacturing practice (GMP) for medicinal products (i.e. Vol. IV of 'the *Rules Governing Medicinal Products in the European Union*')

1	Manufacture of sterile medicinal products
2	Manufacture of biological medicinal products for human use
3	Manufacture of radiopharmaceuticals
4	Manufacture of veterinary medicinal products other than immunologicals
5	Manufacture of immunological veterinary medicinal products
6	Manufacture of medicinal gases
7	Manufacture of herbal medicinal products
8	Sampling of starting and packaging materials
9	Manufacture of liquids, creams and ointments
10	Manufacture of pressurized metered dose aerosol preparations for inhalation
11	Computerized systems
12	Use of ionizing radiation in the manufacture of medicinal products
13	Good manufacturing practice for investigational medicinal products
14	Manufacture of products derived from human blood or human plasma

Table 3.4. Some of the 'Points to Consider' publications available from the FDA. Many of these can now be downloaded directly from the FDA Center for Biologics Evaluation and Research (CBER) home page, the address of which is: http://WWW.fda.gov/cber/

Points to Consider in the Manufacture and Testing of Monoclonal Antibody Products for Human Use
Points to Consider on Plasmid DNA Vaccines for Preventive Infectious Disease Indications
Points to Consider in the Manufacture and Testing of Therapeutic Products for Human Use Derived from Transgenic Animals
Points to Consider in the Characterization of Cell Lines used to Produce Biologicals
Points to Consider in the Production and Testing of New Drugs and Biologicals Produced by Recombinant DNA Technology
Points to Consider in Human Somatic Cell Therapy and Gene Therapy

implementation of the exacting standards laid down in these publications ensures total quality assurance in the drug manufacturing process.

THE MANUFACTURING FACILITY

Appropriate design and layout of the pharmaceutical facility is an issue central to the production of safe, effective medicines. In common with many other manufacturing facilities, pharmaceutical facilities contain specific production, quality control (QC) and storage areas, etc. However, certain aspects of facility design and operation are unique to this industry, in particular with regard to manufacturers of parenteral (injectable) products. Incorporation of these features is rendered mandatory by guides to pharmaceutical GMP. Particularly noteworthy features, including clean room technology and generation of ultra pure water, are reviewed below.

While the majority of critical manufacturing operations of injectable pharmaceuticals (e.g. most biopharmaceuticals) occurs in specialized clean areas, proper design and maintenance of non-critical areas (e.g. storage, labelling and packing areas) is also vital to ensure overall product safety. Strict codes of hygiene also apply to these non-critical areas.

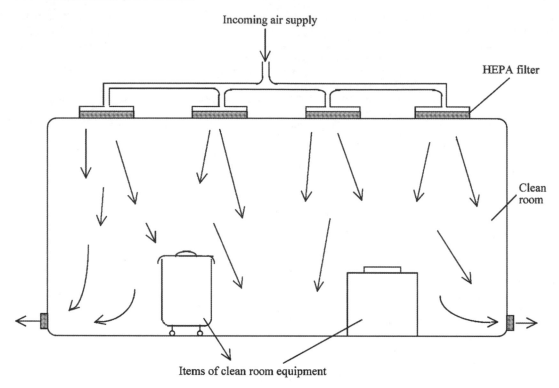

Figure 3.1. Diagrammatic illustration of the flow pattern of HEPA-filtered air through a typical clean room. Air is pumped into the room through HEPA filters (see text) located in the ceiling, and exits via extract units, normally located at floor level. Although the air flow is non-unidirectional (i.e. not true laminar flow), it generates a constant downward sweeping motion, which helps remove air-borne particulate matter from the room

Clean rooms

Clean rooms are environmentally controlled areas within the pharmaceutical facility in which critical manufacturing steps for injectable/sterile (bio)pharmaceuticals must be undertaken. The rooms are specifically designed to protect the product from contamination. Common potential contaminants include microorganisms and particulate matter. These contaminants can be airborne, or derived from process equipment, personnel, etc.

Clean rooms are designed in a manner that allows tight control of entry of all substances (e.g. equipment, personnel, in-process product, and even air; Figures 3.1 and 3.2). In this way, once a clean environment is generated in the room, it can easily be maintained.

A basic feature of clean room design is the presence in their ceilings of high-efficiency particulate air (HEPA) filters. These depth filters, often several inches thick, are generally manufactured from layers of high-density glass fibre. Air is pumped into the room via the filters, generating a constant downward sweeping motion. The air normally exits via exhaust units, generally located near ground level. This motion promotes continued flushing from the room of any particulates generated during processing (Figure 3.1).

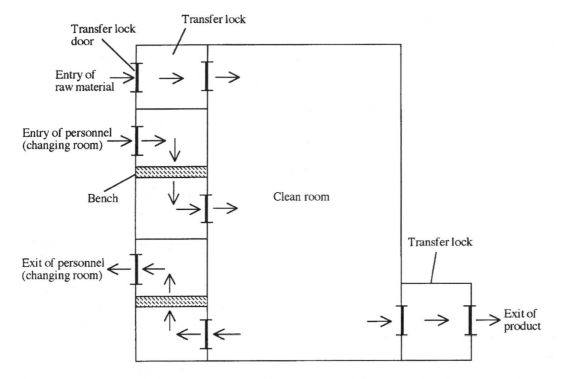

Figure 3.2. Generalized clean room design. Entry of personnel occurs via changing rooms, where the operators first remove their outer garments and subsequently put on suitable clean room clothing (see e.g. Figure 3.3). All raw materials, portable equipment, etc. enters the clean room via a transfer lock. After being placed in the transfer lock, such items are sanitized (where possible) by, for example, being rubbed down with a disinfectant solution. They are then transferred into the clean room proper, by clean room personnel. Processed product usually exits the clean room via an exit transfer lock and personnel often exit the room via a changing room separate from the one they entered (in some cases, the same changing room is used as an entry and exit route). Note that, in practice, product may be processed in a number of different (adjacent) clean rooms

HEPA filters of different particulate-removing efficiency are available, allowing the construction of clean rooms of various levels of cleanliness (Table 3.5). Such rooms are classified on the basis of the number of (a) airborne particles and (b) viable microorganisms present in the room. In Europe clean rooms are classified as grade A, B, C or D (in order of decreasing cleanliness). In the USA, where approximately similar specifications are used, cleanrooms are classified as class 100 (equivalent to grade A/B), class 10 000 (grade C) or class 100 000 (grade D).

HEPA filters in grade B, C and D clean rooms are normally spaced evenly in the ceiling, occupying somewhere in the region of 20–25% of total ceiling area. Generation of class A clean room conditions generally requires a modified design. The use of high-specification HEPA filters, along with the generation of a unidirectional downward air distribution pattern (i.e. laminar flow), is essential. This is only achieved if filter occupancy of ceiling space is 100%. Most commonly, portable (horizontal or vertical) laminar flow cabinets placed in class B cleanrooms are used to generate localized class A conditions. In more extensive facilities, however, an entire class A room may be constructed.

Table 3.5. Specifications laid down (in the *EC Guide to Good Manufacturing Practice for Medicinal Products*) for class A, B, C and D clean rooms, as used in the pharmaceutical industry

Grade	Maximum permitted number of particles per m³ of clean room air		Maximum permitted number of viable microorganisms per m³ of clean room air
	0.5 μm particle diameter	5.0 μm particle diameter	
A	3500	0	Statistically <1
B	3500	0	5
C	350 000	2000	100
D	3 500 000	20 000	500

While an effective HEPA air-handling system is essential to the generation of clean room conditions, many additional elements are equally important in maintaining such conditions. Clean room design is critical in this regard. All exposed surfaces should have a smooth, sealed impervious finish in order to minimize accumulation of dirt/microbial particles and to facilitate effective cleaning procedures. Floors, walls and ceilings can be coated with durable, chemical-resistant materials, such as epoxy resins, polyester or PVC coatings. Alternatively, such surfaces may be completely overlaid with smooth vinyl-based sheets, thermally welded to ensure a smooth, unbroken surface.

Fixtures within the room (e.g. work benches, chairs, equipment, etc.) should be kept to a minimum, and ideally be designed and fabricated from material that facilitates effective cleaning (e.g. polished stainless steel). The positioning of such fixtures should not hinder effective cleaning processes. Pipework should be installed in such a way as to allow effective cleaning around them and the presence of uncleanable recesses must be avoided. All corners and joints between walls and ceilings or floors are rounded, and equipment with movable parts (e.g. motors, pumps) should be encased.

The transfer of processing materials, or entry of personnel into clean areas, carries with it the risk of reintroduction of microorganisms and particulate matter. The principles of GMP minimizes such risks by stipulating that entry of all substances/personnel into a clean room must occur via air-lock systems (Figure 3.2). Such air-locks, with separate doors opening into the clean room and the outside environment, act as a buffer zone. All materials/process equipment entering the clean area are cleaned, sanitized, (or autoclaved if practicable) outside this area, and then passed directly into the transfer lock, from where it is transferred into the clean room by clean room personnel.

An interlocking system ensures that both doors of the transfer lock are never simultaneously open, thus precluding formation of a direct corridor between the uncontrolled area and the clean area. Transfer locks are also positioned between adjacent clean rooms of different grades of cleanliness.

Personnel represent a major potential source of process contaminants (e.g. microorganisms, particulates, etc.), hence they are required to wear specialized protective clothing when working in clean areas. Operators enter the clean area via a separate air lock, which serves as a changing area. They remove their outer clothing at one end of the area, and put on (usually pre-sterilized) gowns, face masks and gloves at the other end of the changing area. Clean room clothing is made from non-shedding material, and covers most of the operator's body (Figure 3.3).

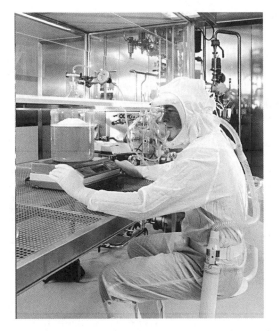

Figure 3.3. Operator wearing clean room clothing suitable for working under aseptic conditions. Note that his entire body is covered. This precludes the possibility of the operator shedding skin, microorganisms or other particulate matter into the product. Photo courtesy of SmithKline Beecham Biological Services s.a., Belgium

A high standard of operator personal hygiene is also of critical importance, and all personnel should receive appropriate training in this regard. Only the minimum number of personnel required should be present in the clean area at any given time. This is facilitated by a high degree of process automation. The installation in clean room walls of windows that serve as observational decks, coupled with intercom systems, also helps by facilitating a certain degree of supervision from outside the clean area.

Cleaning, decontamination and sanitation (CDS)

Essential to the production of a safe, effective product is the application of an effective cleaning, decontamination and sanitation (CDS) regime in the manufacturing facility. Cleaning involves the removal of 'dirt', i.e. miscellaneous organic and inorganic material which may accumulate in process areas or equipment during production. Decontamination refers to the inactivation and removal of undesirable substances, which generally exhibit some specific biological activity likely to be detrimental to the health of patients receiving the drug. Examples include endotoxins, viruses, or prions. Sanitation refers specifically to the destruction and removal of viable microorganisms (i.e. bioburden).

Effective CDS procedures are routinely applied to:

- surfaces in the immediate manufacturing area which do not come into direct contact with the product (e.g. clean room walls and floors, work tops, ancillary equipment);
- surfaces coming into direct contact with the product (e.g. manufacturing vessels, chromatographic columns, product filters, etc.).

CDS of the general manufacturing area

Primary cleaning generally entails scrubbing/rinsing the target surface with water or a detergent solution. Subsequent decontamination/sanitation procedures vary, often involving application of disinfectants or other bacteriocidal agents. Thorough cleaning prior to disinfectant application is essential, as dirt can inactivate many disinfectants or shield microorganisms from disinfectant action. A range of suitable disinfectants are commercially available, containing active ingredients including alcohols, phenol, chlorine and iodine. Different disinfectants are often employed on a rotating basis, to minimize the likelihood of the development of disinfectant-resistant microbial strains.

CDS of clean room walls, floors and accessible surfaces of clean room equipment is routinely undertaken between production runs. The final CDS step often entails 'fogging' the room. This is achieved by placing some of the disinfectant in an aerosol-generating device (a 'fogging machine'). This generates a fine disinfectant mist, or fog, within the clean room, capable of penetrating areas difficult to reach in any other manner.

CDS of process equipment

CDS of surfaces/equipment coming into direct contact with the product requires special consideration. While CDS procedures of guaranteed efficiency must be applied, it is imperative that no trace of the CDS agents subsequently remain on such surfaces, as this would result in automatic product contamination. The final stage of most CDS procedures, as applied to such process equipment, involves exhaustive rinsing with highly pure water (water for injections; WFI). This is followed if at all possible by autoclaving.

CDS of processing and holding vessels, as well as equipment that is easily detachable/dismantled (e.g. homogenizers, centrifuge rotors, flexible tubing filter housing, etc.), is usually relatively straightforward. However, CDS of large equipment/process fixtures can be more challenging, due to the impracticality/undesirability of their dismantling. Examples include the internal surfaces of fermentation equipment, large processing/storage tanks, process-scale chromatographic columns, fixed piping through which product is pumped, etc. Specific 'cleaning in place' (CIP) procedures can generally be used to accommodate such equipment. A detergent solution can be pumped through fixed pipework, followed by WFI and then the passage of sterilizing 'live' steam generated from WFI. Internal surfaces of fermentation/processing vessels can be scrubbed down. Such vessels are generally jacketed (Figure 3.4), thus allowing temperature control of their contents by passage of cooling water/steam through the jacket, as appropriate. Passage of steam through the jacket of the empty vessel facilitates sterilization of its internal surfaces by dry heat.

The cleaning of process-scale chromatography systems used in the purification of biopharmaceuticals can also present challenges. Although such systems are disassembled periodically, this is not routinely undertaken after each production run. CIP protocols must thus be applied periodically to such systems. The level and frequency of CIP undertaken will depend largely on the level and type of contaminants present in the product-stream applied. Columns used during the earlier stages of purification may require more frequent attention than systems used as a final 'clean-up' step of a nearly pure protein product. While each column is flushed with buffer after each production run, a full-scale CIP procedure may be required only after every 3–10 column runs. Most of the contaminants present in such columns are acquired from these previous production runs.

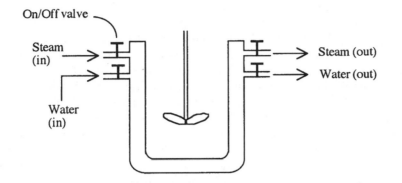

Figure 3.4. Diagram of a typical jacketed processing vessel. Such vessels are usually made from high grade stainless steel. By opening/closing the appropriate valves, steam or cold water can be circulated through the jacket. In this way, the vessel's contents can be heated or cooled, as appropriate. In addition, passage of steam through the jacket of the empty vessel will effectively sanitize its internal surfaces

Processing of product derived from microbial sources can result in contamination of chromatographic media with lipid, endotoxins, nucleic acids and other biomolecules. Application of plant-derived extracts can result in column fouling with pigments and negatively charged polyphenolics, as well as various substances released from plant cell vacuoles (many of which are powerful protein precipitants/denaturants). In addition, some plant-derived enzymes are capable of degrading certain carbohydrate-based (e.g. dextran) chromatographic media. Chromatography of extracts from animal/human tissue can result in column contamination with infectious agents or biomolecules, such as lipids. Furthermore, buffer components may sometimes precipitate out of solution within the column.

Fortunately, most types of modern chromatographic media are resistant to a range of harsh physicochemical influences that may be employed in CIP protocols (Table 3.6). CIP protocols for chromatography columns are normally multistep, consisting of sequential flushing of the gel with a series of CDS agents.

Table 3.6. The range of CIP agents often used to clean/sanitize chromatographic columns. Most CIP protocols would make use of two or more of these agents, allowing them to sequentially percolate through the column at a slow flow rate. Contact time can range from several minutes to overnight. NaOH is particularly effective at removing most contaminant types

0.5–2.0 M NaCl
Non-ionic detergents (0.1–1.0%)
NaOH (0.1–1.0 M)
Acetic acid (20–50%)
Ethanol (~20%)
EDTA (~1.0 mM)
Protease solution
Dilute buffer

Application of concentrated solutions of neutral salts (e.g. KCl or NaCl) is often effective in removing precipitated/aggregated proteins, or other material retained in the column via ionic interaction with the media. The use of buffers containing EDTA or other chelating agents helps remove any metal ions associated with the gel. Use of (dilute) detergent solutions is effective in removing lipid and a whole range of other contaminants. Solvent-containing (e.g. ethanol, butanol, isopropanol) buffers may also be used in this regard. Increasing the column temperature to 50–60°C may sometimes be considered, particularly if lipid appears to be a major column contaminant (most lipids liquefy at such temperatures).

Sodium hydroxide is one of the most extensively used chromatography CIP agents. It is readily available, inexpensive and effective. It is usually applied to a column at strengths of up to 1.0 M. At such concentrations, it quickly removes/destroys most contaminants, including microorganisms and viruses. It will also degrade endotoxin (discussed later) within minutes.

Most types of chromatographic media can withstand incubation with NaOH for prolonged periods. This allows CDS efficiency to be maximized by retaining NaOH in the column for time periods of the order of 30–60 minutes (silica gel is an exception, as it is quickly destroyed at pH values greater than 8). The chromatographic column is subsequently rinsed exhaustively by pumping WFI (or buffer made with WFI) through, until the column effluent is free from all traces of NaOH. Prolonged exposure of the chromatographic media/column parts to residual NaOH could promote column deterioration, and obviously could contaminate/inactivate the protein stream in the next production run.

Chromatographic systems are also designed to facilitate effective CIP. Internal surfaces of the column, its valves and piping, are smooth, impervious and devoid of recesses which could harbour microorganisms or other contaminants.

Periodic system disassembly allows more extensive CDS procedures to be undertaken. Most columns are manufactured from glass, or more usually, tough plastic or stainless steel. After a thorough cleaning of all disassembled components, sterilization by autoclaving is usually undertaken prior to re-assembly. Most chromatographic media likewise can be autoclaved before column re-pouring.

CIP of the ring main systems used to store and circulate WFI and purified water around the pharmaceutical plant is also routinely undertaken (see next section). This normally entails emptying the ring main systems (including reservoirs), opening all the outlet valves, and subsequently pumping sterile steam through all pipework. This is generally sufficient to physically dislodge any traces of trapped particulate matter or biological agents harboured in the system.

Water for biopharmaceutical processing

Water represents one of the most important raw materials used in biopharmaceutical manufacture. It is used as a basic ingredient of fermentation media, and in the manufacture of buffers used throughout product extraction and purification. It represents the solvent in which biopharmaceutical products sold in liquid form are dissolved, and in which freeze-dried biopharmaceuticals will be reconstituted immediately prior to use. It is also used for ancillary processes, such as the cleaning of equipment, piping and product-holding tanks. It is additionally used to clean/rinse the vials into which the final product is filled.

It has been estimated that up to 30 000 litres of water is required to support the production of 1 kg of a recombinant biopharmaceutical produced in a microbial system. It is not surprising, therefore, that the generation of water of suitable purity for processing is central to the successful operation of any (bio)pharmaceutical facility. The use of potable water (i.e. water of drinking standard) is limited to tasks such as routine cleaning of non-critical areas/process equipment. Such water must be subject to further in-house purification prior to its use in the manufacturing process. Water of two different levels of quality is usually required. These are termed 'purified water' and 'water for injections' (WFI). These are distinguished on the basis of the range and quantity of allowable contaminants, with WFI being the most pure. Specific criteria defining levels and types of contaminants permissible in both (along with guidelines as to how the water must be produced) are outlined in international pharmacopoeias.

Purified water has a number of limited uses in pharmaceutical manufacturing. It is often used as the solvent in the manufacture of aqueous-based oral products (e.g. cough mixtures, veterinary de-wormers, etc.). It is not intended to be used as a solvent in the downstream processing of parenteral products — the category into which almost all biopharmaceuticals fall. It is used for primary cleaning of some process equipment/clean room floors, particularly in class D or C clean areas, and for the generation of steam in the facilities' autoclaves. In biopharmaceutical processing, purified water is often used in the generation of fermentation media used to culture biopharmaceutical-producing recombinant microorganisms. Its use in subsequent downstream processing is precluded, as its specifications allows the presence of many contaminants which downstream processing aims to minimize or eliminate from the product.

Water for injection finds extensive application in biopharmaceutical manufacturing. Although there is no regulatory requirement to do so, some manufacturers use WFI when making microbial fermentation media. It is also commonly used in making culture media used in the process-scale propagation of biopharmaceutical-producing mammalian cell lines. Low initial bioburden in WFI renders its sterilization by filtration more straightforward. Furthermore, mammalian cells can be particularly sensitive to some potential water contaminants. The presence of even low concentrations of heavy metals, for example, can adversely effect the growth/product-producing characteristics of these cells.

WFI is the grade of water used exclusively in all downstream biopharmaceutical processing procedures, ranging from making extraction/homogenization/chromatography buffers to rinsing process equipment coming into direct contact with the product.

Generation of purified water and water for injections (WFI)

Purified water and WFI are generated from potable water. While the main techniques by which they are produced are specified by pharmacopoeias, pre-treatment of the incoming potable water will vary, and is often dictated by the range of contaminants found in this water.

While some companies may have a private source of potable water, most obtain incoming water from local municipal authorities. This water is sure to contain various levels of several potential contaminants (Table 3.7). A multi-step purification procedure is then undertaken, which usually contains some or all of the following steps (see also Figure 3.5):

- the incoming water is collected in a storage or 'break' tank, from where it is pumped through a depth filter, organic trap and carbon filter. The depth filter often contains a mixture of granular anthracite, washed sand, and gravel. Solids and colloidal material are retained as the water percolates through the filter bed. The bed may be regenerated every few days by backwashing (i.e. reversing the direction of water flow through the bed). The organic trap

Table 3.7. Range of impurities found in potable water. Even extremely low levels of any such impurities renders this grade of water unacceptable for pharmaceutical processing purposes. Reproduced by permission of John Wiley & Co Ltd from Walsh & Headon (1994)

Particulate matter	Soil particles
	Dirt particles
	Particles derived from decaying organic matter, such as leaves
	Particles derived from leaching of internal surfaces of water pipes
Various dissolved substances	Substances derived from decaying organic matter
	Traces of agricultural run-off
	Minerals, leached into the source water
	Various polluting substances
Viable organisms	Various microorganisms

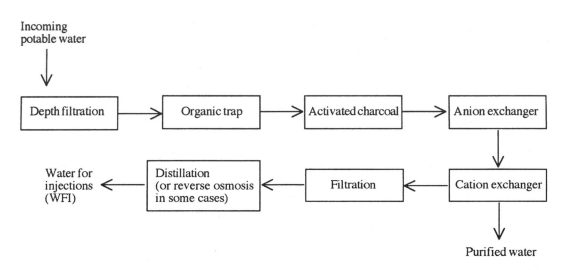

Figure 3.5. Overview of a generalized procedure by which purified water and WFI are generated in a pharmaceutical facility. Refer to text for specific details

contains a resin to which much organic matter will bind, while the carbon (activated charcoal) will absorb residual organics (e.g. humic acid) as well as chlorine and other disinfectants often added by the municipal authorities to control drinking water bioburden;

- a deionization step is normally undertaken next, entailing sequential passage of water through a cation exchanger and anion exchanger. Cations in the water (e.g. Na^+, Ca^{2+}, Mg^{2+}) are retained on the cation exchanger, by displacing H^+ ions off the exchanger. Anions (e.g. Cl^-, SO_3^{2-} are exchanged with the hydroxyl (OH^-)) counter-ions of the anion exchanger. In some instances the water will then be fed directly into a smaller, mixed-bed ion exchanger (e.g. containing both cation and anion exchangers), as a final polishing step.

The efficiency of these steps can be conveniently monitored by continuous in-line measurement of the resistivity of the water (deionization results in increased resistivity, typically to levels of 1–10 MΩ). If the resistivity of the deionized water falls below a value of approximately 1 MΩ, automatic system shut-off, followed by regeneration of the anion and cation exchange beds (with NaOH and HCl respectively), is initiated.

Deionizers fail to remove microbial contaminants, and exchange resin beds can often actually harbour microorganisms, contaminating the water. For this reason, filtration or UV treatment often constitutes the next purification step. One such treatment configuration entails pumping the deionized water through a 0.45 µm filter, followed by exposure to UV (at 254 nm). This may be followed by yet another filtration step through a 0.22 µm filter to remove UV-inactivated microorganisms. In some systems the 0.22 µm filter may even be replaced by ultrafilters capable of retaining molecules whose molecular mass is significantly greater than 10 kDa. Such systems will remove not only bacteria but also many bacterial products, including endotoxin and additional organic and colloidal material.

Deionized water often meets the pharmacopoeial criteria laid down for 'purified water'. Sometimes, however, further purification may be necessary to attain this standard. This often entails a distillation or reverse-osmosis step. Deionized water will, however, not meet the pharmacopoeial requirements for WFI. WFI is best generated by distillation of deionized water. Distillation entails converting water to vapour by heat, followed by passing over a condenser, which results in condensation of pure water. Dissolved minerals and most organics are not volatile at 100°C.

Reverse osmosis (RO) entails the use of a semi-permeable membrane (permeable to the solvent, i.e. water molecules, but impermeable to solutes, i.e. contaminants). Osmosis describes the movement of solvent molecules across such a membrane from a solution of lower solute concentration to one of higher solute concentration. The force promoting this movement is termed 'osmotic pressure'. During reverse osmosis, a pressure greater than the natural osmotic pressure is applied to the system from the higher solute concentration side, causing solvent molecules to flow in the opposite direction.

RO membranes are manufactured from polymers such as cellulose acetate or polyamides. A single pass of water through such membranes can remove 95% of all dissolved solids and 99% of microorganisms and endotoxins. Double RO systems are often employed, increasing the efficiency of the process still further, and providing some element of protection against the consequences of puncture of one of the membranes. While RO systems are less expensive than distillation, many regard distillation as being a safer option. Pin-head punctures of RO membranes can be hard to detect. Membranes are also susceptible to microbial colonization and cannot be exposed to high temperatures, which renders effective sanitation more difficult.

Distribution system for WFI

Upon its manufacture, WFI is fed into a sealed storage vessel, often made from stainless steel. The water is circulated via a series of pipework throughout the building, and from which a number of outlet valves are available. The pipework leads back to the storage tank, allowing constant recirculation of the water throughout the facility. Because of this it is known as a ring main or loop system (Figure 3.6).

As pharmacopoeial specifications preclude the addition of sanitizing agents such as chlorine, maintenance of WFI within microbiological specifications requires special attention. While circulating, the WFI is maintained at a flow rate of the order 9 ft/s. This ensures constant turbulent flow, discouraging microbial attachment to internal surfaces of the distribution pipes. The WFI is also constantly maintained at temperatures of the order of 85°C, again to discourage microbial growth.

Water collected from the WFI hot loop is generally allowed to cool before use for biopharmaceutical processing (hot buffers would not only potentially denature the protein

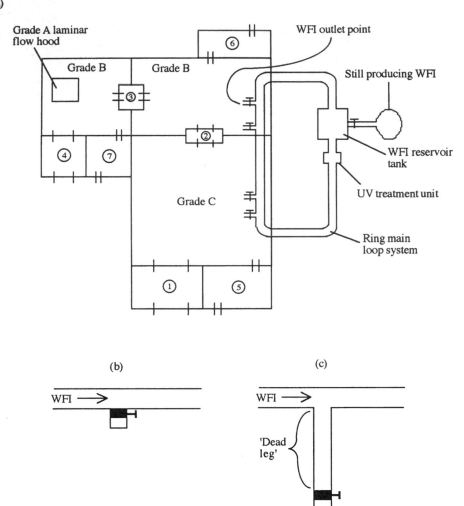

(a)

(b)

(c)

① ② ③ = transfer locks into grade C, B (and grade B with portable grade A laminar flow hood)
clean rooms, respectively

④ = product exit transfer lock

⑤ ⑥ ⑦ = changing rooms servicing indicated clean rooms

Figure 3.6. (a) Generalized diagram of how WFI is distributed throughout a typical pharmaceutical facility. One or more outlet valves from the ring main system are in place in the clean rooms in which product manufacture is undertaken. Note that no such outlet is present in the clean room where final product fill will take place (i.e. the grade B cleanroom housing the grade A laminar flow hood in the above example). (b) Illustration of an acceptable valve design at a WFI outlet point. This design prevents stagnation of water, which could occur if such an outlet point was poorly designed, as illustrated in (c). Refer to text for specific details

product, but their pH values could change quite dramatically when cooled from 85°C to 25°C). In some instances a separate loop system is constructed in which WFI is circulated at ambient temperature allowing its immediate use in processing operations. To maintain water quality, however, this entire circulating system must be emptied and sanitized every 24 h.

Careful design of circulating systems also helps to maintain the microbiological quality of WFI. Circulating pipework lengths are fused together by welding, as opposed to the use of threaded fittings, which could harbour bacteria. 'Dead-legs' (areas where water could stagnate, e.g. at water outlet points), are avoided, and bends in pipes are smooth and curving, as opposed to the use of abrupt T-junctions. UV cells are also fitted on-line in the system, subjecting circulating water to their continual bactericidal influence.

Upon initial installation, the pipework is cleaned by passage of detergent or other cleaning agents, followed by a water rinse. 'Passivation' (exposure of the internal pipework surfaces to chemical agents, rendering the surface less reactive subsequently) is then undertaken, usually by oxidation using nitric acid or certain organic acids.

WFI is quite corrosive, especially at 85°C, and it can promote leeching from even high-grade stainless steel piping. Addition of ozone to the WFI can alleviate this, as the ozone's microcidal properties facilitate prolonged storage/circulation of the water at 25°C. Other innovations in this field include replacement of stainless steel pipework with chemically inert plastics. However, extensive tests need to be undertaken in order to prove that WFI cannot leach potentially dangerous substances from these plastics before their use will become routine.

Loop systems distributing purified water also exist in most facilities, with their design being somewhat similar to WFI systems. The more relaxed microbiological specifications relating to purified water renders the design and operation of such systems less complex. Purified water is generally circulated at ambient temperatures, via stainless steel or sometimes plastic-based tubing.

Samples of WFI and purified water are usually collected daily by quality control personnel, and tested for conformance to specification. Failure to meet specification results in the system being emptied and fully sanitized, before generation of fresh water.

Documentation

Adequate documentation forms an essential part of good manufacturing practice. For this reason, every aspect of pharmaceutical manufacture is characterized by the existence of extensive associated documentation. This is essential in order to:

- help prevent errors/misunderstandings associated with verbal communication;
- facilitate the tracing of the manufacturing history of any batch of product;
- ensure reproducibility in all aspects of pharmaceutical manufacture.

Most documents associated with pharmaceutical manufacturing fall into one of four categories:

- standard operating procedures (SOPs);
- specifications;
- manufacturing formulae, processing and packaging instructions;
- records.

Great care is taken when initially preparing such documents to ensure they are written/ worded in a clear and unambiguous fashion. They are usually written by supervisory personnel, and inspected by senior technical personnel (often the production or QC manager or both), before their final approval for general use. Such documents are reviewed regularly, and updated as required.

SOPs are documents which detail how staff should undertake particular procedures or processes. These procedures/processes are usually of a general nature, often being independent of any one pharmaceutical product. Many SOPs fall into one of several general categories, including:

- SOPs detailing step-by-step operational procedures for specific items of equipment (e.g. autoclaves, homogenizers, freeze-dryers, pH meters, product labelling machines, etc.);
- SOPs detailing maintenance/validation procedures for specific items of equipment or facility areas, e.g. SOPs detailing CDS of clean rooms;
- SOPs relating directly to personnel (e.g. step-by-step procedures undertaken when gowning-up before entering a clean room);
- SOPs relating to testing/analysis (e.g. procedures detailing how to properly sample raw materials/finished product for QC analysis, SOPs relating to the routine sampling and testing of WFI from the ring main system, etc.).

Specifications

Specifications are normally written by QC personnel. They detail the exact qualitative and quantitative requirements to which individual raw materials or product must conform. For example, specifications for chemical raw materials will set strict criteria relating to the percentage active ingredients present, permitted levels of named contaminants, etc. Specifications for packing materials will, for example, lay down exact dimensions of product packaging cartons; specifications for product labels will detail label dimensions and exact details of label text, etc. Specifications for all raw materials are sent to raw material suppliers and, upon their delivery, QC personnel will ensure that these raw materials meet their specifications before being released to production (the raw materials are held in 'quarantine' prior to their approval). Final product specifications will also be prepared. As most products are manufactured to conform with pharmacopoeial requirements, many of the specifications set for raw materials/finished product are simply transcribed from the appropriate pharmacopoeia.

Manufacturing formulae, processing and packaging instructions

Manufacturing formulae should clearly indicate the product name, potency or strength, and exact batch size. It lists each of the starting raw materials required, and the quantity in which each is required. The processing instructions should contain step-by-step manufacturing instructions. The detail given should be sufficient to allow a technically competent person, unfamiliar with the process, to successfully undertake the manufacturing procedure.

The processing instructions should also indicate the principal items of equipment utilized during manufacture, and the precise location in which each step should be undertaken (e.g. in a specific clean room, etc.). It will also list any specific precautions which must be observed during manufacture (e.g. precautions to protect the product from, perhaps, excessive heating, or to protect the operator from any potentially dangerous product constituent). Each product will also have its own labelling and packing instructions, indicating:

- the label to be used, and its exact text;

- exact packing instructions (e.g. how many units of product per pack, how may packs per shipping carton, etc.).

A copy of the label to be used is generally attached to the documents, to allow the supervisor and operators to verify easily that the correct label has been dispensed for the product in question.

Records

Maintenance of adequate and accurate records forms an essential part of GMP. For any given batch of product, records relating to every aspect of manufacture of that batch will be retained. These records will include:

- specification results obtained on all raw materials;
- batch manufacturing, processing and packaging records;
- QC analysis results of bulk and finished product.

These records, along with samples of finished product, must be retained in the facility for at least 1 year after the expiry of that batch. Should any difficulty arise regarding the finished product, the records should allow tracing back of all direct manufacturing steps, as well as indirect procedures which might influence the quality/safety of the product. During inspections, regulatory inspectors usually examine the records relating to a number of randomly chosen batches in detail, in order to help them assess ongoing adherence to GMP in the facility.

Generation of manufacturing records

Prior to commencement of the manufacturing of a specific product, production personnel will print/photocopy the manufacturing formulae, processing and packaging instructions associated with that product. The responsible individual fills in the batch number in the space provided (a batch number is a unique combination of numbers and/or letters assigned to that batch, in order to distinguish it from all other batches). This photocopied document forms the blueprint for manufacture of that batch. A space is provided after each manufacturing/packing instruction. When that step is completed, the responsible operator initials the space and includes the exact time and date undertaken. This forms a detailed record of manufacture.

Additional supporting documents are also included in the manufacturing records. These may include computerized print-outs from weighing equipment used to dispense chemical raw materials, or recorder charts obtained, e.g. from a freeze-drier upon completion of freeze-drying that batch of product.

QC records relating to raw materials, in-process and final product are generated in much the same way — by printing/photocopying originals and filling in the test results obtained.

Advances in information technology are now impacting upon the pharmaceutical industry. Many documents are now maintained in electronic format. In fact, some regard it as likely that in the future 'paperless facilities' will become commonplace, with all documentation being computerized. Several aspects of such electronic document maintenance deserve special attention. Adequate back-up files should always be retained. Also, restricted access to computerized systems is required to ensure that data/documentation is only entered/amended by persons authorized to do so.

SOURCES OF BIOPHARMACEUTICALS

The bulk of biopharmaceuticals currently on the market are produced by genetic engineering using various recombinant expression systems. While a wide range of potential protein production systems are available (Table 3.8), most of the recombinant proteins that have gained marketing approval to date are produced either in recombinant *Eschericia coli* or in recombinant mammalian cell lines (Table 3.9). Such recombinant systems are invariably constructed by the introduction of a gene or cDNA coding for the protein of interest into a well-characterized strain of the chosen producer cell. Examples include *E. coli* K12 and Chinese hamster ovary strain K1 (CHO-K1). Gene/cDNA transfer is normally achieved by using an appropriate expression plasmid, or other standard gene-manipulating techniques. Each recombinant production system displays its own unique set of advantages and disadvantages, as described below.

E. coli as a source of recombinant, therapeutic proteins

Many microorganisms represent attractive potential production systems for therapeutic proteins. They can usually be cultured in large quantities, inexpensively and in a short time, by standard methods of fermentation. Production facilities can be constructed in any world region, and the scale of production can be varied as required.

The expression of recombinant proteins in cells in which they do not naturally occur is termed 'heterologous protein production'. By far the most common microbial species used to produce

Table 3.8. Expression systems that are/could potentially be used for the production of recombinant biopharmaceutical products (CHO=Chinese hamster ovary; BHK=baby hamster kidney)

E. coli (and additional prokaryotic systems, e.g. Bacilli)
Yeast (particularly *Saccharomyces cerevisiae*)
Fungi (particularly *Aspergillus*)
Animal cell culture (particularly CHO and BHK cell lines)
Transgenic animals (focus thus far is upon sheep and goats)
Plant-based expression systems (various)
Insect cell culture systems

Table 3.9. Some biopharmaceuticals currently on the market that are produced by genetic engineering in either *E. coli* or animal cells. CHO=Chinese hamster ovary cells; BHK=baby hamster kidney cells

Biopharmaceutical product	Source	Biopharmaceutical product	Source
Tissue plasminogen activator (tPA)	*E. coli*, CHO	Follicle-stimulating hormone (FSH)	CHO
Insulin	*E. coli*	Interferon-β	CHO
		Erythropoietin	CHO
Interferon-α	*E. coli*	Glucocerebrosidase	CHO
Interferon-γ	*E. coli*	Factor VIIa	BHK
Interleukin-2 (IL-2)	*E. coli*		
Granulocyte colony-stimulating factor (G-CSF)	*E. coli*		
Human growth hormone (hGH)	*E. coli*		

Table 3.10. Levels of expression of various biopharmaceuticals produced in recombinant *E. coli* cells

Biopharmaceutical	Level of expression (% of total cellular protein)
Interferon-γ	25
Insulin	20
Interferon-β	15
Tumour necrosis factor	15
α_1-Antitrypsin	15
Interleukin 2	10
Human growth hormone	5

heterologous proteins of therapeutic interest is *Eschericia coli*. The first biopharmaceutical produced by genetic engineering to gain marketing approval (in 1982) was recombinant human insulin (trade name Humulin), produced in *E. coli*. An example of a more recently approved biopharmaceutical which is produced in *E. coli* is that of Ecokinase, a recombinant tissue plasminogen activator (tPA, Chapter 9), approved for sale in the EU in 1996. Many additional examples are provided in subsequent chapters.

As a recombinant production system, *E. coli* displays a number of advantages, which include:

- *E. coli* has long served as the model system for studies relating to prokaryotic genetics. Its molecular biology is thus well characterized;
- high levels of expression of heterologous proteins can be achieved in recombinant *E. coli* (Table 3.10). Modern, high-expression promoters can routinely ensure that levels of expression of the recombinant protein reach up to 30% total cellular protein;
- *E. coli* cells grow rapidly on relatively simple and inexpensive media, and the appropriate fermentation technology is well established.

These advantages, particularly the ease of genetic manipulation, rendered *E. coli* the primary biopharmaceutical production system for many years. However, *E. coli* also displays a number of drawbacks as a biopharmaceutical producer, including:

- heterologous proteins accumulate intracellularly;
- inability to undertake post-translational modifications (particularly glycosylation) of proteins;
- the presence of lipopolysaccharide on its surface.

The vast bulk of proteins synthesized naturally by *E. coli* (i.e. its homologous proteins) are intracellular. Few are exported to the periplasmic space, or are released as true extracellular proteins. Heterologous proteins expressed in *E. coli* thus invariably accumulate in the cell cytoplasm. Intracellular protein production complicates downstream processing (relative to extracellular production) because:

- additional primary processing steps are required, i.e. cellular homogenization, with subsequent removal of cell debris by centrifugation or filtration;
- more extensive chromatographic purification is required in order to separate the protein of interest from the several thousand additional homologous proteins produced by the *E. coli* cells.

An additional complication of high-level intracellular heterologous protein expression is inclusion body formation. Inclusion bodies (refractile bodies) are insoluble aggregates of partially folded heterologous product. Because of their dense nature, they are easily observed by dark field microscopy. Presumably, when expressed at high levels, heterologous proteins overload the normal cellular protein-folding mechanisms. Under such circumstances, it would be likely that hydrophobic patches, normally hidden from the surrounding aqueous phase in fully folded proteins, would remain exposed in the partially folded product. This, in turn, would promote aggregate formation via intermolecular hydrophobic interactions.

However, the formation of inclusion bodies displays one processing advantage — it facilitates the achievement of a significant degree of subsequent purification by a single centrifugation step. Because of their density, inclusion bodies sediment even more rapidly than cell debris. Low-speed centrifugation thus facilitates the easy and selective collection of inclusion bodies directly after cellular homogenization. After collection, inclusion bodies are generally incubated with strong denaturants, such as detergents, solvents or urea. This promotes complete solubilization of the inclusion body (i.e. complete denaturation of the proteins therein). The denaturant is then removed by techniques such as dialysis or diafiltration. This facilitates re-folding of the protein, a high percentage of which will generally fold into its native, biologically active, conformation.

Various attempts have been made to prevent inclusion body formation when expressing heterologous proteins in *E. coli*. Some studies have shown that a simple reduction in the temperature of bacterial growth (from 37°C to 30°C) can significantly decrease the incidence of inclusion body formation. Other studies have shown that expression of the protein of interest as a fusion partner with thioredoxin will eliminate inclusion body formation in most instances. Thioredoxin is a homologous *E. coli* protein, expressed at high levels. It is localized at the adhesion zones in *E. coli*, and is a heat-stable protein. A plasmid vector has been engineered which facilitates expression of a fusion protein, consisting of thioredoxin linked to the protein of interest via a short peptide sequence, recognized by the protease enterokinase (Figure 3.7). The fusion protein is invariably expressed at high levels, while remaining in soluble form. Congregation at adhesion zones facilitates its selective release into the media by simple osmotic shock. This can greatly simplify its subsequent purification. After its release, the fusion protein is incubated with enterokinase, thus releasing the protein of interest (Figure 3.7)

An alternative means of reducing/potentially eliminating inclusion body accumulation entails the high-level co-expression of molecular chaperones, along with the protein of interest. Chaperones are themselves proteins which promote proper and full folding of other proteins into their biologically active, native three-dimensional shape. They usually achieve this by transiently binding to the target protein during the early stages of its folding and guiding further folding by preventing/correcting the occurrence of improper hydrophobic associations.

The inability of prokaryotes such as *E. coli* to carry out post-translational modifications (particularly glycosylation) can limit their usefulness as production systems for some therapeutically useful proteins. Many such proteins, when produced naturally in the body, are glycosylated (Table 3.11). However, the lack of the carbohydrate component of some glycoproteins has little, if any, negative influence upon their biological activity. The unglycosylated form of interleukin-2, for example, displays essentially identical biological activity to that of the native glycosylated molecule. In such cases, *E. coli* can serve as a satisfactory production system.

Another concern with regard to the use of *E. coli* is the presence on its surface of lipopolysaccharide (LPS) molecules. The pyrogenic nature of LPS (see later) renders essential its

Plasmid
vector
(pTrxFus)

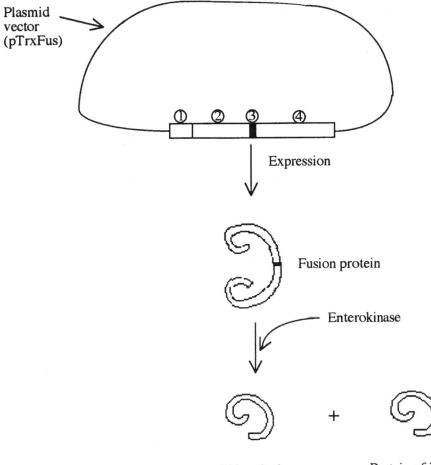

Expression

Fusion protein

Enterokinase

Thioredoxin   +   Protein of interest

Key: ① = strong promoter

       ② = thioredoxin gene

       ③ = nucleotide sequence coding for the peptide sequence which
            serves as cleavage site for the protease (enterokinase)

       ④ = gene/cDNA coding for the protein of interest

Figure 3.7.   High level expression of a protein of interest in *E. coli* in soluble form by using the engineered
'thiofusion' expression system. Refer to text for specific details

Table 3.11. Proteins of actual or potential therapeutic use that are glycosylated when produced naturally in the body (or by hydridoma technology in the case of monoclonal antibodies). These proteins are discussed in detail in various subsequent chapters

Most interleukins (interleukin-1 being an important exception)
Interferon-β and -γ (most interferon-αs are unglycosylated)
Colony stimulating factors
Tumour necrosis factors
Gonadotrophins (follicle stimulating hormone, luteinizing hormone and human chorionic gonadotrophin)
Blood factors (e.g. factors VII, VIII and IX)
Erythropoietin
Thrombopoietin
Tissue plasminogen activator
α_1-Antitrypsin
Intact monoclonal antibodies

removal from the product stream. Fortunately, several commonly employed downstream processing procedures achieve such a separation without any great difficulty.

Expression of recombinant proteins in animal cell culture systems

Technical advances facilitating genetic manipulation of animal cells now allow routine production of therapeutic proteins in such systems. The major advantage of these systems is their ability to carry out post-translational modification of the protein product. As a result, many biopharmaceuticals that are naturally glycosylated are now produced in animal cell lines (Table 3.9). Chinese hamster ovary (CHO) and baby hamster kidney (BHK) cells have become particularly popular in this regard.

While their ability to carry out post-translational modifications renders their use desirable/ essential for producing many biopharmaceuticals, animal cell-based systems do suffer from a number of disadvantages. When compared to *E. coli*, animal cells display very complex nutritional requirements, grow more slowly and are far more susceptible to physical damage. In industrial terms, this translates into increased production costs.

In addition to recombinant biopharmaceuticals, animal cell culture is used to produce various other biologically-based pharmaceuticals. Chief amongst these are a variety of vaccines and hybridoma cell-produced monoclonal antibodies (Chapter 10). Earlier interferon preparations were also produced in culture by a particular lymphoblastoid cell line (the Namalwa cell line), which was found to naturally synthesize high levels of several interferon-αs (Chapter 4).

Additional production systems: yeasts

Attention has also focused upon a variety of additional production systems for recombinant biopharmaceuticals. Yeast cells (particularly *Saccharomyces cerevisiae*) display a number of characteristics that make them attractive in this regard. These characteristics include:

- their molecular biology has been studied in detail, facilitating their genetic manipulation;
- most are GRAS-listed organisms ('generally regarded as safe'), and have a long history of industrial application (e.g. in brewing and baking);

- they grow relatively quickly in relatively inexpensive media, and their tough outer cell wall protects them from physical damage;
- suitable industrial scale fermentation equipment/technology is already available;
- they possess the ability to carry out post-translational modifications of proteins.

The practical potential of yeast-based production systems has been confirmed by the successful expression of a whole range of proteins of therapeutic interest in such systems. However, a number of disadvantages relating to heterologous protein production in yeast have been recognized. These include:

- although capable of glycosylating heterologous human proteins, the glycosylation pattern usually varies somewhat from the pattern observed in the native glycoprotein (when isolated from its natural source, or when expressed in recombinant animal cell culture systems);
- in most instances, expression levels of heterologous proteins remain less than 5% of total cellular protein. This is significantly lower than expression levels typically achieved in recombinant *E. coli* systems.

Despite such potential disadvantages, several recombinant biopharmaceuticals now approved for general medical use are produced in yeast (*S. cerevisiae*)-based systems (Table 3.12). Interestingly, most such products are not glycosylated. The oligosaccharide component of glycoproteins produced in yeasts generally contain high levels of mannose. Such high mannose-type glycosylation patterns generally trigger their rapid clearance from the blood stream. Such products, therefore, would be expected to display a short half-life when parenterally administered to man.

Fungal production systems

Fungi have elicited interest as heterologous protein producers, as many have a long history of use in the production of various industrial enzymes, such as α-amylase and glucoamylase. Suitable fermentation technology therefore already exists. In general, fungi are capable of high-level expression of various proteins, many of which they secrete into their extracellular media. The extracellular production of a biopharmaceutical would be distinctly advantageous in terms of subsequent downstream processing. Fungi also possess the ability to carry out

Table 3.12. Recombinant therapeutic proteins approved for general medical use that are produced in *Saccharomycese cerevisiae*. All are subsequently discussed in the chapter indicated

Trade name	Description	Use	Refer to Chapter
Novolog	Engineered short-acting insulin	Diabetes mellitus	8
Leukine	Colony stimulating factor (GM-CSF)	Bone marrow transplantation	6
Recombivax, Comvax, Engerix B, Tritanrix-HB, Infanrix, Twinrix, Primavax, Hexavax	All vaccine preparations containing rHBsAg as one component	Vaccination	10
Revasc, Refludan	Hirudin	Anticoagulant	9
Fasturtec	Urate oxidase	Hyperuricaemia	9
Regranex	Platelet-derived growth factor	Diabetic ulcers	7

post-translational modifications. Patterns of glycosylation achieved can, however, differ from typical patterns obtained when a glycoprotein is expressed in a mammalian cell line.

Most fungal host strains also naturally produce significant quantities of extracellular proteases, which can potentially degrade the recombinant product. This difficulty can be partially overcome by using mutant fungal strains secreting greatly reduced levels of proteases. Although researchers have produced a number of potential therapeutic proteins in recombinant fungal systems, no biopharmaceutical produced by such means has thus far sought or gained marketing approval.

Transgenic animals

The production of heterologous proteins in transgenic animals has gained much attention in the recent past. The generation of transgenic animals is most often undertaken by directly microinjecting exogenous DNA into an egg cell. In some instances, this DNA will be stably integrated into the genetic complement of the cell. After fertilization, the ova may be implanted into a surrogate mother. Each cell of the resultant transgenic animal will harbour a copy of the transferred DNA. As this includes the animal's germ cells, the novel genetic information introduced can be passed on from one generation to the next.

A transgenic animal harbouring a gene coding for a pharmaceutically useful protein could become a live bioreactor, producing the protein of interest on an ongoing basis. In order to render such a system practically useful, the recombinant protein must be easily removable from the animal, in a manner which would not be injurious to the animal (or the protein). A simple way of achieving this is to target protein production to the mammary gland. Harvesting of the protein thus simply requires the animal to be milked.

Mammary-specific expression can be achieved by fusing the gene of interest with the promoter-containing regulatory sequence of a gene coding for a milk-specific protein. Regulatory sequences of the whey acid protein (WAP), β-casein and α- and β-lactoglobulin genes have all been used to date to promote production of various pharmaceutical proteins in the milk of transgenic animals (Table 3.13).

One of the earliest successes in this regard entailed the production of human tissue plasminogen activator (tPA) in the milk of transgenic mice. The tPA gene was fused to the upstream regulatory sequence of the mouse whey acidic protein—the most abundant protein found in mouse milk. More practical from a production point of view was the subsequent production of tPA in the milk of transgenic goats, again using the murine WAP gene regulatory sequence to drive expression (Figure 3.8). Goats and sheep have proved to be the most attractive host systems, as they exhibit a combination of attractive characteristics. These include:

- high milk production capacities (Table 3.14);
- ease of handling and breeding, coupled to well-established animal husbandry techniques.

A number of additional general characteristics may be cited which render attractive the production of pharmaceutical proteins in the milk of transgenic farm animals. These include:

- ease of harvesting of crude product—which simply requires the animal to be milked;
- pre-availability of commercial milking systems, already designed with maximum process hygiene in mind;
- low capital investment (i.e. relatively low-cost animals replace high-cost traditional fermentation equipment) and low running costs;

Table 3.13. Proteins of actual/potential therapeutic use that have been produced in the milk of transgenic animals

Protein	Animal species	Expression levels in milk
tPA	Goat	6 g/l
Interleukin-2	Rabbit	0.5 mg/l
Factor VIII	Pig	3 mg/l
Factor IX	Sheep	1 g/l
α1-Antitrypsin	Goat	20 g/l
Fibrinogen	Sheep	5 g/l
Erythropoietin	Rabbit	50 mg/l
Antithrombin III	Goat	14 g/l
Human α-lactalbumin	Cow	2.5 g/l
Insulin-like growth factor I	Rabbit	1 g/l
Protein C	Pig	1 g/l
Growth hormone	Rabbit	50 mg/l

- high expression levels of proteins are potentially attained. In many instances, the level of expression exceeds 1 g protein/litre milk. In one case, initial expression levels of 60 g/l were observed, which stabilized at 35 g/l as lactation continued (the expression of the α_1-antitrypsin gene, under the influence of the ovine β-lactoglobulin promoter, in a transgenic sheep). Even at expression levels of 1 g/l, one transgenic goat would produce a similar quantity of product in 1 day as would likely be recoverable from a 50–100 l bioreactor system;
- ongoing supply of product is guaranteed (by breeding);
- milk is biochemically well characterized, and the physicochemical properties of the major native milk proteins of various species are well known. This helps rational development of appropriate downstream processing protocols (Table 3.15).

Despite the attractiveness of this system, a number of issues remain to be resolved before it is broadly accepted by the industry. These include:

- variability of expression levels. While in many cases expression levels of heterologous proteins exceed 1 g/l, in some instances expression levels as low as 1.0 mg/l have been obtained;
- characterization of the exact nature of the post-translational modifications the mammary system is capable of undertaking, e.g. the carbohydrate composition of tPA produced in this system differs from the recombinant enzyme produced in murine cell culture systems;
- significant time lag between the generation of a transgenic embryo and commencement of routine product manufacture. Once a viable embryo containing the inserted desired gene is generated, it must firstly be brought to term. This gestation period ranges from 1 month for rabbits to 9 months for cows. The transgenic animal must then reach sexual maturity before breeding (5 months for rabbits, 15 months for cows). Before they begin to lactate (i.e. produce the recombinant product), they must breed successfully and bring their offspring to term. The overall time lag to routine manufacture can, therefore, be almost 3 years in the case of cows or 7 months in the case of rabbits. Furthermore, if the original transgenic embryo turns out to be male, a further delay is encountered as this male must breed in order to pass

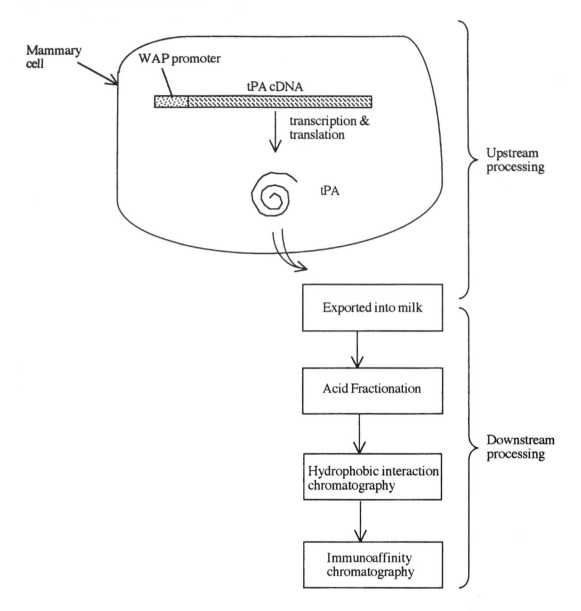

Figure 3.8. The production and purification of tPA from the milk of transgenic goats (WAP = murine whey acid). The downstream processing procedure yielded in excess of an 8000-fold purification factor with an overall product yield of 25%. The product was greater than 98% pure, as judged by SDS-electrophoresis

on the desired gene to daughter animals—who will then eventually produce the desired product in their milk.

Another general disadvantage of this approach relates to the use of the micro-injection technique to introduce the desired gene into the pronucleus of the fertilized egg. This approach

Table 3.14. Typical annual milk yields (litres) as well as time lapse between generation of the transgene embryo and first product harvest (first lactation) of indicated species

Species	Annual milk yield (l)	Time to first production batch (months)
Cow	6000–9000	33–36
Goat	700–800	18–20
Sheep	400–500	18–20
Pig	250–300	16–17
Rabbit	4–5	7

Table 3.15. Some physicochemical properties of the major (bovine) milk proteins

Protein	Caseins	β-Lactoglobulin	α-Lactalbumin	Serum albumin	IgG
Concentration (g/l)	25 (Total)	2–4	0.5–1.5	0.4	0.5–1.0
Mass (kDa)	20–25	18	14	66	150
Phosphorylated?	Yes	No	No	No	No
Isoelectric point	Vary	5.2	4.2–4.8	4.7–4.9	5.5–8.3

is inefficient and time-consuming. There is no control over issues such as if/where in the host genomes the injected gene will integrate. Overall, only a modest proportion of manipulated embryos will culminate in the generation of a healthy biopharmaceutical-producing animal.

A number of alternative approaches are being developed which may overcome some of these issues. Replication-defective retroviral vectors are available which will more consistently (a) deliver a chosen gene into cells and (b) ensure chromosomal integration of the gene. A second innovation is the application of nuclear transfer technology.

Nuclear transfer entails substituting the genetic information present in an unfertilized egg with donor genetic information. The best-known product of this technology is 'Dolly' the sheep, produced by substituting the nucleus of a sheep egg with a nucleus obtained from an adult sheep cell (genetically, therefore, Dolly was a clone of the original 'donor' sheep). An extension of this technology applicable to biopharmaceutical manufacture entails using a donor cell nucleus previously genetically manipulated so as to harbour a gene coding for the biopharmaceutical of choice. The technical viability of this approach was proved in the late 1990s upon the birth of two transgenic sheep, 'Polly' and 'Molly'. The donor nucleus used to generate these sheep harboured an inserted (human) blood factor IX gene under the control of a milk protein promoter. Both now produce significant quantities of human factor IX in their milk.

At the time of writing, no therapeutic protein produced in the milk of transgenic animals had been approved for general medical use. A number of companies, however, continue to pursue this strategy. These include GTC Biotherapeutics USA (formerly Genzyme Transgenics) and PPL Therapeutics (Scotland). α_1-Antitrypsin, antithrombin and a range of monoclonal antibody-based products produced via transgenic technology continue to be evaluated by these companies.

In addition to milk, a range of recombinant proteins have been expressed in various other targeted tissues/fluids of transgenic animals. Antibodies and other proteins have been produced in the blood of transgenic pigs and rabbits. This mode of production is, however, unlikely to be pursued industrially for a number of reasons:

- only relatively low volumes of blood can be harvested from the animal at any given time point;
- serum is a complex fluid, containing a variety of native proteins. This renders purification of the recombinant product more complex;
- many proteins are poorly stable in serum;
- the recombinant protein could have negative physiological side effects on the producer animal.

Therapeutic proteins have also been successfully expressed in the urine and seminal fluid of various transgenic animals. Again, issues of sample collection, volume of collected fluid and the appropriateness of these systems renders unlikely their industrial-scale adoption. One system, however, that does show industrial promise is the targeted production of recombinant proteins in the egg white of transgenic birds. Targeted production is achieved by choice of an appropriate egg white protein promoter sequence. Large quantities of recombinant product can potentially accumulate in the egg, which can then be collected and processed with relative ease.

Transgenic plants

The production of pharmaceutical proteins using transgenic plants has also gained some attention over the last decade. The introduction of foreign genes into plant species can be undertaken by a number of means of which *Agrobacterium*-based vector-mediated gene transfer is most commonly employed. *Agrobacterium tumefaciens* and *A. rhizogenes* are soil-based plant pathogens. Upon infection, a portion of *Agrobacterium* Ti plasmid is translocated to the plant cell and is integrated into the plant cell genome. Using such approaches, a whole range of therapeutic proteins have been expressed in plant tissue (Table 3.16). Depending upon the specific promoters used, expression can be achieved uniformaly throughout the whole plant or can be limited, e.g. to expression in plant seeds.

Plants are regarded as potentially attractive recombinant protein producers for a number of reasons, including:

- cost of plant cultivation is low;
- harvest equipment/methodologies are inexpensive and well established;
- ease of scale-up;

Table 3.16. Some proteins of potential/actual therapeutic interest that have been expressed (at laboratory level) in transgenic plants

Protein	Expressed in	Production levels achieved
Erythropoietin	Tobacco	0.003% of total soluble plant protein
Human serum albumin	Potato	0.02% of soluble leaf protein
Glucocerebrosidase	Tobacco	0.1% of leaf weight
Interferon-α	Rice	Not listed
Interferon-β	Tobacco	0.00002% of fresh weight
GM-CSF	Tobacco	250 ng/ml extract
Hirudin	Canola	1.0% of seed weight
Hepatitis B surface antigen	Tobacco	0.007% of soluble leaf protein
Antibodies/antibody fragment	Tobacco	Various

- proteins expressed in seeds are generally stable in the seed for prolonged periods of time (often years);
- plant-based systems are free of human pathogens (e.g. HIV).

However, a number of potential disadvantages are also associated with the use of plant-based expression systems, including:

- variable/low expression levels sometimes achieved;
- potential occurrence of post-translational gene silencing (a sequence-specific mRNA degradation mechanism);
- glycosylation patterns achieved differ significantly from native human protein glycosylation patterns;
- seasonal/geographical nature of plant growth.

For these reasons, as well as the fact that additional tried and tested expression systems are already available, production of recombinant therapeutic proteins in transgenic plant systems has not as yet impacted significantly on the industry.

The most likely focus of future industry interest in this area concerns the production of oral vaccines in edible plants or fruit, such as tomatoes and bananas. Animal studies have clearly shown that ingestion of transgenic plant tissue expressing recombinant sub-unit vaccines (see Chapter 10 for a discussion of sub-unit vaccines) induces the production of antigen-specific antibody responses, not only in mucosal secretions but also in the serum. The approach is elegant in that direct consumption of the plant material provides an inexpensive, efficient and technically straightforward mode of large-scale vaccine delivery, particularly in poorer world regions. However, several hurdles hindering the widespread application of this technology include:

- the immunogenicity of orally administered vaccines can vary widely;
- the stability of antigens in the digestive tract varies widely;
- the genetics of many potential systems remain poorly characterized, leading to inefficient transformation systems and low expression levels.

Insect cell-based systems

A wide range of proteins have been produced at laboratory scale in recombinant insect cell culture systems. The approach generally entails the infection of cultured insect cells with an engineered baculovirus (a viral family that naturally infects insects) carrying the gene coding for the desired protein, placed under the influence of a powerful viral promoter. Amongst the systems most commonly employed are:

- the silkworm virus *Bombyx mori* nuclear polyhedrovirus (BmNPV), in conjunction with cultured silkworm cells (i.e. *Bombyx mori* cells) or;
- the virus *Autographa californica* nuclear polyhedrovirus (AcNPV), in conjunction with cultured armyworm cells (*Spodoptera frugiperda* cells).

Baculovirus/insect cell-based systems are cited as having a number of advantages, including:

- high-level intracellular recombinant protein expression. The use of powerful viral promoters such as promoters derived from the viral polyhedrin or P10 genes can drive recombinant protein expression levels to 30–50% of total intracellular protein;

- insect cells can be cultured more rapidly and using less expensive media than mammalian cell lines;
- human pathogens (e.g. HIV) do not generally infect insect cell lines.

However, a number of disadvantages are also associated with this production system, including:

- targeted extracellular recombinant production generally results in low-level extracellular accumulation of the desired protein (often in the mg/l range). Extracellular production simplifies subsequent downstream processing, as discussed later in this chapter;
- post-translational modifications, in particular glycosylation patterns, can be incomplete and/ or can differ very significantly from the patterns associated with native human glycoproteins.

Therapeutic proteins successfully produced on a laboratory scale in insect cell lines include hepatitis B surface antigen, interferon-γ and tissue plasminogen activator (tPA). To date, no therapeutic product produced by such means has been approved for human use. Two veterinary vaccines, however, have; 'Bayovac CSF E2' and 'Porcilis Pesti' are both subunit vaccines (Chapter 10) containing the E2 surface antigen protein of classical swine fever virus as active ingredient. The vaccines are administered to pigs in order to immunize against classical swine fever and an overview of their manufacture is provided in Figure 3.9.

An alternative insect cell-based system used to achieve recombinant protein production entails the use of live insects. Most commonly, live caterpillars or silkworms are injected with the engineered baculovirus vector, effectively turning the whole insect into a live bioreactor. One veterinary biopharmaceutical, Vibragen Omega, is manufactured using this approach and an overview of its manufacture is outlined in Figure 3.10. Briefly, whole live silkworms are introduced into pre-sterilized cabinets and reared on laboratory media. After 2 days, each silkworm is innoculated with engineered virus, using an automatic microdispenser. This engineered silkworm polyhedrosis virus harbours a copy of cDNA coding for feline interferon-ω. During the subsequent 5 days of rearing, a viral infection is established and hence recombinant protein synthesis occurs within the silkworms. After acid extraction, neutralization and clarification, the recombinant product is purified chromatographically. A two-step affinity procedure using blue sepharose dye affinity and copper chelate sepharose chromatography is employed (see later in this chapter). After a gel-filtration step, excipients (sorbitol and gelatin) are added and the product is freeze-dried after filling into glass vials.

PRODUCTION OF FINAL PRODUCT

This section briefly overviews how biopharmaceutical substances are produced in a biopharmaceutical/biotech manufacturing facility. As the vast bulk of biopharmaceuticals are proteins synthesized in recombinant prokaryotic (e.g. *E. coli*) or eukaryotic (e.g. mammalian cells) production systems, attention will focus specifically upon these.

As defined in this text, the production process is deemed to commence when a single vial of the working cell bank system (see later) is taken from storage, and the cells therein cultured in order to initiate the biosynthesis of a batch of product (Figure 3.11). The production process is deemed to be complete only when the final product is filled in its final containers and those containers have been labelled and placed in their final product packaging.

Production can be divided into 'upstream' and 'downstream' processing (Figure 3.11). Upstream processing refers to the initial fermentation process, which results in the initial generation of product. Downstream processing refers to the actual purification of the protein

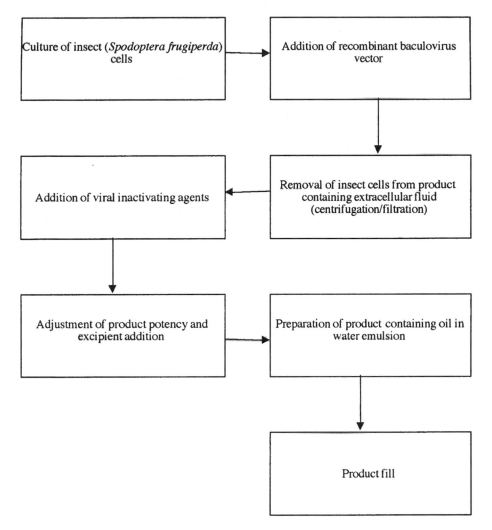

Figure 3.9. Generalized overview of the industrial-scale manufacture of recombinant E2 classical swine fever-based vaccine, using insect cell culture production systems. Clean (uninfected) cells are initially cultured in 500–1000 litre bioreactors for several days, followed by viral addition. Upon product recovery, viral inactivating agents such as β-propiolactone or 2-bromoethyl-iminebromide are added in order to destroy any free viral particles in the product stream. No chromatographic purification is generally undertaken as the product is substantially pure; the cell culture media is protein-free and the recombinant product is the only protein exported in any quantity by the producer cells. Excipients added can include liquid paraffin and polysorbate 80 (required to generate an emulsion). Thiomersal may also be added as a preservative. The final product generally displays a shelf-life of 18 months when stored refrigerated

product and generation of finished product format (i.e. filling into its final product containers, freeze-drying if a dried product format is required), followed by sealing of the final product containers. Subsequent labelling and packaging steps represent the very final steps of finished product manufacture.

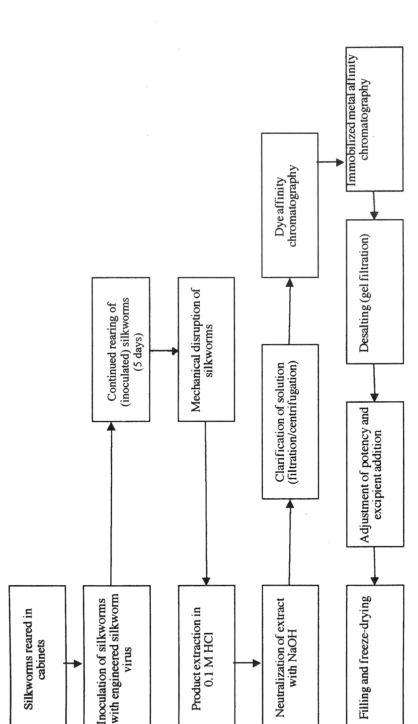

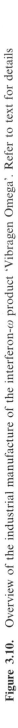

Figure 3.10.   Overview of the industrial manufacture of the interferon-ω product 'Vibragen Omega'. Refer to text for details

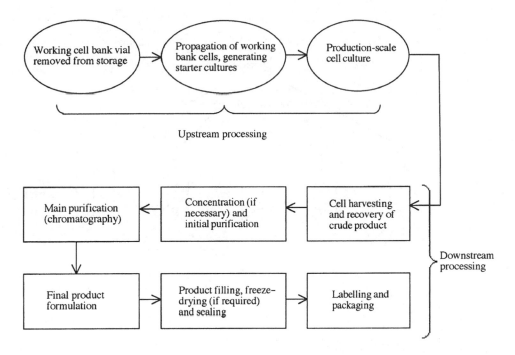

Figure 3.11. Overview of the production process for a biopharmaceutical product. Refer to text for specific details

Cell banking systems

Recombinant biopharmaceutical production cell lines are most often initially constructed by the introduction into these cells of a plasmid housing a nucleotide sequence coding for the protein of interest. After culture, the resultant product-producing cell line is generally aliquoted into small amounts, which are placed in ampoules and subsequently immersed in liquid nitrogen. The content of all the ampoules is therefore identical, and the cells are effectively preserved for indefinite periods when stored under liquid nitrogen. This batch of cryopreserved ampoules form a 'cell bank' system, whereby one ampoule is thawed and the cells therein cultured in order to seed, for example, a single production run. This concept is applied to both prokaryotic and eukaryotic biopharmaceutical-producing cells.

The cell bank's construction design is normally two-tiered, consisting of a 'master cell bank' and a 'working cell bank' (Figure 3.12). The master cell bank is constructed first, directly from a culture of the newly constructed production cell line. It can consist of several hundred individually stored ampoules. These ampoules are not used to directly seed a production batch. Instead, they are used, as required, to generate a working cell bank. The generation of a single working cell bank normally entails thawing a single master cell bank ampoule, culturing of the cells therein, with their subsequent aliquoting into multiple ampoules. These ampoules are then cryopreserved and form the working cell bank. When a single batch of new product is required, one ampoule from the working cell bank is thawed and used to seed that batch. When all the

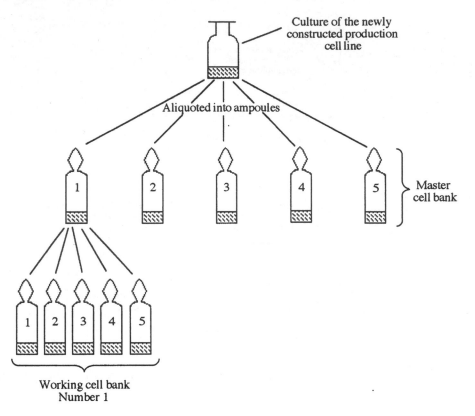

Figure 3.12. The master cell bank/working cell bank system. For simplicity each bank shown above contains only five ampoules. In reality, each bank would likely consist of several hundred ampoules. Working cell bank number 2 will be generated from master cell bank vial number 2 only when working cell bank number 1 is exhausted, and so on

vials composing the first working cell bank are exhausted, a second vial of the master cell bank is used to generate a second working cell bank, and so on.

The rationale behind this master cell bank/working cell bank system is to ensure an essentially indefinite supply of the originally developed production cells for manufacturing purposes. This is more easily understood by example. If only a single-tier cell-bank system existed, containing 250 ampoules, and 10 ampoules were used per year to manufacture 10 batches of product, the cell bank would be exhausted after 25 years. However, if a two-tier system exists, where a single master cell bank ampoule is expanded as required, to generate a further 250 ampoule working cell bank, the entire master cell bank would not be exhausted for 6250 years.

Upstream processing

The upstream processing element of the manufacture of a batch of biopharmaceutical product begins with the removal of a single ampoule of the working cell bank. This vial is used to inoculate a small volume of sterile growth medium, with subsequent incubation under

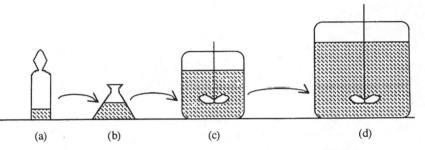

Figure 3.13.   Outline of the upstream processing stages involved in the production of a single batch of product. Initially, the contents of a single ampoule of the working cell bank (a) is used to inoculate a few hundred ml of medium (b). After growth, this lab-scale starter culture is used to inoculate several litres/tens of litres of medium present in a small bioreactor (c). This production scale starter culture is used to inoculate the production-scale bioreactor (d), which often contains several thousands/tens of thousands litres of medium. This process is equally applicable to prokaryotic or eukaryotic-based producer cell lines, although the bioreactor design, conditions of growth, etc. will differ in these two instances

appropriate conditions. This describes the growth of lab-scale starter cultures of the producer cell line. This starter culture is in turn used to inoculate a production-scale starter culture, which is used to inoculate the production-scale bioreactor (Figure 3.13). The medium composition and fermentation conditions required to promote optimal cell growth/product production will have been established during initial product development, and routine batch production is a highly repetitive, highly automated process. Bioreactors are generally manufactured from high-grade stainless steel, and can vary in size from a few tens of litres to several tens of thousands of litres (Figure 3.14). At the end of the production-scale fermentation process, the crude product is harvested, which signals commencement of downstream processing.

Microbial cell fermentation

Over half of all biopharmacuticals thus far approved are produced in recombinant *E. coli* or *S. cerevisiae*. Industrial-scale bacterial and yeast fermentation systems share many common features, an overview of which is provided below. Most remaining biopharmaceuticals are produced using animal cell culture, mainly by recombinant BHK or CHO cells (or hybridoma cells in the case of some monoclonal antibodies; Appendix 1). While industrial-scale animal cell culture shares many common principles with microbial fermentation systems, it also differs in several respects, as subsequently described. Microbial fermentation/animal cell culture is a vast speciality area in its own right. As such, only a summary overview can be provided below and the interested reader is referred to the Further Reading section.

Microbial cell fermentation has a long history of use in the production of various biological products of commercial significance (Table 3.17). As a result, a wealth of technical data and experience has accumulated in the area. A generalized microbial fermenter design is presented in Figure 3.15. The impeller, driven by an external motor, serves to ensure even distribution of nutrients and cells in the tank. The baffles (stainless steel plates attached to the side walls) serve to enhance impeller mixing by preventing vortex formation. Various ports are also present through which probes are inserted which monitor pH, temperature and sometimes the concentration of a critical metabolite (e.g. the carbon source). Additional ports serve to

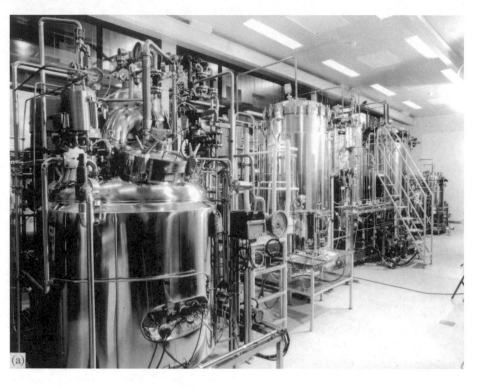

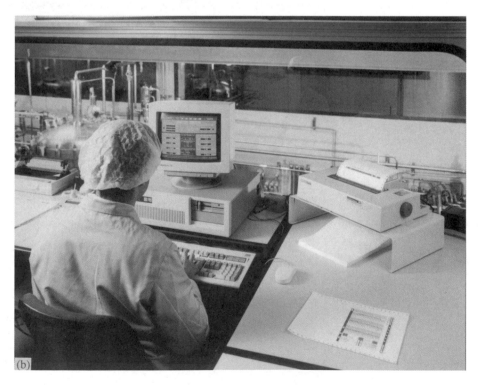

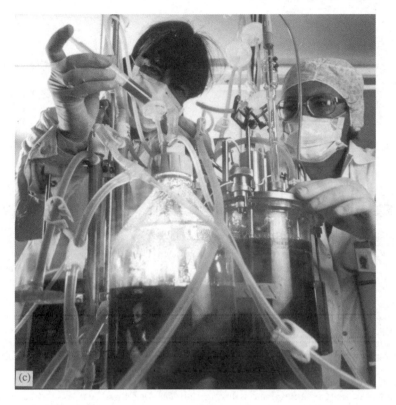

Figure 3.14. (a) Typical industrial-scale fermentation equipment as employed in the biopharmaceutical sector. (b) Control of the fermentation process is highly automated, with all fermentation parameters being adjusted by computer. (b). Photos (a) and (b) courtesy of SmithKline Beecham Biological Services, s.a., Belgium. Photo (c) illustrates the inoculation of a lab-scale fermenter with recombinant microorganisms used in the production of a commercial interferon preparation. Photo (c) courtesy of Pall Life Sciences, Ireland

facilitate addition of acid/base (pH adjustment) or, if required, addition of nutrients during the fermentation process.

Typically, the manufacture of a batch of biopharmaceutical product entails filling the production vessel with the appropriate quantity of WFI. Heat-stable nutrients required for producer cell growth are then added and the resultant media is sterilized *in situ*. This can be achieved by heat and many fermenters have inbuilt heating elements or, alternatively, outer jackets (see also Figure 3.4) through which steam can be passed in order to heat the vessel contents. Heat-labile ingredients can be sterilized by filtration and added to the fermenter after the heat step. Media composition can vary from simple defined media (usually glucose and some mineral salts) to more complex media, using yeast extract and peptone. Choice of media depends upon factors such as:

- exact nutrient requirements of producer cell line to maximize cell growth and product production;
- economics (total media cost);
- extracellular or intracellular nature of product. If the biopharmaceutical is an extracellular

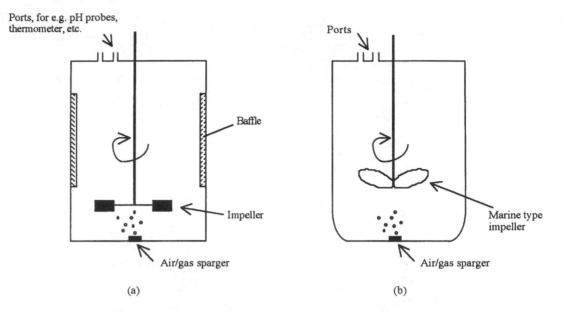

Figure 3.15.   Design of a generalized microbial cell fermentation vessel (a) and an animal cell bioreactor (b). Animal cell bioreactors display several structural differences as compared to microbial fermentation vessels. Note in particular (i) the use of a marine-type impeller (some animal cell bioreactors—air lift fermenters—are devoid of impellers, and use sparging of air-gas as the only means of media agitation); (ii) the absence of baffles and; (iii) curved internal surfaces at the bioreactor base. These modifications aim to minimize damage to the fragile animal cells during culture. Note that various additional bioreactor configurations are also commercially available. Reprinted by permission of John Wiley & Sons Ltd from Walsh (2002)

Table 3.17.   Various products (non-biopharmaceutical) of commercial significance manufactured industrially using microbial fermentation systems

Product type	Example	Example producer
Simple organic molecules	Ethanol	*Saccharomyces cerevisiae Pachysolen tannophilus*, some *Clostridium* spp.
	Butanol	*Clostridium acetobutylicum, C. saccharoacetobutylicum*
	Acetone	*Clostridium acetobutylicum, C. saccharoacetobutylicum*
	Acetic acid	Various acetic acid bacteria
	Lactic acid	*Lactobacillus* spp.
Amino acids	Lysine	*Corynebacterium glutamicum*
	Glutamic acid	*Corynebacterium glutamicum*
Enzymes	Proteases	Various Bacilli, e.g. *Bacillus licheniformis*
	Amylases	*Bacillus subtilis, Aspergillus oryzae*
	Cellulases	*Trichoderma viride, Penicillium pinophilum*
Antibiotics	Penicillin	*Penicillium chrysogenum*
	Bacitracin	*Bacillus licheniformis*

product, then the less complex the media composition, the better in order to render subsequent product purification as straightforward as possible.

Fermentation follows for several days subsequent to inoculation with the production-scale starter culture (Figure 3.13). During this process, biomass (i.e. cell mass) accumulates. In most cases, product accumulates intracellulary and the cells are harvested when maximum biomass yields are achieved. This 'feed batch' approach is the one normally taken during biopharmaceutical manufacture, although reactors can also be operated on a continuous basis, where fresh nutrient media is continually added and a fraction of the media/biomass continually removed and processed. During fermentation, air (sterilized by filtration) is sparged into the tank to supply oxygen and the fermenter is also operated at a temperature appropriate to optimal cell growth (usually between 25–37°C, depending upon the producer cell type). In order to maintain this temperature, cooling rather than heating is required in some cases. Large-scale fermentations, in which cells grow rapidly and to a high cell density, can generate considerable heat due to (a) microbial metabolism and (b) mechanical activity, e.g. stirring. Cooling is achieved by passing the coolant (cold water or glycol) through a circulating system associated with the vessel jacket or sometimes via internal vessel coils.

Mammalian cell culture systems

Mammalian cell culture is more technically complex and more expensive than microbial cell fermentation. It is, therefore, usually only used in the manufacture of therapeutic proteins that show extensive and essential post-translational modifications. In practice, this usually refers to glycosylation and the use of animal cell culture would be appropriate where the carbohydrate content and pattern is essential either to the protein's biological activity, stability or serum half-life. Therapeutic proteins falling into this category include erythropoietin (Chapter 6), the gonadotrophins (Chapter 8), some cytokines (Chapters 4–7) and intact monoclonal antibodies (Chapter 10).

The culture of animal cells differs from that of microbial cells in several generalized respects, including:

- they require more complex media;
- extended duration of fermentation due to slow growth of animal cells;
- they are more fragile than microbial cells due to the absence of an outer cell wall.

Basic animal cell culture media generally contains:

- most L-amino acids;
- many/most vitamins;
- salts (e.g. NaCl, KCl, $CaCl_2$);
- carbon source (often glucose);
- antibiotics (e.g. penicillin or streptomycin);
- supplemental serum;
- buffering agent (often CO_2-based).

Antibiotics are required to prevent microbial growth consequent to accidental microbial contamination. Supplemental serum (often bovine or fetal calf serum, or synthetic serum composed of a mixture of growth factors, hormones and metabolites typically found in serum) is required as a source of the often ill-defined growth factors required by some animal cell lines.

The media constituents, several of which are heat-labile, are generally dissolved in WFI and filter-sterilized into the pre-sterile animal cell reactor. Reactor design (and operation) differs somewhat from microbial fermentations, mainly with a view to minimizing damage to the more fragile cells during cell culture (Figure 3.15). Although the generalized reactor design presented in Figure 3.15 is commonly employed on industrial scale, alternative reactor configurations are also available. These include hollow-fibre systems as well as the classical roller-bottle systems. Roller bottles are still used in the industrial production of some vaccines, erythropoietin and growth hormone-based products. Roller bottles are cylindrical bottles which are partially filled with media, placed on their sides and mechanically rolled during cell culture. This system is gentle on the cells and the rolling action ensures homogeneity in the culture media and efficient oxygen transfer. The major disadvantage associated with applying roller-bottle technology on an industrial scale is that many thousands of bottles are required to produce a single batch of product.

Different animal cell types display different properties pertinent to their successful culture. Those used to manufacture biopharmaceuticals are invariably continuous (transformed) cell lines. Such cells will grow relatively vigorously and easily in submerged culture systems, be they roller bottle- or bioreactor-based.

Unlike transformed cell lines, non-continuous cell lines generally:

- *display anchorage dependence* (i.e. will only grow and divide when attached to a solid substratum; continuous cell lines will grow in free suspension);
- *grow as a monolayer*;
- *exhibit contact inhibition* (physical contact between individual cells inhibits further division);
- *display a finite lifespan*, i.e. die, generally after 50–100 cell divisions, even when cultured under ideal conditions;
- *display longer population doubling times* and grow to lower cell densities when compared to continuous cell lines;
- *usually have more complex media requirements*.

Many of these properties would obviously limit applicability of non-continuous cell lines in the industrial-scale production of recombinant proteins. However, such cell types are routinely cultured for research purposes, toxicity testing, etc.

The anchorage-dependent growth properties of such non-continuous cell lines impacts upon how they are cultured, both at lab and industrial scale. If grown in roller bottles/other low-volume containers, cells grow attached to the internal walls of the vessel. Large-scale culture can be undertaken in submerged-type vessels, such as that described in Figure 3.15(b) in conjunction with the use of microcarrier beads. Microcarriers are solid or sometimes porous spherical particles approximately $200\,\mu\mathrm{m}$ in diameter, manufactured from such materials as collagen, dextran or plastic. They display densities slightly greater than water, such that gentle mixing within the animal cell bioreactor is sufficient to maintain the beads in suspension and evenly distributed throughout the media. Anchorage-dependent cells can attach to, and grow on, the beads' outer surfaces/outer pores.

Downstream processing

An overview of the steps normally undertaken during downstream processing is presented in Figure 3.16. Details of the exact steps undertaken during the downstream processing of any specific biopharmaceutical product are usually considered highly confidential by the

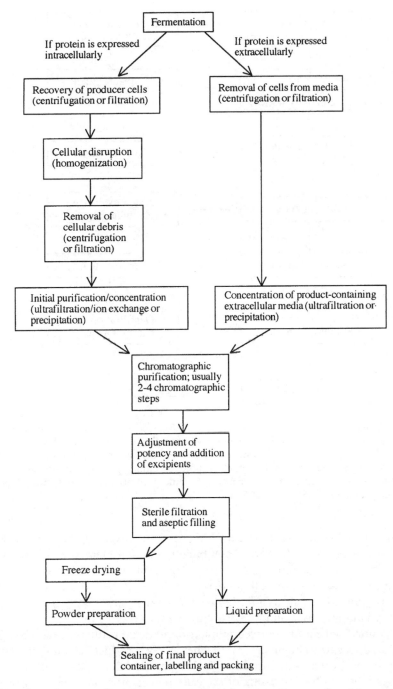

Figure 3.16. Overview of a generalized downstream processing procedure employed to produce a finished product (protein) biopharmaceutical. Quality control also plays a prominent role in downstream processing. QC personnel collect product samples during/after each stage of processing. These samples are analysed to ensure that various in-process specifications are met. In this way, the production process is tightly controlled at each stage

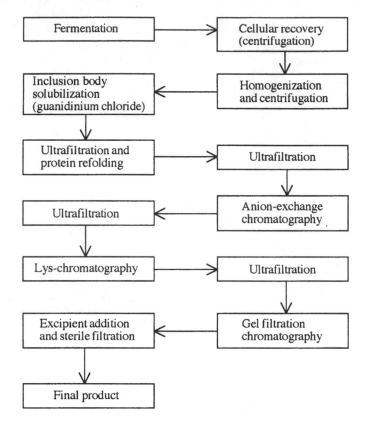

Figure 3.17. A likely purification procedure for tPA produced in recombinant *E. coli* cells. The heterologous product accumulates intracellularly in the form of inclusion bodies. In this particular procedure, an ultrafiltration step is introduced on several occasions to concentrate the product stream, particularly prior to application to chromatographic columns. Lysine affinity chromatography (Lys-chromatography) is employed as tPA is known to bind immobilized lysine molecules. Adapted with permission from Datar *et al.* (1993)

manufacturer. Such details are thus rarely made generally available. However, a potential downstream processing procedure for recombinant tPA is presented in Figure 3.17, and other examples are provided at various stages through the remainder of this text.

Downstream processing is normally undertaken under clean room conditions, with the final steps (e.g. sterile filtration and aseptic filling into final product containers) being undertaken under Grade A laminar flow conditions (Figure 3.18).

In general, animal cell culture-derived biopharmaceutical products are secreted into the media (i.e. are produced as extracellular proteins), whereas the product accumulates intracellularly in many recombinant prokaryotic producer cell types. In the case of intracellular proteins, fermentation is followed by harvesting of the cells. This is normally achieved by centrifugation (Figure 3.19) or sometimes filtration. Recovery of cells is followed by their disruption in order to release their intracellular contents, including the protein of interest. A variety of means may be used to disrupt cells. Amongst the most popular microbial cell disrupters are homogenizers. During homogenization, a suspension of cells is forced under high pressure through an orifice of

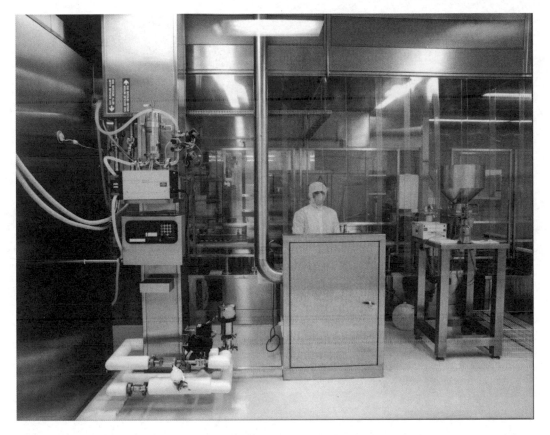

Figure 3.18. Photograph illustrating a typical pharmaceutical clean room and some of the equipment usually therein. Note the presence of a curtain of (transparent) heavy-gauge polyethylene strips (most noticeable directly in front of the operator). These strips box off a grade A laminar flow work station. Product filling into final product containers is undertaken within the grade A zone. The filling process is highly automated, requiring no direct contact between the operator and the product. This minimizes the chances of accidental product contamination by production personnel. Photo courtesy of SmithKline Beecham Biological Services s.a., Belgium

narrow internal diameter. This generates high shear forces. As the cells emerge from the outlet point, they also experience an instantaneous drop in pressure, to normal atmospheric pressure. The combination of high shear forces and drop in pressure serves to rupture most microbial cells with relative ease. Additional disruption methods include agitation in the presence of abrasives, such as glass beads.

After cellular disruption, the cell debris is generally removed by centrifugation, leaving behind a dilute solution of crude (unpurified) protein product. If the producer cell secretes the product, the initial stages of downstream processing are less complex. After fermentation, the cells are removed by centrifugation or filtration, leaving behind the product-containing fermentation media.

The next phase of downstream processing usually entails concentration of the crude protein product. This yields smaller product volumes, which are more convenient to work with and can subsequently be processed with greater speed. Concentration may be achieved by inducing

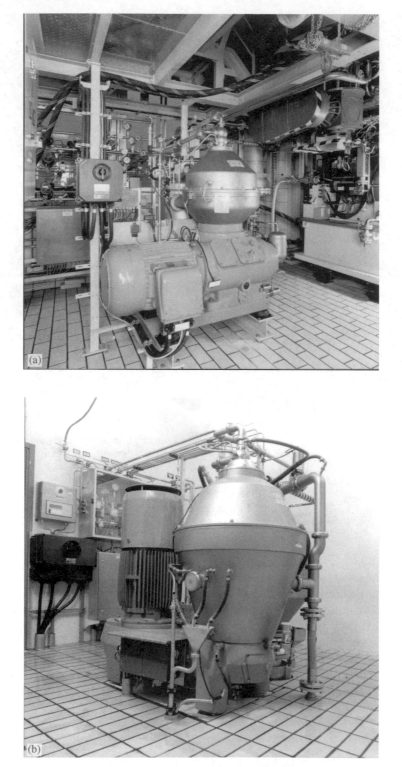

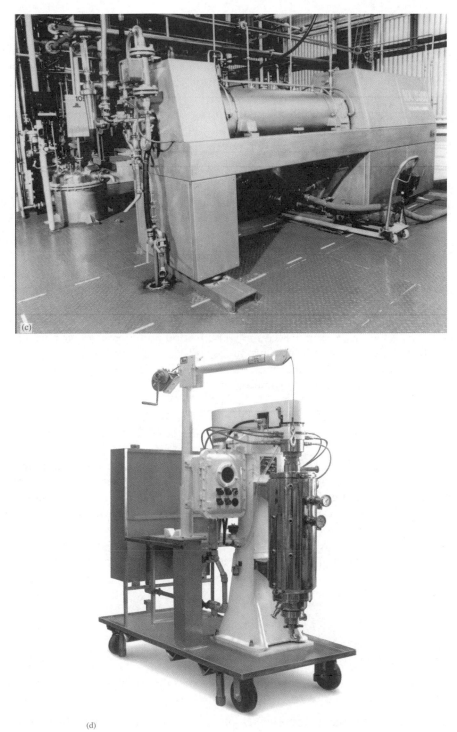

Figure 3.19. (a–d) Photographic representation of various industrial-scale centrifuges. Photos courtesy of Alfa Laval Separation AB, Sweden

product precipitation using, for example, salts such as ammonium sulphate or solvents such as ethanol. However, ultrafiltration is the more usual method employed (Figure 3.20).

Ultrafiltration membranes are usually manufactured from tough plastic-based polymers, such as polyvinyl chloride or polycarbonate. A range of membranes are available which display different cut-off points (Figure 3.20). Membranes displaying cut-off points of 3, 10, 30, 50 and 100 kDa are most commonly used. Thus, if the protein of interest displays a molecular mass of 70 kDa, it may be concentrated effectively by using an ultrafilter membrane displaying a molecular mass cut-off point of 50 kDa. Ultrafiltration is a popular method of concentration because:

- high product recovery rates may be attained (typically of the order of 99%);
- processing times are rapid;
- process-scale ultrafiltration equipment is readily available, and running costs are relatively modest.

After concentration, high-resolution chromatographic purification is usually undertaken. A variety of different chromatographic techniques are available, which separate proteins from each other on the basis of differences in various physiochemical characteristics (Table 3.18.) Detailed description of the theory and practice underlining these systems go far beyond the scope of this text, and are freely available in the scientific literature.

In general, a combination of two to four different chromatographic techniques are employed in a typical downstream processing procedure. Gel filtration and ion exchange chromatography are amongst the most common. Affinity chromatography is employed wherever possible, as its high biospecificity facilitates the achievement of a very high degree of purification. Examples include the use of immunoaffinity chromatography to purify blood factor VIII and lysine affinity chromatography to purify tPA. A selection of affinity systems are presented in Table 3.19. In addition to separation of contaminant proteins from the protein of interest, most such high-resolution chromatographic steps will also facilitate the removal of non-proteinaceous contaminants, as discussed later.

As with most aspects of downstream processing, the operation of chromatographic systems is highly automated and is usually computer-controlled. While medium-sized process-scale chromatographic columns (e.g. 5–15 litres) are manufactured from toughened glass or plastic, larger processing columns are available that are manufactured from stainless steel. Process-scale chromatographic separation is generally undertaken under low pressure, but production-scale high-pressure systems (e.g. process-scale high pressure liquid chromatography (HPLC)) are sometimes used, as long as the protein product is not adversely affected by the high pressure experienced. A HPLC-based 'polishing step' is sometimes employed, e.g. during the production of highly purified insulin preparations.

Final product formulation

High-resolution chromatography normally yields a protein that is 98–99% pure. The next phase of downstream processing entails formulation into final product format. This generally involves:

- addition of various excipients (substances other than the active ingredient(s) which, for example, stabilize the final product or enhance the characteristics of the final product in some other way);

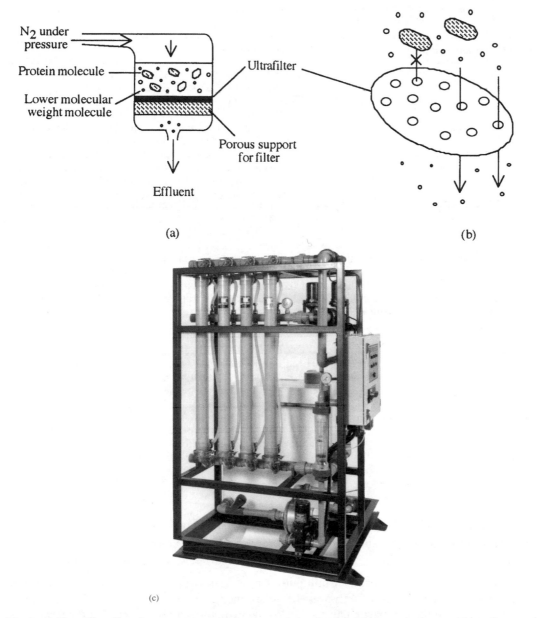

(a)

(b)

(c)

Figure 3.20. Ultrafiltration separates molecules on the basis of size and shape. (a) a diagramatic representation of a typical laboratory-scale ultrafiltration system. The sample (e.g. crude protein solution) is placed in the ultrafiltration chamber, where it sits directly above the ultrafilter membrane. The membrane in turn sits on a macroporous support which provides it with mechanical strength. Pressure is then applied (usually in the form of an inert gas), as shown. Molecules larger than the pore diameter (e.g. large proteins) are retained on the upstream side of the ultrafilter membrane. However, smaller molecules — particularly water molecules — are easily forced through the pores, thus effectively concentrating the protein solution [see also (b)]. Membranes can be manufactured that display different pore sizes, i.e. have different molecular mass cut-off points. (c) An industrial-scale ultrafiltration system. Photo courtesy of Elga Ltd, UK

Table 3.18. Various chromatographic techniques that may be used to separate proteins from each other. The basis upon which separation is achieved is also listed

Chromatographic technique	Basis of separation
Ion-exchange	Differences in protein surface charge at a given pH
Gel-filtration	Differences in size/shape of different proteins
Hydrophobic interaction chromatography (HIC)	Differences in the size and extent of hydrophobic patches on the surface of proteins
Affinity chromatography	Ability of a protein to bind in a bio-specific (selective) manner to a chosen immobilized ligand
Metal chelate chromatography	Ability of certain proteins to complex with zinc and copper
Hydroxyapatite chromatography	Mechanism not fully understood. Involves ability of some proteins to bind to calcium and phosphate ions on the surface of hydroxyapatite crystals

Table 3.19. Some forms of affinity chromatography that may be employed to purify a selected protein. Virtually all proteins carry out their biological effects by interacting in some way with other molecules, which can be given the general title 'ligands'. This interaction is often quite biospecific. Immobilization of such ligands (or molecules which mimic ligands) onto chromatographic beads thus facilitates selective purification of the molecule of interest

Affinity system	Application
Protein A chromatography	Protein A, produced by *Staphylococcus aureus*, binds IgG. It is used extensively in antibody purification protocols
Lectin affinity chromatography	Lectins are a group of proteins capable of binding carbohydrates. Lectin affinity chromatography may be used to purify glycoproteins
Immunoaffinity chromatography	Immobilized antibodies may be used as affinity absorbants for the antigen that stimulated their production (e.g. purification of factor VIII using immobilized anti-factor VIII antibodies)
Dye affinity chromatography	Purification of proteins that display ability to interact tightly with selected dyes

- filtration of the final product through a 0.22 μm absolute filter in order to generate sterile product, followed by its aseptic filling into final product containers;
- freeze-drying (lyophilization) if the product is to be marketed in a powdered format.

The decision to market the product in liquid or powder form is often dictated by how stable the protein is in solution. This in turn must be determined experimentally, as there is no way to predict the outcome for any particular protein. Some proteins may remain stable for months or even years in solution, particularly if stabilizing excipients are added and the solution is refrigerated. Other proteins, particularly when purified, may retain biological activity for only a matter of hours or days when in aqueous solution.

Some influences that can alter the biological activity of proteins

A number of different influences can denature or otherwise modify proteins, rendering them less active/inactive. As all protein products are marketed on an activity basis, every precaution must

Table 3.20. The various molecular alterations that usually result in loss of a protein's biological activity

---

Non-covalent alterations
   Partial/complete protein denaturation
Covalent alterations
  Hydrolysis
  Deamidation
  Imine formation
  Racemization
  Oxidation
  Disulphide exchange
  Isomerization
  Photodecomposition

---

be taken to minimize loss of biological activity during downstream processing and subsequent storage. Disruptive influences can be chemical (e.g. oxidizing agents, detergents, etc.), physical (e.g. extremes of pH, elevated temperature, vigorous agitation) or biological (e.g. proteolytic degradation). Minimization of inactivation can be achieved by minimizing the exposure of the product stream to such influences, and undertaking downstream processing in as short a time as possible. In addition, it is possible to protect the protein from many of these influences by the addition of suitable stabilizing agents. The addition of such agents to the final product is often essential in order to confer upon the product an acceptably long shelf-life. During initial development, considerable empirical study is undertaken by the formulators to determine what excipients are most effective in enhancing a product's stability. Detailed treatment of the topic of protein stability and stabilizers is in itself worthy of a complete book. Only a summary overview is provided below and the interested reader is referred to the Further Reading section at the end of this chapter.

A number of different molecular mechanisms can underpin the loss of biological activity of any protein. These include both covalent and non-covalent modification of the protein molecule, as summarized in Table 3.20. Protein denaturation, for example, entails a partial or complete alteration of the protein's 3-D shape. This is underlined by the disruption of the intramolecular forces that stabilize a protein's native conformation, viz hydrogen bonding, ionic attractions and hydrophobic interactions. Covalent modifications of protein structure that can adversely effect its biological activity are summarized below.

Proteolytic degradation

Proteolytic degradation of a protein is characterized by hydrolysis of one or more peptide (amide) bonds in the protein backbone, generally resulting in loss of biological activity. Hydrolysis is usually promoted by the presence of trace quantities of proteolytic enzymes, but can also be caused by some chemical influences.

Proteases belong to one of six mechanistic classes:

- serine proteases I (mammalian) or II (bacterial);
- cysteine proteases;
- aspartic proteases;
- metalloproteases I (mammalian) and II (bacterial).

Table 3.21. Some of the most commonly employed protease inhibitions and the specific classes of proteases they inhibit

Inhibitor	Protease class inhibited
PMSF	Serine proteases, some cysteine proteases
Benzamidine	Serine proteases
Pepstatin A	Aspartic proteases
EDTA	Metallo-proteases

PMSF = Phenylmethylsulphonyl fluoride.   EDTA = Ethylenediaminetetra-acetic acid

The classes are differentiated on the basis of groups present at the protease active site known to be essential for activity; e.g. a serine residue forms an essential component of the active site of serine proteases. Both exo-proteases (catalysing the sequential cleavage of peptide bonds beginning at one end of the protein) and endo-proteases (cleaving internal peptide bonds, generating peptide fragments) exist. Even limited endo- or exo-proteolytic degradation of biopharmaceuticals usually alters/destroys their biological activity.

Proteins differ greatly in their intrinsic susceptibility to proteolytic attack. Resistance to proteolysis seems to be dependent upon higher levels of protein structure (i.e. secondary and tertiary structure), as tight packing often shields susceptible peptide bonds from attack. Denaturation thus renders proteins very susceptible to proteolytic degradation.

A number of strategies may be adopted in order to minimize the likelihood of proteolytic degradation of the protein product, these include:

- minimizing processing times;
- processing at low temperatures;
- use of specific protease inhibitors.

Minimizing processing times obviously limits the time during which proteases may come into direct contact with the protein product. Processing at low temperatures (often 4°C) reduces the rate of proteolytic activity. Inclusion of specific proteolytic inhibitors in processing buffers, in particular homogenization buffers, can be very effective in preventing uncontrolled proteolysis. While no one inhibitor will inhibit proteases of all mechanistic classes, a number of effective inhibitors for specific classes are known (Table 3.21). The use of a cocktail of such inhibitors is thus most effective. However, the application of many such inhibitors in biopharmaceutical processing is inappropriate due to their toxicity.

In most instances, the instigation of precautionary measures protecting proteins against proteolytic degradation is of prime importance during the early stages of purification. During the later stages, most of the proteases present will have been removed from the product stream. A major aim of any purification system is the complete removal of such proteases, as the presence of even trace amounts of these catalysts can result in significant proteolytic degradation of the finished product over time.

Protein deamidation

Deamidation and imide formation can also negatively influence a protein's biological activity. Deamidation refers to the hydrolysis of the side-chain amide group of asparagine and/or

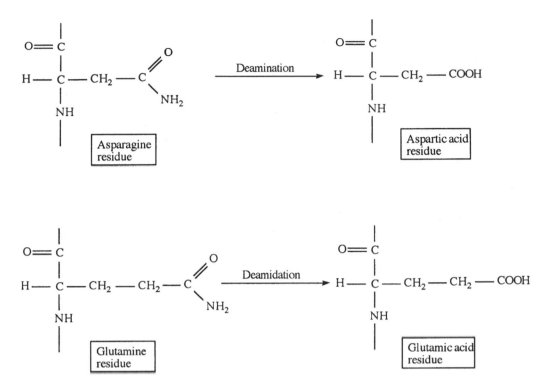

Figure 3.21. Deamidation of asparagine and glutamine, yielding aspartic acid and glutamic acids, respectively. This process can often be minimized by reducing the final product pH to 4–5

glutamine, yielding aspartic and glutamic acid, respectively (Figure 3.21). This reaction is promoted especially at elevated temperatures and extremes of pH. It represents the major route by which insulin preparations usually degrade. Imide formation occurs when the α-amino nitrogen of either asparagine, aspartic acid, glutamine or glutamic acid attacks the side-chain carbonyl group of these amino acids. The resultant structures formed are termed aspartimides or glutarimides, respectively. These cyclic imide structures are, in turn, prone to hydrolysis.

Oxidation and disulphide exchange

The side chains of a number of amino acids are susceptible to oxidation by air. Although the side chains of tyrosine, tryptophan and histidine can be oxidized, the sulphur atoms present in methionine or cysteine are by far the most susceptible. Methionine can be oxidized by air or more potent oxidants, initially forming a sulphoxide and, subsequently, a sulphone (Figure 3.22). The sulphur atom of cysteine is readily oxidized, forming either a disulphide bond or (in the presence of potent oxidizing agents) sulphonic acid (Figure 3.22). Oxidation by air normally results only in disulphide bond formation. The oxidation of any constituent amino acid residue can (potentially) drastically reduce the biological activity of a polypeptide.

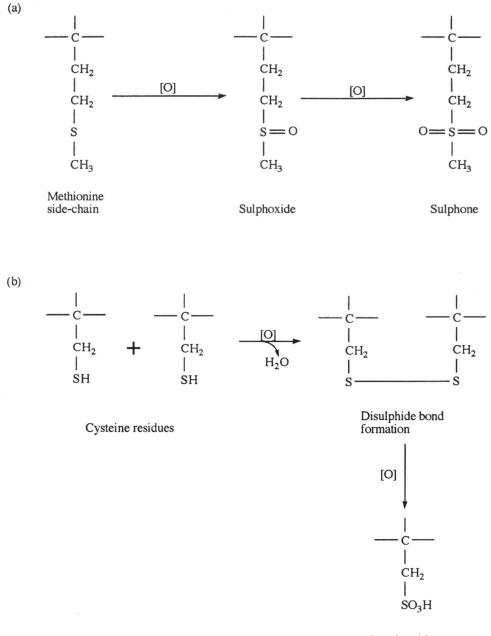

Figure 3.22. Oxidation of (a) methionine and (b) cysteine side-chains, as can occur upon exposure to air or more potent oxidizing agents (e.g. peroxide, superoxide, hydroxyl radicals or hypochlorite). Refer to text for specific details

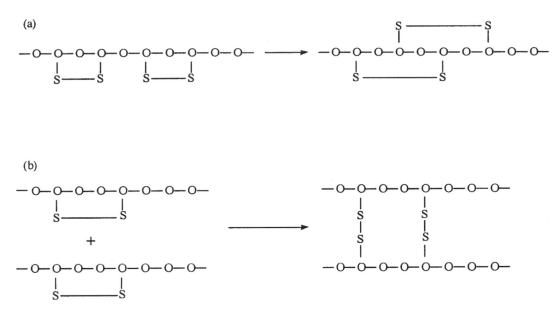

Figure 3.23. Diagram representing the molecular process of intra-chain (a) and inter-chain (b) disulphide exchange. Refer to text for specific details. (-O-=amino acid residues in polypeptide)

Oxidation of methionine is particularly favoured under conditions of low pH, and in the presence of various metal ions. Methionine residues on the surface of a protein are obviously particularly susceptible to oxidation. Those buried internally in the protein are less accessible to oxidants. Human growth hormone (hGH) contains three methionine residues (at positions 14, 125 and 170). Studies have found that oxidation of methionine 14 and 125 (the more readily accessible ones) does not greatly effect hGH activity; however, oxidation of all three methionine residues results in almost total inactivation of the molecule.

Oxidation can be best minimized by replacing the air in the head space of the final product container with an inert gas such as nitrogen, and/or the addition of antioxidants to the final product.

Disulphide exchange can also sometimes occur and prompt a reduction in biological activity (Figure 3.23). Intermolecular disulphide exchange can result in aggregation of individual polypeptide molecules.

Alteration of glycoprotein glycosylation patterns

Many proteins of therapeutic value are glycoproteins, i.e. display one or more oligosaccharide chains covalently attached to the polypeptide backbone. Examples of such proteins include immunoglobulins, blood clotting factors, α_1-antitrypsin and some interferons. Analysis of the carbohydrate composition of glycoproteins reveals the presence of a variety sugars, including D-galactose, D-mannose and L-fucose (neutral sugars), the amino-sugars; N-acetylglucosamine

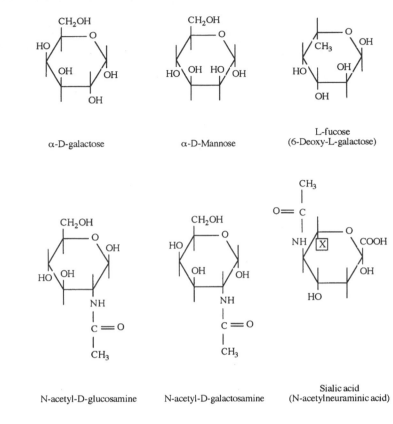

Figure 3.24. Monosaccharides that commonly constitute the carbohydrate portion of glycoproteins. Refer to text for details. Note that individual hydrogen atoms attached to the core ring structure are omitted for clarity of presentation

and *N*-acetylgalactosamine, and acidic sugars (e.g. sialic acid) (Figure 3.24). These sugar chains are attached to the protein backbone via two common covalent bond types (Figure 3.25):

1. *O*-glycosidic linkages, in which the sugar side chain is attached via the hydroxyl group of serine or threonine, or sometimes modified amino acids such as hydroxylysine.
2. *N*-glycosidic linkages, in which attachment is via the amino group of asparagine (rarely, attachment via an *S*-glycosidic linkage involving cysteine residues can also occur).

Carbohydrate side chains are synthesized by a family of enzymes known as glycosyltransferases. For any glycoprotein, the exact composition and structure of the carbohydrate side-

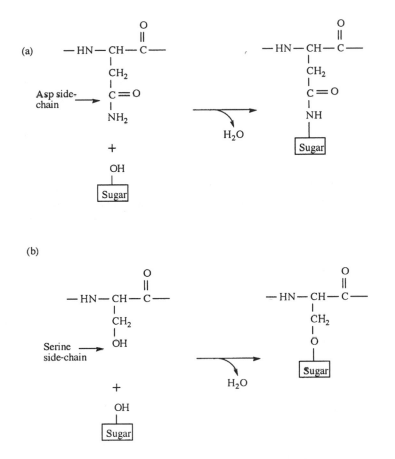

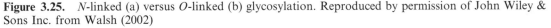

Figure 3.25. *N*-linked (a) versus *O*-linked (b) glycosylation. Reproduced by permission of John Wiley & Sons Inc. from Walsh (2002)

chain can vary slightly from one molecule of that glycoprotein to the next. This results in micro-heterogeneity, which can be directly visualized, e.g. by isoelectric focusing (discussed later). Virtually all therapeutic glycoproteins, even when produced naturally in the body, exhibit such heterogeneity; e.g. two species of human interferon-γ, of molecular mass 20 and 25 kDa, respectively, differ from each other only in the degree and sites of (*N*-linked) glycosylation.

The sugar chains on glycoproteins can serve a number of different functions, including:

- in some cases the carbohydrate component plays a direct role in mediating the glycoprotein's biological activity, e.g. removal (or extensive alteration) of the carbohydrate component of human chorionic gonadotrophin (hCG; Chapter 8) significantly decreases its ability to induce characteristic responses in sensitive cells. Desialylated erythropoietin (EPO; Chapter 6) also exhibits very little biological activity *in vivo*;
- the carbohydrate component may play a recognition role in some cases, e.g. sugar residues of some glycoproteins can play an essential role in processes such as lysosomal targeting and cell adhesion events;

- the carbohydrate component serves to substantially increase the solubility of several glycoproteins;
- the carbohydrate component helps regulate the biological half-life of some serum glycoproteins. It increases the serum half-life of some glycoproteins by decreasing the rate of clearance from the serum. Furthermore, modification/partial degradation (i.e. asialoglycoproteins) of the carbohydrate component can accelerate removal of the protein from the serum;
- the carbohydrate component probably exerts a direct stabilizing influence upon the conformation of many glycoproteins.

Alteration of its carbohydrate component can therefore potentially affect the biological activity of the glycoprotein, or alter its immunological properties. In practice, however, expression of many normally glycosylated proteins in *E. coli* generates a protein product whose biological characteristics are indistinguishable from the native product. Furthermore, the glycosylation patterns obtained when human glycoproteins are expressed in non-human eukaryotic expression systems (e.g. animal cell culture) are usually distinct from the glycosylation pattern associated with the native human protein. The glycosylation pattern of human tPA produced in transgenic animals, for example, is different from the pattern obtained when the same gene is expressed in a recombinant mouse cell line. Both these patterns are in turn different from the native human pattern. The tPA from all sources is, however, safe and effective. The clinical significance of altered glycosylation patterns/micro-heterogeneity is best determined by clinical trials. If the product is found to be safe and effective, then routine end-product QC analysis for carbohydrate-based micro-heterogeneity is carried out, more to determine batch-to-batch consistency (which is desirable) than to detect microheterogeneity *per se*.

Most glycoprotein biopharmaceuticals will exhibit microheterogeneity. Isoelectric focusing of typical batches of the therapeutic monoclonal antibody OKT-3 (Chapter 10) reveals at least four bands, representing four product variations that differ slightly in their carbohydrate content. Likewise, isoelectric focusing of batches of erythropoietin (40 kDa glycoprotein hormone, up to 50% of which is carbohydrate; Chapter 6) typically reveals up to six bands, which again differ only in their carbohydrate content. In any such instance, batch rejection would only be considered if strongly atypical heterogeneity was observed.

Large deviations from normal batch-to-batch glycosylation pattern is most likely caused by the presence of a glycosidase capable of enzymatic degradation of the carbohydrate side-chains. The likelihood of such eventualities may be minimized by carrying out downstream processing at low temperatures, and as quickly as possible.

Stabilizing excipients used in final product formulations

A range of various substances may be added to a purified (polypeptide) biopharmaceutical product in order to stabilize that product (Table 3.22). Such agents can stabilize proteins in a number of different ways. Specific examples include:

- *serum albumin*. Addition of serum albumin has been shown to stabilize various different polypeptides (Table 3.23). Human serum albumin (HSA) is often employed in the case of biopharmaceuticals destined for parenteral administration to humans. In many cases, it is used in combination with additional stabilizers, including amino acids (mainly glycine) and carbohydrates. Serum albumin itself is quite a stable molecule, capable of withstanding

Table 3.22. Some major excipient groups that may be added to protein-based biopharmaceuticals in order to stabilize the biological activity of the finished product

Serum albumin
Various individual amino acids
Various carbohydrates
Alcohols and polyols
Surfactants

Table 3.23. Various biopharmaceutical preparations for which human serum albumin (HSA) has been described as a potential stabilizer

α- and β-Interferons	Tissue plasminogen activator
γ-Interferon	Tumour necrosis factor
Interleukin-2	Monoclonal antibody preparations
Urokinase	γ-Globulin preparations
Erythropoietin	Hepatitis B surface antigen

conditions of low pH or elevated temperature (it is stable for over 10 h at 60°C). It also displays excellent solubility characteristics. It is postulated that albumin stabilizers exert their stabilizing influences by both direct and indirect means. Certainly, it helps decrease the level of surface adsorption of the active biopharmaceutical to the internal walls of final product containers. It also could act as an alternative target, e.g. for traces of proteases or other agents that could be deleterious to the product. It may also function to directly stabilize the native conformation of many proteins. It has been shown to be an effective cryoprotectant for several biopharmaceuticals (e.g. IL-2, tPA and various interferon preparations), helping to minimize potentially detrimental effects of the freeze-drying process on the product. However, the use of HSA is now discouraged, due to the possibility of accidental transmission of blood-borne pathogens. The use of recombinant HSA would overcome such fears.

- *Various amino acids* are also used as stabilizing agents for some biopharmaceutical products (Table 3.24). Glycine is most often employed and it (as well as other amino acids) has been found to help stabilize various interferon preparations, as well as erythropoietin, factor VIII,

Table 3.24. Amino acids, carbohydrates and polyols that have found most application as stabilizers for some biopharmaceutical preparations

Amino acids	Carbohydrates	Polyols
Glycine	Glucose	Glycerol
Alanine	Sucrose	Mannitol
Lysine	Trehalose	Sorbitol
Threonine	Maltose	Polyethylene glycol

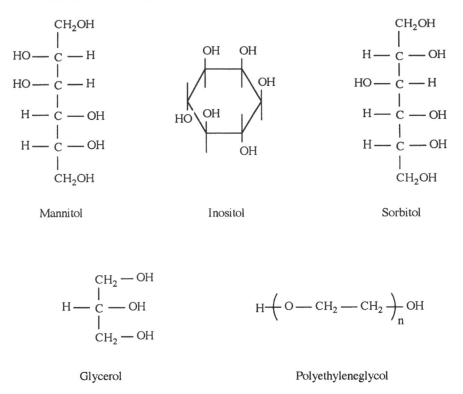

Figure 3.26.   Structure of some polyols sometimes used to stabilize proteins

urokinase and arginase. Amino acids are generally added to final product at concentrations of 0.5–5%. They appear to exert their stabilizing influence by various means, including reducing surface adsorption of product, inhibiting aggregate formation, as well as directly stabilizing the conformation of some proteins, particularly against heat denaturation. The exact molecular mechanisms by which such effects are achieved remain to be elucidated.

- *Several polyols* (i.e. molecules displaying multiple hydroxyl groups) have found application as polypeptide-stabilizing agents. Polyols include substances such as glycerol, mannitol, sorbitol and polyethylene glycol, as well as inositol (Table 3.24 and Figure 3.26). A subset of polyols are the carbohydrates, which are listed separately (and thus somewhat artificially) from polyols in Table 3.24. Various polyols have been found to directly stabilize proteins in solution, while carbohydrates in particular are also often added to biopharmaceutical products prior to freeze-drying, in order to provide physical bulk to the freeze-dried cake.

- *Surfactants* are well-known protein denaturants. However, when sufficiently dilute, some surfactants (e.g. polysorbate) exert a stabilizing influence on some protein types. Proteins display a tendency to aggregate at interfaces (air–liquid or liquid–liquid), a process which often promotes their denaturation. Addition of surfactant reduces the surface tension of aqueous solutions and often increases the solubility of proteins dissolved therein. This helps to reduce the rate of protein denaturation at interfaces. Polysorbate, for example, is included in some γ-globulin preparations and in the therapeutic monoclonal antibody, OKT-3 (Chapter 10).

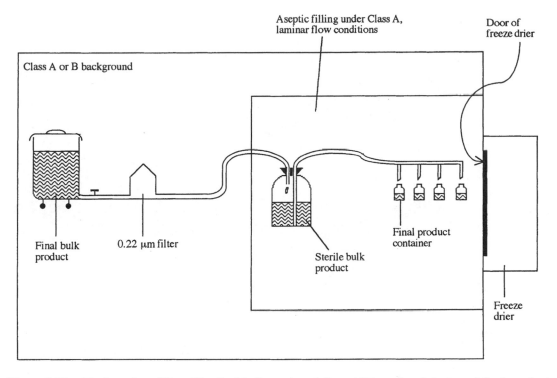

Figure 3.27. Final product filling. The final bulk product (after addition of excipients and final product QC testing) is filter sterilized by passing through a 0.22 μm filter. The sterile product is aseptically filled into (pre-sterilized) final product containers under grade A laminar flow conditions. Much of the filling operation uses highly automated filling equipment. After filling, the product container is either sealed (by an automated aseptic sealing system) or freeze-dried first, followed by sealing

Final product fill

An overview of a typical final product filling process is presented in Figure 3.27. The bulk final product firstly undergoes QC testing to ensure its compliance with bulk product specifications. While implementation of GMP during manufacturing will ensure that the product carries a low microbial load, it will not be sterile at this stage. The product is then passed through a (sterilizing) 0.22 μm filter, Figure 3.28. The sterile product is housed (temporarily) in a sterile product-holding tank, from where it is aseptically filled into pre-sterilized final product containers (usually glass vials). The filling process normally employs highly automated liquid filling systems. All items of equipment, pipework, etc. with which the sterilized product comes into direct contact must obviously themselves be sterile. Most such equipment items may be sterilized by autoclaving, and be aseptically assembled prior to the filling operation (which is undertaken under Grade A laminar flow conditions). The final product containers must also be pre-sterilized. This may be achieved by autoclaving, or passage through special equipment which subjects the vials to a hot WFI rinse, followed by sterilizing dry heat and UV treatment. If the product can be filled into plastic-based containers, alternative 'blow–fill–seal' systems may be used, Figure 3.29; as its name suggests, such equipment first moulds plastic into the final product container (the moulding conditions ensure container sterility), followed immediately by

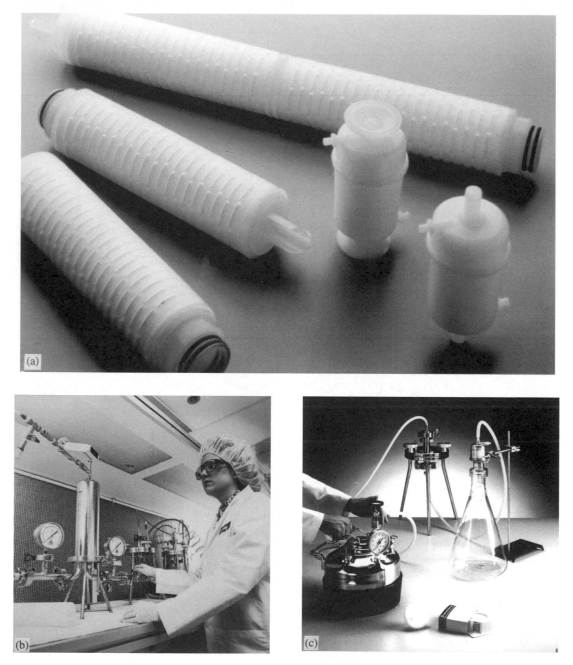

Figure 3.28.   Photographic representation of a range of filter types and their stainless steel housing. Most filters used on an industrial scale are of a pleated cartridge design which facilitates housing of maximum filter area within a compact space (a). These are generally housed in stainless steel housing units (b). Some process operations, however, still make use of flat (disc) filters, which are housed in a tripod-based stainless steel housing (c). Photos courtesy of Pall Life Sciences, Ireland

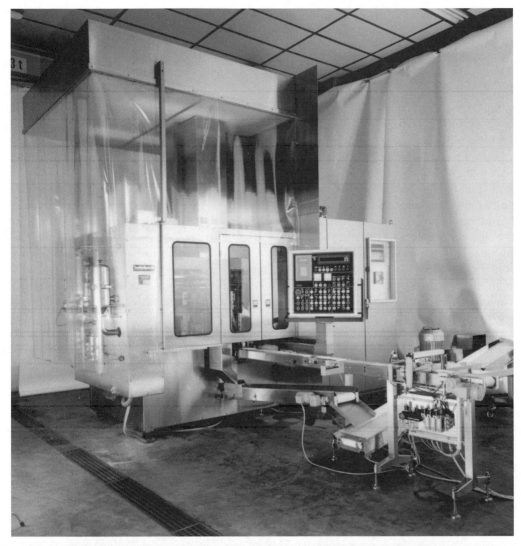

Figure 3.29. Photographic representation of a blow–fill–seal machine, which can be particularly useful in the aseptic filling of liquid products (refer to text for details). While used fairly extensively in facilities manufacturing some traditional parenteral products, this system has not yet found application in biopharmaceutical manufacture. This is due mainly to the fact that many biopharmaceutical preparations are sold not in liquid, but in freeze-dried format. Also, some proteins display a tendancy to adsorb onto plastic surfaces. Photo courtesy of Rommelag a.g., Switzerland

automated filling of sterile product into the container and its subsequent sealing. In this way operator intervention in the filling process is minimized.

Freeze-drying

Freeze-drying (lyophilization) refers to the removal of solvent directly from a solution while in the frozen state. Removal of water directly from (frozen) biopharmaceutical products via lyophilization yields a powdered product, usually displaying a water content of the order of 3%. In general, removal of the solvent water from such products greatly reduces the likelihood of chemical/biological-mediated inactivation of the biopharmaceutical. Freeze-dried biopharmaceutical products usually exhibit longer shelf-lives than products sold in solution. Freeze drying-is also recognized by the regulatory authorities as being a safe and acceptable method of preserving many parenteral products.

Freeze-drying is a relatively gentle way of removing water from proteins in solution. However, this process can promote the inactivation of some protein types and specific excipients (cryoprotectants) are usually added to the product in order to minimize such inactivation. Commonly used cryoprotectants include carbohydrates, such as glucose and sucrose; proteins, such as human serum albumin; and amino acids, such as lysine, arginine or glutamic acid. Alcohols/polyols have also found some application as cryoprotectants.

The freeze-drying process is initiated by the freezing of the biopharmaceutical product in its final product containers. As the temperature is decreased, ice crystals begin to form and grow. This results in an effective concentration of all the solutes present in the remaining liquid phase, including the protein and all added excipients, e.g. the concentration of salts may increase to levels as high as 3 M. Increased solute concentration alone can accelerate chemical reactions damaging to the protein product. In addition, such concentration effectively brings individual protein molecules into more intimate contact with each other, which can prompt protein–protein interactions and, hence, aggregation.

As the temperature drops still lower, some of the solutes present may also crystallize, thus being effectively removed from the solution. In some cases, individual buffer constituents can crystallize out of solution at different temperatures. This will dramatically alter the pH values of the remaining solution and, in this way, can lead to protein inactivation.

As the temperature is further lowered, the viscosity of the unfrozen solution increases dramatically until molecular mobility effectively ceases. This unfrozen solution will contain the protein, as well as some excipients and (at most) 50% water. As molecular mobility has

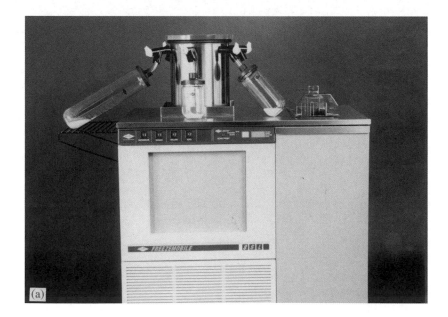

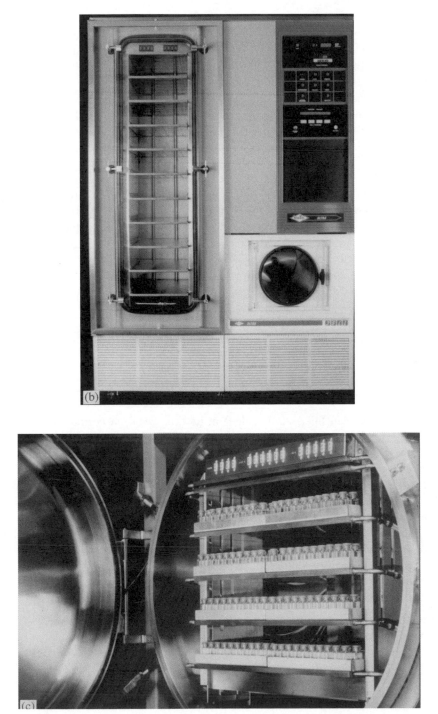

Figure 3.30. Photographic representation of (a) lab-scale, (b) pilot-scale and (c) industrial-scale freeze driers. Refer to text for details. Photo courtesy of Virtis, USA

effectively stopped, chemical reactivity also all but ceases. The consistency of this 'solution' is that of glass, and the temperature at which this is attained is called the glass transition temperature, Tg'. For most protein solutions, Tg' values reside between $-40°C$ and $-60°C$. The primary aim of the initial stages of the freeze-drying process is to decrease the product temperature below that of its Tg' value as quickly as possible.

The next phase of the freeze-drying process entails the application of a vacuum to the system. When the vacuum is established, the temperature is increased, usually to temperatures slightly in excess of $0°C$. This promotes sublimation of the crystalline water, leaving behind a powdered cake of dried material. Once satisfactory drying has been achieved, the product container is sealed.

The drying chamber of industrial-scale freeze-dryers usually opens into a clean room (Figure 3.27). This facilitates direct transfer of the product-containing vials into the chamber. Immediately prior to filling, rubber stoppers are usually partially inserted into the mouth of each vial in such a way as not to hinder the outward flow of water vapour during the freeze-drying process. The drying chamber normally contains several rows of shelves, each of which can accommodate several thousand vials (Figure 3.30). These shelves are wired to allow their electrical heating and cooling and their upward or downward movement. After the freeze-drying cycle is complete (which can take 3 days or more), the shelves are then moved upwards. As each shelf moves up, the partially-inserted rubber seals are inserted fully into the vial mouth as they come in contact with the base plate of the shelf immediately above them. After product recovery, the empty chamber is closed and is then heat-sterilized (using its own chamber-heating mechanism). The freeze-drier is then ready to accept its next load.

Labelling and packing

After the product has been filled (and sealed) in its final product container, it is immediately placed under quarantine. QC personnel then remove representative samples of the product and carry out tests to ensure conformance to final product specification. The most important specifications will relate to product potency, sterility and final volume fill, as well as the absence of endotoxin or other potentially toxic substances. Detection and quantification of excipients added will also be undertaken.

Only after QC personnel are satisfied that the product meets these specifications will it be labelled and packed. These operations are highly automated. Labelling, in particular, deserves special attention. Mislabelling of product remains one of the most common reasons for product recall. This can occur relatively easily, particularly if the facility manufactures several different products, or even a single product at several different strengths. Information presented on a label should normally include:

● name and strength/potency of the product;
● specific batch number of the product;
● date of manufacture and expiry date;
● storage conditions required.

Additional information often presented includes the name of the manufacturer, a list of excipients included and a brief summary of the correct mode of product usage.

When a batch of product is labelled and packed, and QC personnel are satisfied that labelling and packing are completed to specification, the QC manager will write and sign a Certificate of Analysis. This details the pre-defined product specifications and confirms conformance of the actual batch of product in question to these specifications. At this point, the product, along with its Certificate of Analysis, may be shipped to the customer.

ANALYSIS OF THE FINAL PRODUCT

All pharmaceutical finished products undergo rigorous QC testing, in order to confirm their conformance to pre-determined specifications. Potency testing is of obvious importance, ensuring that the drug will be efficacious when administered to the patient. A prominent aspect of safety testing entails analysis of product for the presence of various potential contaminants.

The range and complexity of analytical testing undertaken for recombinant biopharmaceuticals far outweighs those undertaken with regard to 'traditional' pharmaceuticals manufactured by organic synthesis. Not only are proteins (or additional likely biopharmaceuticals, such as nucleic acids; Chapter 11) much larger and more structurally complex than traditional low molecular mass drugs, their production in biological systems renders the range of potential contaminants far broader (Table 3.25). Recent advances in analytical techniques renders practical the routine analysis of complex biopharmaceutical products. An overview of the range of finished-product tests of recombinant protein biopharmaceuticals is outlined below. Explanation of the theoretical basis underpinning these analytical methodologies is not undertaken, as this would considerably broaden the scope of the text. Appropriate references are provided in Further Reading at the end of the chapter for the interested reader.

Protein-based contaminants

Most of the chromatographic steps undertaken during downstream processing are specifically included to separate the protein of interest from additional contaminant proteins. This task is not an insubstantial one, particularly if the recombinant protein is expressed intracellularly.

In addition to protein impurities emanating directly from the source material, other proteins may be introduced during upstream or downstream processing. For example, animal cell culture media is typically supplemented with bovine serum/fetal calf serum (2–25%), or with a defined cocktail of various regulatory proteins required to maintain and stimulate growth of these cells. Downstream processing of intracellular microbial proteins often requires the addition of endonucleases to the cell homogenate to degrade the large quantity of DNA liberated upon

Table 3.25. The range and medical significance of potential impurities present in biopharmaceutical products destined for parenteral administration. Reproduced by permission of John Wiley & Sons Ltd from Walsh & Headon (1994)

Impurity	Medical consequence
Microorganisms	Potential establishment of a severe microbial infection — septicaemia
Viral particles	Potential establishment of a severe viral infection
Pyrogenic substances	Fever response which, in serious cases, culminates in death
DNA	Significance is unclear — could bring about an immunological response
Contaminating proteins	Immunological reactions. Potential adverse effects if the contaminant exhibits an unwanted biological activity

cellular disruption (DNA promotes increased solution viscosity, rendering processing difficult; viscosity, being a function of the DNA's molecular mass, is reduced upon nuclease treatment).

Minor amounts of protein could also potentially enter the product stream from additional sources, e.g. protein shed from production personnel. Implementation of GMP should, however, minimize contamination from such sources.

The clinical significance of protein-based impurities relates to: (a) their potential biological activities; and (b) their antigenicity. While some contaminants may display no undesirable biological activity, others may exhibit activities deleterious to either the product itself (e.g. proteases which could modify/degrade the product) or the recipient patient (e.g. the presence of contaminating toxins).

Their inherent immunogenicity also renders likely an immunological reaction against protein-based impurities upon product administration to the recipient patient. This is particularly true in the case of products produced in microbial or other recombinant systems (i.e. most biopharmaceuticals). While the product itself is likely to be non-immunogenic (being coded for by a human gene), contaminant proteins will be endogenous to the host cell, and hence foreign to the human body. Administration of the product can elicit an immune response against the contaminant. This is particularly likely if a requirement exists for ongoing, repeat product administration (e.g. administration of recombinant insulin). Immunological activation of this type could also potentially (and more seriously) have a sensitizing effect on the recipient against the actual protein product.

In addition to distinct gene products, modified forms of the protein of interest are also considered impurities, rendering desirable their removal from the product stream. While some such modified forms may be innocuous, others may not. Modified product 'impurities' may compromise the product in a number of ways, e.g:

- biologically inactive forms of the product will reduce overall product potency;
- some modified product forms remain biologically active but exhibit modified pharmacokinetic characteristics (i.e. timing and duration of drug action);
- modified product forms may be immunogenic.

Altered forms of the protein of interest can be generated in a number of ways by covalent and non-covalent modifications (see e.g. Table 3.20).

Removal of altered forms of the protein of interest from the product stream

Modification of any protein will generally alter some aspect of its physicochemical characteristics. This facilitates removal of the modified form by standard chromatographic techniques during downstream processing. Most downstream procedures for protein-based biopharmaceuticals include both gel-filtration and ion-exchange steps. Aggregated forms of the product will be effectively removed by gel-filtration (because they now exhibit a molecular mass greater by several orders of magnitude than the native product). This technique will equally efficiently remove extensively proteolysed forms of the product. Glycoprotein variants whose carbohydrate moieties have been extensively degraded will also likely be removed by gel-filtration (or ion-exchange) chromatography. Deamidation and oxidation will generate product variants with altered surface charge characteristics, often rendering their removal by ion-exchange relatively straightforward. Incorrect disulphide bond formation, partial denaturation and limited proteolysis can also alter the shape and surface charge of proteins, facilitating their

Table 3.26. Methods used to characterize (protein-based) finished product biopharmaceuticals. An overview of most of these methods is presented over the next several sections of this chapter

---

Non-denaturing gel electrophoresis
Denaturing (SDS) gel electrophoresis
2-D electrophoresis
Capillary electrophoresis
Peptide mapping
HPLC (mainly reverse phase — HPLC)
Isoelectric focusing
Mass spectrometry
Amino acid analysis
N-terminal sequencing
Circular dichromism studies
Bioassays and immunological assays

---

removal from the product by ion-exchange or other techniques, such as hydrophobic interaction chromatography.

The range of chromatographic techniques now available, along with improvements in the resolution achievable using such techniques, renders possible the routine production of protein biopharmaceuticals that are in excess of 97–99% pure. This level of purity represents the typical industry standard with regard to biopharmaceutical production.

A number of different techniques may be used to characterize protein-based biopharmaceutical products, and to detect any protein-based impurities that may be present in that product (Table 3.26). Analyses for non-protein-based contaminants are described in subsequent sections.

Product potency

Any biopharmaceutical must obviously conform to final product potency specifications. Such specifications are usually expressed in terms of 'units of activity' per vial of product (or per therapeutic dose, or per mg of product). A number of different approaches may be undertaken to determine product potency. Each exhibits certain advantages and disadvantages.

Bioassays represent the most relevant potency-determining assay, as they directly assess the biological activity of the biopharmaceutical. Bioassay involves applying a known quantity of the substance to be assayed to a biological system which responds in some way to this applied stimulus. The response is measured quantitatively, allowing an activity value to be assigned to the substance being assayed.

All bioassays are comparative in nature, requiring parallel assay of a 'standard' preparation against which the sample will be compared. Internationally accepted standard preparations of most biopharmaceuticals are available from organizations such as the World Health Organization (WHO) or the *US Pharmacopoeia*.

An example of a straightforward bioassay is the traditional assay method for antibiotics. Bioassays for modern biopharmaceuticals are generally more complex. The biological system used can be whole animals, specific organs or tissue types, or individual mammalian cells in culture.

Bioassays of related substances can be quite similar in design. Specific growth factors, for example, stimulate the accelerated growth of specific animal cell lines. Relevant bioassays can be undertaken by incubation of the growth factor-containing sample with a culture of the relevant sensitive cells and radiolabelled nucleotide precursors. After an appropriate time period, the level of radioactivity incorporated into the DNA of the cells is measured. This is a measure of the bioactivity of the growth factor.

The most popular bioassay of erythropoietin (EPO) involves a mouse-based bioassay [EPO stimulates red blood cell (RBC) production, making it useful in the treatment of certain forms of anaemia; Chapter 6]. Basically, the EPO-containing sample is administered to mice, along with radioactive iron (^{57}Fe). Subsequent measurement of the rate of incorporation of radioactivity into proliferating RBCs is undertaken (the greater the stimulation of RBC proliferation, the more iron is taken up for haemoglobin synthesis).

One of the most popular bioassays for interferons is termed the 'cytopathic effect inhibition assay'. This assay is based upon the ability of many interferons to render animal cells resistant to viral attack. It entails incubation of the interferon preparation with cells sensitive to destruction by a specific virus. That virus is then subsequently added, and the percentage of cells that survive thereafter is proportional to the levels of interferon present in the assay sample. Viable cells can assimilate certain dyes, such as neutral red. Addition of the dye, followed by spectrophotometric quantitation of the amount of dye assimilated, can thus be used to quantitfy percentage cell survival. This type of assay can be scaled down to run in a single well of a microtitre plate. This facilitates automated assay of a large number of samples with relative ease.

While bioassays directly assess product potency (i.e. activity), they suffer from a number of drawbacks, including:

- *Lack of precision*. The complex nature of any biological system, be it an entire animal or an individual cell, often results in the responses observed being influenced by factors such as the metabolic status of individual cells, or (in the case of whole animals) sub-clinical infections, stress levels induced by human handling, etc.
- *Time*. Most bioassays take days, and in some cases weeks, to run. This can render routine bioassays difficult, and impractical to undertake as a quick QC potency test during downstream processing.
- *Cost*. Most bioassay systems, particularly those involving whole animals, are extremely expensive to undertake.

Because of such difficulties, alternative assays have been investigated, and sometimes are used in conjunction with, or instead of, bioassays. The most popular alternative assay systems are the immunoassays.

Immunoassays employ monoclonal or polyclonal antibody preparations to detect and quantify the product. The specificity of antibody–antigen interaction ensures good assay precision. The use of conjugated radiolabels (radioimmunoassay; RIA) or enzymes (enzyme immunoassay: EIA) to allow detection of antigen–antibody binding renders such assays very sensitive. Furthermore, when compared to bioassays, immunoassays are rapid (undertaken in minutes to hours), inexpensive and straightforward to undertake.

The obvious disadvantage of immunoassays is that immunological reactivity cannot be guaranteed to correlate directly with biological activity. Relatively minor modifications of the protein product, while having a profound influence on its biological activity, may have little or no influence on its ability to bind antibody.

Table 3.27. Common assay methods used to quantify proteins. The principle upon which each method is based is also listed

Method	Principle
Absorbance at 280 nm (A$_{280}$; UV method)	The side chain of selected amino acids (particularly tyrosine and tryptophan) absorbs UV at 280 nm
Absorbance at 205 nm (far UV method)	Peptide bonds absorb UV at 190–220 nm
Biuret method	Binding of copper ions to peptide bond nitrogen under alkaline conditions generates a purple colour
Lowry method	Lowry method uses a combination of the Biuret copper-based reagent and the 'Folin–Ciocalteau' reagent, which contains phosphomolybdic-phosphotungstic acid. Reagents react with protein, yielding a blue colour which displays an absorbance maximum at 750 nm
Bradford method	Bradford reagent contains the dye, Coomassie blue G-250, in an acidic solution. The dye binds to protein, yielding a blue colour which absorbs maximally at 595 nm
Bicinchonic acid method	Copper-containing reagent which, when reduced by protein, reacts with bicinchonic acid yielding a complex that displays an absorbance maximum at 562 nm
Peterson method	Essentially involves initial precipitation of protein out of solution by addition of trichloroacetic acid (TCA). The protein precipitate is redissolved in NaOH and the Lowry method of protein determination is then performed
Silver-binding method	Interaction of silver with protein — very sensitive method

For such reasons, while immunoassays may provide a convenient means of tracking product during downstream processing, performance of a bioassay on at very least the final product is often considered necessary to prove that potency falls within specification.

Determination of protein concentration

Quantification of total protein in the final product represents another standard analysis undertaken by QC. A number of different protein assays may be potentially employed (Table 3.27).

Detection and quantification of protein by measuring absorbency at 280 nm is perhaps the simplest such method. This approach is based on the fact that the side-chains of tyrosine and tryptophan absorb at this wavelength. The method is popular, as it is fast, easy to perform and is non-destructive to the sample. However, it is a relatively insensitive technique, and identical concentrations of different proteins will yield different absorbance values if their contents of tyrosine and tryptophan vary to any significant extent. For these reasons, this method is rarely used to determine the protein concentration of the final product, but it is routinely used during downstream processing to detect protein elution off chromatographic columns, and hence track the purification process.

Measuring protein absorbance at lower wavelengths (205 nm) increases the sensitivity of the assay considerably. Also, as it is the peptide bonds that are absorbing at this wavelength, the assay is subject to much less variation due to the amino acid composition of the protein. The most common methods used to determine protein concentration are the dye-binding procedure using Coomassie brilliant blue, and the bicinchonic acid-based procedure. Various dyes are known to bind quantitatively to proteins, resulting in an alteration of the characteristic absorption spectrum of the dye. Coomassie brilliant blue G-250, for example, becomes protonated when dissolved in phosphoric acid, and has an absorbance maximum at 450 nm. Binding of the dye to a protein (via ionic interactions) results in a shift in the dye's absorbance spectrum, with a new major peak (at 595 nm) being observed. Quantification of proteins in this case can thus be undertaken by measuring absorbance at 595 nm. The method is sensitive, easy and rapid to undertake. Also it exhibits little quantitative variation between different proteins.

Protein determination procedures using bicinchonic acid were developed by Pierce chemicals, who hold a patent on the product. The procedure entails the use of a copper-based reagent containing bicinchonic acid. Upon incubation with a protein sample, the copper is reduced. In the reduced state it reacts with bicinchonic acid, yielding a purple colour which absorbs maximally at 562 nm.

Silver also binds to proteins, an observation which forms the basis of an extremely sensitive method of protein detection. This technique is used extensively to detect proteins in electrophoretic gels, as discussed in the next section.

Detection of protein-based product impurities

Sodium dodecyl sulphate polyacrylamide gel electrophoresis (SDS–PAGE) represents the most commonly used analytical technique in the assessment of final product purity (Figure 3.31). This technique is well established and easy to perform. It provides high-resolution separation of polypeptides on the basis of their molecular mass. Bands containing as little as 100 ng protein can be visualized by staining the gel with dyes such as Coomassie blue. Subsequent gel analysis by scanning laser densitometry allows quantitative determination of the protein content of each band (thus allowing quantification of protein impurities in the product).

The use of silver-based stains increases the detection sensitivity up to 100-fold, with individual bands containing as little as 1 ng protein usually staining well. However, because silver binds to protein non-stoichiometrically, quantitative studies using densitometry cannot be undertaken.

SDS–PAGE is normally run under reducing conditions. Addition of a reducing agent such as β-marceptoethanol or dithiothreitol (DTT) disrupts inter-chain (and intra-chain) disulphide linkages. Individual polypeptides held together via disulphide linkages in oligomeric proteins will thus separate from each other on the basis of their molecular mass.

The presence of bands additional to those equating to the protein product generally represent protein contaminants. Such contaminants may be unrelated to the product, or may be variants of the product itself (e.g. differentially glycosylated variants, proteolytic fragments, etc.). Further characterization may include Western blot analysis. This involves eluting the protein bands from the electrophoretic gel onto a nitrocellulose filter. The filter can then be probed using antibodies raised against the product. Binding of the antibody to the 'contaminant' bands suggests that they are variants of the product.

One concern relating to SDS–PAGE-based purity analysis is that contaminants of the same molecular mass as the product will go undetected, as they will co-migrate with it. 2-dimensional (2-D) electrophoretic analysis would overcome this eventuality in most instances.

2-D electrophoresis is normally run so that proteins are separated from each other on the basis of a different molecular property in each dimension. The most commonly utilized method entails separation of proteins by isoelectric focusing (see below) in the first dimension, with

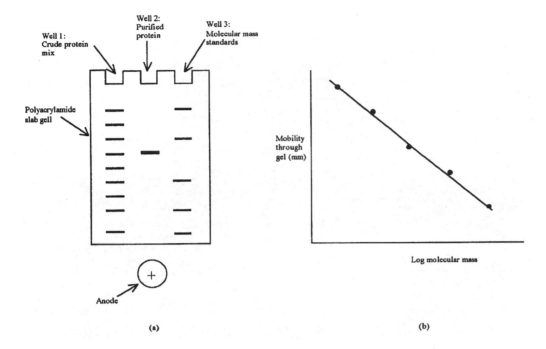

Figure 3.31. Separation of proteins by SDS–PAGE. Protein samples are incubated with SDS (as well as reducing agents, which disrupt disulphide linkages). The electric field is applied across the gel after the protein samples to be analysed are loaded into the gel wells. The rate of protein migration towards the anode is dependent upon protein size. After electrophoresis is complete, individual protein bands may be visualized by staining with a protein-binding dye (a). If one well is loaded with a mixture of proteins, each of known molecular mass, a standard curve relating distance migrated to molecular mass can be constructed (b). This allows estimation of the molecular mass of the purified protein. Reproduced by permission of John Wiley & Sons Inc. from Walsh (2002)

separation in the second dimension being undertaken in the presence of SDS, thus promoting band separation on the basis of protein size. Modified electrophoresis equipment which renders 2-D electrophoretic separation routine is freely available. Application of biopharmaceutical finished products to such systems allows rigorous analysis of purity.

Isoelectric focusing (IEF) entails setting up a pH gradient along the length of an electrophoretic gel. Applied proteins will migrate under the influence of an electric field, until they reach a point in the gel at which the pH equals the protein's isoelectric point (pI; the pH at which the protein exhibits no overall net charge—only species with a net charge will move under the influence of an electric field). IEF thus separates proteins on the basis of charge characteristics.

This technique is also utilized in the biopharmaceutical industry to determine product homogeneity. Homogeneity is best indicated by the appearance in the gel of a single protein band, exhibiting the predicted pI value. Interpretation of the meaning of multiple bands, however, is less straightforward, particularly if the protein is glycosylated (the bands can also be stained for the presence of carbohydrates). Glycoproteins varying slightly in their carbohydrate content will vary in their sialic acid content, and hence exhibit slightly different pI values. In

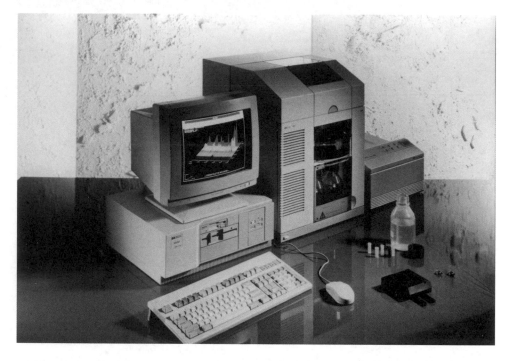

Figure 3.32. Photograph of a capillary electrophoresis system (the HP-3D capillary electrophoresis system manufactured by Hewlett-Packard). Refer to text for details. Photo courtesy of Hewlett Packard GmbH, Germany

such instances IEF analysis seeks to establish batch-to-batch consistency in terms of the banding pattern observed.

IEF also finds application in analysing the stability of biopharmaceuticals over the course of their shelf-life. Repeat analysis of samples over time will detect deamidation or other degradative processes which alter protein charge characteristics.

Capillary electrophoresis

Capillary electrophoresis systems are also likely to play an increasingly prominent analytical role in the QC laboratory (Figure 3.32). As with other forms of electrophoresis, separation is based upon different rates of protein migration upon application of an electric field.

As its name suggests, in the case of capillary electrophoresis, this separation occurs within a capillary tube. Typically, the capillary will have a diameter of 20–50 mm and be up to 1 m long (it is normally coiled to facilitate ease of use and storage). The dimensions of this system yield greatly increased surface area:volume ratio (when compared to slab gels), hence greatly increasing the efficiency of heat dissipation from the system. This in turn allows operation at a higher current density, thus speeding up the rate of migration through the capillary. Sample analysis can be undertaken in 15–30 min, and on-line detection at the end of the column allows automatic detection and quantification of eluting bands.

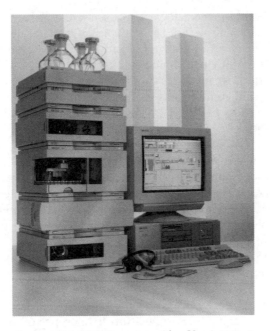

Figure 3.33. Photograph of a typical HPLC system (the Hewlett-Packard HP1100 system). Photo courtesy of Hewlett-Packard GmbH, Germany

The speed, sensitivity, high degree of automation and ability to directly quantify protein bands renders this system ideal for biopharmaceutical analysis.

High-pressure liquid chromatography (HPLC)

HPLC occupies a central analytical role in assessing the purity of low molecular mass pharmaceutical substances (Figure 3.33). It also plays an increasingly important role in analysis of macromolecules such as proteins. Most of the chromatographic strategies used to separate proteins under 'low pressure' (e.g. gel filtration, ion-exchange, etc.) can be adapted to operate under high pressure. Reverse phase, size exclusion and, to a lesser extent, ion-exchange-based HPLC chromatography systems are now used in the analysis of a range of biopharmaceutical preparations. On-line detectors (usually a UV monitor set at 220 nm or 280 nm) allows automated detection and quantification of eluting bands.

HPLC is characterized by a number of features which render it an attractive analytical tool. These include:

- excellent fractionation speeds (often just minutes per sample);
- superior peak resolution;
- high degree of automation (including data analysis);
- ready commercial availability of various sophisticated systems.

Reverse-phase HPLC (RP-HPLC) separates proteins on the basis of differences in their surface hydrophobicity. The stationary phase in the HPLC column normally consists of silica or a polymeric support to which hydrophobic arms (usually alkyl chains such as butyl, octyl or octadecyl groups) have been attached. Reverse-phase systems have proved themselves to be a particularly powerful analytical technique, capable of separating very similar molecules, displaying only minor differences in hydrophobicity. In some instances, a single amino acid substitution or the removal of a single amino acid from the end of a polypeptide chain can be detected by RP-HPLC. In most instances modifications such as deamidation will also cause peak shifts. Such systems, therefore, may be used to detect impurities, be they related or unrelated to the protein product. RP-HPLC finds extensive application in analysis of insulin preparations. Modified forms or insulin polymers are easily distinguishable from native insulin on reverse-phase columns.

While RP-HPLC has proved its analytical usefulness, its routine application to analysis of specific protein preparations should be undertaken only after extensive validation studies. HPLC in general can have a denaturing influence on many proteins (especially larger, complex proteins). Reverse-phase systems can be particularly harsh, as interaction with the highly hydrophobic stationary phase can induce irreversible protein denaturation. Denaturation would result in the generation of artifactual peaks on the chromatogram.

Size exclusion HPLC (SE-HPLC) separates proteins on the basis of size and shape. As most soluble proteins are globular (i.e. roughly spherical in shape), in most instances separation is essentially achieved on the basis of molecular mass. Commonly used SE-HPLC stationary phases include silica-based supports and cross-linked agarose of defined pore size. Size exclusion systems are most often used to analyse product for the presence of dimers or higher molecular mass aggregates of itself, as well as proteolysed product variants.

Calibration with standards allows accurate determination of the molecular mass of the product itself, as well as any impurities. Batch-to-batch variation can also be assessed by comparison of chromatograms from different product runs.

Ion-exchange chromatography (both cation and anion) can also be undertaken in HPLC format. Although not as extensively employed as RP or SE systems, ion-exchange-based systems are of use in analysing for impurities unrelated to the product, as well as detecting and quantifying deamidated forms.

Mass spectrometry

Recent advances in the field of mass spectrometry now extends the applicability of this method to the analysis of macromolecules, such as proteins. Using electrospray mass spectrometry, it is now possible to determine the molecular mass of many proteins to within an accuracy of $\pm 0.01\%$. A protein variant missing a single amino acid residue can easily be distinguished from the native protein in many instances. Although this is a very powerful technique, analysis of the results obtained can sometimes be less than straightforward. Glycoproteins, for example, yield extremely complex spectra (due to their natural heterogeneity), making the significance of the findings hard to interpret.

Immunological approaches to detection of contaminants

Most recombinant biopharmaceuticals are produced in microbial or mammalian cell lines. Thus, although the product is derived from a human gene, all product-unrelated contaminants will be derived from the producer organism. These non-self-proteins are likely to be highly immunogenic in humans, rendering their removal from the product stream especially important. Immunoassays may be conveniently used to detect and quantify non-product-related impurities in the final preparation (immunoassays generally may not be used to determine levels of product-related impurities, as antibodies raised against such impurities would almost certainly cross-react with the product itself).

The strategy usually employed to develop such immunoassays is termed the 'blank run approach'. This entails constructing a host cell identical in all respects to the natural producer cell, except that it lacks the gene coding for the desired product. This blank producer cell is then subjected to upstream processing procedures identical to those undertaken with the normal producer cell. Cellular extracts are subsequently subjected to the normal product purification process, but only to a stage immediately prior to the final purification steps. This produces an array of proteins which could co-purify with the final product. These proteins (of which there may be up to 200, as determined by 2-D electrophoric analysis) are used to immunize horses, goats or other suitable animals. Polyclonal antibody preparations capable of binding specifically to these proteins are therefore produced. Purification of the antibodies allows their incorporation in radioimmunoassay or enzyme-based immunoassay systems, which may subsequently be used to probe the product. Such multi-antigen assay systems will detect the sum total of host cell-derived impurities present in the product. Immunoassays identifying a single potential contaminant can also be developed.

Immunoassays have found widespread application in detecting and quantifying product impurities. These assays are extremely specific and very sensitive, often detecting target antigen down to p.p.m. levels. Many immunoassays are available commercially and companies exist which will rapidly develop tailor-made immunoassay systems for biopharmaceutical analysis.

Application of the analytical techniques discussed thus far focuses upon detection of proteinaceous impurities. A variety of additional tests are undertaken which focus upon the active substance itself. These tests aim to confirm that the presumed active substance observed by electrophoresis, HPLC, etc. is indeed the active substance, and that its primary sequence (and to a lesser extent, higher orders of structure) conform to licensed product specification. Tests performed to verify the product identity include amino acid analysis, peptide mapping, N-terminal sequencing and spectrophotometric analyses.

Amino acid analysis

Amino acid analysis remains a characterization technique undertaken in many laboratories, particularly if the product is a peptide or small polypeptide (molecular mass $\leqslant 10\,000$ Da). The strategy is simple — determine the range and quantity of amino acids present in the product and compare the results obtained with the expected (theoretical) values. The results should be comparable.

The peptide/polypeptide product is usually hydrolysed by incubation with 6 N HCl at elevated temperatures (110°C), under vacuum, for extended periods (12–24 h). The constituent amino acids are separated from each other by ion-exchange chromatography, and identified by comparison with standard amino acid preparations. Reaction with ninhydrin allows subsequent quantification of each amino acid present.

While this technique is relatively straightforward and automated amino acid analysers are commercially available, it is subject to a number of disadvantages that limit its usefulness in biopharmaceutical analysis. These include:

- hydrolysis conditions can destroy/modify certain amino acid residues, particularly tryptophan, but also serine, threonine and tyrosine;

- the method is semi-quantitative rather than quantitative;
- sensitivity is at best moderate; low-level contaminants may go undetected (i.e. not significantly alter the amino acid profile obtained), particularly if the product is a high molecular mass protein.

These disadvantages, along with the availability of alternative characterization methodologies, limit application of this technique in biopharmaceutical analysis.

Peptide mapping

A major concern relating to biopharmaceuticals produced in high-expression recombinant systems is the potential occurrence of point mutations in the product's gene, leading to an altered primary structure (i.e. amino acid sequence). Errors in gene transcription or translation could also have similar consequences. The only procedure guaranteed to detect such alterations is full sequencing of a sample of each batch of the protein; a considerable technical challenge. Although partial protein sequencing is normally undertaken (see later) the approach most commonly used to detect alterations in amino acid sequence is peptide (fingerprint) mapping.

Peptide mapping entails exposure of the protein product to a reagent which promotes hydrolysis of peptide bonds at specific points along the protein backbone. This generates a series of peptide fragments. These fragments can be separated from each other by a variety of techniques, including one- or two-dimensional electrophoresis and, in particular, RP-HPLC. A standardized sample of the protein product, when subjected to this procedure, will yield a characteristic peptide fingerprint, or map, with which the peptide maps obtained with each batch of product can subsequently be compared. If the peptides generated are relatively short, a change in a single amino acid residue is likely to alter the peptide's physicochemical properties sufficiently to alter its position within the peptide map (Figure 3.34). In this way single (or multiple) amino acid substitutions, deletions, insertions or modifications can usually be detected. This technique plays an important role in monitoring batch-to-batch consistency of the product, and also obviously can confirm the identity of the actual product.

The choice of reagent used to fragment the protein is critical to the success of this approach. If a reagent generates only a few very large peptides, a single amino acid alteration in one such peptide will be more difficult to detect than if it occurred in a much smaller peptide fragment. On the other hand, generation of a large number of very short peptides can be counter-productive, as it may prove difficult to resolve all the peptides from each other by subsequent chromatography. Generation of peptide fragments containing an average of 7–14 amino acids is most desirable.

The most commonly utilized chemical cleavage agent is cyanogen bromide (it cleaves the peptide bond on the carboxyl side of methionine residues). V8 protease, produced by certain staphylococci, along with trypsin, are two of the more commonly used proteolytic-based fragmentation agents.

Knowledge of the full amino acid sequence of the protein usually renders possible predetermination of the most suitable fragmentation agent for any protein. The amino acid sequence of human growth hormone, for example, harbours 20 potential trypsin cleavage sites. Under some circumstances it may be possible to use a combination of fragmentation agents to generate peptides of optimal length.

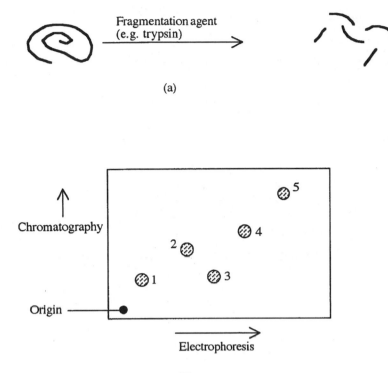

(a)

(b)

Figure 3.34. Generation of a peptide map. In this simple example, the protein to be analysed is treated with a fragmentation agent, e.g. trypsin (a). In this case, five fragments are generated. The digest is then applied to a sheet of chromatography paper (b) at the point marked 'origin'. The peptides are then separated from each other in the first (vertical) dimension by paper chromatography. Subsequently, electrophoresis is undertaken (in the horizontal direction). The separated peptide fragments may be visualized, e.g. by staining with ninhydrin. 2-D separation of the peptides is far more likely to completely resolve each peptide from the others. In the case above, for example, chromatography (in the vertical dimension) alone would not have been sufficient to fully resolve peptides 1 and 3. During biopharmaceutical production, each batch of the recombinant protein produced should yield identical peptide maps. Any mutation which alters the protein's primary structure (i.e. amino acid sequence) should result in at least one fragment adopting an altered position in the peptide map

N-terminal sequencing

N-terminal sequencing of the first 20–30 amino acid residues of the protein product has become a popular quality control test for finished biopharmaceutical products. The technique is useful as it:

- positively identifies the protein;
- confirms (or otherwise) the accuracy of the amino acid sequence of at least the N-terminus of the protein;
- readily identifies the presence of modified forms of the product in which one or more amino acids are missing from the N-terminus.

N-terminal sequencing is normally undertaken by Edman degradation (Figure 3.35). Although this technique was developed in the 1950s, advances in analytical methodologies now facilitate

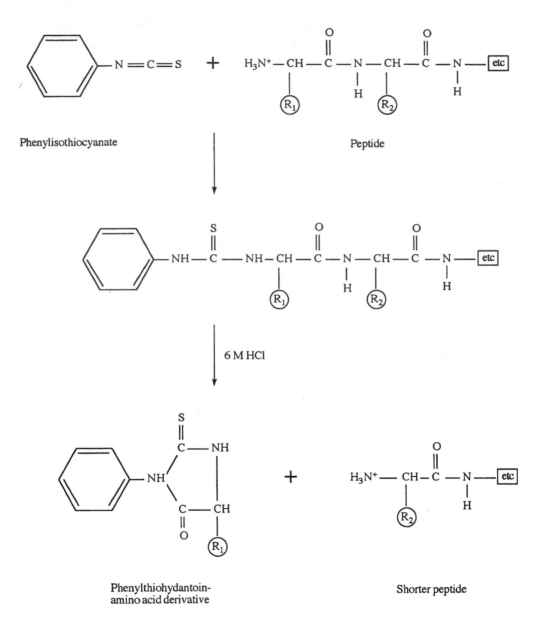

Figure 3.35. The Edman degradation method, by which the sequence of a peptide/polypeptide may be elucidated. The peptide is incubated with phenylisothiocyanate, which reacts specifically with the N-terminal amino acid of the peptide. Addition of 6 M HCl results in liberation of a phenylthiohydantoin-amino acid derivative and a shorter peptide, as shown. The phenylthiohydantoin derivative can then be isolated and its constituent amino acids identified by comparison to phenylthiohydantion derivatives of standard amino acid solutions. The shorter peptide is then subjected to a second round of treatment, such that its new amino terminus may be identified. This procedure is repeated until the entire amino acid sequence of the peptide has been established

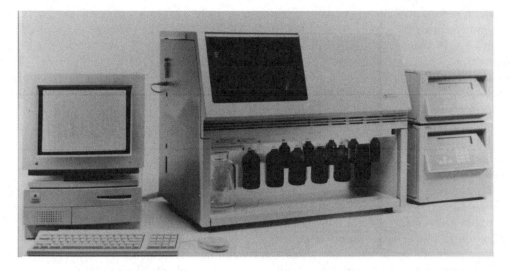

Figure 3.36.   Photo of a modern protein sequencing system. Photo courtesy of Perkin-Elmer Applied Biosystems Ltd, UK

fast and automated determination of up to the first 100 amino acids from the N-terminus of most proteins, and usually requires a sample size of less than $1 \mu M$ to do so (Figure 3.36).

Analogous techniques facilitating sequencing from a polypeptide's C-terminus remain to be satisfactorily developed. The enzyme carboxypeptidase C sequentially removes amino acids from the C-terminus, but often only removes the first few such amino acids. Furthermore, the rate at which it hydrolyses bonds can vary, depending on which amino acids have contributed to bond formation. Chemical approaches based on principles similar to the Edman procedure have been attempted. However, poor yields of derivitized product and the occurrence of side reactions have prevented widespread acceptance of this method.

Analysis of secondary and tertiary structure

Analyses such as peptide mapping, N-terminal sequencing or amino acid analysis yield information relating to a polypeptide's primary structure, i.e. its amino acid sequence. Such tests yield no information relating to higher-order structures (i.e. secondary and tertiary structure of polypeptides, along with quaternary structure of multi-subunit proteins). While a protein's 3-D conformation may be studied in great detail by X-ray crystallography or NMR spectroscopy, routine application of such techniques to biopharmaceutical manufacture is impractical from both a technical and economic standpoint. Limited analysis of protein secondary and tertiary structure can, however, be more easily undertaken using spectroscopic methods, particularly far-UV circular dichroism. More recently proton-NMR has also been applied to studying higher orders of protein structure.

Endotoxin and other pyrogenic contaminants

Pyrogens are substances which, when they enter the blood stream, influence hypothalamic regulation of body temperature, usually resulting in fever. Medical control of pyrogen-induced fever proves very difficult, and in severe cases results in patient death.

Pyrogens represent a diverse group of substances, including various chemicals, particulate matter and endotoxin (lipopolysaccharide, LPS — a molecule derived from the outer membrane of Gram-negative bacteria). Such Gram-negative organisms harbour 3–4 million LPS molecules on their surface, representing in the region of 75% of their outer membrane surface area. Gram-negative bacteria clinically significant in human medicine include *E. coli*, *Haemophilus influenzae*, *Salmonella enterica*, *Klebsiella pneumoniae*, *Bordetella pertussis*, *Pseudomonas aeruginosa*, *Chylamydia psittaci* and *Legionella pneumophila*.

In many instances the influence of pyrogens on body temperature is indirect, e.g. entry of endotoxin into the bloodstream stimulates the production of interleukin 1 (IL-1; Chapter 5) by macrophages. It is the IL-1 that directly initiates the fever response (hence its alternative name, 'endogenous pyrogen').

While entry of any pyrogenic substance into the bloodstream can have serious medical consequences, endotoxin receives most attention because of its ubiquitous nature. It is therefore the pyrogen most likely to contaminate parenteral (bio)pharmaceutical products. Effective implementation of GMP minimizes the likelihood of product contamination by pyrogens, e.g. GMP dictates that chemical reagents used in the manufacture of process buffers be extremely pure. Such raw materials are therefore unlikely to contain chemical contaminants displaying pyrogenic activity. Furthermore, GMP encourages filtration of virtually all parenteral products through a 0.45 µm or 0.22 µm filter at points during processing and prior to filling in final product containers (even if the product can subsequently be sterilized by autoclaving). Filtration ensures removal of all particulate matter from the product. In addition, most final product containers are rendered particle-free immediately prior to filling by an automatic pre-rinse using WFI. As an additional safeguard, the final product will usually be subject to a particulate matter test by QC before final product release. The simplest format for such a test could involve visual inspection of vial contents, although specific particle detecting and counting equipment is more routinely used.

Contamination of the final product with endotoxin is more difficult to control because:

- many recombinant biopharmaceuticals are produced in Gram-negative bacterial systems, thus the product source is also a source of endotoxin;
- despite rigorous implementation of GMP, most biopharmaceutical preparations will be contaminated with low levels of Gram-negative bacteria at some stage of manufacture. These bacteria shed endotoxin into the product stream, which is not removed during subsequent bacterial filtration steps. This is one of many reasons why GMP dictates that the level of bioburden in the product stream should be minimized at all stages of manufacture;
- the heat-stability exhibited by endotoxin (see next section) means that autoclaving of process equipment will not destroy endotoxin present on such equipment;
- adverse medical reactions caused by endotoxin are witnessed in humans at dosage rates as low as 0.5 ng/kg body weight.

Endotoxin, the molecule

The structural detail of a generalized endotoxin (LPS) molecule is presented in Figure 3.37. As its name suggests, LPS consists of a complex polysaccharide component linked to a lipid (lipid A) moiety. The polysaccharide moiety is generally composed of 50 or more monosaccharide units linked by glycosidic bonds. Sugar moieties often found in LPS include glucose, glucosamine, mannose and galactose, as well as more extensive structures such as

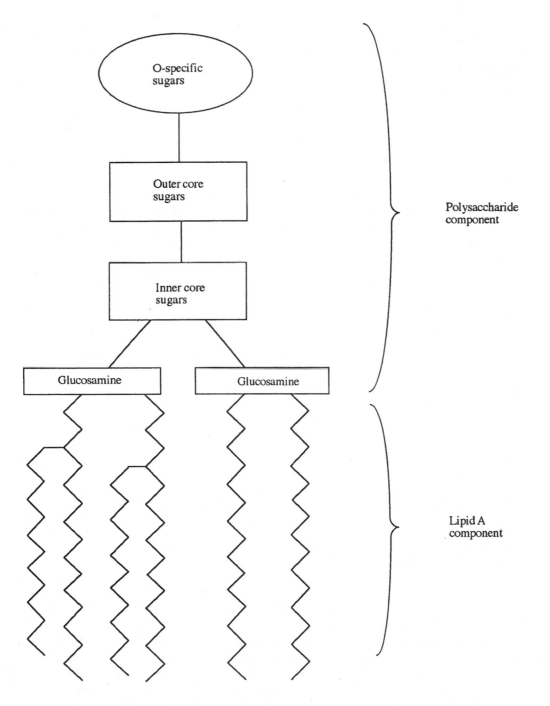

Figure 3.37. Structure of a generalized lipopolysaccharide (LPS) molecule. LPS consitutes the major structural component of the outer membrane of Gram-negative bacteria. Although LPS of different Gram-negative organisms differ in their chemical structure, each consists of a complex polysacharide component, linked to a lipid component. Refer to text for specific details

L-glycero-mannoheptose. The polysaccharide component of LPS may be divided into several structural domains. The inner (core) domains vary relatively little between LPS molecules isolated from different Gram-negative bacteria. The outer (O-specific) domain is usually bacterial strain-specific.

Most of the LPS biological activity (pyrogenicity) is associated with its lipid A moiety. This usually consists of six or more fatty acids attached directly to sugars such as glucosamine. Again, as is the case in relation to the carbohydrate component, lipid A moieties of LPS isolated from different bacteria can vary somewhat. The structure of *E. coli*'s lipid A has been studied in greatest detail. Its exact structure has been elucidated, and it can be chemically synthesized.

Pyrogen detection

Pyrogens may be detected in parenteral preparations (or other substances) by a number of methods. Two such methods are widely employed in the pharmaceutical industry.

Historically, the rabbit pyrogen test constituted the most widely used method. This entails parenteral administration of the product to a group of healthy rabbits, with subsequent monitoring of rabbit temperature using rectal probes. Increased rabbit temperature above a certain point suggests the presence of pyrogenic substances. The basic rabbit method, as outlined in the *European Pharmacopoeia*, entails initial administration of the product to three rabbits. The product is considered to have passed the test if the total (summed) increase of the temperature of all three animals is less than 1.15°C. If the total increase recorded is greater than 2.65°C the product has failed. However, if the response observed falls between these two limits, the result is considered inconclusive, and the test must be repeated using a further batch of animals.

This test is popular because it detects a wide spectrum of pyrogenic substances. However, it is also subject to a number of disadvantages, including:

- it is expensive (there is a requirement for animals, animal facilities and animal technicians);
- excitation/poor handling of the rabbits can affect the results obtained, usually prompting a false-positive result;
- sub-clinical infection/poor overall animal health can also lead to false-positive results;
- use of different rabbit colonies/breeds can yield variable results.

Another issue of relevance is that certain biopharmaceuticals (e.g. cytokines such as 1L-1 and TNF; Chapter 5), themselves, induce a natural pyrogenic response. This rules out use of the rabbit-based assay for detection of exogenous pyrogens in such products. Such difficulties have led to the increased use of an *in vitro* assay; the *Limulus* amoebocyte lysate (LAL) test. This is based upon endotoxin-stimulated coagulation of amoebocyte lysate obtained from horseshoe crabs. This test is now the most widely used assay for the detection of endotoxins in biopharmaceutical and other pharmaceutical preparations.

Development of the LAL assay was based upon the observation that the presence of Gram-negative bacteria in the vascular system of the American horseshoe crab, (*Limulus polyphemus*), resulted in the clotting of its blood. Tests on fractionated blood showed the factor responsible for coagulation resided within the crab's circulating blood cells, the amoebocytes. Further research revealed that the bacterial agent responsible for initiation of clot formation was endotoxin.

The endotoxin molecule activates a coagulation cascade quite similar in design to the mammalian blood coagulation cascade (Figure 3.38). Activation of the cascade also requires the

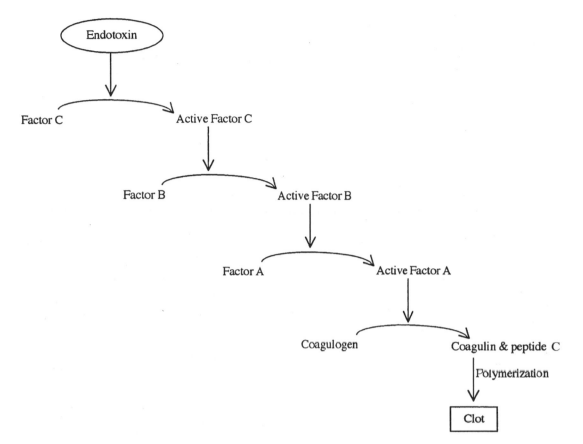

Figure 3.38. Activation of clot formation by endotoxin. The presence of endotoxin causes stepwise, sequential activation of various clotting factors present naturally within the amoebocytes of the American horseshoe crab. The net result is the generation of the polypeptide fragment coagulin, which polymerizes, thus forming a gel or clot

presence of divalent cations such as calcium or magnesium. The final steps of this pathway entail the proteolytic cleavage of the polypeptide coagulogen, forming coagulin, and a smaller peptide fragment. Coagulin molecules then interact non-covalently, forming a 'clot' or 'gel'.

The LAL-based assay for endotoxin became commercially available in the 1970s. The LAL reagent is prepared by extraction of blood from the horseshoe crab, followed by isolation of its amoebocytes by centrifugation. After a washing step, the amoebocytes are lysed, and the lysate dispensed into pyrogen-free vials. The assay is normally performed by making a series of 1:2 dilutions of the test sample using (pyrogen-free) WFI (and pyrogen-free test tubes; see later). A reference standard endotoxin preparation is treated similarly. LAL reagent is added to all tubes, incubated for 1 h, and these tubes are then inverted to test for gel (i.e. clot) formation, which would indicate presence of endotoxin.

More recently a colorimetric-based LAL procedure has been devised. This entails addition to the LAL reagent of a short peptide, susceptible to hydrolysis by the LAL clotting enzyme. This synthetic peptide contains a chromogenic tag (usually paranitroaniline, pNA) which is released free into solution by the clotting enzyme. This allows spectrophotometric analysis of the test sample, facilitating more accurate end-point determination.

The LAL system displays several advantages when compared to the rabbit test, most notably:

- *sensitivity* — endotoxin levels as low as a few picograms (pg) per ml of sample assayed will be detected;
- *cost* — the assay is far less expensive than the rabbit assay;
- *speed* — depending upon the format used, the LAL assay may be conducted within 15–60 min.

Its major disadvantage is its selectivity — it only detects endotoxin-based pyrogens. In practice, however, endotoxin represents the pyrogen by far the most likely to be present in pharmaceutical products. The LAL method is used extensively within the industry. It is used not only to detect endotoxin in finished parenteral preparations, but also in WFI and in biological fluids such as serum or cerebrospinal fluid.

Before the LAL assay is routinely used to detect/quantify endotoxin in any product, its effective functioning in the presence of that product must be demonstrated by validation studies. Such studies are required to prove that the product (or, more likely, excipients present in the product) do not interfere with the rate/extent of clot formation (i.e. are neither inhibitors nor activators of the LAL-based enzymes). LAL enzyme inhibition could facilitate false-negative results upon sample assay. Validation studies entail, for example, observing the effect of spiking endotoxin-negative product with known quantities of endotoxin, or spiking endotoxin with varying quantities of product, before assay with the LAL reagents.

All ancillary reagents used in the LAL assay system (e.g. WFI, test tubes, pipette tips for liquid transfer, etc.) must obviously be endotoxin-free. Such items can be rendered endotoxin-free by heat. Its heat-stable nature, however, renders necessary very vigorous heating in order to destroy contaminant endotoxin. A single autoclave cycle is insufficient, with total destruction requiring three consecutive autoclave cycles. Dry heat may also be used (180°C for 3 h or 240°C for 1 h).

GMP requires that, where practicable, process equipment coming into direct contact with the biopharmaceutical product stream should be rendered endotoxin-free (depyrogenated) before use. Autoclaving, steam or dry heat can effectively be used on many process vessels, pipework, etc., which are usually manufactured from stainless steel or other heat-resistant material. Such an approach is not routinely practicable in the case of some items of process equipment, such as chromatographic systems. Fortunately, endotoxin is sensitive to strongly alkaline conditions, thus routine CIP of chromatographic systems using 1 M NaOH represents an effective depyrogenation step. More gentle approaches, such as exhaustive rinsing with WFI (until an LAL test shows the eluate to be endotoxin-free) can also be surprisingly effective.

It is generally unnecessary to introduce specific measures aimed at endotoxin removal from the product during downstream processing. Endotoxin present in the earlier stages of production are often effectively removed from the product during chromatographic fractionation. The endotoxin molecule's highly negative charge often facilitates its effective removal from the product stream by ion-exchange chromatography. Gel filtration chromatography also serves to remove endotoxin from the product. While individual lipopolysaccharide molecules exhibit an average molecular mass of less than 20 kDa, these molecules aggregate in aqueous environments, generating supramolecular structures of molecular mass 100–1 000 kDa.

The molecular mass of most biopharmaceuticals is considerably less than 100 kDa (Table 3.28). The proteins would thus elute from gel-filtration columns much later than contaminating

Table 3.28. The molecular mass of some polypeptide biopharmaceuticals. Many are glycosylated, thereby exhibiting a range of molecular masses due to differential glycosylation

Protein	Molecular mass (kDa)	Protein	Molecular mass (kDa)	Protein	Molecular mass (kDa)
IFN-α	20–27	TNF-α	52*	EGF	6
IFN-β	20	GM-CSF	22	NGF	26
IFN-γ	20–25	G-CSF	21	Insulin	5.7
IL-2	15–20	EPO	36	hGH	22
IL-1	17.5	TPO	60	FSH	34
IL-12	30–35	IGF-1	7.6	LH	28.5

*Biologically active, trimeric form. IFN=interferon; IL=interleukin; TNF=tumour necrosis factor; GM-CSF= granulocyte macrophage colony stimulating factor; G-CSF=granulocyte colony stimulating factor; EPO= erythropoietin; TPO=thrombopoietin; IGF=insulin-like growth factor; EGF=epidermal growth factor; NGF= nerve growth factor; hGH=human growth hormone; FSH=follicle stimulating hormone; LH=leuteinizing hormone

endotoxin aggregates. Should the biopharmaceutical exhibit a molecular mass approaching or exceeding 100 kDa, effective separation can still be achieved by inclusion of a chelating agent, such as EDTA, in the running buffer. This promotes depolymerization of the endotoxin aggregates into monomeric (20 kDa) form.

Additional techniques capable of separating biomolecules on the basis of molecular mass (e.g. ultrafiltration) may also be used to remove endotoxin from the product stream.

DNA

The clinical significance of DNA-based contaminants in biopharmaceutical products remains unclear. Many traditional biological-based preparations, especially those such as vaccines produced in cell culture systems, have been found to consistently contain host cell-derived DNA. No adverse clinical effects related to the presence of such DNA has been reported.

The concerns relating to the presence of DNA in modern biopharmaceuticals focuses primarily upon the presence of active oncogenes in the genome of several producer cell types (e.g. monoclonal antibody production in hybridoma cell lines). Parenteral administration of DNA contaminants containing active oncogenes to patients is considered undesirable. The concern is that uptake and expression of such DNA in human cells could transform those cells, leading to cancer. There is some evidence to suggest that naked DNA can be assimilated by some cells at least, under certain conditions (Chapter 11). Guidelines to date state that an acceptable level of residual DNA in recombinant products is of the order of 10 pg per therapeutic dose.

DNA hybridization studies (e.g. the 'dot-blot' assay) utilizing radiolabelled DNA probes allows detection of DNA contaminants in the product, to levels in the nanogram (ng) range. The process begins with isolation of the contaminating DNA from the product. This can be achieved, for example, by phenol and chloroform extraction and ethanol precipitation. The isolated DNA is then applied as a spot (i.e. a 'dot') onto nitrocellulose filter paper, with subsequent baking of the filter at 80°C under vacuum. This promotes (a) DNA denaturation, yielding single strands, and (b) binding of the DNA to the filter.

A sample of total DNA derived from the cells in which the product is produced is then radiolabelled with ^{32}P using the process of nick translation. It is heated to 90°C (promotes denaturation, forming single strands) and incubated with the baked filter for several hours at 40°C. Lowering the temperature allows re-annealing of single strands via complementary base-pairing to occur. Labelled DNA will re-anneal with any complementary DNA strands immobilized on the filter. After the filter is washed (to remove non-specifically bound radiolabelled probe) it is subjected to autoradiography, which allows detection of any bound probe.

Quantification of the DNA isolated from the product involves concurrent inclusion in the dot-blot assay of a set of spots, containing known quantities of DNA and derived from the producer cell. After autoradiography, the intensity of the test spot is compared with the standards.

In many instances there is little need to incorporate specific DNA removal steps during downstream processing. Endogenous nucleases liberated upon cellular homogenization come into direct contact with cellular DNA, resulting in its degradation. Commercial DNases are sometimes added to crude homogenate to reduce DNA-associated product viscosity. Most chromatographic steps are also effective in separating DNA from the product stream. Ion-exchange chromatography is particularly effective, as DNA exhibits a large overall negative charge (due to the phosphate constituent of its nucleotide backbone).

Microbial and viral contaminants

Finished-product biopharmaceuticals, along with other pharmaceuticals intended for parenteral administration, must be sterile (the one exception being live bacterial vaccines). The presence of microorganisms in the final product is unacceptable for a number of reasons:

- parenteral administration of contaminated product would likely lead to the establishment of a severe infection in the recipient patient;
- microorganisms may be capable of metabolizing the product itself, thus reducing its potency. This is particularly true of protein-based biopharmaceuticals, as most microbes produce an array of extracellular proteases;
- microbial-derived substances secreted into the product could adversely effect the recipient's health. Examples include endotoxin secreted from Gram-negative bacteria, or microbial proteins which would stimulate an immune response.

Terminal sterilization by autoclaving guarantees product sterility. Heat sterilization, however, is not a viable option in the case of biopharmaceuticals. Sterilization of biopharmaceuticals by filtration, followed by aseptic filling into a sterile final-product container, inherently carries a greater risk of product contamination. Finished-product sterility testing of such preparations thus represents one of the most critical product tests undertaken by QC. Specific guidelines relating to sterility testing of finished products are given in international pharmacopoeias.

Biopharmaceutical products are also subjected to screening for the presence of viral particles prior to final product release. Although viruses could be introduced, e.g. via infected personnel during downstream processing, proper implementation of GMP minimizes such risk. Any viral particles found in the finished product are most likely derived from raw material sources. Examples could include HIV or hepatitis viruses present in blood used in the manufacture of blood products. Such raw materials must be screened before processing for the presence of likely viral contaminants.

A variety of murine (mouse) and other mammalian cell lines have become popular host systems for the production of recombinant human biopharmaceuticals. Moreover, most monoclonal antibodies used for therapeutic purposes are produced by murine-derived hybridoma cells. These cell lines are sensitive to infection by various viral particles. Producer cell lines are screened during product development studies to ensure freedom from a variety of pathogenic advantageous agents, including various species of bacteria, fungi, yeasts, mycoplasma, protozoa, parasites, viruses and prions. Suitable microbiological precautions must subsequently be undertaken to prevent producer cell banks from becoming contaminated with such pathogens.

Removal of viruses from the product stream can be achieved in a number of ways. The physicochemical properties of viral particles differ greatly from most proteins, ensuring that effective fractionation is automatically achieved by most chromatographic techniques. Gel-filtration chromatography, for example, effectively separates viral particles from most proteins on the basis of differences in size.

In addition to chromatographic separation, specific downstream processing steps may be undertaken which are specifically aimed at removal or inactivation of viral particles potentially present in the product stream. Significantly, many are 'blanket' procedures, equally capable of removing known or potentially likely viral contaminants, and any uncharacterized/undetected viruses. Filtration through a $0.22\,\mu m$ filter effectively removes microbial agents from the product stream, but fails to remove most viral types. Repeat filtration through a $0.1\,\mu m$ filter appears more effective in this regard. Alternatively, incorporation of an ultrafiltration step (preferably at the terminal stages of downstream processing) also proves effective.

Incorporation of downstream processing steps known to inactivate a wide variety of viral types provides further assurance that the final product is unlikely to harbour active virus. Heating and irradiation are amongst the two most popular such approaches. Heating the product to $40{-}60°C$ for several hours inactivates a broad range of viruses. Many biopharmaceuticals can be heated to such temperatures without being denatured themselves. Such an approach has been used extensively to inactivate blood-borne viruses in blood products. Exposure of product to controlled levels of UV radiation can also be quite effective, while having no adverse effect on the product itself.

Viral assays

A range of assay techniques may be used to detect and quantify viral contaminants in both raw materials and finished biopharmaceutical products. No generic assay exists that is capable of detecting all viral types potentially present in a given sample. Viral assays currently available will detect only a specific virus, or at best a family of closely related viruses. The strategy adopted, therefore, usually entails screening product for viral particles known to be capable of infecting the biopharmaceutical source material. Such assays will not normally detect newly evolved viral strains, or uncharacterized/unknown viral contaminants. This fact underlines the importance of including at least one step in downstream processing which is likely to indiscriminately inactivate or remove viruses from the product. This acts as a safety net.

Current viral assays fall into one of three categories:

- immunoassays;
- assays based on viral DNA probes;
- bioassays.

Generation of antibodies that can recognize and bind to specific viruses is straightforward. A sample of live or attenuated virus, or a purified component of the viral caspid, can be injected into animals to stimulate polyclonal antibody production (or to facilitate monoclonal antibody production by hybridoma technology). Harvested antibodies are then employed to develop specific immunoassays which can be used to routinely screen test samples for the presence of that specific virus. Immunoassays capable of detecting a wide range of viruses are available commercially. The sensitivity, ease, speed and relative inexpensiveness of these assays render them particularly attractive.

An alternative assay format entails the use of virus-specific DNA probes. These can be used to screen the biopharmaceutical product for the presence of viral DNA. The assay strategy is similar to the dot-blot assays used to detect host cell derived DNA contaminants, as discussed earlier.

Viral bioassays of various different formats have also been developed. One format entails incubation of the final product with cell lines sensitive to a range of viruses. The cells are subsequently monitored for cytopathic effects or other obvious signs of viral infection.

A range of mouse, rabbit or hamster antibody production tests (MAPs, RAPs or HAPs) may also be undertaken. These bioassays entail administration of the product to a test animal. Any viral agents present will elicit the production of anti-viral antibodies in that animal. Serum samples (withdrawn from the animal approximately 4 weeks after product administration) are screened for the presence of antibodies recognizing a range of viral antigens. This can be achieved by enzyme immunoassay, in which immobilized antigen is used to screen for the virus-specific antibodies. These assay systems are extremely sensitive, as minute quantities of viral antigen will elicit strong antibody production. A single serum sample can also be screened for antibodies specific to a wide range of viral particles. Time and expense factors, however, militate against this particular assay format.

Miscellaneous contaminants

In addition to those already discussed, biopharmaceutical products may harbour other contaminants, some of which may be intentionally added to the product-stream during the initial stages of downstream processing. Examples could include buffer components, precipitants (ethanol or other solvents, salts, etc.), proteolytic inhibitors, glycerol, anti-foam agents, etc. In addition to these, other contaminants may enter the product during downstream processing in a less controlled way. Examples could include metal ions leached from product-holding tanks/pipework, or breakdown products leaking from chromatographic media. The final product containers must also be chosen carefully. They must be chemically inert, and be of suitable quality to eliminate the possibility of leaching of any substance from the container during product storage. For this reason high-quality glass vials are often used.

In some instances it may be necessary to demonstrate that all traces of specific contaminants have been removed prior to final product filling. This would be true, for example, of many proteolytic inhibitors added during the initial stages of downstream processing to prevent proteolysis by endogenous proteases. Some such inhibitors may be inherently toxic, and many could (inappropriately) inhibit endogenous proteases of the recipient patient.

Demonstration of the absence (from the product) of breakdown products from chromatographic columns may be necessary in certain instances. This is particularly true with regard to some affinity chromatography columns. Various chemical-coupling methods may be used to attach affinity ligands to the chromatographic support material. Some such procedures entail the use of toxic reagents which, if not entirely removed after coupling, could leach into the product. In some cases, ligands can also subsequently leach from the columns, particularly after sustained usage or over-vigorous sanitation procedures. Improvements in the chemical stability of modern chromatographic media have, however, reduced such difficulties, and most manufacturers have carried out extensive validation studies regarding the stability of their products.

Sophisticated analytical methodologies facilitate detection of vanishingly low levels of many contaminants in biopharmaceutical preparations. The possibility exists, however, that uncharacterized contaminants may persist, remaining undetected in the final product. As an additional safety measure, finished products are often subjected to 'abnormal toxicity' or 'general safety' tests. Standardized protocols for such tests are outlined in various international pharmacopoeias. These normally entail parenteral administration of the product to at least five healthy mice. The animals are placed under observation for 48 h, and should exhibit no ill-effects (other than expected symptoms). The death or illness of one or more animals signals a requirement for further investigation, usually using a larger number of animals. Such toxicity testing represents a safety net, designed to expose any unexpected activities in the product which could compromise the health of the recipient.

Validation studies

Validation can be defined as 'the act of proving that any procedure, process, equipment, material, activity or system leads to the expected results'. Routine and adequate validation studies form a core principle of GMP as applied to (bio)pharmaceutical manufacture, as such studies help assure the overall safety of the finished product (Box 3.1).

All validation procedures must be carefully designed and fully documented in written format (Box 3.1). The results of all validation studies undertaken must also be documented, and retained in the plant files. As part of their routine inspection of manufacturing facilities, regulatory personnel will usually inspect a sample of these records, to ensure conformance to GMP.

Validation studies encompass all aspects of (bio)pharmaceutical manufacture. All new items of equipment must be validated before being routinely used. Initial validation studies should be comprehensive, with follow-up validation studies being undertaken at appropriate time intervals (e.g. daily, weekly or monthly). It is considered judicious to validate older items of equipment with increased frequency. Such studies can forewarn the manufacturer of impending equipment failure. Some validatory studies are straightforward, e.g. validation of weighing equipment simply entails weighing standardized weights. Autoclaves may be validated by placing external temperature probes at various points in the autoclave chamber during a routine autoclave run. Validation studies should confirm that all areas within the chamber reach the required temperature for the required time.

Periodic validation of clean room HEPA filters is also an essential part of GMP. After their installation, HEPA filters are subjected to a leak test. Particle counters are also used to validate clean room conditions. A particle counter is a vacuum cleaner-like machine capable of sucking air from its surroundings at constant velocity, and passing it through a counting chamber. The number of particles per m^3 of air tested can easily be determined. Furthermore, passage of the air through a $0.2 \mu m$ filter housed in the counter will trap all airborne microorganisms. By placing the filter on the surface of a nutrient agar-containing Petri dish, trapped microorganisms will grow as colonies, allowing determination of the microbial load per m^3 of air.

In addition to equipment, many processes/procedures undertaken during pharmaceutical manufacture are also subject to periodic validation studies. Validation of biopharmaceutical

---

Box 3.1.   Validation studies: a glossary of some important terms

Validation master plan: document that serves as an overall guide for a facility's validation programme. It identifies all items/procedures etc. which must be subjected to validation studies, describes the nature of testing in each instance and defines the responsibilities of those engaged in validation activities.

Validation protocol: document describing the specific item to be validated, the specific validation protocol to be carried out and acceptable results, as per acceptance criteria.

Prospective validation: validation undertaken prior to commencement of routine product manufacture.

Concurrent validation: validation undertaken while routine manufacture of product is also taking place.

Retrospective validation: validation carried out by review of historical records.

Qualification: how an individual element of an overall validation programme performs. When validation of that specific element is complete, it is 'qualified'. When all elements are (satisfactorily) completed, the system is validated.

Design qualification: auditing the design of a facility (or element of a facility, such as a clean room) to ensure that it is compliant with the specifications laid down and that it is therefore capable of meeting GMP requirements.

Installation qualification: auditing/testing to ensure that specific items of equipment have been correctly installed in accordance with the design specifications laid down.

Operational qualification: auditing/testing process which elevates the system being tested to make sure it is fully operational and will perform within operating specifications.

Performance qualification: demonstration that equipment/processes operate satisfactorily and consistently during the manufacture of actual product.

---

aseptic filling procedures is amongst the most critical. The aim is to prove that the aseptic procedures devised are capable of delivering a sterile finished product, as intended.

Aseptic filling validation entails substituting a batch of final product with nutrient broth. The broth is subject to sterile filtration and aseptic processing. After sealing the final product containers, they are incubated at 30–37°C, which encourages growth of any contaminant microorganisms (growth can be easily monitored by subsequently measuring the absorbance at 600 nm). Absence of growth validates the aseptic procedures developed.

Contaminant-clearance validation studies are of special significance in biopharmaceutical manufacture. As discussed in the previous section, downstream processing must be capable of removing contaminants such as viruses, DNA and endotoxin from the product stream. Contaminant-clearance validation studies normally entails spiking the raw material (from which the product is to be purified) with a known level of the chosen contaminant, and subjecting the contaminated material to the complete downstream processing protocol. This allows determination of the level of clearance of the contaminant achieved after each purification step, and the contaminant reduction factor for the overall process.

Viral clearance studies, for example, are typically undertaken by spiking the raw material with a mixture of at least three different viral species, preferably ones that represent likely product contaminants, and for which straightforward assay systems are available. Loading levels of up to 1×10^{10} viral particles are commonly used. The cumulative viral removal/inactivation observed should render the likelihood of a single viral particle remaining in a single therapeutic dose of product being greater than one in a million.

A similar strategy is adopted when undertaking DNA clearance studies. The starting material is spiked with radiolabelled DNA and then subjected to downstream processing. The level of residual DNA remaining in the product stream after each step can easily be determined by monitoring for radioactivity.

The quantity of DNA used to spike the product should ideally be somewhat in excess of the levels of DNA normally associated with the product prior to its purification. However, spiking of the product with a vast excess of DNA is counter-productive in that it may render subsequent downstream processing unrepresentative of standard production runs.

For more comprehensive validation studies, the molecular mass profile of the DNA spike should roughly approximate to the molecular mass range of endogenous contaminant DNA in the crude product. Obviously, the true DNA clearance rate attained by downstream processing procedures (e.g. gel-filtration) will depend to some extent on the molecular mass characteristics of the contaminant DNA.

Other manufacturing procedures requiring validation include cleaning, decontamination and sanitation (CDS) procedures developed for specific items of equipment/processing areas. Of particular importance is the ability of such procedures to remove bioburden. This may be assessed by monitoring levels of microbial contamination before and after application of CDS protocols, to the equipment item in question.

FURTHER READING

Books

Butler, M. (1996). *Animal Cell Culture and Technology. The Basics*. IRL Press, Oxford.

Carpenter, J. (2002). *Rational Design of Stable Protein Formulations*. Kluwer Academic, Dordrecht.

Dass, C. (2000). *Principles and Practice of Biological Mass Spectrometry*. Wiley, Chichester.

Desai, M. (2000). *Downstream Protein Processing Methods*. Humana, New York.

Flickinger, M. (1999). *The Encyclopedia of Bioprocess Technology*. Wiley, Chichester.

Frokjaer, S. (2000). *Pharmaceutical Formulation Development of Peptides and Proteins*. Taylor and Francis, London.

Grindley, J. & Ogden, J. (2000). *Understanding Biopharmaceuticals. Manufacturing and Regulatory Issues*. Interpharm Press, Denver, CO.

Harris, E. (2000). *Protein Purification Applications*. Oxford University Press, Oxford.

Janson, J. (1998). *Protein Purification*. Wiley, Chichester.

Kellner, R. (1999). *Microcharacterization of Proteins*. Wiley, Chichester.

Martindale, The Extra Pharmacopoeia, 31st edn (1996). Rittenhouse Book Distributors, USA.

Merten, O. (2001). *Recombinant Protein Production with Prokaryotic and Eucaryotic Cells*. Kluwer Academic, Dordrecht.

Oxender, D. & Post, L. (1999). *Novel Therapeutics from Modern Biotechnology*. Springer-Verlag, Berlin.

Ramstorp, M. (2000). *Contamination Control and Cleanroom Technology*. Wiley, Chichester.

Roe, S. (2001). *Protein Purification Techniques*. Oxford University Press, Oxford.

The European Pharmacopoeia, Vol. 4 (2002). Council of Europe, Strasbourg.

The Pharmaceutical Codex, Vol. 12 (1994). Pharmaceutical Press, Wallingford, UK.

The Rules Governing Medicinal Products in the European Community. (a multi-volume work; various publication dates). European Commission, Brussels.

The United States Pharmacopoeia, 26-NF 21 (2003). United States Pharmacopoeial Convention, USA.

Venn, R. (2000). *Principles and Practice of Bioanalysis*. Taylor and Francis, London.

Walsh, G. & Headon, D. (1994). *Protein Biotechnology*. Wiley, Chichester.

Walsh, G. (2002). *Proteins: Biochemistry and Biotechnology*. Wiley, Chichester.
Whyte, W. (2001). *Cleanroom Technology*. Wiley, Chichester.

Articles

Sources of biopharmaceuticals and upstream processing

Baneyx, F. (1999). Recombinant protein expression in *E. coli*. *Curr. Opin. Biotechnol.* **10**, 411–421.

Carrio, M. & Villaverde, A. (2002). Construction and deconstruction of bacterial inclusion bodies. *J. Biotechnol.* **96**(1), 3–12.

Datar, R. *et al.* (1993). Process economics of animal cell and bacterial fermentations: a case study analysis of tissue plasminogen activator. *Bio/Technology* **11**, 340–357.

Fischer, R. *et al.* (1999). Towards molecular farming in the future: using plant cell suspension cultures as bioreactors. *Biotechnol Appl. Biochem.* **30**, 109–112.

Helmrich, A. & Barnes, D. (1998). Animal cell culture equipment and techniques. *Methods Cell Biol.* **57**, 3–17.

Houdebine, L. (2000). Transgenic animal bioreactors. *Transgen. Res.* **9**(4–5), 305–320.

Hu, W. & Peshwa, M. (1993). Mammalian cells for pharmaceutical manufacturing. *Am. Soc. Microbiol. News* **59**, 65–68.

Larrick, J. & Thomas, D. (2001). Producing proteins in transgenic plants and animals. *Curr. Opin. Biotechnol.* **12**(4), 411–418.

La Vallie, E. *et al.* (1993). A thioredoxin gene fusion expression system that circumvents inclusion body formation in the *E. coli* cytoplasm. *Bio/Technology* **11**, 187–193.

Mason, H. *et al.* (2002). Edible plant vaccines: applications for prophylactic and therapeutic molecular medicine. *Trends Mol. Med.* **8**(7), 324–329.

Punt, P. *et al.* (2002). Filamentous fungi as cell factories for heterologous protein production. *Trends Biotechnol.* **20**, 5, 200–206.

Rosen, J. *et al.* (1996). The mammary gland as a bioreactor: factors resulting in the efficient expression of milk protein-based transgenes. *Am. J. Clin. Nutr.* **63**, 627S–632S.

Varley, J & Birch, J. (1999). Reactor design for large scale suspension animal cell culture. *Cytotechnology* **29**(3), 177–205.

Wright, G. *et al.* (1991). High level expression of active human α_1-antitrypsin in the milk of transgenic sheep. *Bio/Technology* **9**, 830–834.

Purification, characterization, formulation

Arakawa, T. *et al.* (2001). Factors effecting short-term and long-term stabilities of proteins. *Adv. Drug Delivery Rev.* **46**, 307–326.

Bernard, A. *et al.* (1996). Downstream processing of insect cultures. *Cytotechnology* **20**(1–3), 239–257.

Cleland, J. *et al.* (1993). The development of stable protein formulations: a close look at protein aggregation, deamidation and oxidation. *Crit. Rev. Therapeut. Drug Carrier Syst.* **10**(4), 307–377.

Ding, J. & Ho, B. (2001). A new era in pyrogen testing. *Trends Biotechnol.* **18**(8), 277–280

Geisow, M. (1991). Characterizing recombinant proteins. *Bio/Technology* **9**, 921–924.

Hoglund, M. (1998). Glycosylated and non-glycosylated recombinant human granulocyte colony stimulating factor (rhG-CSF)—what is the difference? *Med. Oncol.* **15**(4), 229–233.

Hu, S. & Dovichi, N. (2002). Capillary electrophoresis for the analysis of biopolymers. *Anal. Chem.* **74**(12) 2833–2850.

Kakehi, K. *et al.* (2002). Analysis of glycoproteins and the oligosaccharides thereof by high performance capillary electrophoresis—significance in regulatory studies on biopharmaceutical products. *Bio Chromatogr.* **16**(2), 103–115.

Keller, K. *et al.* (2001). The bioseparation needs for tomorrow. *Trends Biotechnol.* **19**(11), 438–441.

Lee, J. (2000). Biopharmaceutical formulation. *Curr. Opin. Biotechnol.* **11**(1), 81–84.

Mann, M. *et al.* (2001). Analysis of proteins and proteomes by mass spectrometry. *Ann Rev. Biochem.* **70**, 437–473.

Ullao-Aguirre, A. *et. al.* (1999). Role of glycosylation in function of follicle-stimulating hormone. *Endocrinology* **11**(3), 205–215.

Wang, W. (2000). Lyophilization and development of solid protein pharmaceuticals. *International J. Pharmaceut.* **203**(1–2), 1–60.

Wei, W. (1999). Instability, stabilization and formulation of liquid protein pharmaceuticals. *Int. J. Pharmaceut.* **185**(2), 129–188.

Willey, K. (1999). An elusive role for glycosylation in the structure and function of reproductive hormones. *Hum. Reprod. Update* **5**(4), 330–335.

Regulation and validation

Chew, N. (1993). Validation of biopharmaceutical processes. *Pharmaceut. Technol. Eur.* **5**(11), 34–39.

Dabbah, R. & Grady, L. (1998). Pharmacopoeial harmonization in biotechnology. *Curr. Opin. Biotechnol.* **9**, 307–311.

Darling, A. (2002). Validation of biopharmaceutical purification processes for virus clearance evaluation. *Mol. Biotechnol.* **21**(1), 57–83.

Glennon, B. (1997). Control system validation in multipurpose biopharmaceutical facilities. *J. Biotechnol.* **59**(1–2), 53–61.

Lubiniecki, A. (1998). Biopharmaceutical regulation—progress and challenges. *Curr. Opin. Biotechnol.* **9**, 305–306.

Seamon, K. (1998). Specifications for biotechnology-derived protein drugs. *Curr. Opin. Biotechnol.* **9**, 319–325.

Chapter 4

The cytokines — the interferon family

CYTOKINES

Cytokines are a diverse group of regulatory proteins or glycoproteins whose classification remains somewhat confusing, (Table 4.1). These molecules are normally produced in minute quantities by the body. They act as chemical communicators between various cells, inducing their effect by binding to specific cell surface receptors, thereby triggering various intracellular signal transduction events.

Most cytokines act upon or are produced by leukocytes (white blood cells), which constitute the immune and inflammatory systems (Box 4.1). They thus play a central role in regulating both immune and inflammatory function and related processes, such as haematopoiesis (the production of blood cells from haematopoietic stem cells in the adult bone marrow) and wound healing. Indeed, several immunosuppressive and anti-inflammatory drugs are now known to induce their biological effects by regulating the production of several cytokines.

The term 'cytokine' was first introduced in the mid-1970s. It was applied to polypeptide growth factors controlling the differentiation and regulation of cells of the immune system. The interferons (IFNs) and interleukins (ILs) represented the major polypeptide families classified as cytokines at that time. Additional classification terms were also introduced, including; lymphokines [cytokines such as interleukin-2 (IL-2) and interferon-γ (IFN-γ), produced by lymphocytes] and monokines [cytokines such as tumour necrosis factor-α (TNF-α) produced by monocytes]. However, classification on the basis of producing cell types also proved inappropriate, as most cytokines are produced by a range of cell types, e.g. both lymphocytes and monocytes produce IFN-α.

Initial classification of some cytokines was also undertaken on the basis of the specific biological activity by which the cytokine was first discovered, e.g. TNF exhibited cytotoxic effects on some cancer cell lines, colony stimulating factors (CSFs) promoted the growth *in vitro* of various leukocytes in clumps or colonies. This, too, proved an unsatisfactory classification mechanism, as it was subsequently shown that most cytokines display a range of biological

Biopharmaceuticals: Biochemistry and Biotechnology, Second Edition by Gary Walsh
John Wiley & Sons Ltd: ISBN 0 470 84326 8 (ppc), ISBN 0 470 84327 6 (pbk)

Table 4.1. The major proteins/protein families that constitute the cytokine group of regulatory molecules

---

The interleukins (IL-1 to IL-15)
The interferons (IFN-α, -β, -γ, -τ, -ω)
Colony stimulating factors (G-CSF, M-CSF, GM-CSF)
Tumour necrosis factors (TNF-α, -β)
The neurotrophins (NGF, BDNF, NT-3, NT-4/5)
Ciliary neurotrophic factor (CNTF)
Glial cell-derived neurotrophic factor (GDNF)
Epidermal growth factor (EGF)
Erythropoietin (EPO)
Fibroblast growth factor (FGF)
Leukaemia inhibitory factor (LIF)
Macrophage inflammatory proteins (MIP-1α, -1β, -2)
Platelet-derived growth factor (PDGF)
Transforming growth factors (TGF-α, -β)
Thrombopoietin (TPO)

Note: G-CSF = granulocyte colony stimulating factor; M-CSF = macrophage colony stimulating factor; GM-CSF = granulocyte-macrophage colony stimulating factor; NGF = nerve growth factor; BDNF = brain-derived neurotrophic factor; NT = neurotrophin.

activities, e.g. the major biological function of TNF is believed to be as a regulator of both the immune and the inflammatory response. More recently, primary sequence analysis of cytokines coupled to determination of secondary and tertiary structure reveal that most cytokines can be grouped into one of six families (Table 4.2).

As a consequence of the various approaches adopted in naming and classifying cytokines, it is hardly surprising to note that many are known by more than one name, e.g. interleukin-1 (IL-1) is also known as lymphocyte activating factor (LAF), endogenous pyrogen, leukocyte endogenous mediator, catabolin and mononuclear cell factor. This has led to even further confusion in this field.

During the 1980s, rapid developments in the areas of recombinant DNA technology and monoclonal antibody technology contributed to a greater depth of understanding of cytokine biology:

- genetic engineering allowed production of large quantities of most cytokines. These could be used for structural and functional studies of the cytokine itself, and its receptor;
- analysis of cytokine genes established the exact evolutionary relationships between these molecules;
- detection of cytokine mRNA and cytokine receptor mRNA allowed identification of the full range of sources and target cells of individual cytokines;
- hybridoma technology facilitated development of immunoassays capable of detecting and quantifying cytokines;
- inhibition of cytokine activity *in vivo* by administration of monoclonal antibodies, and more recently by gene knockout studies, continues to elucidate the physiological and pathophysiological effect of various cytokines.

The cytokine family continues to grow and often a decision to include a regulatory protein in this category is not a straightforward one. The following generalizations may be made with regard to most cytokines:

THE CYTOKINES—THE INTERFERON FAMILY 191

Box 4.1.   Leukocytes, their range and function

Leukocytes (white blood cells) encompass all blood cells that contain a nucleus, and these cells basically constitute the cells of the immune system. They thus function to protect the body by inactivating and destroying foreign agents. Certain leukocytes are also capable of recognizing and destroying altered body cells, such as cancer cells. Most are not confined exclusively to blood, but can circulate/exchange between blood, lymph and body tissues. This renders them more functionally effective by facilitating migration and congregation at a site of infection.

Leukocytes have been sub-classified into three families: mononuclear phagocytes, lymphocytes and granulocytes. These can be differentiated from each other on the basis of their interaction with a dye known as Romanowsky stain.

Mononuclear phagocytes consist of monocytes and macrophages and execute their defence function primarily by phagocytosis. Like all leukocytes, they are ultimately derived from bone marrow stem cells. Some such stem cells differentiate into monocytes, which enter the bloodstream from the bone marrow. From there, they migrate into most tissues in the body, where they settle and differentiate (mature) to become macrophages (sometimes called histocytes). Macrophages are found in all organs and connective tissue. They are given different names, depending upon in which organ they are located (hepatic macrophages are called Kupffer cells, CNS macrophages are called microglia, while lung macrophages are termed alveolar macrophages). All macrophages are effective scavenger cells, engulfing and destroying (by phagocytosis) any foreign substances they encounter. They also play an important role in other aspects of immunity by producing cytokines, and acting as antigen-presenting cells.

Lymphocytes are responsible for the specificity of the immune response. They are the only immune cells that recognize and respond to specific antigens, due to the presence on their surface of high-affinity receptors. In addition to blood, lymphocytes are present in high numbers in the spleen and thymus. They may be sub-categorized into antibody-producing B lymphocytes, T lymphocytes, which are involved in cell-mediated immunity, and null cells.

T lymphocytes may be sub-categorized on a functional basis into T helper, T cytoxic and T suppressor cells. T helper cells can produce various cytokines, which can stimulate and regulate the immune response. T cytotoxic cells can induce the lysis of cells exhibiting foreign antigen on their surfaces. As such, their major target cells are body cells infected by viruses or other intracellular pathogens (e.g. some protozoa). T suppressor cells function to dampen or suppress an activated immune response, thus functioning as an important 'off' switch.

Most T helper cells express a membrane protein termed CD4 on their surface. Most T cytotoxic and T suppressor cells produce a different cell surface protein, termed CD8. Monoclonal antibodies specifically recognizing CD4 or CD8 proteins can thus be used to differentiate between some T cell types.

Null cells are also known as 'large granular lymphocytes' but are best known as 'natural killer' (NK) cells. These represent a third lymphocyte sub-group. They are capable of directly lysing cancer cells and virally infected cells.

Box 4.1. Leukocytes, their range and function *(continued)*

The third leukocyte cell type are termed granulocytes, due to the presence of large granules in their cytoplasm. Granulocytes, many of which can be activated by cytokines, play a direct role in immunity and also in inflammation. Granulocytes can be sub-divided into three cell types, of which neutrophils (also known as polymorphonuclear leukocytes; PMN leukocytes) are the most abundant. Attracted to the site of infection, they mediate acute inflammation and phagocytose opsonized antigen efficiently due to the presence of an IgG Fc receptor on their surface. Eosinophils display a cell surface IgE receptor and thus seems to specialize in destroying foreign substances that specifically elicit an IgE response (e.g. parasitic worms). These cells also play a direct role in allergic reactions. Basophils also express IgE receptors. Binding of antigen–IgE complex prompts these cells to secrete their granule contents, which mediate hypersensitivity reactions.

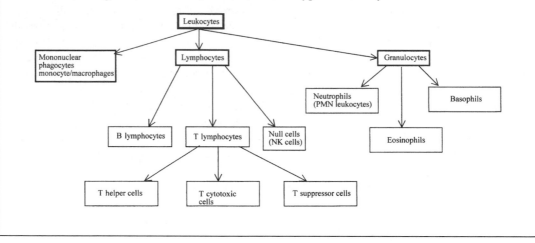

Table 4.2. Cytokines, as grouped on a structural basis

Cytokine family	Members
'β-Trefoil' cytokines	Fibroblast growth factors
	Interleukin-1
Chemokines	Interleukin-8
	Macrophage inflammatory proteins
'Cysteine knot' cytokines	Nerve growth factor
	Transforming growth factors
	Platelet-derived growth factor
EGF family	Epidermal growth factor
	Transforming growth factor-α
Haematopoietins	Interleukins 2–7, -9, -13
	Granulocyte colony stimulating factor
	Granulocyte-macrophage colony stimulating factor
	Leukaemia inhibitory factor
	Erythropoietin
	Ciliary neurotrophic factor
TNF family	Tumour necrosis factor-α and -β

- They are very potent regulatory molecules, inducing their characteristic effects at nanomolar (nM) to picomolar (pM) concentrations.
- Most cytokines are produced by a variety of cell types, which may be leukocytes or non-leukocytes, e.g. IL-1 is produced by a wide range of cells including leukocytes such as monocytes, macrophages, natural killer cells (NK cells), B and T lymphocytes, and non-leukocytes such as smooth muscle cells, vascular endothelial cells (a single layer of cells lining blood vessels), fibroblasts (cells found in connective tissue that produce ground substance and collagen fibre precursors), astrocytes (non-neural cells found in the central nervous system) and chondrocytes (cells embedded in the matrix of cartilage).
- Many cell types can produce more than one cytokine, e.g. lymphocytes produce a wide range of ILs, CSFs, TNF, IFN-α and IFN-γ. Fibroblasts can produce IL-1, IL-6, IL-8, and IL-11, CSFs, INF-β and TNF.
- Many cytokines play a regulatory role in processes other that immunity and inflammation. Neurotrophic factors such as nerve growth factor (NGF) and brain derived neurotrophic factor (BDNF) regulate growth, development and maintenance of various neural populations in the central and peripheral nervous system. Erythropoietin stimulates the production of red blood cells from erythroid precursors in the bone marrow.
- Most cytokines are pleiotropic, i.e. can effect a variety of cell types. Moreover, the effect a cytokine has on one cell type may be the same or different to its effect on a different cell type, e.g. IL-1 can induce fever, hypotension and an acute phase response. Granulocyte-colony stimulating factor (G-CSF) is a growth factor for neutrophils, but is also involved in stimulating migration of endothelial cells and growth of haematopoietic cells. IFN-γ stimulates activation and growth of T and B lymphocytes, macrophages, NK cells, fibroblasts and endothelial cells. It also displays weak anti-proliferative activity with some cell types.
- Most cytokines are inducable, and are secreted by their producer cell, e.g. induction of IL-2 synthesis and release by T-lymphocytes is promoted by binding of IL-1 to its receptor on the surface of T cells. IFN-αs are induced by viral intrusion into the body. In general, potent cytokine inducers include infectious agents, tissue injury and toxic stimuli. The body's main defence against such agents, of course, lies with the immune system and inflammation. Upon binding to target cells, cytokines can often induce the target cell to synthesize and release a variety of additional cytokines.
- In contrast, some cytokines (e.g. some CSFs and erythropoietin) appear to be expressed constitutively. In yet other instances, cytokines such as platelet-derived growth factor and transforming growth factor (TGF)-β are stored in cytoplasmic granules and can be rapidly released in response to appropriate stimuli. Other cytokines (mainly ones with growth factor activity, e.g. TGF-β, fibroblast growth factor and IL-1) are found bound to the extracellular matrix in connective tissue, bone and skin. These are released, bringing about a biological response upon tissue injury.
- Many cytokines exhibit redundancy, i.e. two or more cytokines can induce a similar biological effect. Examples include TNF-α and -β, both of which bind to the same receptor and induce very similar if not identical biological responses. This is also true of the interferon-α family of proteins and interferon-β, all of which bind the same receptor.

Although all cytokines are polypeptide regulatory factors, not all polypeptide regulatory factors are classified as cytokines. Classical polypeptide hormones such as insulin, follicle stimulating hormone (FSH) and growth hormone (GH) are not considered members of the cytokine family. The distinguishing features between these two groups are ill-defined and in many ways artificial. Originally, one obvious distinguishing feature was that hormones were produced by a multicellular, anatomically distinguishable gland (e.g. the pancreas, the pituitary, etc.) and functioned in a true endocrine fashion — affecting cells far distant from the site of their production. Many initially described cytokines are produced by white blood cells (which do not constitute a gland in the traditional sense of the word) and often function in an autocrine/paracrine manner. However, even such distinguishing characteristics have become blurred. Erythropoietin (EPO), for example, is produced in the kidney and liver and acts in an endocrine manner — promoting production of red blood cells in the bone marrow. EPO could thus also be considered to be a true hormone.

Cytokine receptors

Recombinant DNA technology has also facilitated detailed study of cytokine receptors. Based upon amino acid sequence homology, receptors are usually classified as belonging to one of six known superfamilies (Table 4.3). Individual members of any one superfamily characteristically display 20–50% homology. Conserved amino acids normally occur in discrete bands or clusters, which usually correspond to a discrete domain in the receptor. Most receptors exhibit multiple domains. In some cases a single receptor may contain domains characteristic of two or more superfamilies, e.g. the IL-6 receptor contains domains characteristic of both the haematopoietic and immunoglobulin superfamilies, making it a member of both.

Some cytokine receptors are composed of a single transmembrane polypeptide (e.g. receptors for IL-8, IL-9 and IL-10). Many contain two polypeptide components (including IL-3, IL-4 and IL-5 receptors), while a few contain three or more polypeptide components, e.g. the IL-2 receptor contains three polypeptide chains. In some instances a single cytokine may be capable of initiating signal transduction by binding two or more distinct receptors, e.g. IL-1 has two distinct receptors (types I and II), both of which are transmembrane glycoproteins.

Table 4.3. The cytokine receptor superfamilies. Refer to text for further details (see Table 4.1 for explanation of cytokine abbreviations)

Receptor superfamily name	Alternative name	Main members
The haematopoietic receptor superfamily	The cytokine receptor superfamily	Receptors for IL-2–7, -9, -12, G-CSF, GM-CSF, EPO, LIF, CNTF, GH
The Interferon receptor superfamily	Cytokine receptor type II family	Receptors for IFN-α, -β, -γ , IL-10
The immunoglobulin superfamily	–	Receptors for IL-1, IL-6, FGF, PDGF, M-CSF
Protein tyrosine kinase receptor superfamily	–	Receptors for EGF, insulin, insulin-like growth factor-1 (IGF-1)
The nerve growth factor superfamily	–	Receptors for NGF, TGF
The seven transmembrane spanning receptor superfamily	–	Receptors for various chemokines, including IL-8 and MIP
The complement control protein superfamily	–	IL-2 receptor (α-chain)

In many cases where a receptor consists of multiple polypeptides, one of those polypeptides (which will be unique to that receptor) will interact directly with the ligand. The additional polypeptide(s), responsible for initiation of signal transduction, may be shared by a number of receptors. This explains the pleiotrophy exhibited by many cytokines (Figure 4.1).

Some cytokine receptors can directly initiate signal transduction upon binding of ligand. In other cases additional elements are involved. For many receptors the exact intracellular events triggered upon ligand binding remain unelucidated. However, the molecular details of signal transduction pathways for others are now understood. Specific details of several cytokine receptors, along with their modes of signal transduction, will be discussed in the following chapters.

Cytokines as biopharmaceuticals

Cytokines constitute the single most important group of biopharmaceutical substances. As coordinators of the immune and inflammatory response, manipulation of cytokine activity can have a major influence on the body's response to a variety of medical conditions. Administration of certain cytokines can enhance the immune response against a wide range of infectious agents and cancer cells. Erythropoietin has proved effective in stimulating red blood cell production in anaemic persons. Growth factors have obvious potential in promoting wound healing. Neurotrophic factors display some clinical promise in the abatement of certain neurodegenerative diseases.

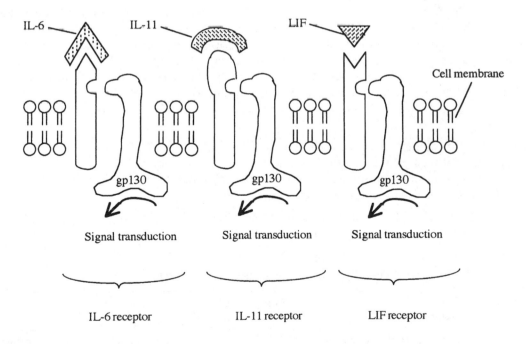

Figure 4.1. Cytokine receptors usually display a unique cytokine ('ligand')-binding domain, but share additional receptor components, which are normally responsible for signal transduction. This explains the molecular basis of pleiotropy. IL-6, IL-11 and leukaemia inhibitory factor (LIF), for example, are all composed of a distinct ligand-specific binding domain, and a separate subunit (gp130). gp130 is responsible for initiating signal transduction and is identical in all three receptors. This is depicted schematically above

A better understanding of the molecular principles underlining cytokine biology may also provide new knowledge-based strategies aimed at defeating certain viral pathogens. These pathogens appear to successfully establish an infection, at least in part, by producing specific proteins which thwart the normal cytokine-based immunological response. The Cowpox virus, for example, produces an IL-1-binding protein, while Shope fibroma virus produces a TNF-binding protein. The Epstein–Barr virus, on the other hand, produces a protein homologous to IL-10.

A variety of medical conditions are now believed to be caused or exacerbated by overproduction of certain cytokines in the body. A variety of pro-inflammatory cytokines, including IL-6 and IL-8 as well as TNF, have been implicated in the pathogenesis of both septic shock and rheumatoid arthritis. Inhibiting the biological activity of such cytokines may provide effective therapies for such conditions. This may be achieved by administration of monoclonal antibodies raised against the target cytokine, or administration of soluble forms of its receptor which will compete with cell surface receptors for cytokine binding.

Some cytokines have already gained approval for medical use. Many more are currently undergoing clinical or pre-clinical trials. Over the next few chapters, the biology and potential medical applications of these cytokines will be discussed in detail. The remainder of this chapter concerns itself with the prototypic cytokine family — the interferons.

THE INTERFERONS

Interferons (IFNs) were the first family of cytokines to be discovered. In 1957 researchers observed that if susceptible animal cells were exposed to a colonizing virus, these cells immediately become resistant to attack by other viruses. This resistance was induced by a substance secreted by virally-infected cells, which was named 'interferon' (IFN). Subsequently it has been shown that most species actually produce a whole range of interferons. Humans produce at least three distinct classes, IFN-α, IFN-β and IFN-γ (Table 4.4). These interferons are produced by a variety of different cell types, and exhibit a wide range of biological effects, including:

- induction of cellular resistance to viral attack;
- regulation of most aspects of immune function;
- regulation of growth and differentiation of many cell types;
- sustenance of early phases of pregnancy in some animal species.

No one IFN will display all of these biological activities. Effects are initiated by the binding of the IFN to its specific cell surface receptor present in the plasma membrane of sensitive cells.

Table 4.4. Human interferons (IFNs) and the cells that produce them

Interferon family	Additional name	No of distinct IFNs in family	Producing cells
IFN-α	Leukocyte IFN, B cell IFN, lymphoblast IFN	>15	Lymphocytes, monocytes, macrophages
IFN-β	Fibroblast IFN, IFN-β-1*	1	Fibroblasts, some epithelial cells
IFN-γ	Immune IFN, T cell IFN	1	T-lymphocytes, NK cells

*Originally a second cytokine was called IFN-β-2, but this was subsequently found to be actually IL-6.

IFN-α and -β display significant amino acid sequence homology (30%), bind to the same receptor, induce similar biological activities and are acid-stable. For these reasons, IFN-α and IFN-β are sometimes collectively referred to as 'type I interferons', or 'acid-stable interferons'. IFN-γ is evolutionarily distinct from the other interferons; it binds to a separate receptor and induces a different range of biological activities, and it is thus often referred to as type II interferon.

Due to their biological activities, most interferons are of actual or likely use in the treatment of many medical conditions, including:

- augmentation of the immune response against infectious agents (viral, bacterial, protozoan, etc.);
- treatment of some autoimmune conditions;
- treatment of certain cancer types.

Interferons may be detected and quantified using various bioassays or by immunoassay systems. While such assays were available, subsequent purification, characterization and medical utilization of IFNs initially proved difficult due to the tiny quantities in which these regulatory proteins are produced naturally by the body. By the early 1970s, advances in animal cell culture technology, along with the identification of cells producing increased concentrations of IFNs, made some (mostly IFN-αs) available in reasonable quantities. It was not until the advent of genetic engineering, however, that all IFNs could be produced in quantities sufficient to satisfy demand for both pure and applied purposes.

The biochemistry of interferon-α

For many years after its initial discovery, it was assumed that IFN-α represented a single gene product. It is now known that virtually all species produced multiple, closely related IFN-αs. Purification studies from the 1970s using high-resolution chromatographic techniques (mainly ion-exchange and gel-filtration chromatography, immunoaffinity chromatography and isoelectric focusing) first elucidated this fact.

In humans at least 24 related genes or pseudo-genes exist, which code for the production of at least 16 distinct mature IFN-αs. These can be assigned to one of two families, types I and II. Humans are capable of synthesizing at least 15 type I IFN-αs and a single type II IFN-α.

Most mature type I IFN-αs contain 166 amino acids (one contains 165), while type II IFN-α is composed of 172 amino acids. All are initially synthesized containing an additional 23 amino acid signal peptide. Based upon amino acid sequence data, the predicted molecular mass of all IFN-αs is in the 19–20 kDa range. SDS–PAGE analysis, however, reveals observed molecular masses up to 27 kDa. Isoelectric points determined by isoelectric focusing range between 5 and 6.5. The heterogeneity observed is most likely due to O-linked glycosylation, although several IFN-αs are not glycosylated. Some IFN-αs also exhibit natural heterogeneity due to limited proteolytic processing at the carboxyl terminus.

Individual IFN-αs generally exhibit in excess of 70% amino acid homology with each other. They are rich in leucine and glutamic acid, and display conserved cysteines (usually at positions 1, 29, 99 and 139). These generally form two disulphide bonds in the mature molecule. Their tertiary structures are similar, containing several α-helical segments, but appear devoid of β-sheets.

Individual members of the IFN-α family each have an identifying name. In most cases names were assigned by placing a letter after the 'α', (i.e. IFN-αA, IFN-αB, etc.). However, some exceptions exist, which contain a number or a number and letter, e.g. IFN-α7, IFN-α8, IFN-α2B. Just to ensure total confusion, several are known by two different names, e.g. IFN-α7 is also known as IFN-αJ1.

Interferon-β

IFN-β, normally produced by fibroblasts, was the first interferon to be purified. Humans synthesize a single IFN-β molecule containing 166 amino acid residues, which exhibits 30% sequence homology to IFN-αs. The mature molecule exhibits a single disulphide bond, and is a glycoprotein of molecular mass in excess of 20 kDa. The carbohydrate side-chain is attached via an N-linked glycosidic bond to asparigine residue 80. The carbohydrate moiety facilitates partial purification by lectin affinity chromatography. Immunoaffinity chromatography using monoclonal antibodies raised against IFN-β, as well as dye affinity chromatography, has also been employed in its purification. IFN-β's tertiary structure is dominated by five α-helical segments, three of which lie parallel to each other, with the remaining two being anti-parallel to these.

Interferon-γ

IFN-γ is usually referred to as 'immune' interferon. It was initially purified from human peripheral blood lymphocytes using techniques including concanavalin-A and dye affinity chromatography, as well as gel filtration chromatography. This IFN is produced predominantly by lymphocytes. Its synthesis by these cells is reduced when they come into contact with presented antigen. Additional cytokines, including IL-2 and IL-12 can also induce IFN-γ production under certain circumstances. A single IFN-γ gene exists, located on human chromosome number 12. It displays little evolutionary homology to type I IFN genes. The mature polypeptide contains 143 amino acids with a predicted molecular mass of 17 kDa. SDS–PAGE analysis reveals three bands of molecular mass 16–17, 20 and 25 kDa, arising because of differential glycosylation. The 20 kDa band is glycosylated at asparagine 97, while the 25 kDa species is glycosylated at asparagines 25 and 97. In addition, mature IFN-γ exhibits natural heterogeneity at its carboxyl terminus due to proteolytic processing (five truncated forms have been identified). The molecule's tertiary structure consists of six α-helical segments linked by non-helical regions.

Gel filtration analysis reveals bands of molecular mass 40–70 kDa. These represent dimers (and some multimers) of the IFN-γ polypeptide. Its biologically active form appears to be a homodimer in which the two subunits are associated in an anti-parallel manner.

Interferon signal transduction

All interferons mediate their biological effect by binding to high-affinity cell surface receptors. Binding is followed by initiation of signal transduction, culminating in an altered level of expression of several IFN-responsive genes. While both positive and negative regulation exists, thus far positive regulation (upregulation) of gene expression has been studied in greatest detail.

All IFN-stimulated genes are characterized by the upstream presence of an interferon-stimulated response element (ISRE). Signal transduction culminates in the binding of specific regulatory factors to the ISRE, which stimulates RNA polymerase II-mediated transcription of the IFN-sensitive genes. The induced gene products then mediate the anti-viral, immuno-modulatory and other effects characteristically induced by IFNs.

The interferon receptors

The availability of large quantities of purified IFNs facilitates detailed study of the interferon receptors. Binding studies using radiolabelled interferons can be undertaken, and photoaffinity crosslinking of labelled IFN to its receptor facilitates subsequent purification of the ligand–receptor complex. Recombinant DNA technology has also facilitated direct cloning of IFN receptors. Binding studies using radiolabelled type I IFNs reveals that they all compete for binding to the same receptor, whereas purified IFN-γ does not compete. Partial purification of the IFN-α receptor was undertaken by a number of means. One approach entailed covalent attachment of radiolabelled IFN-α to the receptor using bifunctional crosslinking agents, followed by purification of the radioactive complex. An alternative approach utilized an immobilized IFN-α ligand for affinity purification. The receptor has also been cloned, and the gene is housed on human chromosome number 21.

Studies have actually revealed two type I IFN receptor polypeptides. Sequence data from cloning studies place both in the class II cytokine receptor family. Both are transmembrane N-linked glycoproteins. Studies using isolated forms of each show that one polypeptide (called the α/β-receptor) is capable of binding all type I IFNs. The other one (the $\alpha\beta$-receptor) is specific for IFN-αB (a specific member of the IFN-α family). Both receptors are present on most cell types.

The IFN-γ receptor (the type II receptor) displays a more limited cellular distribution than that of the type I receptors (Table 4.5). This receptor is a transmembrane glycoprotein of molecular mass 50 kDa, which appears to function as a homodimer. The extracellular IFN-γ-binding region consists of approximately 200 amino acid residues folded into two homologous domains. Initiation of signal transduction also requires the presence of a second transmembrane glycoprotein, known as AF-1 (accessory factor 1), which associates with the extracellular region of the receptor.

The intracellular events triggered upon binding of type I or II IFNs to their respective receptors are quite similar. The sequence of events, known as the JAK–STAT pathway, has been elucidated only in the last few years. It has quickly become apparent that this pathway plays a prominent role in mediating signal transduction, not only for IFN but also for many cytokines.

The JAK–STAT pathway

Cytokine receptors can be divided into two groups; those whose intracellular domains exhibit intrinsic protein tyrosine kinase (PTK) activity, and those whose intracellular domains are

Table 4.5. Cell types that display an IFN-γ receptor on their surfaces

Haematopoietic cells	T lymphocytes
	B lymphocytes
	Macrophages
	Polymorphonuclear leukocytes
	Platelets
Somatic cells	Endothelial cells
	Epithelial cells
	Various tumour cells

devoid of such activity. Many of the latter group of receptors, however, activate intracellular soluble PTKs upon ligand binding.

Janus kinases (JAKs) represent a recently discovered family of PTKs that seem to play a central role in mediating signal transduction of many cytokines, and probably many non-cytokine regulatory molecules. These enzymes harbour two potential active sites and were thus named after Janus, the Roman god with two faces. It is likely that only one of those 'active' sites is functional. Four members of the JAK family have been best characterized to date: Jak 1, Jak 2, Jak 3 and Tyk 2. They all exhibit molecular masses in the region of 130 kDa and approximately 40% amino acid sequence homology. They appear to be associated with the cytoplasmic domain of many cytokine receptors, but remain catalytically inactive until binding of the cytokine to the receptor (Figure 4.2).

In most instances, ligand binding appears to promote receptor dimerization, bringing their associated JAKs into close proximity (Figure 4.2). The JAKs then phosphorylate — and hence activate — each other (transphosphorylation). The activated kinases subsequently phosphorylate specific tyrosine residues on the receptor itself. This promotes direct association between one or more members of a family of cytoplasmic proteins (STATs) and the receptor. Once docked at the receptor surface, the STATs are in turn phosphorylated (and hence activated) by the JAKs (Figure 4.2). As described below, activated STATs then translocate to the nucleus and directly regulate expression of IFN and other cytokine-sensitive genes.

STAT stands for 'signal transducers and activators of transcription'. As the name suggests, these proteins (a) form an integral part of cytoplasmic signal transduction initiated by certain regulatory molecules and (b) activate transcription of specific genes in the nucleus. Thus far, at least six distinct mammalian STATs (STAT 1–STAT 6) have been identified, in size ranging from 84–113 kDa. Some may be differentially spliced, increasing the number of functional proteins in the family, e.g. STAT 1 exists in two forms: STAT 1α contains 750 amino acid residues and exhibits a molecular mass of 91 kDa (it is sometimes called STAT 91); STAT 1β is a splicing variant of the same gene product, which lacks the last 38 amino acid residues at the C terminal of the protein and exhibits a molecular mass of 84 kDa (hence it is sometimes called STAT 84). Similar variants have been identified for STATs 3 and 5. STATs have also been located in non-mammalian species, such as the fruit fly. All STATs exhibit significant sequence homology and are composed of a number of functional domains (Figure 4.3). The SH2 domain functions to bind phosphotyrosine, thus docking the STAT at the activated receptor surface. As detailed below, this domain is also required for STAT interaction with JAKs (which then phosphorylates the STAT) and to promote subsequent dimerization of the STATs. An essential tyrosine is located towards the STAT C-terminus (around residue 700), which in turn is then phosplorylated by PTK. STATs are differentially distributed in various cells/tissues. STATs 1, 2 and 3 seem to be present in most cell types, allbeit at varying concentrations. Tissue distribution of STAT 4 and 5 is more limited.

Not surprisingly, different ligands activate different members of the STAT family (Table 4.6). Some, e.g. STAT 1 and 3, are activated by many ligands, while others respond to far fewer ligands, e.g. STAT 2 appears to be activated only by type I IFNs.

STAT phosphorylation ensures its binding to the receptor, with subsequent disengagement from the receptor in dimeric form. STAT dimerization is believed to involve intermolecular associations between the SH2 domain of one STAT and phosphotyrosine of its partner. Dimerization appears to be an essential prerequisite for DNA binding. Dimers may consist of two identical STATs, but STAT 1–STAT 2 and STAT 1–STAT 3 heterodimers are also frequently formed in response to certain cytokines. The STAT dimers then translocate to the

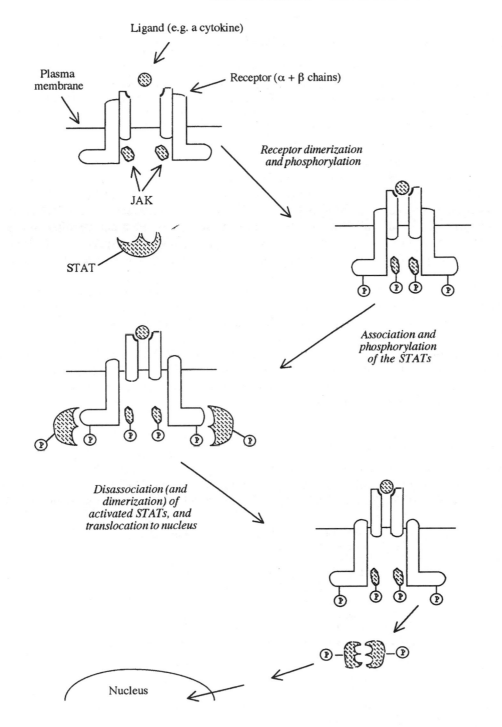

Figure 4.2. Simplified overview of the signal transduction process mediated by the JAK–STAT pathway. Refer to text for specific details

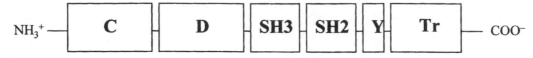

Figure 4.3. Schematic representation of the general domain structure of a STAT protein. A conserved ('C' or 'con') domain is located at the N-terminus, followed by the DNA-binding domain (D). Y represents a short sequence that contains the tyrosine residue phosphorylated by the Janus kinase. The carboxyl terminus domain (T_r) represents a transcriptional activation domain

nucleus, where they bind to specific DNA sequences (STAT 2-dependent signalling represents a partial exception; this STAT forms a complex with STAT 1 and a non-STAT cytoplasmic protein (p48) and this complex translocates to the nucleus and binding of this complex to the DNA is believed not to directly involve STAT-2). STATs bind specific sequences of DNA which approach symmetry or are palindromic (often TTCC X GGAA, where X can be different bases). These sequences are normally present in upstream regulatory regions of specific genes. Binding of the STAT complex enhances transcription of these genes, and the gene products mediate the observed cellular response to cytokine binding.

A number of proteins which inhibit JAK–STAT function have also been identified. These include members of the so-called SOCS/Jab/Cis family and the PIAS family of regulatory proteins. Several appear to function by inhibiting the activation of various STATs, although the mechanisms by which this is achieved remain to be elucidated in detail. The JAK–STAT pathway probably does not function in isolation within the cell. JAKs are believed to activate elements of additional signalling pathways, while STATs are also likely activated by factors other than JAKs. As such, there may be considerable cross-talk between various JAK- and/or STAT-dependent signalling pathways.

The interferon JAK–STAT pathway

Binding of type I interferons to the IFN-α/β (type I) receptor results in the phosphorylation and hence activation of two members of the JAK family; Tyk2 and JAK 1. These kinases then phosphorylate STAT 1α (also called STAT 91), STAT 1β (STAT 84) and STAT 2 (STAT 113).

Table 4.6. Ligands which, upon binding to their cell surface receptors, are known to promote activation of one or more STATs (the STATs activated are also shown). This list, while representative, is not exhaustive

Ligand	STAT-activated
IFN-α	1, 2, 3
IFNγ	1
IL-2	1, 3, 5
IL-3	5
IL-6	1, 3
GM-CSF	5
EGF	1, 3
GH	1, 3, 5

The three activated STATs disengage from the receptor and bind to the cytoplasmic protein, p48. This entire complex translocates to the nucleus, where it interacts directly with upstream regulatory regions of IFN-sensitive genes. These nucleotide sequences are termed interferon-stimulated response elements (ISREs). This induces/augments expression of specific genes, as discussed later.

The essential elements of the signal transduction pathway elicited by IFN-γ is even more straightforward. IFN-γ binding to the type II receptor induces receptor dimerization with consequent activation of JAK 1 and JAK 2. The JAKs phosphorylate the receptor and subsequently the associated STAT 1α. STAT 1α is then released and forms a homodimer which translocates to the nucleus. It regulates expression of IFN-γ-sensitive genes by binding to a specific upstream regulatory sequence of the gene (the IFN-γ-activated sequence, GAS). The PIAS-1 protein appears to play an inhibitory role in this pathway. By complexing with (phosphorylated) STAT 1 proteins, it inhibits DNA binding and transactivation.

The biological effects of interferons

Interferons induce a wide range of biological effects. Generally, type I IFNs induce similar effects, which are distinct from the effects induced by IFN-γ. The most pronounced effect of type I IFNs relates to their anti-viral activity, as well as their anti-proliferative effect on various cell types, including certain tumour cell types. Anti-tumour effects are likely due not only to a direct anti-proliferative effect on the tumour cells themselves but also due to the ability of type I IFNs to increase natural killer (NK) cell and T cytotoxic cell activity. These cells can recognize and destroy cancer cells.

Not all type I IFNs induce exactly the same range of responses, and the anti-viral:anti-proliferative activity ratio differs from one type I IFN to another. As all bind the same receptor, the molecular basis by which variation in biological activities is achieved, is poorly understood as yet.

IFN-γ exhibits at best weak anti-viral and anti-proliferative activity. When co-administered with type I IFNs, however, it potentates these IFN-α/β activities. IFN-γ is directly involved in regulating most aspects of the immune and inflammatory responses. It promotes activation, growth and differentiation of a wide variety of cell types involved in these physiological processes (Table 4.7).

IFN-γ represents the main macrophage activating factor, thus enhancing macrophage-mediated effects, including:

Table 4.7. Cell types participating in the immune, inflammatory or other responses whose activation, growth and differentiation is promoted by IFN-γ

Macrophages/monocytes
Polymorphonuclear neutrophils
T lymphocytes
B lymphocytes
NK cells
Fibroblasts
Endothelial cells

- destruction of invading microorganisms;
- destruction of intracellular pathogens;
- tumour cell cytotoxicity;
- increased major histocompatibility complex (MHC) antigen expression, leading to enhanced activation of lymphocytes via antigen presentation.

Binding of IFN-γ to its surface receptor on polymorphonuclear neutrophils induces increased expression of the gene coding for a neutrophil cell surface protein capable of binding the Fc portion (i.e. the constant region: see also Box 10.2) of immunoglobulin (IgG). This greatly increases the phagocytotic and cytotoxic activities of these cells.

IFN-γ also directly modulates the immune response by affecting growth, differentiation and function of both T and B lymphocytes. These effects are quite complex, and are often influenced by additional cytokines. IFN-γ acts as a growth factor in an autocrine manner for some T cell sub-populations, while it is capable of suppressing growth of other T cell types. It appears to have an inhibitory effect on development of immature B lymphocyte populations but may support mature B cell survival. It can both upregulate and downregulate antibody production under various circumstances.

All IFNs promote increased surface expression of class I MHC antigens. Class II MHC antigen expression is stimulated mainly by IFN-γ (MHC proteins are found on the surface of various cell types. They play an essential role in triggering an effective immune response, not only against foreign antigen but also against altered host cells). While many IFNs promote synergistic effects, some instances are known where two or more IFNs can oppose each other's biological activities. IFN-αJ, for example, can inhibit the IFN-αA-mediated stimulation of NK cells.

The molecular basis by which IFNs promote their characteristic effects, particularly anti-viral activity, is understood at least in part. IFN stimulation of the JAK–STAT pathway induces synthesis of at least 30 different gene products, many of which cooperate to inhibit viral replication. These anti-viral gene products are generally enzymes, the most important of which are 2'-5' oligoadenylate synthetase (2, 5-A_n synthetase) and the eIF-2α protein kinase.

These intracellular enzymes remain in an inactive state after their initial induction. They are activated only when the cell comes under viral attack, and their activation can inhibit viral replication in that cell. The 2'-5' A_n, synthetase acts in concert with two additional enzymes — an endoribonuclease and a phosphodiesterase — to promote and regulate the anti-viral state (Figure 4.4).

Several active forms of the synthetase seem to be inducable in human cells; 40 kDa and 46 kDa variants have been identified which differ only in their carboxyl terminus ends. They are produced as a result of differential splicing of mRNA transcribed from a single gene found on chromosome 11. A larger 85–100 kDa form of the enzyme has been detected, which may represent a heterodimer composed of the 40 and 46 kDa variants.

The synthetase is activated by double-stranded RNA (dsRNA). Although not normally present in human cells, dsRNA is often associated with commencement of replication of certain viruses. The activated enzyme catalyses the synthesis of oligonucleotides of varying length in which the sole base is adenine (2'-5'A_n). This oligonucleotide differs from oligonucleotides present naturally in the cell in that the phosphodiester bonds present are 2'-5' bonds (Figure 4.5). The level of synthesis and average polymer length of the oligonucleotide products appear to depend upon the exact inducing IFN type, as well as the growth state of the cell.

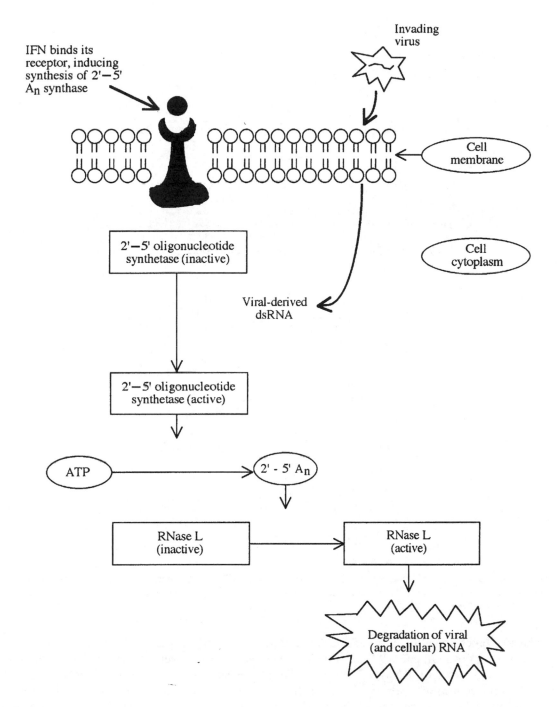

Figure 4.4. Outline of how the $2'–5'$ synthetase system promotes its anti-viral effect. The $2'–5'$ phosphodiesterase 'off switch' is omitted for clarity. Refer to text for details

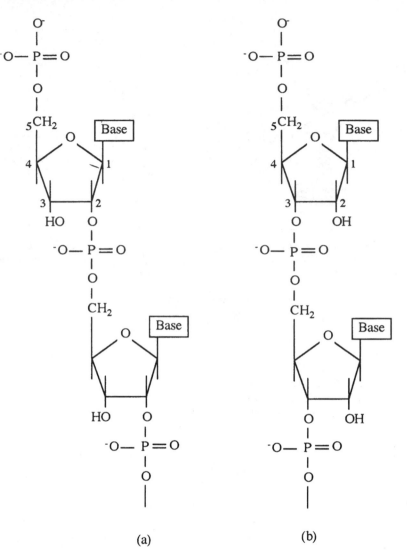

Figure 4.5. (a) Structural detail of the $2'-5'$ oligonucleotides ($2'-5'A_n$) generated by $2'-5'$ A_n synthetase. Compare the $2'-5'$ phosphodiester linkages with the $3'-5'$ linkages characteristic of normal cellular oligonucleotides, such as mRNA (b)

The sole biochemical function of $2'-5'A_n$ (and hence $2'-5'$ A_n synthetase) appears to be as an activator of a dormant endo-RNase, which is expressed constitutively in the cell. This RNase, known as RNase L or RNase F, cleaves all types of single-stranded RNA (ssRNA). This inhibits production of both viral and cellular proteins, thus paralyzing viral replication. Presumably cellular destruction of the invading ssRNA will be accompanied by destruction of any additional viral components. Removal of dsRNA would facilitate deactivation of the endo RNase, allowing translation of cellular mRNA to resume. A $2'-5'$-phosphodiesterase represents a third enzymatic component of this system. It functions as an off switch, as it rapidly degrades the $2'$-$5'$ A_n oligonucleotides. Although this enzyme also appears to be expressed constitutively, IFN binding appears to increase its expression levels in most cells.

The eIF-2α protein kinase system

Intracellular replication of viral particles entirely depends upon successful intracellular transcription of viral genes with subsequent translation of the viral mRNA. Translation of viral or cellular mRNA is dependent upon ribosome formation. Normally several constituent molecules interact with each other on the mRNA transcript, forming the smaller ribosomal subunit. Subsequent formation/attachment of the larger subunit facilitates protein synthesis.

Exposure of cells to IFN normally results in the induction of a protein kinase termed eIF-2α protein kinase. The enzyme, which is synthesized in a catalytically inactive form, is activated by exposure to dsRNA. The activated kinase then phosplorylates its substrate, eIF-2α, which is the smallest subunit of initiation factor 2 (eIF$_2$). This in turn blocks construction of the smaller ribosomal sub-unit, thereby preventing translation of all viral (and cellular) mRNA (Figure 4.6).

Induction of eIF-2α protein kinase is dependent upon both IFN type and cell type. IFN-α, -β and -γ are all known to induce the enzyme in various animal cells. However, in human epithelial cells the kinase is induced only by type I IFNs, while none of the IFNs seems capable of inducing synthesis of the enzyme in human fibroblasts. The purified kinase is highly selective for initiation factor eIF-2, which it phosplorylates at a specific serine residue.

Interferon, in particular type I IFN, is well adapted to its anti-viral function. Upon entry into the body, viral particles are likely to quickly encounter IFN-α/β-producing cells, including macrophages and monocytes. This prompts IFN synthesis and release. These cells act like sentries, warning other cells of the viral attack. Most body cells express the type I IFN receptor, thus the released IFN-α or -β will induce an anti-viral state in such cells.

The ability of IFNs (especially type I IFNs) to induce an anti-viral state is unlikely to be solely dependent upon the enzymatic mechanisms discussed above. Furthermore, the $2'$-$5'A_n$ synthetase and eIF-2α kinase systems may play important roles in mediating additional IFN actions. The ability of such systems to stall protein synthesis in cells may play a role in IFN-induced alterations of cellular differentiation or cell cycle progression. They may also be involved in mediating IFN-induced anti-proliferative effects on various transformed cells.

Major histocompatibility complex (MHC) antigens and β2-macroglobulin are amongst the best known proteins whose synthesis is also induced in a variety of cell types in response to various interferons.

Additional studies focus upon identification and characterization of gene products whose cellular levels are decreased in response to IFN binding, e.g. studies using various human and animal cell lines found that IFN-α and -β can induce a significant decrease in the level of c-myc and c-fos mRNA in some cells. IFN-γ has also been shown to inhibit collagen synthesis in fibroblasts and chondrocytes. Such studies, elucidating the function of gene products whose cellular levels are altered by IFNs, will eventually lead to a more complete picture of how these regulatory molecules induce their characteristic effects.

Interferon biotechnology

The anti-viral and anti-proliferative activity of IFNs, as well as their ability to modulate the immune and inflammatory response, renders obvious their potential medical application. This has culminated in the approval for clinical use of several interferon preparations (Table 4.8).

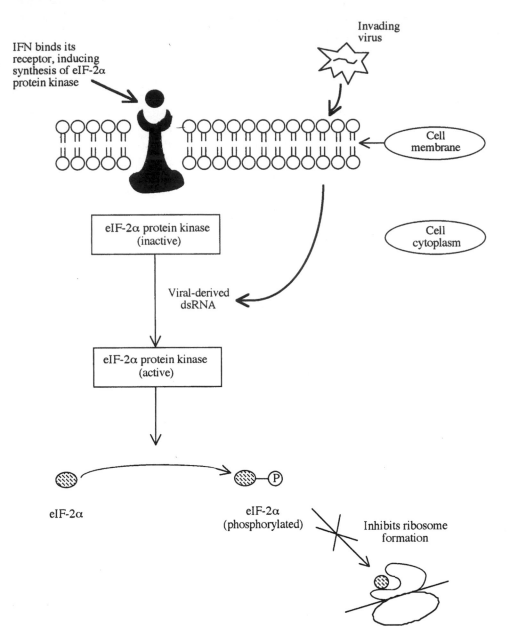

Figure 4.6.   Outline of how the eIF-2α protein kinase system promotes an anti-viral effect

Ongoing clinical trials are likely to expand considerably the medical uses of these regulatory molecules over the next few years.

While at least some of these potential therapeutic applications were appreciated as far back as the late 1950s, initial therapeutic application was rendered impractical due to the extremely low

Table 4.8.   Interferon-based biopharmaceuticals approved to date for general medical use

Product	Company	Indication
Intron A (rIFN-α-2B)	Schering Plough	Cancer, genital warts, hepatitis
PegIntron A (PEGylated rIFN-α-2B)	Schering Plough	Chronic hepatitis C
Viraferon (rIFN-α-2B)	Schering Plough	Chronic hepatitis B and C
ViraferonPeg (PEGylated rIFN-α-2B)	Schering Plough	Chronic hepatitis C
Roferon A (rhIFN-α-2A)	Hoffman–La-Roche	Hairy cell leukaemia
Actimmune (rhIFN-γ-IB)	Genentech	Chronic granulomatous disease
Betaferon (rIFN-β-1B, differs from human protein in that Cys 17 is replaced by Ser)	Schering AG	Multiple sclerosis
Betaseron (rIFN-β-1B, differs from human protein in that Cys 17 is replaced by Ser)	Berlex Laboratories and Chiron	Relapsing, remitting multiple sclerosis
Avonex (rhIFN-β-1A)	Biogen	Relapsing multiple sclerosis
Infergen (rIFN-α, synthetic type I interferon)	Amgen (USA) Yamanouchi Europe (EU)	Chronic hepatitis C
Rebif (rh IFN-β-1A)	Ares Serono	Relapsing/remitting multiple sclerosis
Rebetron (combination of ribavirin and rhIFN-α-2B)	Schering Plough	Chronic hepatitis C
Alfatronol (rhIFN-α-2B)	Schering Plough	Hepatitis B, C and various cancers
Virtron (rhIFN-α-2B)	Schering Plough	Hepatitis B and C
Pegasys (PEGinterferon α-2A)	Hoffman La Roche	Hepatitis C
Vibragen Omega (rFeline interferon-ω)	Virbac	Veterinary (reduce mortality/ clinical signs of canine parvovirusis)

levels at which they are normally produced in the body. Large-scale purification from sources such as blood was non-viable. Furthermore, IFNs exhibit species preference, and in some cases, strict species specificity. This rendered necessary the clinical use of only human-derived interferons in human medicine.

Up until the 1970s, IFN was sourced, in small quantities, directly from human leukocytes obtained from transfused blood supplies. This 'interferon' preparation actually consisted of a mixture of various IFN-αs, present in varying amounts, and was only in the regions of 1% pure. However, clinical studies undertaken with such modest quantities of impure IFN preparations produced encouraging results.

The production of IFN in significant quantities first became possible in the late 1970s, by means of mammalian cell culture. Various cancer cell lines were found to secrete IFNs in greater than normal quantities, and were amenable to large-scale cell culture due to their transformed nature. Moreover, hybridoma technology facilitated development of sensitive IFN immuno-assays. The Namalwa cell line (a specific strain of human lymphoblastoid cells) became the major industrial source of IFN. The cells were propagated in large animal cell fermenters (up to 8000 litres) and subsequent addition of an inducing virus (usually the Sendai virus) resulted in production of significant quantities of leukocyte interferon. Subsequent analysis showed this to consist of at least eight distinct IFN-α subtypes.

Wellferon is the trade name given to one such approved product. Produced by large-scale mammalian (lymphoblastoid) cell cultures, the crude preparation undergoes extensive chromatographic purification, including two immuno-affinity steps. The final product contains nine IFN-α subtypes.

Recombinant DNA technology also facilitated the production of IFNs in quantities large enough to satisfy potential medical needs. The 1980s witnessed the cloning and expression of most IFN genes in a variety of expression systems. The expression of specific genes obviously yielded a product containing a single IFN (sub)-type.

Most IFNs have now been produced in a variety of expression systems including *E. coli*, fungi, yeast and also some mammalian cell lines such as Chinese hamster ovary (CHO) cell lines and monkey kidney cell lines. Most IFNs currently in medical use are recombinant human (rh) products produced in *E. coli*. The inability of *E. coli* to carry out post-translational modifications is in most instances irrelevant, as the majority of human IFN-αs, as well as IFN-β, are not normally glycosylated. While IFN-γ is glycosylated, the *E. coli*-derived unglycosylated form displays a biological activity identical to the native human protein.

The production of IFN in recombinant microbial systems obviously means that any final product contaminants will be microbial in nature. A high degree of purification is thus required to minimize the presence of such non-human substances. Most IFN final product preparations are in the region of 99% pure. Such purity levels are achieved by extensive chromatographic purification. While standard techniques such as gel filtration and ion-exchange are extensively used, reported IFN purification protocols have also entailed the use of various affinity techniques, e.g. using anti-IFN monoclonal antibodies, reactive dyes or lectins (for glycosylated IFNs). Hydroxyapatite, metal-affinity and hydrophobic interaction chromatography have also been employed in purification protocols. Many production columns are run in fast protein or high-performance liquid chromotography (FPLC or HPLC) format, yielding improved and faster resolution. Immunoassays are used to detect and quantify the IFNs during downstream processing, although the product (particularly the finished product) is also usually subjected to a relevant bioassay. The production and medical uses of selected IFNs are summarized in the sections below.

Production and medical uses of IFN-α

Clinical studies undertaken in the late 1970s, with multi-component, impure IFN-α preparations, clearly illustrated the therapeutic potential of such interferons as an anti-cancer agent. These studies found that IFN-α could induce regression of tumours in significant numbers of patients suffering from breast cancer, certain lymphomas (malignant tumour of the lymph nodes) and multiple myeloma (malignant disease of the bone marrow). The IFN preparations could also delay recurrence of tumour growth after surgery in patients suffering from osteogenic sarcoma (cancer of connective tissue involved in bone formation).

The first recombinant IFN to become available for clinical studies was IFN-α2A, in 1980. Shortly afterwards the genes coding for additional IFN-αs were cloned and expressed, allowing additional clinical studies. The anti-viral, anti-tumour and immuno-modulatory properties of these IFNs assured their approval for a variety of medical uses. rhIFN-αs manufactured/ marketed by a number of companies (Table 4.8) are generally produced in *E. coli*.

Clinical trials have shown the recombinant IFNs to be effective in the treatment of various cancer types, with rhIFN-α2A and -α2B both approved for treatment of hairy cell leukaemia. This is a rare B lymphocyte neoplasm for which few effective treatments were previously available. Administration of the rIFNs promotes significant regression of the cancer in up to 90% of patients.

Table 4.9. Some of the indications (i.e. medical conditions) for which intron A is approved. Note that the vast majority are either forms of cancer or viral infections

Hairy cell leukaemia	Laryngeal papillomatosis*
Renal cell carcinoma	Mycosis fungoides**
Basal cell carcinoma	Condyloma acuminata ***
Malignant melanoma	Chronic hepatitis B
AIDS-related Kaposi's sarcoma	Hepatitis C
Multiple myeloma	Chronic hepatitis D
Chronic myelogenous leukaemia	Chronic hepatitis, non-A,
Non-Hodgkin's lymphoma	non-B/C hepatitis

*Benign growths (papillomas) in the larynx.
**A fungal disease.
***Genital warts.

Schering Plough's rhIFN α-2B (Intron A) was first approved in the USA in 1986 for treatment of hairy cell leukaemia, but is now approved for use in more than 50 countries for up to 16 indications (Table 4.9). The producer microorganism is *E. coli*, which harbours a cytoplasmic expression vector (KMAC-43) containing the IFN gene. The gene product is expressed intracellularly and in soluble form. Intron A manufacturing facilities are located in New Jersey and Brinny, County Cork, Ireland.

Upstream processing (fermentation) and downstream processing (purification and formulation) are physically separated by being undertaken in separate buildings. Fermentation is generally undertaken in specially designed 42 000 litre stainless steel vessels. After recovery of the product from the cells, a number of chromatographic purification steps are undertaken, essentially within a large cold room adapted to function under clean room conditions. Crystallization of the IFN-α-2B is then undertaken as a final purification step. The crystalline product is redissolved in phosphate buffer, containing glycine and human albumin as excipients. After aseptic filling, the product is normally freeze-dried. Intron A is usually sold at five commercial strengths (3, 5, 10, 25 and 50 million IU/vial).

More recently, a number of modified recombinant interferon products have also gained marketing approval. These include PEGylated interferons (PEG IntronA and Viraferon Peg (Table 4.8) and the synthetic IFN product, Infergen). PEGylated interferons are generated by reacting purified α-IFNs with a chemically activated form of polyethylene glycol (Chapter 3). Activated methoxypolyethylene glycol is often used, which forms covalent linkages with free amino groups on the IFN molecule. Molecular mass analysis of PEGylated IFNs (e.g. by mass spectroscopy, gel filtration or SDS–PAGE) indicate that the approved PEGylated products consist predominantly of monoPEGylated IFN molecules, with small amounts of both free and diPEGylated species also being present.

The intrinsic biological activity of PEGylated and non-PEGylated IFNs are essentially the same. The PEGylated product, however, displays a significantly prolonged plasma half-life (13–25 h as compared to 4 h for unPEGylated species). The prolonged half-life appears to be mainly due to slower elimination of the molecule, although PEGylation also appears to decrease systemic absorption from the site of injection following subcutaneous administration.

Infergen (interferon αcon-1, or consensus interferon) is an engineered IFN recently approved for the treatment of hepatitis C (Table 4.8). The development of Infergen entailed initial sequence comparisons between a range of IFN-αs. The product's amino acid sequence reflects the most frequently occurring amino acid residue in each corresponding position of these native IFNs. A DNA sequence coding for the product was synthesized and inserted into *E. coli*. The recombinant product accumulates intracellularly as inclusion bodies (Chapter 3).

Large-scale manufacture entails an initial fermentation step. After harvest, the *E. coli* cells are homogenized and the inclusion bodies recovered via centrifugation. After solubilization and re-folding, the interferon is purified to homogeneity by a combination of chromatographic steps. The final product is formulated in the presence of a phosphate buffer and sodium chloride. It is presented as a 30 μg/ml solution in glass vials and displays a shelf-life of 24 months when stored at 2–8°C. When compared on a mass basis, the synthetic interferon displays higher antiviral, antiproliferative and cytokine-inducing activity than do native type I interferons.

Ongoing clinical trials continue to assess the efficacy of rIFN preparations in treating a variety of cancers. Some trials suggest that treatments are most effective when administered in the early stages of cancer development. rhIFN-αs have also proved effective in the treatment of various viral conditions, most notably viral hepatitis. Hepatitis refers to an inflammation of the liver. It may be induced by toxic substances, immunological abnormalities or by viruses (infectious hepatitis). The main viral causative agents are:

- hepatitis A virus (hepatitis A);
- hepatitis B virus (hepatitis B, i.e. classical serum hepatitis);
- hepatitis C virus (hepatitis C, formerly known as classical non-A, non-B hepatitis);
- hepatitis D virus (hepatitis D, i.e. delta hepatitis);
- hepatitis E virus (hepatitis E, i.e. endemic non-A, non-B hepatitis);
- hepatitis GB agent.

This disease may be acute (rapid onset, often accompanied by severe symptoms but of brief duration) or chronic (very long duration).

Hepatitis A is common, particularly in areas of poor sanitation, and is transmitted by food or drink contaminated by a sufferer/carrier. Clinical symptoms include jaundice, and are usually mild. A full recovery is normally recorded. Hepatitis B is transmitted via infected blood. Symptoms of acute hepatitis B include fever, chill, weakness and jaundice. Most sufferers recover from such infection, although acute liver failure and death sometimes occur; 5–10% of sufferers go on to develop chronic hepatitis B. Acute hepatitis C is usually mild and asymptomatic. However, up to 90% of infected persons go on to develop a chronic form of the condition. Hepatitis D is unusual in that it requires the presence of hepatitis B in order to replicate. It thus occurs in some persons concomitantly infected with hepatitis B virus. Its clinical symptoms are usually severe, and can occur in acute or chronic form.

Chronic forms of hepatitis (in particular B, C and D) can result in liver cirrhosis and/or hepatocellular carcinoma. This occurs in up to 20% of chronic hepatitis B sufferers, and up to 30% of chronic hepatitis C sufferers. The scale of human suffering caused by hepatitis on a worldwide basis is enormous. Approximately 5% of the global population suffer from chronic hepatitis B. An estimated 50 million new infections occur each year. Over 1.5 million of the 300 million carriers worldwide die annually from liver cirrhosis and hepatocellular carcinoma.

IFN-α2B is now approved in the USA for the treatment of hepatitis B and C. Clinical studies undertaken with additional IFN-α preparations indicate their effectiveness in managing such conditions, and several such products are also likely to gain regulatory approval.

IFN-α2A, when administered three times weekly for several weeks/months, was found effective in treating several forms of hepatitis. Remission is observed in 30–45% of patients suffering from chronic hepatitis B, while a complete recovery is noted in up to 20% of cases. The drug induces sustained remission in up to 30% of patients suffering from chronic hepatitis C, but can ease clinical symptoms of this disease in up to 75% of such patients. Ongoing studies also indicate its efficacy in treating chronic hepatitis D, although relapse is frequently observed upon cessation of therapy. The drug is normally administered by the intramuscular (i.m.) or subcutaneous (s.c.—directly beneath the skin) injection. Peak plasma concentrations of the IFN are observed more quickly upon i.m. injection (4 h versus 7.5 h). The elimination half-life of the drug ranges from 2.5 to 3.5 h.

IFN-α preparations have also proved efficacious in the treatment of additional viral-induced medical conditions. rhIFN-α2B, as well as IFN-αn3 are already approved for the treatment of sexually transmitted genital warts, caused by a human papilloma virus. While this condition is often unresponsive to various additional therapies, direct injection of the IFN into the wart causes its destruction in up to 70% of patients. Another member of the papilloma virus family is associated with the development of benign growths in the larynx (laryngeal papillomatosis). This condition can be successfully treated with IFN-α preparations, as can certain papilloma-related epithelial cell cancers, such as cervical intraepithelial neoplasm (epithelial cells are those that cover all external surfaces of the body, and line hollow structures—with the exception of blood and lymph vessels). IFN-α's ability to combat a range of additional virally-induced diseases, including AIDS, is currently being appraised in clinical trials.

Medical uses of IFN-β

RhIFN-β has found medical application in the treatment of relapsing–remitting multiple sclerosis (MS), a chronic disease of the nervous system. This disease normally presents in young adults (more commonly women) aged 20–40. It is characterized by damage to the myelin sheath, which surrounds neurons of the central nervous system, and in this way compromises neural function. Clinical presentations include shaky movement, muscle weakness, paralysis, defects in speech, vision and other higher mental functions. The most predominant form of the condition is characterized by recurrent relapses followed by remission. MS appears to be an autoimmune disease, in which elements of immunity (mainly lymphocytes and macrophages) cooperate in the destruction of the myelin. What triggers onset of the condition is unknown, although genetic and environmental factors (including viral infection) have been implicated.

IFN-β preparations approved for medical use to date include Betaferon, Betaseron, Avonex and Rebif (Table 4.8). The former two products are produced in recombinant *E. coli* cells, whereas the latter two are produced in CHO cell lines. Manufacture using *E. coli* generates a non-glycosylated product, although lack of native glycosylation does not negatively affect its therapeutic efficacy. Typically, IFN-β-based drugs reduce the frequency of relapses by about 30% in many patients. In some instances, a sustained reduction in the accumulation of MS brain lesions (as measured by magnetic resonance imaging) is also observed. However, there is little evidence that IFN-β significantly alters overall progression of the disease. A summary overview of the production of one such product (Betaferon) is presented in Figure 4.7.

The molecular mechanism by which IFN-β induces its therapeutic effect is complex and not fully understood. It is believed that the pathology of multiple sclerosis is linked to the activation and proliferation of T lymphocytes specific for epitopes found on specific myelin antigens. Upon migration to the brain, these lymphocytes trigger an inflammatory response mediated by the production of pro-inflammatory cytokines, most notably IFN-γ, IL-1, IL-2 and TNF-α. The inflammatory response, in addition to other elements of immunity (e.g. antibodies and

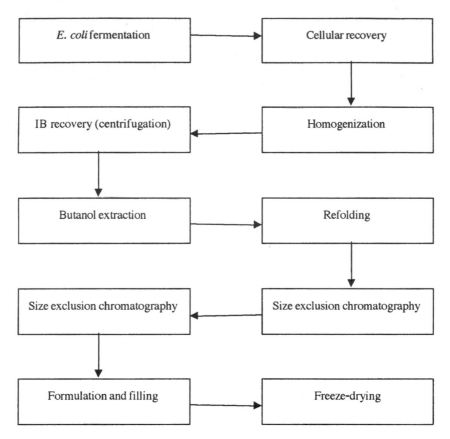

Figure 4.7. Overview of the manufacture of Betaferon, a recombinant human IFN-β produced in *E. coli*. The product differs from native human IFN-β in that it is unglycosylated and cysteine residue 17 had been replaced by a serine residue. *E. coli* fermentation is achieved using minimal salts/glucose media and product accumulates intracellularly in inclusion body (IB) form. During downstream processing, the IBs are solubilized in butanol, with subsequent removal of this denaturant to facilitate product re-folding. After two consecutive gel filtration steps excipients are added, the product is filled into glass vials and freeze-dried. It exhibits a shelf-life of 18 months when stored at 2–8°C

complement activation), results in the destruction of myelin surrounding neuronal axons. IFN-β probably counteracts these effects in part at least by inhibiting production of IFN-γ and TNF-α and hence mediating downregulation of the pro-inflammatory response.

Medical applications of IFN-γ

The most notable medical application of IFN-γ relates to the treatment of chronic granulomatous disease (CGD), a rare genetic condition, with a population incidence of 1 in 250 000–1 in a million. Phagocytic cells of patients suffering from CGD are poorly capable or incapable of ingesting or destroying infectious agents such as bacteria or protozoa. As a result, patients suffer from repeated infections (Table 4.10), many of which can be life-threatening.

Table 4.10. Some pathogens (bacterial, fungal and protozoal) whose phagocyte-mediated destruction is impaired in persons suffering from chronic granulomatous disease (CGD). Administration of IFN-γ, in most cases, enhances the phagocytes' ability to destroy these pathogens. These agents can cause hepatic and pulmonary infections, as well as genito-urinary tract, joint and other infections

Staphylococcus aureus	*Plasmodium falciparum*
Listeria monocytogenes	*Leishmania donovani*
Chlamydia psittaci	*Toxoplasma gondii*
Aspergillus fumigatus	

Phagocytes from healthy individuals are normally capable of producing highly reactive oxidative substances, such as hydrogen peroxide and hypochlorous acid, which are lethal to pathogens. Production of these oxidative species occurs largely via a multi-component NADPH oxidase system (Figure 4.8). CGD is caused by a genetic defect in any component of this oxidase system which compromises its effective functioning.

In addition to recurrent infection, CGD sufferers also exhibit abnormal inflammatory responses, which include granuloma formation at various sites of the body (granuloma refers to

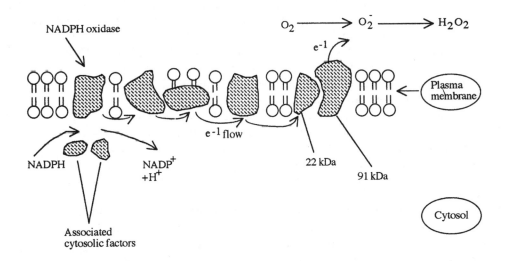

Figure 4.8. Production of reactive oxygen species (ROS) by phagocytes. In addition to degrading foreign substances via phagocytosis, phagocytes secrete ROS into their immediate environment. These can kill microorganisms (and, indeed, damage healthy tissue) in the vicinity, thus helping control the spread of infection. The ROS are produced by an NADPH oxidase system, the main feature of which is a plasma membrane-based electron transport chain. NADPH represents the electron donor. The first membrane carrier is NADPH oxidase, which also requires interaction with at least two cytosolic proteins for activation. The electrons are passed via a number of carriers, including a flavoprotein, to cytochrome b_{558}. This is a haem protein consisting of two subunits (22 kDa and 91 kDa). The cytochrome, in turn, passes the electrons to oxygen, generating a superoxide anion (O^-). The superoxide can be converted to hydrogen peroxide (H_2O_2) spontaneously, or enzymatically, by superoxide dismutase (SOD). A genetic defect affecting any element of this pathway will result in a compromised ability/inability to generate ROS, normally resulting in chronic granulomatous disease (CGD). Over 50% of CGD sufferers display a genetic defect in the 91 kDa subunit of cytochrome b_{558}

a tissue outgrowth which is composed largely of blood vessels and connective tissue). This can lead to obstruction of various ducts, e.g. in the urinary and digestive tract.

Traditionally, treatment of CGD entailed prophylactic administration of anti-microbial agents in an attempt to prevent occurrence of severe infection. However, affected individuals still experience life-threatening infections, requiring hospitalization and intensive medical care, as often as once a year. Attempts to control these infections rely on strong anti-microbial agents and leukocyte transfusions.

Long-term administration of IFN-γ to CGD patients has proved effective in treating/moderating the symptoms of this disease. The recombinant human IFN-γ used therapeutically is produced in *E. coli*, and is termed IFN-γ1B. It displays identical biological activity to native human IFN-γ, although it lacks the carbohydrate component. The product, usually sold in liquid form, is manufactured by Genentech, who market it under the tradename Actimmune. The product is administered on an ongoing basis, usually by s.c. injection three times weekly. In clinical trials its administration, when compared to a control group receiving a placebo, resulted in:

- a reduction in the incidence of life-threatening infections by 50% or more;
- a reduction in the incidence of total infections by 50% or more;
- a reduction in the number of days of hospitalization by three-fold and even, when hospitalization was required, the average stay was halved.

The molecular basis by which IFN-γ induces these effects is understood, at least in part. In healthy individuals this cytokine is a potent activator of phagocytes. It potentiates their ability to generate toxic oxidative products (via the NADPH oxidase system), which they then use to kill infectious agents. In CGD sufferers IFN-γ boosts flux through the NADPH oxidative system. As long as the genetic defect has not totally inactivated a component of the system, this promotes increased synthesis of these oxidative substances. IFN-γ also promotes increased expression of IgG Fc receptors on the surface of phagocytes. This would increase the phagocytes' ability to destroy opsonized infectious agents via phagocytosis (Figure 4.9).

Additional molecular mechanisms must also mediate IFN-γ effects, as it promotes a marked clinical improvement in some CGD patients, without enhancing phagocyte activity. IFN-γ's demonstrated ability to stimulate aspects of cellular and humoral immunity (e.g. via T and B lymphocytes), as well as NK cell activity, is most likely responsible for these observed improvements.

IFN-γ may also prove valuable in treating a variety of other conditions, and clinical trials for various indications are currently under way. This cytokine shows promise in treating leishmaniasis, a disease common in tropical and sub-tropical regions. The causative agent is a parasitic protozoan of the genus *Leishmania*. The disease is characterized by the presence of these protozoa inside certain immune cells, particularly macrophages. IFN-γ appears to stimulate the infected macrophage to produce nitric oxide, which is toxic for the parasite.

Additional studies illustrate that IFN-γ stimulates phagocytic activity in humans suffering from various cancers, AIDS and lepromatous leprosy (leprosy is caused by the bacterium *Mycobacterium leprae*; lepromatous leprosy is a severe contagious form of the disease, leading to disfigurement). IFN-γ may thus prove useful in treating such conditions.

Interferon toxicity

Like most drugs, administration of IFNs can elicit a number of unwanted side effects. Unfortunately, in some instances the severity of such effects can limit the maximum

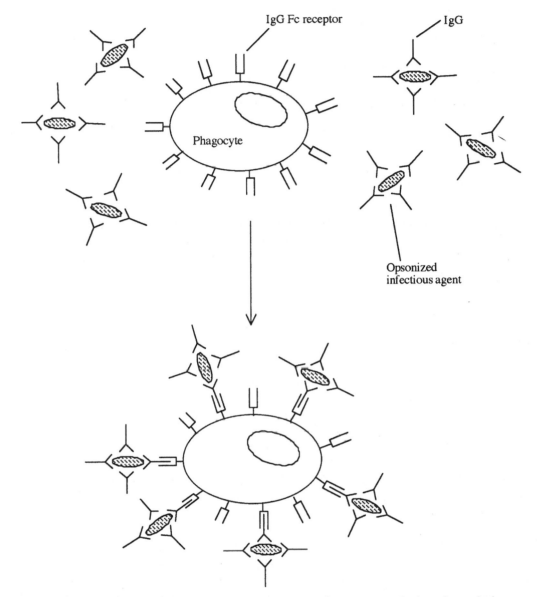

Figure 4.9. Increased expression of IgG Fc receptors on phagocytes results in enhanced phagocytosis. These receptors will retain opsonized (i.e. antibody-coated) infectious agents at their surface by binding the Fc portion of the antibody. This facilitates subsequent phagocytosis

recommended therapeutic dose to a level below that which might have maximum therapeutic effect. Administration of IFNs (in addition to many other cytokines) characteristically induces flu-like symptoms in many recipients. Such symptoms are experienced by most patients within 8 h of IFN-α administration. However, they are usually mild and are alleviated by concurrent administration of paracetamol. Tolerance of such effects also normally develops within the first few weeks of commencing treatment.

Table 4.11. Side effects sometimes associated with therapeutic administration of IFN-αs. In most cases, only minor side effects are noted. However, more serious effects, necessitating cessation of treatment, may occur in up to 17% of patients

Minor side effects	Serious potential side effects
Range of flu-like symptoms, e.g. fever, headache, chills	Anorexia Strong fatigue Insomnia Cardiovascular complications Autoimmune reactions Hepatic decompression

In some instances more severe side effects are noted (Table 4.11), while in a few cases very serious side effects, such as the induction of autoimmune reactions, central nervous system or cardiovascular disturbances, renders necessary immediate withdrawal of treatment.

Administration of IFN-β also characteristically causes flu-like symptoms. More serious side effects, however, are sometimes noted, including:

- hypersensitivity reactions;
- menstrual disorders;
- anxiety and emotional liability;
- depression, which in rare instances may prompt suicidal thoughts.

The only common side effect associated with IFN-γ is the characteristic flu-like symptoms. However, in rare instances and at high doses, adverse clinical reactions have been noted. These have included heart failure, CNS complications (confusion disorientation, parkinsonian-like symptoms), metabolic complications (e.g. hyperglycemia) and various other symptoms.

Prediction of the range or severity of side effects noted after administration of any IFN preparation is impossible. Careful monitoring of the patients, particularly in the earliest stages of treatment, soon reveals the onset of any side effects which might warrant suspension of treatment.

Additional interferons

In the last few years additional members of the IFN family has been discovered. Amino acid sequence analysis of a protein called trophoblastin—which is found in many ruminants—revealed that it was closely related to IFN-α. This result was surprising because, in sheep and several other ruminants, the primary function (and until recently the only known function) of trophoblastin is to sustain the corpus luteum during the early stages of pregnancy. The 172 amino acid protein is produced by the trophoblast (an outer layer of cells which surround the cells that constitute the early embryo) for several days immediately preceding implantation. In many ruminants, therefore, trophoblastin plays an essentially similar role to hCG in humans (Chapter 8).

If amino acid analysis hinted that trophoblastin was in fact an IFN, functional studies have proved it. These studies show that trophoblastin:

- displays the same anti-viral activity as type I IFNs;

- displays anti-proliferative activity against certain tumour cells, *in vitro* at least;
- binds the type I IFN receptor.

Trophoblastin has therefore been named interferon-tau (IFN-τ), and is classified as a type I IFN. There are at least three or four functional IFN-τ genes in sheep and cattle. The molecule displays a molecular mass of 19 kDa and an isoelectric point of 5.5–5.7, in common with other type 1 interferons. Interestingly, the molecule can also promote inhibition of reverse transcriptase activity in cells infected with the HIV virus.

IFN-τ is currently generating considerable clinical interest. While it induces effects similar to type I IFN, it appears to exhibit significantly lower toxicity. Thus it may prove possible to safely use this IFN at dosage levels far greater than the maximum dosage levels applied to currently used type I IFNs; however, this can only be elucidated by future clinical trials.

Interferon-omega (IFN-ω) represents an additional member of the IFN (type I) family. This 170 amino acid glycoprotein exhibits 50–60% amino acid homology to IFN-αs, and appears even more closely related to IFN-τ.

IFN-ω genes have been found in man, pigs and a range of other mammals, but not in dogs or rodents. The IFN induces its antiviral, immunoregulatory and other effects by binding the type I IFN receptor, although the exact physiological relevance of this particular IFN remains to be elucidated. Recently, a recombinant form of feline IFN-ω has been approved within the EU for veterinary use. Its approved indication is for the reduction of mortality and clinical symptoms of parvoviral infections in young dogs. The recombinant product is manufactured using a novel expression system, which entails direct inoculation of silkworms with an engineered silkworm nuclear polyhedrosis virus housing the feline IFN-ω gene. Overviewed in Figure 3.10, the production process begins by (automatically) inoculating silkworms (typically 8000 worms/batch) with the recombinant virus. Infection of silkworm cells results in high-level IFN-ω production, which is subsequently acid-extracted from silkworm body parts. After clarification, the product is purified by a two-step affinity chromatographic process (dye affinity chromatography, using blue sepharose, followed by a metal affinity step, using a copper-chelated sepharose column). A final gel filtration step is undertaken before addition of excipients (sodium chloride, D-sorbitol and gelatin). After filling, the product is freeze-dried.

CONCLUSION

Interferons represent an important family of biopharmaceutical products. They have a proven track record in the treatment of selected medical conditions, and their range of clinical applications continue to grow. It is also likely that many may be used to greater efficacy in the future by their application in combination with additional cytokines.

While it is premature to speculate upon the likely medical applications of IFN-τ, the reduced toxicity exhibited by this molecule will encourage its immediate medical appraisal. The classification of τ as an IFN also raises the intriguing possibility that other IFNs may yet prove useful in the treatment of some forms of reproductive dysfunctions in veterinary and human medicine.

FURTHER READING

Books

Abbas, A. (2003). *Cellular and Molecular Immunology*. W. B. Saunders, London.
Aggarwal, B. (1998). *Human Cytokines*. Blackwell Scientific, Oxford.

Estrov, Z. (1993). *Interferons, Basic Principles and Clinical Applications*. R. G. Landes, Florence, KY.
Fitzgerald, K. (2001). *The Cytokine Facts Book*. Academic Press, London.
Karupiah, G. (1997). *Gamma Interferon in Antiviral Defence*. Landes Bioscience, Lewisville, TX.
Mantovani, A. (2000). *Pharmacology of Cytokines*. Oxford University Press, Oxford.
Mire-Sluis, A. (1998). *Cytokines*. Academic Press, London.
Reder, A. (1996). *Interferon Therapy of Multiple Sclerosis*. Marcel Dekker, New York.

Articles

Cytokines — general

Aringer, M. *et al.* (1999). Interleukin/interferon signalling — a 1999 perspective. *Immunologist* **7**(5), 139–146.
Baggiolini, M. *et al.* (1997). Human chemokines — an update. *An. Rev. Immunol.* **15**, 675–705.
Dardenne, M. & Savino, W. (1996). Interdependence of the endocrine and immune systems. *Adv. Neuroimmunol.* **6**(4), 297–307.
Debetes, R. & Savelkoul, H. (1996). Cytokines as cellular communicators. *Mediat. Inflamm.* **5**(6), 417–423.
Henderson, B. & Wilson, M. (1996). Cytokine induction by bacteria — beyond lipopolysaccharide. *Cytokine* **8**(4), 269–282.
Ihle, J. (1996). STATs: signal transducers and activators of transcription. *Cell* **84**, 331–334.
Kishimoto, T. *et al.* (1994). Cytokine signal transduction. *Cell* **76**, 253–262.
Lau, F. & Horvath, C. (2002). Mechanisms of type I interferon cell signalling and STAT-mediated transcriptional responses. *Mt Sinai J. Med.* **69**(3), 156–168.
Liu, L. *et al.* (1997). Ship, a new player in cytokine-induced signalling. *Leukaemia* **11**(2), 181–184.
Mire-Sluis, A. (1999). Cytokines: from technology to therapeutics. *Trends Biotechnol.* **17**, 319–325.
O'Shea, J.J. *et al.* (2002). Cytokine signalling in 2002: new surprises in the JAK–STAT pathway. *Cell* **109**, S121–S131.
Piscitelli, S. *et al.* (1997). Pharmacokinetic studies with recombinant cytokines — scientific issues and practical considerations. *Clin. Pharmacokinet.* **32**(5), 368–381.
Poole, S. (1995). Cytokine therapeutics. *Trends Biotechnol.* **13**, 81–82.
Proost, P. *et al.* (1996). The role of chemokines in inflammation. *Int. J. Clin. Lab. Res.* **26**(4), 211–223.
Schooltink, H. & Rose, J. (2002). Cytokines as therapeutic drugs. *J. Interferon Cytokine Res.* **22**(5), 505–516.
Takatsu, K. (1997). Cytokines involved in B cell differentiation and their sites of action. *Proc. Soc. Exp. Biol. Med.* **215**(2), 121–133.
Taniguchi, T. (1995). Cytokine signalling through non-receptor protein tyrosine kinases. *Science* **268**, 251–255.

Interferons

Alberti, A. (1999). Interferon αcon-1. A novel interferon for the treatment of chronic hepatitis C. *Biodrugs* **12**(5), 343–357.
Belardelli, F. *et al.* (2002). Interferon-α in tumor immunity and immunotherapy. *Cytokine Growth Factor Rev.* **13**(2), 119–134.
Boehm, U. *et al.* (1997). Cellular responses to interferon-γ. *Ann. Rev. Immunol.* **15**, 749–795.
Brassard, D. *et al.* (2002). Interferon-α as an immunotherapeutic protein. *J. Leukocyte Biol.* **71**(4), 565–581.
Cencic, A. & La Bonnardiere, C. (2002). Trophoblastic interferon-γ: current knowledge and possible role in early pig pregnancy. *Vet. Res.* **33**(2), 139–157.
Chelmonska-Soyta, A. (2002). Interferon-τ and its immunological role in ruminant reproduction. *Arch. Immunol. Ther. Exp.* **50**(1), 47–52.
Colonna, M. *et al.* (2002). Interferon-producing cells: on the front line in immune responses against pathogens. *Curr. Opin. Immunol.* **14**(3), 373–379.
Haria, M. & Benfield, P. (1995). Interferon-α2A. *Drugs* **50**(5), 873–896.
Jonasch, E. & Haluska, F. (2001). Interferon in oncological practice: review of interferon biology, clinical applications and toxicities. *Oncologist* **6**(1), 34–55.
Katre, N. (1993). The conjugation of proteins with polyethylene glycol and other polymers — altering properties of proteins to enhance their therapeutic potential. *Adv. Drug Delivery Rev.* **10**(1), 91–114.
Kirkwood, J. (2002). Cancer immunotherapy: the interferon-α experience. *Semin. Oncol.* **29**(3), 18–26.
Leaman, D. *et al.* (1996). Regulation of STAT-dependent pathways by growth factors and cytokines. *FASEB J.* **10**(14), 1578–1588.
Li, J. & Roberts, M. (1994). Interferon-τ and interferon-α interact with the same receptors in bovine endometrium. *J. Biol. Chem.* **269**(18), 13544–13550.
Lyseng-Williamson, K. & Plosker, G. (2002). Management of relapsing–remitting multiple sclerosis — defining the role of subcutaneous recombinant interferon-β-1a (Rebif). *Dis. Managem. Health Outcomes* **10**(5), 307–325.

Meager, A. (2002). Biological assays for interferons. *J. Immunol. Methods* **261**(1–2), 21–36.

Pestka, S. & Langer, J. (1987). Interferons and their actions. *Ann. Rev. Biochem.* **56**, 727–777.

Simko, R. & Nagy, K. (1996). Interferon-α in childhood hematological malignancies. *Postgrad. Med. J.* **72**(854), 709–713.

Soos, J. & Johnson, H. (1999). Interferon-τ. Prospects for clinical use in autoimmune disorders. *BioDrugs* **11**(2), 125–135.

Todd, P. & Goa, K. (1992). Interferon-γ-1b. *Drugs* **43**(1), 111–122.

Tossing, G. (2001). New developments in interferon therapy. *Eur. J. Med. Res.* **6**(2), 47–65.

Wang, Y. *et al.* (2002). Structural and biological characterization of PEGylated recombinant interferon-α2B and its therapeutic implications. *Adv. Drug Delivery Rev.* **54**(4), 547–570.

Woo, M. & Burnakis, T. (1997). Interferon-α in the treatment of chronic viral hepatitis B and viral hepatitis C. *Ann. Pharmacother.* **31**(3), 330–337.

Younes, H. & Amsden, B. (2002). Interferon-γ therapy: evaluation of routes of administration and delivery systems. *J. Pharmaceut. Sci.* **91**(1), 2–17.

Young, H. & Hardy, K. (1995). Role of interferon-γ in immune cell regulation. *J. Leukocyte Biol.* **58**, 373–379.

Zavyalov, V. & Zavyalova, G. (1997). Interferons α/β and their receptors—place in the hierarchy of cytokines. *APMIS* **105**(3), 161–186.

Chapter 5

Cytokines: interleukins and tumour necrosis factor

The interleukins (ILs) represent another large family of cytokines, with at least 25 different constituent members (IL-1 to IL-25) having been characterized thus far. Most of these polypeptide regulatory factors are glycosylated (a notable exception being IL-1) and display a molecular mass in the range 15–30 kDa. A few interleukins display a higher molecular mass, e.g. the heavily glycosylated, 40 kDa, IL-9.

Most of the interleukins are produced by a number of different cell types. At least 17 different cell types are capable of producing IL-1 (see Table 5.5), while IL-8 is produced by at least 10 distinct cell types. On the other hand, IL-2, -9 and -13 are produced only by T lymphocytes.

Most cells capable of synthesizing one IL are capable of synthesizing several, and many prominent producers of ILs are non-immune system cells (Table 5.1). Regulation of IL synthesis is exceedingly complex and only partially understood. In most instances, induction or repression of any one IL is prompted by numerous regulators—mostly additional cytokines, e.g. IL-1 promotes increased synthesis and release of IL-2 from activated T lymphocytes. It is highly unlikely that cells capable of synthesizing multiple ILs concurrently synthesize them all at high levels.

Nearly all ILs are soluble molecules (one form of IL-1 is cell-associated). They promote their biological response by binding to specific receptors on the surface of target cells. Most ILs exhibit paracrine activity (i.e. the target cells are in the immediate vicinity of the producer cells), while some display autocrine activity (e.g. IL-2 can stimulate the growth and differentiation of the cells that produce it). Other ILs display more systematic endocrine effects (e.g. some activities of IL-1).

The signal transduction mechanisms by which most ILs prompt their biological response are understood, in outline at least. In many cases, receptor binding is associated with intracellular tyrosine phosphorylation events. In other cases, serine and threonine residues of specific intracellular substrates are also phosphorylated. For some ILs, receptor binding triggers alternative signal transduction events, including promoting an increase in intracellular calcium concentration or inducing the hydrolysis of phosphotidylethanolamine with release of diacyl glycerol.

Biopharmaceuticals: Biochemistry and Biotechnology, Second Edition. Gary Walsh
John Wiley & Sons Ltd: ISBN 0 470 84326 8 (ppc), ISBN 0 470 84327 6 (pbk)

Table 5.1. Many cell types are capable of producing a whole range of interleukins. T lymphocytes are capable of producing all the ILs, with the possible exception of IL-7 and IL-15. Many cell types producing multiple ILs can also produce additional cytokines, e.g. both macrophages and fibroblasts are capable of producing several ILs, colony stimulating factors (CSFs) and platelet-derived growth factor (PDGF)

Cell type	Interleukins produced
Macrophages	IL-1, IL-6, IL-10, IL-12
Eosinophils	IL-3, IL-5
Vascular endothelial cells	IL-1, IL-6, IL-8
Fibroblasts	IL-1, IL-6, IL-8, IL-11
Keratinocytes	IL-1, IL-6, IL-8, IL-10

The sum total of biological responses induced by the ILs is large, varied and exceedingly complex. These cytokines regulate a variety of physiological and pathological conditions, including:

- normal and malignant cell growth;
- all aspects of the immune response;
- regulation of inflammation.

Several ILs, particularly those capable of modulating transformed cell growth, as well as those exhibiting immunostimulatory properties, enjoy significant clinical interest. As with other cytokines, the advent of recombinant DNA technology facilitates production of these molecules in quantities sufficient to meet actual/potential medical needs.

The first IL to be approved for medical use was IL-2, approved in 1992 by the FDA for the treatment of renal cell carcinoma. Several additional IL preparations are currently in clinical trials (Table 5.2).

Table 5.2. Some interleukin preparations approved for general medical use (or in clinical trials) and the disease(s) for which they are indicated. The developing company is also listed. The drug status refers to its status in the USA

Product	Drug status	Indication	Developing company
Proleukin (rIL-2)	Approved (1992)	Renal cell carcinoma	Chiron Corp.
Neumega (rIL-11)	Approved (1997)	Prevention of chemotherapy-induced thrombocytopenia	Genetics Institute
IL-2	Clinical trials	HIV	Bayer
IL-2	Clinical trials	HIV and non-Hodgkin's lymphoma	Chiron
IL-4	Clinical trials	Cancer (various)	Schering Plough and National Cancer Institute, USA
IL-4 and IL-13	Clinical trials	Asthma	Regeneron
IL-10	Clinical trials	Inflammatory disease	Schering Plough
IL-18	Clinical trials	Cancer (various)	GlaxoSmithKline
IL-18	Clinical trials	Rheumatoid arthritis, Crohn's disease	Serono

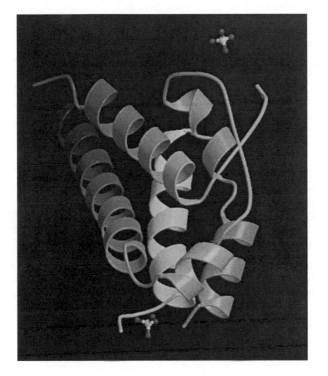

Figure 5.1. 3-D structure of human IL-2. Photo from Arkin *et al.* (in press), by courtesy of the Protein Data Bank: http://www.pdb.org/

INTERLEUKIN-2 (IL-2)

IL-2, also known as T cell growth factor, represents the most studied member of the IL family. It was the first T cell growth factor to be identified and it plays a central role in the immune response. It is produced exclusively by T lymphocytes (especially T helper cells), in response to activation by antigen and mitogens.

Human IL-2 is a single chain polypeptide containing 133 amino acids. It is a glycoprotein, the carbohydrate component being attached via an O-linked glycosidic bond to threonine residue No. 3. The mature molecule displays a molecular mass ranging from 15–20 kDa, depending upon the extent of glycosylation. The carbohydrate moiety is not required for biological activity.

X-ray diffraction analysis shows the protein to be a globular structure, consisting of four α-helical stretches interrupted by bends and loops. It appears devoid of any β-conformation and contains a single stabilizing disulphide linkage involving cysteine numbers 58 and 105 (Figure 5.1).

IL-2 induces its characteristic biological activities by binding a specific receptor on the surface of sensitive cells. The high-affinity receptor complex consists of three membrane-spanning polypeptide chains (α-, β- and γ-; Table 5.3).

The α-chain binds IL-2 with low affinity, with binding being characterized by high subsequent association–disassociation rates. The γ-subunit does not interact directly with IL-2. It is sometimes known as γc (common) as it also appears to be a constituent of the IL-4, -7, -9, -13 and -15 receptors.

Table 5.3. Summary of the polypeptide constituents of the high-affinity human IL-2 receptor

Receptor polypeptide constituent	Additional names	Molecular mass (kDa)
α	P55 Tac CD25	55
β	P75 CD122	75
γ	P64	64

Heterodimeric complexes consisting of $\alpha\gamma$ or $\beta\gamma$ can bind IL-2 with intermediate affinity. The heterotrimeric $\alpha\beta\gamma$ complex represents the cytokine's true high-affinity receptor (Figure 5.2). The exact intracellular signal transduction events triggered by IL-2 are not fully elucidated. The α-receptor chain exhibits a cytoplasmic domain containing only nine amino acids, and is unlikely to play a role in intracellular signalling. Mutational studies reveal that the 286 amino acid β-chain intracellular domain contains at least two regions (a serine-rich region and an acidic region) essential for signal transduction. The β-chain is phosphorylated on a specific tyrosine residue subsequent to IL-2 binding, probably via association of a protein tyrosine kinase essential for generation of intracellular signals. The direct role played by the γ-chain, although unclear, is likely critical. A mutation in the gene coding for this receptor constituent results in severe combined immunodeficiency (X-SCID).

Interestingly, prolonged elevated levels of IL-2 promotes the shedding of the IL-2 receptor α-subunit from the cell surface. Initially, it was suspected that these circulating soluble receptor fragments, capable of binding IL-2, might play a role in inducing immunosuppression (by competing for IL-2 with the cell surface receptor). However, the affinity of IL-2 for the intact receptor ($\alpha\beta\gamma$) is far greater than for the α-subunit, rendering this theory unlikely.

The IL-2 receptor is associated with a number of cell types — mainly cells playing a central role in the immune response (Table 5.4). Binding of IL-2 to its receptor induces growth and differentiation of these cells. This cytokine, therefore, behaves as a central molecular switch, activating most aspects of the immune response.

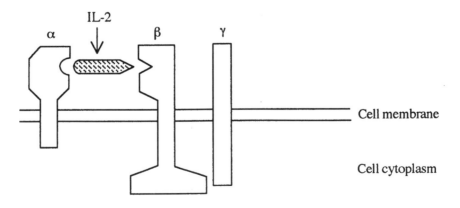

Figure 5.2. Schematic diagram of the high-affinity IL-2 receptor

Table 5.4. The range of cells expressing the IL-2 cell surface receptor. IL-2-stimulated growth and differentiation of these cells forms the molecular basis by which many aspects of the immune response is activated. It thus acts in an autocrine and paracrine manner to mobilize the immune response

T lymphocytes	B lymphocytes
NK cells	LAK cells
Monocytes	Macrophages
Oligodendrocytes	

Quiescent T lymphocytes are stimulated largely by direct binding to an antigen fragment presented on the surface of a macrophage in the context of major histocompatibility complex (MHC) (Figure 5.3). This results in the induction of expression of at least 70 genes whose products are collectively important in immune stimulation. These products include:

- several cytoplasmic proteins capable of inducing T cell growth (i.e. several cellular proto-oncogenes, including C-*fos* and C-*myc*);
- various cytokines, most notably IL-2;
- cytokine receptors, most notably the IL-2 receptor α subunit (the T-lymphocytes appear to constitutively express the β and γ IL-2 receptor polypeptides. Induction of the α gene leads to formation of a high-affinity αβγ receptor complex, thereby rendering the activated T cell highly sensitive to IL-2).

IL-2 acts as a critical autocrine growth factor for T cells, and the magnitude of the T cell response is largely dependent upon the level of IL-2 produced. IL-2 also serves as a growth factor for activated B lymphocytes. In addition to promoting proliferation of these cells, IL-2 (as well as some other ILs) stimulates enhanced antibody production and secretion. In this way it effectively potentates the humoral immune response.

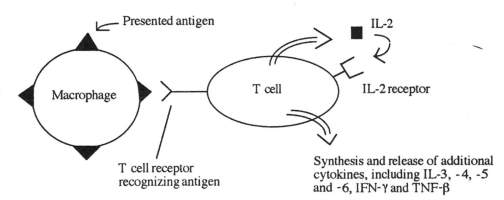

Figure 5.3. Activation of T cells by interaction with macrophage-displayed antigen. Activation results in IL-2 production, which acts in an autocrine manner to stimulate further T cell growth and division. IL-2 thus represents the major regulatory molecule responsible for stimulation of cell-mediated immunity. Note that it was initially believed that binding of presented antigen alone was insufficient to trigger T cell activation. It was thought that co-stimulation with IL-1 was required. However, the assay used to detect the 'co-stimulation' was found not to be specific for IL-1 alone. The role of IL-1 as a co-stimulator of T cell activation is now believed to be minimal at most

A third biological activity of IL-2 pertinent to immunostimulation is its ability to promote the growth of natural killer (NK) cells. It also promotes further differentiation of NK cells, forming lymphokine-activated killer cells (LAKs), which exhibit an enhanced ability to directly kill tumour cells or virally infected cells. NK cells express the β and γ IL-2 receptor subunits only, thus their stimulation by IL-2 requires elevated concentrations of this cytokine. NK cells are also activated by a variety of additional cytokines, including all IFNs as well as tumour necrosis factor (TNF).

The immunopotentative effects of IL-2 rendered it an obvious target for clinical application. At the simplest level, it was hoped that administration of exogenous IL-2 could enhance the immune response to a number of clinical conditions, including:

- cancers;
- T cell and other forms of immunodeficiency;
- infectious diseases.

IL-2 production

As was the case for most other cytokines, medical appraisal/use of IL-2 was initially impractical due to the minute quantities in which it is normally produced. Some transformed cell lines, most notably the Jurkat leukaemia cell line, produces IL-2 in increased quantities and much of the IL-2 used for initial characterization studies was obtained from this source. Large-scale IL-2 production was made possible by rDNA technologies. While the IL-2 gene/cDNA has now been expressed in a wide variety of host systems, it was initially expressed in *E. coli*, and most products being clinically evaluated are obtained from that source. As mentioned previously, the absence of glycosylation on the recombinant product does not alter its biological activity.

Proleukin is the trade name given to the recombinant IL-2 preparation manufactured by Chiron and approved for the treatment of certain cancers. It is produced in engineered *E. coli* and differs from native human IL-2 in that it is non-glycosylated, lacks an N-terminal alanine residue and cysteine 125 has been replaced by a serine residue. After extraction and chromatographic purification, the product is formulated in a phosphate buffer containing mannitol and low levels of the detergent SDS. The product displays typical IL-2 biological activities, including enhancement of lymphocyte mitogenesis and cytotoxicity, induction of LAK/NK cell activity and the induction of IFN-γ production.

IL-2 and cancer treatment

The immunostimulatory activity of IL-2 has proved beneficial in the treatment of some cancer types. An effective anti-cancer agent would prove not only medically valuable but also commercially very successful. In the developed world, an average of one in six deaths is caused by cancer. In the USA alone, the annual death toll from cancer stands in the region of half a million people.

There exists direct evidence that the immune system mounts an immune response against most cancer types. Virtually all transformed cells: (a) express novel surface antigens not expressed by normal cells; or (b) express, at greatly elevated levels, certain antigens present normally on the cell at extremely low levels. These 'normal' expression levels may be so low that they have gone unnoticed by immune surveillance (and thus have not induced immunological tolerance).

The appearance of any such cancer-associated antigen should thus be capable of inducing an immune response which, if successful, should eradicate the transformed cells. The exact elements of immunity responsible for destruction of transformed cells remain to be fully characterized. Both a humoral and cell-mediated response can be induced, although the T cell response appears to be the most significant.

Cytotoxic T cells may play a role in inducing direct destruction of cancer cells, in particular those transformed by viral infection (and who express viral antigen on their surface). *In vitro* studies have shown that cytotoxic T lymphocytes obtained from the blood of persons suffering from various cancer types are capable of destroying those cancer cells.

NK cells are capable of efficiently lysing various cancer cell types and, as already discussed, IL-2 can stimulate differentiation of NK cells forming LAK cells, which exhibit enhanced tumoricidal activity. Macrophages, too, probably play a role. Activated macrophages have been shown to lyse tumour cells *in vitro*, while leaving untransformed cells unaffected. Furthermore, these cells produce TNF and various other cytokines that can trigger additional immunological responses. The production of antibodies against tumour antigens (and the subsequent binding of the antibodies to those antigens) marks the transformed cells for destruction by NK/LAK cells and macrophages — all of which exhibit receptors capable of binding the Fc portion of antibodies.

While immune surveillance is certainly responsible for the detection and eradication of some transformed cells, the prevalence of cancer indicates that this surveillance is nowhere near 100% effective. Some transformed cells obviously display characteristics that allow them to evade this immune surveillance. The exact molecular details of how such 'tumour escape' is achieved remains to be conformed, although several mechanisms have been implicated, including:

- Most transformed cells do not express class II MHC molecules and express lower than normal levels of class I MHC molecules. This renders their detection by immune effector cells more difficult. Treatment with cytokines, such as IFN-γ, can induce increased class I MHC expression which normally promotes increased tumour cell susceptibility to immune destruction.
- Transformed cells expressing tumour-specific surface antigens, which closely resemble normal surface antigens, may not induce an immune response. Furthermore, some tumor antigens, while not usually expressed in adults, were expressed previously during the neonatal period (i.e. just after birth) and are thus believed by the immune cells to be 'self'.
- Some tumours secrete significant quantities of cytokines and additional regulatory molecules which can suppress local immunological activity, e.g. transforming growth factor-β (TGF-β; produced by many tumour types) is capable of inhibiting lymphocyte and macrophage activity.
- Antibody binding to many tumour antigens triggers the immediate loss of the antibody–antigen complex from the transformed cell surface by either endocytosis or extracellular shedding.
- The glycocalyx can possibly shield tumour antigens from the immune system.

Whatever the exact nature of tumour escape, it has been demonstrated, both *in vitro* and *in vivo*, that immunostimulation can lead to enhanced tumour detection and destruction. Several approaches to cancer immunotherapy have thus been formulated, many involving application of IL-2 as the primary immunostimulant.

Experiments conducted in the early 1980s showed that lymphocytes incubated *in vitro* with IL-2 could subsequently kill a range of cultured cancer cell lines, including melanoma and colon cancer cells. These latter cancers do not respond well to conventional therapies. Subsequent investigations showed that cancer cell destruction was mediated by IL-2-stimulated NK cells (i.e. LAK cells). Similar responses were seen in animal models upon administration of LAK cells activated *in vitro* using IL-2.

Clinical studies have shown this approach to be effective in humans. LAK cells originally purified from a patient's own blood, activated *in vitro* using IL-2 and reintroduced into the patient along with more IL-2, promoted complete tumour regression in 10% of patients suffering from melanoma or renal cancer. Partial regression was observed in a further 10–25% of such patients. Administration of high doses of IL-2 alone could induce similar responses but significant side-effects were noted (discussed later).

IL-2-stimulated cytotoxic T cells appear even more efficacious than LAK cells in promoting tumour regression. The approach adopted here entails removal of a tumour biopsy, followed by isolation of T lymphocytes present within the tumour. These tumour-infiltrating lymphocytes (TILs) are cytotoxic T lymphocytes that apparently display a cell surface receptor that specifically binds the tumour antigen in question. They are thus tumour-specific cells. Further activation of these TILs by *in vitro* culturing in the presence of IL-2, followed by reintroduction into the patient along with IL-2, promoted partial/full tumour regression in well over 50% of treated patients.

Further studies have shown additional cancer types, most notably ovarian and bladder cancer, non-Hodgkin's lymphoma and acute myeloid leukaemia, to be at least partially responsive to IL-2 treatment. However, a persistent feature of clinical investigations assessing IL-2 effects on various cancer types, is variability of response. Several trials have yielded conflicting results and no reliable predictor of clinical response is available.

IL-2 and infectious diseases

Although antibiotics have rendered possible medical control of various infectious agents (mainly bacterial), numerous pathogens remain for which no effective treatment exists. Most of these pathogens are non-bacterial (e.g. viral, fungal and parasitic, including protozoan). In addition, the over-use/abuse of antibiotics has hastened the development of antibiotic-resistant 'super-bacteria', which have become a serious medical problem.

The most difficult microbial pathogens to treat are often those that replicate within host cells (e.g. viruses and some parasites), e.g. during the complex life cycle of the malaria parasite in man, this protozoan can infect and destroy liver cells and erythrocytes. Over 2 million people die each year from malaria, with at least 200–300 million people being infected at any given time. Some such agents have even evolved to survive and replicate within macrophages subsequent to uptake via phagocytosis. This is often achieved on the basis that the phagocytosed microbe is somehow capable of preventing fusion of the phagocytosed vesicle with lysozomes. Examples of pathogens capable of survival within macrophages include:

- mycobacteria (e.g. *M. tuberculosis*, the causative agent of tuberculosis, and *M. leprae*, which causes leprosy);

- *Listeria monocytogenes*, a bacterium which, when transmitted to man, causes listeriosis, which is characterized by flu-like symptoms but can cause swelling of the brain and induce abortions;
- *Legionella pneumophila*, the bacterium which causes Legionnaire's disease.

The immunological response raised against intracellular pathogens is largely a T cell response. IL-2's ability to stimulate T cells may render it useful in the treatment of a wide range of such conditions. Clinical trials assessing its efficacy in treating a range of infectious diseases, including AIDS, continue.

A related medical application of IL-2 relates to its potential use as adjuvant material, as discussed in Chapter 10.

Safety issues

Like all other cytokines, administration of IL-2 can induce side effects, which can be dose-limiting. Serious side effects, including cardiovascular, hepatic or pulmonary complications, usually necessitate immediate termination of treatment. Such side effects may be induced not only directly by IL-2 but also by a range of additional cytokines whose synthesis is augmented by IL-2 administration. These cytokines, which can include IL-3, -4, -5 and -6, as well as TNF and IFN-γ, also likely play a direct role in the overall therapeutic benefits accrued from IL-2 administration.

Inhibition of IL-2 activity

A variety of medical conditions exist which are caused or exacerbated by the immune system itself. These are usually treated by administering immunosuppressive agents. Examples include:

- autoimmune diseases in which immunological self-tolerance breaks down and the immune system launches an attack on self-antigens;
- tissue/organ transplantation in which the donor is not genetically identical to the recipient (i.e. in cases other than identical twins). The recipient will mount an immune response against the transplanted tissue, culminating in tissue rejection unless immunosuppressive agents are administered.

Selective immunosuppression in individuals suffering from the above conditions is likely best achieved by preventing the synthesis or functioning of IL-2. Cyclosporin A, one of the foremost immunosuppressive agents currently in use, functions by preventing IL-2 synthesis. A number of alternative approaches are now being considered or tested directly in clinical trials. These include:

- administration of soluble forms of the IL-2 receptor, which would complete with the native (cell surface) receptor for binding of IL-2;
- administration of monoclonal antibodies capable of binding the IL-2 receptor (it must be confirmed that the antibody used is not itself capable of initiating signal transduction upon binding the receptor);
- administration of IL-2 variants which retains their ability to bind the receptor but fail to initiate signal transduction;
- administration of IL-2 coupled to bacterial or other toxins. Binding of the cytokine to its receptor brings the associated toxin into intimate contact with the antigen-activated T cells

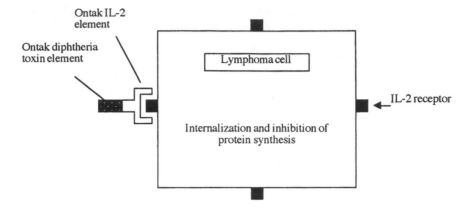

Figure 5.4. Structure and mode of action of the engineered fusion protein 'Ontak'. Refer to text for details

(and other cells, including activated B cells), leading to the destruction of these cells. This would induce selective immunotolerance to whatever specific antigen activated the B/T cells.

Ontak is the tradename given to an IL-2 toxin fusion protein first approved in 1999 in the USA for the treatment of cutaneous T cell lymphoma (Figure 5.4). It is produced in an engineered *E. coli* strain housing a hybrid gene sequence coding for the diphtheria toxin fragments, A and B, fused directly to IL-2. The 58 kDa product is extracted, purified and marketed as a solution (stored frozen), which contains citric acid buffer, the chelating agent EDTA and polysorbate 20. The protein targets cells displaying the IL-2 receptor, found in high levels on the surface of some leukaemic and lymphoma cells, including cutaneous T cell lymphomas. Binding appears to trigger internalization of the receptor–fusion protein complex. Sufficient quantities of the latter escapes immediate cellular destruction to allow diphtheria toxin-mediated inhibition of cellular protein synthesis. Cell death usually results within hours.

INTERLEUKIN-1 (IL-1)

IL-1 is also known as lymphocyte-activating factor (LAF), endogenous pyrogen and catabolin. It displays a wide variety of biological activities and has been appraised clinically in several trials.

Two distinct forms of IL-1 exist: IL-1α and IL-1β. Although different gene products, and exhibiting only 20% amino acid sequence homology, both of these molecules bind the same receptor and induce similar biological activities. The genes coding for IL-1α and -1β both reside on human chromosome No. 2, and display similar molecular organization, both containing seven exons.

IL-1α and -1β are expressed as large (30 kDa) precursor molecules from which the mature polypeptide is released by proteolytic cleavage. Neither IL-1α or -1β possess any known secretory signal peptide and the molecular mechanism by which they exit the cell remains to be characterized. Neither IL appears to be glycosylated.

Table 5.5. The range of cells capable of producing IL-1

T lymphocytes	Vascular endothelial cells
B lymphocytes	Fibroblasts
Monocytes/macrophages	Astrocytes
NK cells	Dendritic cells
Large granular lymphocytes	Microglia
Keratinocytes	Glioma cells
Chondrocytes	

IL-1α is initially synthesized as a 271 amino acid precursor, with the mature form containing 159 amino acids (17.5 kDa). This molecule appears to remain associated with the extracellular face of the cell membrane. IL-1β, initially synthesized as a 269 amino acid precursor, is released fully from the cell. The mature form released contains 153 amino acids and displays a molecular mass in the region of 17.3 kDa.

X-ray diffraction analysis reveals the 3-D structure of both IL-1 molecules to be quite similar. Both are globular proteins, composed of six strands of anti-parallel β-pleated sheet forming a 'barrel', which is closed at one end by a further series of β-sheets.

A wide range of cells are capable of producing IL-1 (Table 5.5). Different cell types produce the different IL-1s in varying ratios. In fibroblasts and endothelial cells, both are produced in roughly similar ratios, whereas in monocytes IL-1β is produced in larger quantities than IL-1α. Activated macrophages appear to represent the major cellular source for IL-1.

The IL-1s induce their characteristic biological activities by binding to specific cell surface receptors present on sensitive cells. Two distinct receptors, types I and II, have been identified. Both IL-1α and IL-1β can bind both receptors. The type I receptor is an 80 kDa transmembrane glycoprotein. It is a member of the IgG superfamily. This receptor is expressed predominantly on fibroblasts, keratinocytes, hepatocytes and endothelial cells. The type II receptor is a 60 kDa transmembrane glycoprotein, expressed mainly on B lymphocytes, bone marrow cells and polymorphonuclear leukocytes. It displays a very short (29 amino acid) intracellular domain and some studies suggest that IL-1s can induce a biological response only upon binding to the type I receptor.

The exact IL-1-mediated mechanism(s) of signal transduction remain to be clarified. A number of different signal transduction pathways have been implicated, including involvement of G proteins. IL-1 has also been implicated in activation of protein kinase C by inducing the hydrolysis of phosphotidylethanolamine.

The biological activities of IL-1

IL-1 mediates a wide variety of biological activities:

- it is a pro-inflammatory cytokine, promoting the synthesis of various substances, such as eicosanoids, as well as proteases and other enzymes involved in generating inflammatory mediators. This appears to be its major biological function;
- it plays a role in activating B lymphocytes, along with additional cytokines and may also play a role in activating T lymphocytes;
- along with IL-6, it induces synthesis of acute phase proteins in hepatocytes;
- it acts as a co-stimulator of haematopoietic cell growth/differentiation.

The relative prominence of these various biological activities depends largely upon the quantities of IL-1 produced in any given situation. At low concentrations, its effects are largely paracrine, e.g. induction of local inflammation. At elevated concentrations, it acts more in an endocrine manner, inducing systematic effects such as the hepatic synthesis of acute phase proteins, but also induction of fever (hence the name, 'endogenous pyrogen') and cachexia (general body wasting, such as that associated with some cancers). Many of these biological activities are also promoted by TNF — another example of cytokine redundancy.

In addition to IL-1α and -1β, a third IL-1-like protein has been identified, termed IL-1 receptor antagonist (IL-1Rα). As its name suggests, this molecule appears to be capable of binding to the IL-1 receptors without triggering an intracellular response.

IL-1 biotechnology

IL-1 continues to be a focus of clinical investigation. This stems from its observed:

- immunostimulatory effects;
- ability to protect/restore the haematopoietic process during, or subsequent to, chemotherapy or radiation therapy;
- anti-proliferative effects against various human tumour cell lines grown *in vitro*, or in animal models.

Most of these effects are most likely mediated not only directly by IL-1 but also by various additional cytokines (including IL-2), induced by IL-1 administration.

The observed effects prompted initiation of clinical trials assessing IL-1's efficacy in treating:

- bone marrow suppression induced by chemo/radiotherapy;
- various cancers.

The initial findings of some such trials (involving both IL-1α and IL-1β) proved disappointing. No significant anti-tumour response was observed in many cases, although side effects were commonly observed. Virtually all patients suffered from fevers, chills and other flu-like symptoms. More serious side effects, including capillary leakage syndrome and hypotension, were also observed and were dose-limiting.

IL-1 thus displays toxic effects comparable to administration of TNF (see later) or high levels of IL-2. However, several clinical studies are still under way and this cytokine may yet prove therapeutically useful, either on its own or, more likely, when administered at lower doses with additional therapeutic agents.

Because of its role in mediating acute/chronic inflammation, (downward) modulation of IL-1 levels may prove effective in ameliorating the clinical severity of these conditions. Again, several approaches may prove useful in this regard, including:

- administration of anti-IL-1 antibodies;
- administration of soluble forms of the IL-1 receptor;
- administration of the native IL-1 receptor antagonist.

Kineret is the trade name given to a recently approved product based on the latter strategy. Indicated in the treatment of rheumatoid arthritis, the product consists of a recombinant form of the human IL-1 receptor antagonist. The 17.3 kDa, 153 amino acid product is produced in engineered *E. coli* and differs from the native human molecule in that it is non-glycosylated and contains an additional N-terminal methionine residue (a consequence of its prokaryotic expression system). The purified product is presented as a solution and contains sodium citrate, EDTA, sodium chloride and polysorbate 80 as excipients. A daily (s.c.) injection of 100 mg is recommended for patients with rheumatoid arthritis. This inflammatory condition is (not surprisingly) characterized by the presence of high levels of IL-1 in the synovial fluid of affected joints. In addition to its pro-inflammatory properties, IL-1 also mediates additional negative influences on joint/bone, including promoting cartilage degradation and stimulation of bone resorption.

An additional approach to IL-1 downregulation could entail development of inhibitors of the proteolytic enzymes that release the active IL from its inactive precursor. Moreover, such inhibitors could probably be taken orally and, thus, would be suitable to treat chronic inflammation (the alternatives outlined above would be administered parenterally).

The enzyme releasing active IL-1β from its 31 kDa precursor has been identified and studied in detail. Termed IL-1β converting enzyme (ICE), it is a serine protease whose only known physiological substrate is the inactive IL-1β precursor. ICE cleaves this precursor between Asp 116 and Ala 117, releasing the active IL-1β.

ICE is an oligomeric enzyme (its active form may be a tetramer). It contains two distinct polypeptide subunits, p20 (20 kDa) and p10 (10 kDa). These two subunit types associate very closely, and the protease's active site spans residues from both. p10 and p20 are proteolytically-derived from a single 45 kDa precursor protein.

INTERLEUKIN-3: BIOCHEMISTRY AND BIOTECHNOLOGY

IL-3 is yet another cytokine whose biotechnological applications have attracted interest. This cytokine is produced primarily by T lymphocytes as well as mast cells and eosinophils. The mature molecule is a 133 amino acid glycoprotein of molecular mass 15–30 kDa. It induces its biological effects by binding a specific receptor—the IL-3 receptor (IL-3R) on sensitive cells. The IL-3R is composed of two subunits, a ligand-binding α-subunit and a β-subunit that appears to mediate signal transduction (Figure 5.5). Binding of IL-3 to its receptor induces phosphorylation of several (mostly unidentified) cellular proteins. These substrates are phosphorylated either on tyrosine residues or threonine and serine residues. The amino acid sequence of the intracellular part of the β-receptor subunit exhibits no homology to any known kinase, suggesting that phosphorylation is mediated by a distinct cytoplasmic kinase that is activated upon ligand binding. The IL-3R β-subunit also forms part of the IL-5 and GM-CSF receptors. Not surprisingly, all of these cytokines share at least some biological activities.

The IL-3 receptor is found on a wide range of haematopoietic progenitor cells (see Chapter 6). They are also present on monocytes and B lymphocytes. Its major biological activity relates to stimulation of growth of various cell types derived from bone marrow cells and which represent the immature precursors to all blood cells (Chapter 6). IL-3 thus appears to play a central role in stimulating the eventual formation of various blood cell types, in particular monocytes, mast cells, neutrophils, basophils and eosinophils, from immature precursor cells in the bone marrow. Several other cytokines (including IL-2, -4, -5, -6, -7, -11, -15 and CSFs) also play important co-stimulatory roles in the maturation of the range of blood cells.

Its growth and differentiation-inducing effects on early haematopoietic progenitor cells forms the basis of clinical interest in IL-3. Its administration to healthy patients results in increased blood leukocyte counts, although the concentration of all white blood cell types is not equally increased.

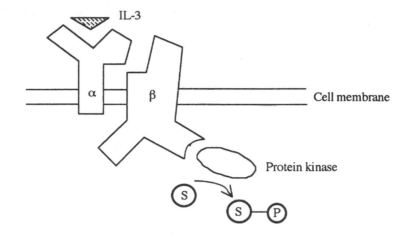

Figure 5.5. The IL-3 receptor. A high-affinity receptor is formed by association of an IL-3-binding α-subunit and a second β-subunit. Although both receptor constituents are transmembrane glycoproteins, the 70 kDa α-subunit exhibits only a minor intracellular domain, and is itself incapable of initiating signal transduction. The β-subunit (also 70 kDa) contains a significant intracellular domain, responsible for signal transduction. Ligand binding likely promotes association and activation of an intracellular kinase(s) which phosphorylates various substrates, including the β-subunit itself

Clinical trials continue to investigate IL-3's ability to stimulate production of blood cells in patients suffering from bone marrow failure induced by, for example, chemotherapy. In some such studies, leukocyte, neutrophil and platelet recovery was significantly improved by i.v. or s.c. IL-3 administration. Additionally, in studies with cancer patients, fewer cycles of chemotherapy had to be postponed because of complications resulting from depressed bone marrow function when IL-3 was concurrently administered to the patient. As with many drugs, however, other trials using IL-3 have shown less encouraging results regarding its efficacy in stimulating blood cell production.

Clinical interest in IL-3 is also sustained due to its low toxicity. Few side effects other than minor bone pain and nausea are witnessed at typical therapeutic doses (usually in the region of 5 μg/kg body weight). Further trials will probably investigate the effects of IL-3 treatment in combination with additional cytokines, such as CSFs. Such approaches may prove to be more effective in stimulating overall blood cell production.

INTERLEUKIN-4

IL-4, also known as B cell stimulating factor, is produced by a variety of cell types, most notably mast cells and T cells. It is a 129 amino acid glycoprotein exhibiting a molecular mass of 15–19 kDa, depending upon the level of glycosylation. The protein forms a compact globular shape and exhibits four α-helical stretches as well as a short stretch of a (two-stranded) β-sheet. The overall conformation is stabilized by three disulphide bonds and the protein exhibits a high pI value, in the region of 10.5 (Figure 5.6).

The IL-4 receptor consists of at least two polypeptides. An 800 amino acid α-chain, which is heavily glycosylated (also known as p140), is primarily responsible for binding IL-4. The second chain is γ(c) which, as discussed earlier, is also a constituent of the IL-2 receptor. The molecular details underlining signal transduction remain to be characterized in detail, although both

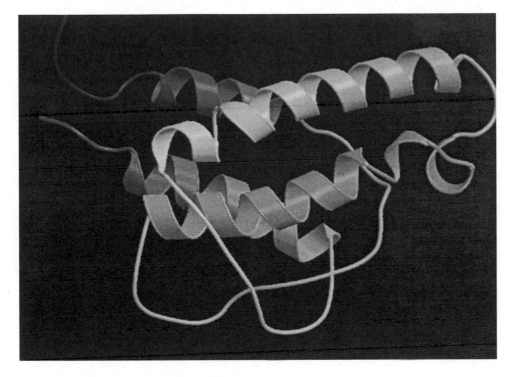

Figure 5.6. 3-D structure of human IL-4. Photo from Powers *et al.* (1992), by courtesy of the Protein Data Bank: http://www.pdb.org/

protein tyrosine kinase and breakdown of PIP_2 (phosphatidylinositol bisphosphate)-mediated mechanisms have been implicated.

IL-4 has various effects on a number of cell types. Its main target cells appear to be B and T lymphocytes and also monocytes, fibroblasts and endothelial cells. Specific biological effects include:

- promotes proliferation of B cells, as well as growth and differentiation of many T cells including T_H2 helper cells, which, in turn, stimulate humoral immunity and cytotoxic T cells. It also stimulates NK cell activity;
- promotes antibody class switching in B cells, resulting in the production of IgE;
- promotes growth of mast cells (along with IL-3);
- inhibits macrophage activation;
- promotes some cell types (especially endothelial cells) to express surface cellular adhesion molecules. These serve as docking sites for monocytes and eosinophils in particular, and thus these cells are attracted to the vicinity of IL-4 production.

Due to its immunostimulatory effects, IL-4 is being assessed clinically for the treatment of various cancer types. Its therapeutic potential in this regard remains unclear until further clinical data is generated. Administration of IL-4 does prompt many characteristic cytokine side effects, the severity of which sometimes equates to IL-1 administration.

In some instances, therapeutic benefit might accrue from inhibition of IL-4 activity. This cytokine plays a central role in the induction of immediate hypersensitivity (i.e. allergic) reactions, through processes such as:

- induction of IgE synthesis—which is a major mediator of many allergic reactions;
- its ability to promote congregation of monocytes and eosinophils, which, again, contain cellular mediators of inflammation;
- its growth-promoting effect on mast cells (which harbour granules filled with inflammatory/ allergic substances, such as histamine).

Blocking of IL-4 activity by strategies previously discussed in the context of other cytokines (e.g. administration of soluble receptor fragments, monoclonal antibodies, etc.) thus may have a potential role to play in treating allergies, especially acute life-threatening episodes associated with asthma or anaphylaxis.

INTERLEUKIN-6

IL-6 is a pleiotropic cytokine, synthesized by a variety of cell types (both leukocyte and non-leukocyte), which induces biological effects in a number of cell types—both leukocyte and non-leukocyte (Table 5.6).

The gene coding for IL-6 consists of five exons separated by four introns, and is present on chromosome 7. IL-6 is initially synthesized as a 26 kDa, 212 amino acid precursor protein. Subsequent removal of a 28 amino acid signal peptide yields the mature 184 amino acid cytokine, whose molecular mass remains at approximately 26 kDa due to glycosylation (removal of the carbohydrate component appears to have no effect on the biological activity of the molecule). Interestingly, IL-6, produced by fibroblasts and monocyte/macrophages at least, is also phosphorylated at several residues.

The IL-6 receptor, present on IL-6-sensitive cells (Table 5.6), consists of two associated transmembrane polypeptides, α and β. The extracellular domains of both are glycosylated. The 449 amino acid, 80 kDa α-chain (IL-6 Rα) binds IL-6 directly, while the 130 kDa β-chain (IL-6 Rβ, gp 130) then initiates intracellular signalling (Figure 5.7).

The exact details of signal transduction remain to be clarified. Binding of IL-6 to the α-chain, however, appears to facilitate direct interaction of the β-chain with a second β-chain. This

Table 5.6. Cells synthesizing and targeted by IL-6. Macrophages, endothelial cells and fibroblasts are probably the major producer cells

Producer cells	IL-6 sensitive cells (i.e. express IL-6 receptor)
T lymphocytes	T lymphocytes
B lymphocytes	Activated B lymphocytes
Macrophages	Monocytes
Fibroblasts	Fibroblasts
Bone marrow stromal cells	Epithelial cells
Endothelial cells	Hepatocytes
Keratinocytes	Neural cells
Astrocytes	

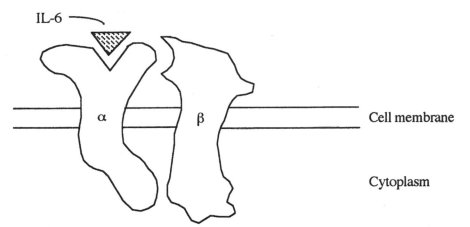

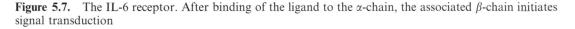

Figure 5.7.   The IL-6 receptor. After binding of the ligand to the α-chain, the associated β-chain initiates signal transduction

β-homodimer initiates signal transduction in which an early step is phosphorylation of the β-chains on specific tyrosine residues.

The main biological activities induced by binding of IL-6 to its receptor include:

- induction of hepatic synthesis of acute phase proteins. Release of these proteins into the blood appears to aid mediation of natural immunity and protect against tissue injury;
- induction of terminal differentiation of activated B lymphocytes, forming antibody-secreting plasma cells and induction of antibody synthesis by these cells;
- the stimulation (e.g. along with IL-1) of T cell activation and proliferation;
- enhances the proliferation of the bone marrow haematopoietic progenitor stem cells, again acting synergistically with other cytokines (including GM-CSF, IL-3 and IL-4).

In addition to these activities, IL-6 has been shown, *in vitro* at least, to regulate the growth and differentiation of various other cells—both normal and transformed. It inhibits the *in vitro* growth of human fibroblasts and endothelial cells. As both these cell types also synthesize IL-6, this may suggest the presence *in vivo* of a negative autocrine feedback loop (Figure 5.8). Plasmacytoma cells (transformed antibody-producing B lymphocytes), on the other hand, also secrete IL-6 and express and IL-6 receptor. In this case, however, the feedback loop is positive.

This cytokine has also been found, *in vitro*, to inhibit the growth of some transformed human cells, including leukaemia, lymphoma and breast carcinoma cell lines. More recently, IL-6 has been implicated in the differentiation of some neuronal cells. Also, when incubated *in vitro* with rat pituitary cells, it stimulates production and release of ACTH (adrenocorticotrophin). This hormone, normally released when the body is under any form of stress, stimulates glucocorticoid synthesis by the adrenal gland. Glucocorticoids suppress synthesis of IL-6, in monocyte macrophages at least. In this way, it is possible that the neuroendocrine and immune systems can communicate regarding regulating IL-6 synthesis.

While the role of IL-6 as a co-stimulator of activated B and T lymphocytes could suggest a medical role in potentiating the immune response, clinical interest has focused upon its ability to inhibit the growth of some cancer cells and stimulate haematopoietic cell growth *in vitro*.

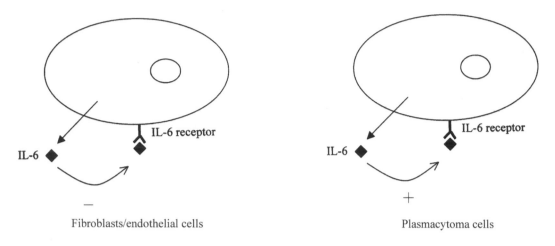

Figure 5.8. IL-6 receptor · IL-6 · Fibroblasts/endothelial cells − · IL-6 receptor · IL-6 · Plasmacytoma cells +

Figure 5.8. Several cells secreting IL-6 also display IL-6 receptors on their surface, thus facilitating autocrine regulation by this interleukin. In the case of fibroblasts and endothelial cells, this regulation appears negative (inhibitory to cell growth). In the case of plasmacytoma cells, however, the autocrine loop is positive, with IL-1 stimulating further growth

Some data are available from limited clinical trials. Thus far, the main haematological effects noted are an increase in blood platelet count (by up to 200%) and a decrease in circulating erythrocyte levels. In fact, at high dosage levels, anaemia was induced in some patients, requiring erythrocyte transfusion. At lower doses, and perhaps in combination with additional cytokines (e.g. CSFs), this IL may prove useful in treating thrombocytopenia, a medical condition characterized by a reduction in blood platelet counts. This results in prolonged bleeding after injury, spontaneous bleeding into the skin and bruising. So far, little hard evidence has been produced showing an anti-tumour effect of IL-6. This illustrates a frequently noted observation. Successful results with experimental drugs *in vitro*, or even in animal studies, do not always translate into successful results when that drug is administered to human patients. However, additional clinical trials are under way and the clinical future of IL-6 still hangs in the balance.

INTERLEUKIN-11

IL-11 is a cytokine that has gained approval for general medical use. This cytokine, produced largely by IL-1-activated bone marrow stromal cells and fibroblasts, functions as a haematopoietic growth factor. It stimulates (a) thrombopoiesis (the production of platelets formed by the shedding of fragments of cytoplasm from large bone marrow cells called megakaryocytes; Chapter 6) and (b) growth/differentiation of bone marrow cells, derived from stem cells that have become committed to differentiate into macrophages.

IL-11 is a 23 kDa, 178-amino acid polypeptide. Its receptor appears to be a single-chain 150 kDa transmembrane protein. Binding of IL-11 results in tyrosine phosphorylation of several intracellular proteins which, in turn, somehow promote the observed biological activities of IL-11.

The rationale for assessing IL-11 as a potential therapeutic agent relates mainly to its ability to induce platelet synthesis. Platelet counts can be significantly lowered due to certain disease conditions, and in patients undergoing cancer chemotherapy. Trials in patients receiving chemotherapy illustrated that s.c. administration of IL-11, at levels above 25 μg/kg body weight/ day, did stimulate platelet production, at least partially offsetting the chemotherapeutic effects. When administered at levels of 50 μg/kg/day, a significant increase in the bone marrow megakaryocyte population was noted. At levels in excess of 75 μg/kg/day, side effects including fatigue and oedema (tissue swelling due to accumulation of fluid) were also noted.

Neumega is the trade name given to the IL-11-based product approved for the prevention of thrombocytopenia. The product is produced in engineered *E. coli* cells and is presented as a purified product in freeze-dried format. Excipients include phosphate buffer salts and glycine. It is reconstituted (with water for injections) to a concentration of 5 mg/ml before s.c. administration.

INTERLEUKIN-5

The biological activities of several other interleukins also render them likely candidates for therapeutic application. IL-5 represents one such candidate. IL-5 is a 115 amino acid glycoprotein produced mainly by activated T lymphocytes and also by mast cells. It functions as a homodimer, exhibiting a molecular mass of 45 kDa. The individual polypeptide chains interact non-covalently and the overall dimeric structure is stabilized by two interchain disulphide linkages between cysteines 42 and 84 of each chain. Removal or alterations of the cytokine's carbohydrate side-chain does not appear to affect its biological activity.

X-ray diffractional analysis of crystalline human IL-5 reveals a two-domain structure, with each domain consisting of four α-helical stretches and one β-stretch consisting of two anti-parallel β-strands.

The human IL-5 receptor consists of two transmembrane glycoprotein subunits. The glycosylated 60 kDa α-chain binds IL-5 but is unable to induce direct signal transduction. A β-chain, unable to bind IL-5 directly, is associated with the α-chain to form an intact receptor complex. This 130 kDa β-chain, which also constitutes part of the IL-3 and GM-CSF receptors, appears to initiate signal transduction. In addition to the form anchored in the plasma membrane, cells are capable of producing a mRNA coding for a soluble form of the receptor α-chain by a process of alternative splicing. The exact physiological significance of this is unclear, as expression/secretion of this alternative mRNA in humans appears very low. When the corresponding cDNA is expressed in animal cell lines, and the soluble receptor purified and subjected to ligand binding studies, it was found to compete effectively with the membrane receptor for IL-5 binding. Clearly, if synthesized and secreted by human cells, this soluble receptor protein could have an antagonistic effect on IL-5 bioactivity. Soluble receptors for a number of additional human cytokines (some already discussed) have also been discovered (Table 5.7).

In humans, IL-5 functions as a growth and differentiation factor for eosinophils. It also stimulates basophil growth and may influence B lymphocyte activity. Eosinophils are leukocytes containing large cytoplasmic granules. The granules contain basic proteins capable of binding to acidic dyes such as eosin. The two main granular proteins are eosinophil cationic protein and major basic protein. Eosinophils play a particularly important role in mediating the destruction

Table 5.7. Cytokines for which soluble receptors have been detected in biological fluids. The exact functional role played by these binding proteins, in modulating cytokine activity, remains to be elucidated in most cases

IL-2	IL-7
IL-4	IFN-γ
IL-6	TNF

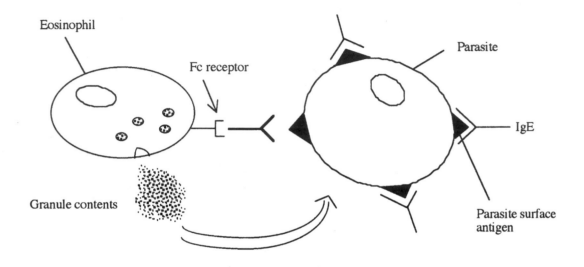

Figure 5.9. The destruction of parasites by eosinophils. Eosinophils bind to opsonized parasites via IgE-Fc receptors expressed on their surface. Binding induces release of granular contents by exocytosis. Major basic protein, the most abundant granular-derived protein, then initiates destruction of the parasite by lysis

of helminth parasites. Helminths stimulate IgE synthesis, which opsonize the parasite by binding to its surface antigens. Eosinophils bind the opsonized particle and secrete their granular contents, which induces destruction of the parasite by lysis (Figure 5.9). While IL-5 may have therapeutic potential in the treatment of some helminth infections, the role it plays in mediating acute inflammatory disease is currently receiving most attention.

Eosinophils are believed to play a major role in many inflammatory and allergic conditions. These effects are mediated by release of their granular contents, which can induce local host cell damage. One common such condition, affecting 10 million people in the USA alone, is asthma. Most forms of asthma are actually immediate hypersensitivity reactions (i.e. inappropriate over-reaction of certain elements of immunity to selected antigens). Asthma can also be characterized as an inflammatory disease, involving certain T helper lymphocytes (which also produce IL-5) and eosinophils in the airway mucosa. The granular eosinophil contents may play an important role in mediating chronic bronchial inflammation.

While eosinophil production can be induced by IL-3, IL-5 and GM-CSF *in vitro*, only IL-5 plays this role effectively *in vivo*. It follows that blocking the biological activity of IL-5 may provide a means of treating or alleviating chronic or inflammatory conditions associated, at least in part, with eosinophilia (increased eosinophil counts).

A number of strategies may be adopted to inhibit IL-5 activity. Methods currently under investigation include:

- inhibition of IL-5 synthesis/release by T-lymphocytes;
- use of anti-IL-5 monoclonal antibodies or soluble IL-5 receptor polypeptides;
- development of a mutant IL-5 capable of binding its receptor but without triggering signal transduction;
- identification of a low molecular mass substance which, by interacting with either IL-5 or its receptor, would prevent direct interaction of the cytokine and its receptor and hence prevent IL-5 signalling.

A soluble receptor has been identified *in vivo* which, when produced by recombinant means and administered at higher levels, does act as an effective receptor antagonist. Fab fragments of a humanized anti-IL-5 monoclonal antibody (Chapter 10) have also been produced, which can reduce IL-5-mediated effects in animal models.

Alanine scans (use of genetic engineering to generate a series of mutant proteins in which each residue in the native protein is systematically changed to alanine) of IL-5 have identified several residues important in ligand–receptor interaction. Replacement of IL-5 residue No. 13 (usually Glu) with alanine, while having no effect upon receptor binding, almost totally prevents subsequent initiation of signal transduction.

The ongoing (chronic) nature of many inflammatory conditions renders most attractive the development of a drug which would:

- exhibit a long circulatory half-life;
- be relatively inexpensive;
- be capable of being administered orally.

All the protein-based potential therapeutics discussed above fail to meet any of these criteria. Low molecular mass antagonists of IL-5 or its receptor may prove of most use. A number of research teams are screening for such substances. The development strategies pursued include:

- computer-aided drug design; attempts are being made to logically design molecules capable of binding to specific regions of IL-5 (or its receptor) and hence blocking their function;
- traditional screening methods; the screening of microbial, plant or other extracts for substances capable of interfering with IL-5 ligand–receptor interaction.

Thus far, at least one class of compound — isothiazolone derivatives — has been identified as potent IL-5 inhibitors. These substances react with a free sulphydryl group on the surface of the IL-5 receptor α-subunit, thereby preventing ligand binding. Isothiazolones are already used as anti-microbial agents, but are quite toxic.

Overall, therefore, inhibition of IL-5-mediated biological activities may be achieved, at least in part, by a number of means. All studies to date, however, have been undertaken *in vitro*. Clinical trials will be necessary to assess whether any of these strategies are effective in treating chronic asthma or other inflammatory conditions.

INTERLEUKIN-12

Interleukin 12 represents a cytokine that has just begun to generate substantial clinical interest. This is due to its ability to generate a very strong cell-mediated immune response. IL-12 is a heterodimeric structure composed of two polypeptide subunits, termed p35 and p40. p35 is a 196 amino acid glycoprotein exhibiting a molecular mass in the 30–35 kDa range. p40, containing 306 amino acids, is also glycosylated and exhibits a molecular mass in the 35–45 kDa range. Neither chain on its own exhibits biological activity . Monocytes/macrophages appear to represent the major cellular source of IL-12. Sensitive cells express a cell surface 180 kDa glycoprotein, which serves as the IL-12 receptor. The mechanism of signal transduction remains to be characterized. Whatever its mechanism of signal transduction, IL-12 induces a number of important biological effects, including:

- stimulation of IFN-γ synthesis and release from T lymphocytes and NK cells;
- activation of NK cells;
- induction of the growth and differentiation of precursor T lymphocytes specifically producing T_H1 cells.

Such biological activities suggest various clinical scenarios in which this cytokine may be positively employed (Table 5.8).

T_H1 cells (i.e. T helper type 1 lymphocytes) are the cellular population that triggers a cell-mediated immune response. This is the most effective means by which the immune system can identify and destroy many foreign agents, particularly viruses, bacteria or parasites, that have entered host cells.

In many instances, the unaided immune response to such infections can be inadequate, leading to prolonged and/or serious illness. Examples include the malaria and tuberculosis agents, the HIV virus (which has infected at least 14 million people worldwide), leishmaniasis (caused by the protozoan *Leishmania*, from which 12 million people suffer) and schistosomiasis, (caused by the *Schistoma mansoni* helminth, which currently infects approximately 250 million people worldwide).

One underlining therapeutic hope for IL-12 is, therefore, that its administration will initiate a strong cell-mediated immune response, thus effectively destroying many infectious agents such as those described above.

IL-12-stimulated IFN-γ production and NK cell activation further potentates the overall immune response, not only to infectious agents but also against transformed cells. Cytotoxic T cells and NK cells represent two of the most important immune effector functions against cancer. IL-12-mediated immunological activity also renders this cytokine a potentially

Table 5.8.   Some potential clinical applications of IL-12. While animal trials and *in vitro* studies have yielded encouraging results, clinical trials in humans must be undertaken to assess the real therapeutic potential of this cytokine

---

Combating infectious diseases (viral, protozoal, fungal, bacterial, helminthic)
Anti-cancer agent
Alleviating allergic reactions
Vaccine adjuvant

---

important vaccine adjuvant. Its inclusion in vaccine preparations should lead to an enhanced T cell response against the injected antigen.

Thus far, *in vitro* and animal studies have confirmed IL-12's ability to enhance many immunological functions. Leishmaniasis is a common protozoan disease in tropical/subtropical regions, including Africa, India, Central and South America and Southern Europe. Animal studies have shown that IL-12 administration initiates a strong T_H1-mediated immune response in infected mice, effective in combating the disease and conferring future immunity.

Similiar animal studies using a malaria model system have also proved successful. Using a strain of mice for which malaria infection is normally lethal, scientists have found that administration of low doses of IL-12 (10–30 ng/day for 5 days) to infected mice offered effective protection against the disease.

IL-12 may also prove useful in the treatment of AIDS. AIDS patients exhibit reduced IL-12 levels and, not surprisingly, reduced T cell-mediated immunological capability. It is hoped that IL-12 administration to HIV-infected individuals might boost the cell-mediated immunological function, thus delaying the onset/progression of full-blown AIDS. IL-12 may also prompt a more efficient immunological response against opportunistic infectious agents to which AIDS patients often succumb due to their immunocompromised state. IL-12 administration to immunodeficient mice generates an effective protective response (largely by activating NK cells) to the protozoan pathogen *Toxoplasma gondii*, a common opportunistic infectious agent of AIDS patients.

IL-12 therapy may yet also play a role in treating or alleviating some allergies. Most allergic/immediate hypersensitivity reactions are predominantly triggered by a T_H2-mediated humoral response, with the production of antibodies such as IgE often triggering inflammation or host cell damage. Administration of IL-12 may alleviate some of the effects by switching the predominant immune response to a T_H1-mediated one.

The potential of IL-12 as an effective vaccine adjuvant has also been confirmed in some animal studies. To be effective, most vaccines must trigger a strong T cell and B cell response. This may not always occur in practice. Co-administration of IL-12 with foreign antigen was found to stimulate a strong T_H1 response in mice, enhancing the protective effect of various vaccines, e.g. co-administration of IL-2 with heat-killed *Listeria monocytogenes* protected mice from a subsequent lethal dose challenge of the live bacteria. Immunization using heat-killed bacteria alone did not afford such complete immunological protection.

Overall, therefore, IL-12 exhibits therapeutic promise in the treatment of a broad range of diseases. However, as is the case with all drugs, *in vitro* activity/animal trials do not guarantee efficacy in humans. The real therapeutic significance of IL-12 can only be appraised by clinical trials. Some studies further investigating the effect of IL-12 in malaria are under way in Rhesus monkeys. Human clinical trials have also been initiated to assess the effects of IL-12 administration in HIV, chronic viral hepatitis and renal cancer. It is interesting to note that biotech companies have initiated clinical trials relating to diseases prevalent in affluent First World regions. IL-12 may, however, show greatest potential in treating protozoan and other infectious agents widespread in poorer world regions.

Clinical trials will also yield the first reliable appraisal of any side effects associated with IL-12 administration. Limited information from animal studies hints that, at high doses, IL-12 may cause toxic shock-like syndromes in recipients, and may also be linked to the development of atherosclerotic plaques.

ILs, therefore, represent a family of proteins of considerable therapeutic promise. While it is likely that several additional IL preparations will gain regulatory approval over the next few years, only comprehensive clinical trials will reveal the true medical significance of this family of cytokines. While emphasis has been placed thus far upon assessing therapeutic applications of individual ILs, it is likely that their use in combination with additional cytokines may display greater therapeutic advantage.

TUMOUR NECROSIS FACTORS (TNFs)

The tumour necrosis factor (TNF) family of cytokines essentially consists of two related regulatory factors: TNF-α (cachectin) and TNF-β (lymphotoxin). Although both molecules bind the same receptor and induce very similar biological activities, they display limited sequence homology. The human TNF-α and -β genes are located adjacent to each other on chromosome 6, being separated by only 1100 base pairs. Both contain three introns and their expression appears to be coordinately regulated. TNF-α, sometimes referred to simply as TNF, has been studied in significantly greater detail than lymphotoxin.

TNF biochemistry

TNF-α is also known as cachectin, macrophage cytotoxic factor, macrophage cytotoxin and necrosin. As some of these names suggest, activated macrophages appear to represent the most significant cellular source of TNF-α, but it is also synthesized by many other cell types (Table 5.9). Producer cells do not store TNF-α, but synthesize it *de novo* following activation.

Human TNF-α is initially synthesized as a 233 amino acid polypeptide, which is anchored in the plasma membrane by a single membrane-spanning sequence. This TNF pro-peptide, which itself displays biological activity, is usually proteolytically processed by a specific extracellular metalloprotease. Proteolytic cleavage occurs between residues 76 (Ala) and 77 (Val), yielding the mature (soluble) 157 amino acid TNF-α polypeptide. Mature human TNF-α appears to be devoid of a carbohydrate component and contains a single disulphide bond.

Monomeric TNF is biologically inactive — the active form is a homotrimer in which the three monomers associate non-covalently about a three-fold axis of symmetry, forming a compact bell-shaped structure. X-ray crystallographic studies reveal that each monomer is elongated and characterized by a large content of anti-parallel β-pleated sheet, which closely resembles subunit proteins of many viral caspids (Figure 5.10).

A number of stimuli are known to act as inducers of TNF production (Table 5.10). Bacterial lipopolysaccharide represents the most important inducer, and TNF mediates the patho-physiological effects of this molecule. TNF biosynthesis is regulated by both transcriptional and post-transcriptional mechanisms. Macrophages appear to constitutively express TNF-α mRNA,

Table 5.9.   The major cellular sources of human TNF-α. As is clearly evident, TNF-α synthesis is not restricted to cells of the immune system, but is undertaken by a wide variety of different cells in different anatomical locations, including the brain

Macrophages	B and T lymphocytes
NK cells	Polymorphonuclear leukocytes
Eosinophils	Astrocytes
Hepatic Kupffer cells	Langerhans cells
Glomerular mesangial cells	Brain microglial cells
Fibroblasts	Various transformed cell lines

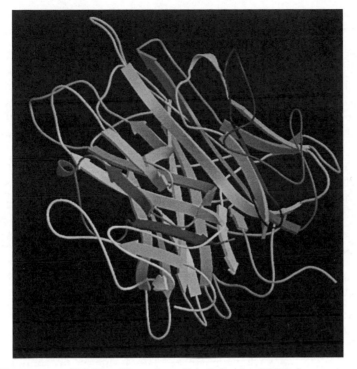

Figure 5.10. 3-D structure of TNF-α. Photo from Eck & Sprang (1989), by courtesy of the Protein Data Bank: http://www.pdb.org/

Table 5.10. Major physiological inducers of TNF-α production

Lipopolysaccharide	Bacterial enterotoxin
Mycobacteria	Various viruses
Fungi	Parasites
Antibody–antigen complexes	Various cytokines (e.g. IL-1)
Inflammatory mediators	TNF-α (autocrine activity)

which is translated only upon their activation. After activation, the rate of gene expression may increase only three-fold, although cellular TNF-α mRNA levels may increase 100-fold and secretion of soluble TNF-α may increase 10 000-fold.

Biological activities of TNF-*a*

The availability of large quantities of recombinant TNF-α facilitates rigorous investigation of the effects of this cytokine on cells *in vitro*, as well as its systemic *in vivo* effects. Like most cytokines, TNF-α exhibits pleiotropic effects on various cell types. The major biological responses induced by this cytokine include:

- activation of certain elements of both non-specific and specific immunity, in particular in response to Gram-negative bacteria;
- induction/regulation of inflammation;

- selective cytotoxic activity against a range of tumour cells;
- mediation of various pathological conditions, including septic shock, cachexia and anorexia.

The exact range of biological effects induced by TNF-α is dependent upon a number of factors, most notably the level at which TNF-α is produced. At low concentrations, TNF-α acts locally in a paracrine and autocrine manner, predominantly influencing white blood cells and endothelial cells. Under such circumstances, TNF-α's major activity relates to regulation of immunity and inflammation. In some situations, however, very large quantities of TNF-α may be produced (e.g. during severe Gram-negative bacterial infections). In such instances, TNF-α enters the blood stream and acts in an endocrine manner. Systemic effects of TNF-α (systemic means relating to the whole body, not just a specific area or organ), which include severe shock, are largely detrimental. Prolonged elevated systemic levels of TNF-α induce additional effects on, for example, whole-body metabolism, as discussed later. Many of TNF-α's biological effects are augmented by interferon-γ.

Immunity and inflammation

At low concentrations, TNF-α activates a range of leukocytes which mediate selected elements of both specific and non-specific immunity. These TNF-α actions include:

- activation of various phagocytic cells, including macrophages, neutrophils and polymorpho-nuclear leukocytes;
- enhanced toxicity of eosinophils and macrophages towards pathogens;
- exerts anti-viral activity somewhat similar to class I interferons, and increases surface expression of class I MHC molecules on sensitive cells;
- enhances proliferation of IL-2-dependent T lymphocytes.

In addition, TNF-α influences immunity indirectly by promoting synthesis and release of a variety of additional cytokines, including interferons, IL-1, IL-6, IL-8 and some CSFs.

TNF-α also plays a prominent role in mediating the inflammatory response and, indeed, this may be its major normal physiological role. It promotes inflammation by a number of means, including:

- promoting activation of neutrophils, eosinophils and other inflammatory leukocytes;
- induction of expression of various adhesion molecules on the surface of vascular endothelial cells. These act as docking sites for neutrophils, monocytes and lymphocytes, facilitating their accumulation at local sites of inflammation;
- displays chemotactic effects, especially for monocytes and polymorphonuclear leukocytes;
- enhances vascular leakness by promoting a reorganization of the cytoskeleton of endothelial cells;
- induction of synthesis of various lipid-based inflammatory mediators, including some prostaglandins and platelet-activating factor (PAF), macrophages and other cells. Many of these promote sustained vasodilation and increased vascular leakage;
- induction of synthesis of pro-inflammatory cytokines, such as IL-1 and IL-8.

TNF-α, therefore, promotes various aspects of immunity and inflammation. Blockage of its activity, e.g. by administration of anti-TNF-α antibodies, has been shown to compromise the body's ability to contain and destroy pathogens.

TNF-α exhibits cytotoxic effects on a wide range of transformed cells. Indeed, initial interest in this molecule (and its naming) stems from its anti-tumour activity. These investigations date back to the turn of the century, when an American doctor, William Coley, noted that tumours regressed in some cancer patients after the patient had suffered a severe bacterial infection. Although such observations prompted pioneering scientists to treat some cancer patients by injection with live bacteria, the approach was soon abandoned, as many patients died due to the resulting uncontrolled bacterial infections — before they could be 'cured' of the cancer. The active tumour agent turned out to be TNF-α (high circulating levels of which were induced by the bacterial-derived LPS).

TNF fails to induce death of all tumour cell types. While many transformed cells are TNF-sensitive, the cytokine exerts, at best, a cytostatic effect on others, and has no effect on yet others. The cytotoxic activity is invariably enhanced by the presence of IFN-γ. The concurrent presence of this interferon increases the range of transformed cell types sensitive to TNF-α, and can upgrade its cytostatic effects to cytotoxic ones. It can also render many untransformed cells, in particular epithelial and endothelial cells, susceptible to the cytotoxic effects of TNF-α.

TNF-α can mediate death of sensitive cells via apoptosis or necrosis (necrotic death is charactertized by clumping of the nuclear chromatin, cellular swelling, disintegration of intracellular organelles and cell lysis. Apoptotic death is characterized by cellular shrinking, formation of dense 'apoptotic' masses and DNA fragmentation).

In addition to its cytotoxic effects, TNF-α appears to regulate the growth of some (non-transformed) cell types. It is capable of stimulating the growth of macrophages and fibroblasts, while suppressing division of haematopoietic stem cells. The systemic effects of this cytokine on cellular growth *in vitro* are thus complex and as yet only poorly appreciated.

TNF receptors

Two TNF receptor types have been characterized. The type I receptor displays a molecular mass of 55 kDa, and is known as TNF-R55 (also P-55, TNFR1 or CD120α). The type II receptor is larger (75 kDa) and is known as TNF-R75 (also P-75, TNFR2 or CD120β). Both receptors bind both TNF-α and TNF-β. A TNF receptor is present on the plasma membrane of almost all nucleated cell types, generally in numbers varying from 100–10 000. Although virtually all cells express TNF-R55, the TNF-R75 cell surface receptor distribution is more restricted — being most prominent on haematopoietic cells. Differential regulation of expression of these two receptor types is also apparent. Generally, low constitutive expression of TNF-R55 is observed, with TNF-R75 expression being inducible.

Both receptor types are members of the nerve growth factor receptor superfamily and exhibit the characteristic four (cysteine-rich) repeat units in their extracellular domain. The extracellular domains of TNF-R55 and TNF-R75 exhibit only 28% homology while their intracellular domains are devoid of any homology, indicating the likely existence of distinct signalling mechanisms.

It appears that TNF-R55 is capable of mediating most TNF activities, while the biological activities induced via the TNF-R75 receptor are more limited. For example, TNF's cytotoxic activity, as well as its ability to induce synthesis of various cytokines and prostaglandins, are all mediated mainly/exclusively by TNF-R55. TNF-R75 appears to play a more prominent role in the induction of synthesis of T lymphocytes. All of the biological activities mediated by TNF-R75 can also be triggered via TNF-R55, and usually at much lower densities of receptors. TNF-R75 thus appears to play more of an accessory role, mainly to enhance effects mediated via TNF-R55.

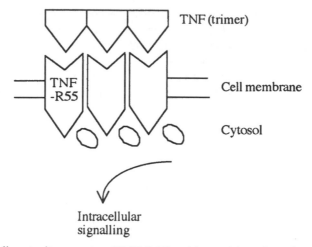

Figure 5.11. TNF binding to its receptor (TNF-R55), with resulting clustering of the receptor and generation of intracellular signals. Binding of TNF to its other receptor (TNF-R75) also induces receptor clustering (see text for details)

Binding of TNF to either receptor type results in oligomerization of the receptor (Figure 5.11). Indeed, antibodies raised against the extracellular domains of the receptors can induce TNF activity, indicating that the major/sole function of the TNF ligand is to promote such clustering of receptors. In most cases, binding of TNF to TNF-R55 results in rapid internalization of the ligand–receptor complex, followed by lysosomal degradation. In contrast, binding of TNF to TNF-R75 does not induce such receptor internalization. In some cases, ligand-binding appears to activate selective cleavage of the extracellular domain, resulting in the release of soluble TNF-R75. Soluble forms of both receptor types have been found in both the blood and urine.

The exact molecular mechanisms by which TNF-induced signal transduction are mediated remain to be characterized in detail. Oligomerization of the receptors is often followed by their phosphorylation — most likely by accessory kinases that associate with the intracellular domain of the receptor (neither receptor type displays intrinsic protein kinase activity). The existence of several phosphoproteins capable of associating with (the intracellular domain of) TNF-R55 and TNF-R75 has also been established. Following clustering of the TNF receptors, these associated proteins are likely to become activated, thus mediating additional downstream events which eventually trigger characteristic TNF molecular responses. The downstream events are complex and varied. Experimental evidence from various studies implicate a variety of mechanisms, including phosphorylation events, as well as activation of various phospholipases, resulting in the generation of messengers such as diacylglycerol, inositol phosphates and arachidonic acid.

TNF: therapeutic aspects

The initial interest in utilizing TNF as a general anti-cancer agent has diminished, largely due to the realization that:

- many tumours are not susceptible to destruction mediated by TNF (indeed, some tumours produce TNF as an autocrine growth factor);
- tumour cell necrosis is not TNF's major biological activity;

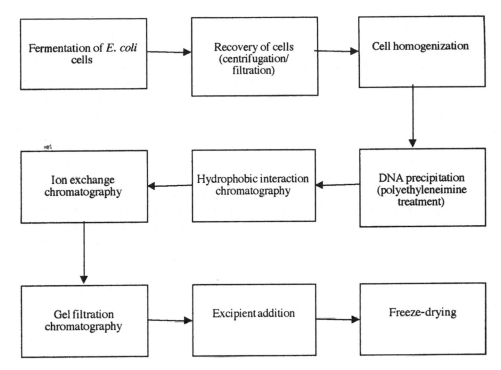

Figure 5.12. Overview of the likely steps undertaken during the manufacture of the recombinant TNF-α product Beromun. Exact details do not appear to be freely available. It is unclear from the publicly available descriptions whether the product accumulates intracellularly in soluble form or in the form of inclusion bodies

Table 5.11. Some diseases in which TNF is known to mediate many of the symptoms

Disease	Symptoms induced by TNF
Cancer	Cachexia
	Stimulation of growth of some tumours
Septic shock	Vascular leakage
	Tissue necrosis
	Hypotension
	Activates blood clotting
Rheumatoid arthritis	Tissue inflammation
	Possible role in destruction of joints
Multiple sclerosis	Inflammation
Diabetes	Death of pancreatic islet cells induces insulin resistance

- severe side-effects usually accompany systemic administration of therapeutically relevant doses of this cytokine.

One such product has, however, been approved for general medical use. Beromun is the trade name given to a TNF-α based product produced by recombinant means in *E. coli*. The recombinant product is identical to the native human protein, with three 17.3 kDa, 157 amino acid polypeptides forming the biologically active homotrimer. An overview of its manufacture is provided in Figure 5.12. Beromun is indicated for the treatment of soft tissue sarcoma in the limbs. It is administered by isolated limb perfusion (i.e. 3–4 mg of product is circulated through the limb over 90 min via a perfusion circuit divorced from general body circulation). As the product does not enter systemic circulation, toxic systemic side effects are avoided. Surgical removal of the tumour mass generally ensues but prior treatment with Beromun prevents/delays the need for whole limb amputation in most patients.

Most clinical interest in TNF now centres around neutralizing its biological effects in situations where overexpression of TNF induces negative clinical effects. TNF has been firmly implicated in mediating many of the adverse effects associated with dozens of diseases (Table 5.11). Administration of anti-TNF monoclonal antibodies or soluble forms of the TNF receptor should help reduce the severity of many of the symptoms of these diseases.

Enbrel is a product now approved for medical use which is based upon this strategy. The product is an engineered hybrid protein consisting of the extracellular domain of the TNF p75 receptor fused directly to the Fc (constant) region of human IgG (see Chapter 10, Box 10.2, for a discussion of antibody structure). The product is expressed in a CHO cell line from which it is excreted as a dimeric soluble protein of approximately 150 kDa. After purification and excipient addition (mannitol, sucrose and trometamol), the product is freeze-dried. It is indicated for the treatment of rheumatoid arthritis and is usually administered as a twice weekly s.c. injection of 25 mg product reconstituted in water for injections. Enbrel functions as a competitive inhibitor of TNF, a major pro-inflammatory cytokine. Binding of TNF to Enbrel prevents it from binding to its true cell surface receptors. Although commercial product literature makes little or no reference to the function of the antibody Fc component, its presence may hasten removal and degradation of the product–TNF complex.

More recently, an additional approach to preventing TNF toxicity has been proposed. Several metalloprotease inhibitors (most notably hydroxamic acid) prevent proteolytic processing (i.e. release) of TNF-α from producer cell surfaces. Such inhibitors may also prove useful in preventing TNF-induced illness. The extent to which TNF (and inhibitors of TNF) will serve as future therapeutic agents remains to be determined by future clinical trials.

FURTHER READING

Books

Balkwill, F. (2000). *The Cytokine Network*. Oxford University Press, Oxford.
Fitzgerald, K. (2001). *Cytokine Factsbook*. Academic Press, London.
Mantovani, A. (2000). *Pharmacology of Cytokines*. Oxford University Press, Oxford.
Mire-Sluis, A. (1998). *Cytokines*. Academic Press, London.

Articles

Interleukins

Arkin, M.A., Randal, M., Delano, W.L. *et al.* (in press). Binding of small molecules to a hot-spot at a protein–protein interface. Protein Data Bank: www.rcsb.org/pdb.
Atkins, M. (2002). Interleukin 2: clinical applications. *Semin. Oncol.* **29**(3), 12–17.
Aulitzky, W. *et al.* (1994). Interleukins. Clinical pharmacology and therapeutic use. *Drugs*, **48**(5), 667–677.
Brown, M. & Hural, J. (1997). Function of IL-4 and control of its expression. *Crit. Rev. Immunol.* **17**(1), 1–32.
Devos, R. *et al.* (1995). Interleukin-5 and its receptor: a drug target for eosinophilia associated with chronic allergic disease. *J. Leukocyte Biol.* **57**, 813–818.

Fehniger, T. *et al.* (2002). Interleukin-2 and interleukin 15: immunotherapy for cancer. *Cytokine Growth Factor Rev.* **13**(2), 169–183.

Fickenscher, H. *et al.* (2002). The interleukin-10 family of cytokines. *Trends Immunol.* **23**(2), 89–96.

Fry, J. & Mackall, C. (2002). Interleukin-7: from bench to clinic. *Blood* **99**(11), 3892–3904.

Jeal, W. & Goa, K. (1997). Aldesleukin (recombinant interleukin-2) — a review of its pharmacological properties, clinical efficacy and tolerability in patients with renal cell carcinoma. *Biodrugs* **7**(4), 285–317.

Komschlies, K. *et al.* (1995). Diverse immunological and haematological effects of interleukin-7: implications for clinical application. *J. Leukocyte Biol.* **58**, 623–631.

Martin, M. & Falk, W. (1997). The interleukin-1 receptor complex and interleukin 1 signal transduction. *Eur. Cytokine Network* **8**(1), 5–17.

Noble, S. & Goa, K. (1997). Aldesleukin (recombinant interleukin-2) — a review of its pharmacological properties, clinical efficacy and tolerability in patients with metastic melanoma. *Biodrugs* **7**(5), 394–422.

Powers, R., Garrett, D.S., March, C.J. *et al.* (1992). Three-dimensional solution structure of human interleukin-4 by multidimensional heteronuclear magnetic resonance spectroscopy. *Science* **256**, 1673.

Renauld, J. *et al.* (1995). Interleukin-9 and its receptor: involvement in mast cell differentiation and T cell oncogenesis. *J. Leukocyte Biol.* **57**, 353–359.

Ryan, J. (1997). Interleukin-4 and its receptor — essential mediators of the allergic response. *J. Allergy Clin. Immunol.* **99**(1), 1–5.

Scott, P. (1993). IL-12: initiation cytokine for cell mediated immunity. *Science* **260**, 496–497.

Simpson, R. *et al.* (1997). Interleukin-6 structure–function relationships. *Protein Sci.* **6**(5), 929–955.

Wigginton, J. & Wiltrout, R. (2002). IL-12/IL-2 combination cytokine therapy for solid tumors: translation from benchside to bedside. *Expert Opin. Biol. Therapy* **2**(5), 513–524.

Tumour necrosis factor

Argiles, J. & Lepezsoriano, F. (1997). Cancer cachexia — a key role for TNF. *Int. J. Oncol.* **10**(3), 565–572.

Bodmer, J. *et al.* (2002). The molecular architecture of the TNF superfamily. *Trends Biochem. Sci.* **27**(1), 19–26.

Bondeson, J. *et al.* (2000). TNF as a therapeutic agent. *Immunologist* **8**(6), 136–140.

Crowe, P. *et al.* (1994). A lymphotoxin-β-specific receptor. *Science* **264**, 707–709.

Darnay, B. & Aggarwal, B. (1997). Early events in TNF signalling — a story of associations and disassociations. *J. Leukocyte Biol.* **61**(5), 559–566.

Dellinger, R. *et al.* (1997). From the bench to the bedside — the future of sepsis research. *Chest* **111**(3), 744–753.

Eck, M.J. & Sprang, S.R. (1989). The structure of tumor necrosis factor-α at 2.6 Å resolution. Implications for receptor binding. *J. Biol. Chem.* **264**, 17595.

Feldmann, M. *et al.* (1997). Anti-tumor necrosis factor-α therapy of rheumatoid arthritis. *Adv. Immunol.* **64**, 283–350.

Hohlfeld, R. (1997). Biotechnological agents for the immunotherapy of multiple sclerosis — principles, problems and perspectives. *Brain* **120**, 865–916.

McDermot, M. (2001). TNF and TNFR biology in health and disease. *Cell. Mol. Biol.* **47**(4), 619–635.

MacEwan, D. (2002). TNF receptor subtype signalling: differences and cellular consequences. *Cell. Signalling* **14**(6), 477–492.

McGeer, E. & McGeer, P. (1997). Inflammatory cytokines in the CNS — possible role in the pathogenesis of neurodegenerative disorders and therapeutic implications. *CNS Drugs* **7**(3), 214–228.

Maini, R. *et al.* (1997). TNF blockade in rheumatoid arthritis — implications for therapy and pathogenesis. *APMIS* **105**(4), 257–263.

Moreland, W. *et al.* (1997). Biological agents for treating rheumatoid arthritis — concepts and progress. *Arthritis Rheumatism* **40**(3), 397–409.

Terranova, P. (1997). Potential roles of tumor necrosis factor-α in follicular development, ovulation and the life-span of the corpus luteum. *Domest. Anim. Endocrinol.* **14**(1), 1–15.

Tracey, K. & Cerami, A. (1994). Tumor necrosis factor: a pleiotropic cytokine and therapeutic target. *Ann. Rev. Med.* **45**, 491–503.

Vandenabeele, P. *et al.* (1995). Two tumor necrosis factor receptors: structure and function. *Trends Cell Biol.* **5**, 392–399.

Chapter 6

Haemopoietic growth factors

Blood consists of red and white cells which, along with platelets, are all suspended in plasma. All peripheral blood cells are derived from a single cell type: the stem cell (also known as a pluripotential, pluripotent or haemopoietic stem cell). These stem cells reside in the bone marrow, alongside additional cell types, including (marrow) stromal cells. Pluripotential stem cells have the capacity to undergo prolonged or indefinite self-renewal. They also have the potential to differentiate, thereby yielding the range of cells normally found in blood (Table 6.1). This process, by which a fraction of stem cells are continually 'deciding' to differentiate (thus continually producing new blood cells and platelets to replace aged cells), is known as haemopoiesis.

The study of the process of haemopoiesis is rendered difficult by the fact that it is extremely difficult to distinguish or separate individual stem cells from their products during the earlier stages of differentiation. However, a picture of the process of differentiation is now beginning to emerge (Figure 6.1). During the haemopoietic process, the stem cells differentiate, producing cells that become progressively more restricted in their choice of developmental options.

The production of many mature blood cells begins when a fraction of the stem cells differentiate, forming a specific cell type termed CFU-S (CFU refers to colony forming unit). These, in turn, differentiate yielding CFU-GEMM cells, a mixed CFU which has the potential to differentiate into a range of mature blood cell types, including granulocytes, monocytes, erythrocytes, platelets, eosinophils and basophils. Note that lymphocytes are not derived from the CFU-GEMM pathway, but differentiate via an alternative pathway from stem cells (Figure 6.1).

The details of haemopoiesis presented thus far prompt two very important questions. How is the correct balance between stem cell self-renewal and differentiation maintained? And what forces exist that regulate the process of differentiation? The answer to both questions, in particular the latter, is beginning to emerge in the form of a group of cytokines termed 'haemopoietic growth factors' (Table 6.2). This group includes:

- several (of the previously described) interleukins (ILs) that primarily affect production and differentiation of lymphocytes;
- colony stimulating factors (CSFs), which play a major role in the differentiation of stem-derived cells into neutrophils, macrophages, megakaryocytes (from which platelets are derived), eosinophils and basophils;

Biopharmaceuticals: Biochemistry and Biotechnology, Second Edition. Gary Walsh
John Wiley & Sons Ltd: ISBN 0 470 84326 8 (ppc), ISBN 0 470 84327 6 (pbk)

Table 6.1. The range of blood cells that are ultimately produced upon the differentiation of pluripotential stem cells (see text for details). (Note that osteoclasts are multinucleated cells often associated with small depressions on the surface of bone; they function to reabsorb calcified bone)

Neutrophils	T and B lymphocytes
Eosinophils	Erythrocytes
Basophils	Monocytes
Megakaryocytes	Osteoclasts

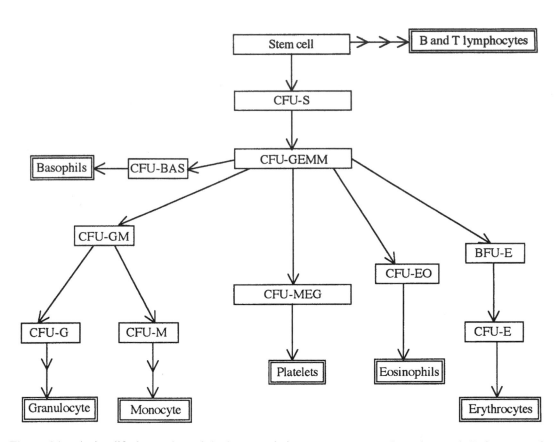

Figure 6.1. A simplified overview of the haemopoietic process as currently understood. Refer to text for details. CFU = colony forming unit; BFU = burst forming unit

- erythropoietin, which is essential in the production of red blood cells;
- thrombopoietin, which is essential in the production of platelets.

Most of these haemopoietic growth factors are glycoproteins, displaying a molecular mass in the region of 14–24 kDa. Most are produced by more than one cell type and several display redundancy in their actions. In general several such regulators can stimulate proliferation of any

Table 6.2. Major haemopoietic growth factors described to date

Various interleukins
Granulocyte-macrophage-colony stimulating factor (GM-CSF)
Granulocyte-colony stimulating factor (G-CSF)
Macrophage-colony stimulating factor (M-CSF)
Leukaemia inhibitory factor (ILF)
Erythropoietin (EPO)
Thrombopoietin (TPO)

one haemopoietic cell lineage. This is due to the presence of receptors for several such factors on their surface. Receptor numbers for any one growth factor are low (less than 500/cell) and proliferation can be stimulated even when only a small proportion of these are occupied.

Genetic engineering has allowed the production of recombinant forms of virtually all of the currently recognized haemopoietic growth factors. This has facilitated development of a greater depth of understanding of the haemopoietic process. When stem cells were treated *in vitro* with various growth factors, only IL-3 was able to sustain/promote their growth and differentiation. Treatment with individual CSFs, or other ILs, failed not only to promote differentiation but, in most cases, even to promote continued survival of the cells. Subsequent experimentation illustrated the requirement for a combination of growth factors in most instances. A combination of granulocyte-colony stimulating factor (G-CSF) and macrophage-colony stimulating factor (M-CSF) was found to promote neutrophil and macrophage differentiation, while similar synergistic interactions were noted when IL-1 and IL-3 or G-CSF and granulocyte-macrophage-colony stimulating factor (GM-CSF) were used in combination. Such requirements for stem cell maintenance and differentiation are also likely to be mirrored *in vivo*.

In vivo, haemopoietic cells are usually found clustered in close association with various types of bone marrow stromal cells. It appears that the stromal cells play a direct role in promoting proliferation/differentiation of the stem cells. Indeed, co-culture of the stromal and stem cells facilitates self-renewal and differentiation of the latter in the absence of exogenously added growth factors. Interestingly, direct contact between the two cell types is required. This appears to indicate that the growth factors are physically associated with the surface of the stromal cell, rather than being released in soluble form. When grown *in vitro*, stromal cells are known to produce various haemopoietic growth factors, including IL-4, -6 and -7, as well as G-CSF.

During normal haemopoiesis, only a small fraction of stem cells undergo differentiation at any given time. The remainder continue to self-renew. The molecular detail underpinning self-renewal is poorly understood. However, it has been shown that certain transformed stem cells can be induced to undergo continuous proliferation *in vitro* under the influence of IL-3. The concentration of IL-3 is critical, with differentiation occurring below certain threshold concentrations of this cytokine. The delicate balance between stem cell renewal and differentiation is probably affected not only by the range of growth factors experienced but also by the concentration of each growth factor.

THE INTERLEUKINS AS HAEMOPOIETIC GROWTH FACTORS

The IL family of cytokines have been discussed in detail in Chapter 5. IL-3 is perhaps the IL that figures most prominently in the haemopoietic process, and appears to stimulate not only

CFU-GEMM, but also the precursor cells of basophils, eosinophils and platelets. The role of IL-11 has been discussed in Chapter 5.

GRANULOCYTE-COLONY STIMULATING FACTOR (G-CSF)

G-CSF is also known as pluripoietin and CSF-β. Two slight variants are known, one consisting of 174 amino acids, the other of 177. These are products of alternative splicing. The smaller polypeptide predominates, and also displays significantly greater biological activity than the larger variant.

G-CSF is a glycoprotein, displaying a single O-linked glycosylation site and an apparent molecular mass in the region of 21 kDa. The molecule is stabilized by the presence of two disulphide linkages. It displays a compact 3-D structure, featuring four α-helical bundles similar to growth hormone and IL-2. It is synthesized by various cell types (Table 6.3), and functions as a growth and differentiation factor for neutrophils and their precursor cells. It also appears to activate mature neutrophils (which are leukocytes capables of ingesting and killing bacteria). G-CSF also appears to act in synergy with additional haemopoietic growth factors to stimulate growth/differentiation of various other haemopoietic progenitor cells. In addition, this cytokine promotes the proliferation and migration of endothelial cells. The G-CSF receptor has been well characterized. It is a single transmembrane polypeptide, found on the surface of neutrophils, as well as various haemopoietic precursor cells, platelets, endothelial cells and, notably, various myeloid leukaemias (myeloid means derived from bone marrow; leukaemia refers to a cancerous condition in which there is uncontrolled overproduction of white blood cells in the bone marrow or other blood-forming organs. The white cells produced are generally immature/abnormal and the condition results in the suppression of production of healthy white blood cells).

The extracellular region of the G-CSF receptor is heavily glycosylated (containing nine potential glycosylation sites) and displays a molecular mass in the region of 150 kDa. Two variants of the receptor in humans have been noted which display differences in the intracellular

Table 6.3. Summary of some of the properties of G-CSF, M-CSF and GM-CSF

	G-CSF	M-CSF	GM-CSF
Molecular mass (kDa)	21	45–90	22
Main producer cells	Bone marrow stromal cells Macrophages Fibroblasts	Lymphocytes Myoblasts Osteoblasts Monocytes Fibroblasts Endothelial cells	Macrophages T lymphocytes Fibroblasts Endothelial cells
Main target cells	Neutrophils Also other haemopoietic progenitors and endothelial cells	Macrophages and their precursor cells	Haematopoietic progenitor cells Granulocytes Monocytes Endothelial cells Megakaryocytes T lymphocytes Erythroid cells

domain. The exact mode of signal transduction remains to be fully detailed. G-CSF binding does appear to prompt the phosphorylation of several cytoplasmic proteins, and an associated JAK 2 kinase has been implicated.

MACROPHAGE COLONY-STIMULATING FACTOR (M-CSF)

M-CSF serves as a growth, differentiation and activation factor for macrophages and their precursor cells. It is also known as CSF-1. This cytokine is produced by various cell types (Table 6.3). The mature form is a glycoprotein (containing three potential N-linked glycosylation sites), and its 3-D structure is stabilized by multiple disulphide linkages. Three related forms of human M-CSF have been characterized. All are ultimately derived from the same gene and share common C- and N-termini. The largest consists of 522 amino acids with the 406 and 224 amino acid forms lacking different lengths of the internal sequence of the 522 form. The molecular masses of these mature M-CSFs are in the range 45–90 kDa.

The biologically active form of M-CSF is a homodimer. These homodimers can exist as integral cell surface proteins, or may be released from their producer cell by proteolytic cleavage, thus yielding the soluble cytokine.

The M-CSF receptor is a single chain, heavily glycosylated, polypeptide of molecular mass 150 kDa. Its intracellular domain displays tyrosine kinase activity which is capable of autophosphorylation, as well as phosphorylating additional cytoplasmic polypeptides.

GRANULOCYTE-MACROPHAGE COLONY STIMULATING FACTOR (GM-CSF)

GM-CSF is also known as CSF-α or pluripoietin-α. It is a 127 amino acid, single chain, glycosylated polypeptide, exhibiting a molecular mass in the region of 22 kDa. Its 3-D structure exhibits a bundle of four α-helices and a two-stranded antiparallel β-sheet (Figure 6.2). It thus resembles the other CSFs. GM-CSF is produced by various cells (Table 6.3) and studies have indicated that its biological activities include:

- Proliferation/differentiation factor of haemopoietic progenitor cells, particularly those yielding neutrophils (a variety of granulocyte) and macrophages, but also eosinophils, erythrocytes and megakaryocytes. *In vivo* studies also demonstrate this cytokine's ability to promote haemopoiesis.
- Activation of mature haemopoietic cells, resulting in:
  – enhanced phagocytic activity;
  – enhanced microbiocidal activity;
  – augmented anti-tumour activity;
  – enhanced leukocyte chemotaxis.

The intact GM-CSF receptor is a heterodimer, consisting of a low-affinity α-chain and a β-chain, which also forms part of the IL-3 and IL-5 receptors (the β-chain alone does not bind GM-CSF). The α-chain is a 80 kDa glycoprotein and exhibits only a short intracellular domain. The larger β-chain (130 kDa) displays a significant intracellular domain. Signal transduction involves the (tyrosine) phosphorylation of a number of cytoplasmic proteins (Figure 6.3).

The multiplicity of activities attributed to GM-CSF (particularly by *in vitro* studies), along with the redundancy exhibited by this cytokine, renders difficult appraisal of its most significant physiological role (this is, of course, also true in the case of many other cytokines). Studies

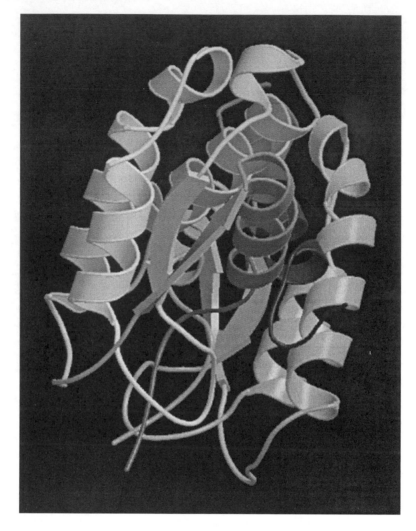

Figure 6.2.   3-D structure of GM-CSF. Photo from Walter *et al.* (1992), by courtesy of the Protein Data Bank: http://www.pdb.org/

designed to elucidate its exact role, by generation of mutant mice lacking GM-CSF, have yielded surprising results. These mice were found to be healthy and fertile, and were capable of sustaining normal steady-state haemopoiesis. In fact, the only physiological abnormality revealed was associated with the lungs, where a major build-up of surfactant was noted (surfactant is a mixture of various phospholipids and proteins, which appears to function mainly to reduce surface tension at the alveolar air–liquid interface). Although GM-CSF can undoubtedly influence haemopoiesis when administered experimentally, the above finding casts serious doubt on the physiological significance of such activity. It also illustrates the power of the technique by which knock-out mice, lacking a specific gene, can be generated, and shows how this technique can help delineate the true physiological role of that gene's product.

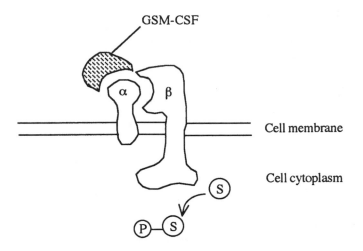

Figure 6.3. The GM-CSF receptor. Ligand binding appears to promote the phosphorylation of various cytoplasmic polypeptide substrates (at least in part via an associated JAK 2 kinase), leading to signal transduction

CLINICAL APPLICATION OF CSFs

As haemopoietic growth factors serve to stimulate the production of mature blood cells, their clinical application in diseases characterized by sub-optimal production of specific blood cell types was obvious. Several CSF preparations have gained regulatory approval, or are currently being assessed in clinical trials (Table 6.4). G-CSF and GM-CSF have proved useful in the treatment of neutropenia. All three CSF types are (or are likely to be) useful in the treatment of infectious diseases, some forms of cancer and the management of bone marrow transplants (Table 6.4), as they stimulate the differentiation/activation of white blood cell types most affected by such conditions.

Table 6.4. Colony-stimulating factors approved for medical use or in clinical trials

Product	Status	Indication	Company
Nepogen (filgrastim; G-CSF)	Approved	Neutropenia caused by chemotherapy Bone marrow transplants	Amgen Inc.
Leukine (sargramostim; GM-CSF)	Approved	Autologous bone marrow transplantation Neutrophil recovery after bone marrow transplantation	Immunex
Neulasta (PEGylated filgrastim)	Approved	Neutropenia	Amgen
GM-CSF	In clinical trials	Immune stimulation in malignant melanoma Crohn's disease	Berlex
GM-CSF	In clinical trials	Myeloid reconstitution following stem cell transplantation	Cangene

Table 6.5.   Some causes of neutropenia

Genetic (particularly in black populations)
Severe bacterial infection
Severe sepsis
Severe viral infection
Aplastic anaemia*
Acute leukaemia
Hodgkin's/non-Hodgkin's lymphoma
Various drugs, especially anti-cancer drugs
Autoimmune neutropenia

---

*Aplastic anaemia describes bone marrow failure characterized by serious reduction in the number of stem cells present

Neutropenia is a condition characterized by a decrease in blood neutrophil count below 1.5×10^9 cells/l (normal blood count $2.0–7.5 \times 10^9$ cells/l). Its clinical symptoms include the occurrence of frequent and usually serious infections, often requiring hospitalization. Neutropenia may be caused by a number of factors (Table 6.5), at least some of which are responsive to CSF treatment. Particularly noteworthy is neutropenia triggered by administration of chemotherapeutic drugs to cancer patients. Chemotherapeutic agents (e.g. cyclophosphamide, doxorubicin and methotrexate), when administered at therapeutically effective doses, often induce the destruction of stem cells and/or compromise stem cell differentiation.

Filgrastim is a recombinant human G-CSF (produced in *E. coli*), approved for chemotherapy-induced neutropenia since 1991. Although the 18.8 kDa recombinant product is not glycosylated and contains an additional N-terminal methionine residue (due to expression in *E. coli*), it displays biological activity indistinguishable from native G-CSF. The product is presented in freeze-dried format and contains buffer elements as well as sorbitol and Tween as excipients.

Administration of filgrastim (0.5 µg/kg/day) to healthy volunteers for six consecutive days resulted in up to a 10-fold increase in their absolute neutrophil count. Daily administration to patients receiving chemotherapy greatly reduced the duration and severity of leucopenia (reduction in the numbers of total white blood cells). The magnitude of the specific neutrophil response depended upon the number of progenitor cells still surviving upon commencement of treatment. Neutrophils from patients with neutropenia treated with filgrastim also display enhanced phagocytosis and chemotaxis, at least transiently.

Filgrastim is used in conjunction with cancer chemotherapy in one of two ways: prophylactic administration aims to prevent onset of neutropenia in the first place, while therapeutic administration aims to reverse neutropenia already established. It is generally effective in both circumstances and in clinical trials it was found to reduce the number of (neutropenia-induced) days of patient hospitalization by up to 50%. Filgrastim administration may also permit modest increases in the maximum dose intensity utilizable in chemotherapeutic regimes.

Filgrastim is usually administered by subcutaneous injection. Dosage levels range from 5–10 µg/kg/day, with peak plasma drug concentrations being observed 2–8 hours after administration. The mechanism by which filgrastim is removed from circulation is unclear, but the drug's elimination half-life ranges from less than 2 h to almost 5 h. The drug is generally well tolerated. The most common adverse reaction is mild bone pain, which occurs in up to 20% of cancer patients receiving treatment. This is easily treated with analgesics.

While filgrastim has proved a useful adjuvant to chemotherapy for many cancers, its administration in cases of myeloid leukaemia would give cause for concern, as these cells express receptors for G-CSF. In such cases, G-CSF could potentially promote accelerated growth of these malignant cells.

Filgrastim also shows therapeutic promise in the treatment of additional conditions characterized by depressed blood neutrophil counts. Such conditions include severe chronic neutropenia, leukaemia and AIDS.

Neulasta is the tradename given to a PEGylated form of filgrastim approved for general medical use in the USA in 2002. Manufacture of this product entails covalent attachment of an activated monomethoxypolyethylene glycol molecule to the N-terminal methionyl residue of filgrastim. The product is formulated in the presence of acetate buffer, sorbitol and polysorbate and is presented in pre-filled syringes for subcutaneous injection. As in the case of PEGylated interferons (IFNs) (Chapter 4), the rationale for PEGylation is to increase the drug's plasma half-life, thereby reducing the frequency of injections required.

G-CSF and GM-CSF have also found application after allogenic or autologous bone marrow transplantation, to accelerate neutrophil recovery (allogenic means that donor and recipient are different individuals, while autologous means that donor and recipient are the same individual).

Bone marrow transplantation, particularly allogenic transplantation, is often a treatment of choice for individuals suffering from acute or chronic leukaemia, aplastic anaemia or various stem cell-related genetic disorders (e.g. thalassaemias).

Allogenic transplantation generally entails removal of approximately 1 l of marrow from a matched donor (usually a sibling, preferably an identical twin). The recipient patient is prepared by intensive chemotherapy (or radiotherapy) to kill residual malignant marrow cells. The donated marrow cells are then administered intravenously to the patient, and they re-populate the marrow cavity. The peripheral blood count normally rises within 2–4 weeks.

Autologous bone marrow transplantation involves initial removal of some marrow from the patient, its storage in liquid nitrogen, followed by its re-introduction into the patient subsequent to chemo- or radiotherapy. Leukine is the tradename given to a recombinant human GM-CSF preparation produced in engineered *S. cerevisiae* (Table 6.4).

LEUKAEMIA INHIBITORY FACTOR (LIF)

LIF is an additional haemopoietic growth factor. It is also known as HILDA (human interleukin for DA cells) and hepatocyte stimulatory factor III. It is produced by a range of cell types, including T cells, liver cells and fibroblasts. LIF is a 180 amino acid, heavily glycosylated, 45 kDa protein. It affects both haemopoietic and non-haemopoietic tissue, often acting in synergy with other cytokines, particularly IL-3. It stimulates the differentiation of macrophages and promotes enhanced platelet formation. It also prompts synthesis of acute phase proteins by the liver and promotes increased bone resorption. The greatest concentrations of LIF receptors are associated with monocytes, embryonic stem cells, liver cells and the placenta. The receptor complex is composed of two transmembrane glycoproteins: the 190 kDa LIFRα-chain which displays affinity for LIF, and a β-chain (gp130), which also forms part of the IL-6 receptor.

ERYTHROPOIETIN (EPO)

Erythropoietin (EPO) is an additional haemopoietic growth factor. It is primarily responsible for stimulating and regulating erythropoiesis (i.e. erythrogenesis, the production of red blood cells) in mammals.

The 'erythron' is a collective term given to mature erythrocytes, along with all stem cell-derived progeny that have committed to developing into erythrocytes. It can thus be viewed as a dispersed organ, whose primary function relates to transport of oxygen and carbon dioxide (haemoglobin constitutes up to one-third of the erythrocyte cytoplasm), as well as maintaining blood pH. An average adult contains in the region of 2.3×10^{13} erythrocytes (weighing up to 3 kg). They are synthesized at a rate of about 2.3 million cells/s, and have a circulatory life of approximately 120 days, during which they travel almost 200 miles.

EPO is an atypical cytokine in that it acts as a true (endocrine) hormone and is not synthesized by any type of white blood cell. It is encoded by a single copy gene, located on (human) chromosome 7. The gene consists of four introns and five exons. The mature EPO gene product contains 166 amino acids and exhibits a molecular mass in the region of 36 kDa (Figure 6.4) EPO is a glycoprotein, almost 40% of which is carbohydrate. Three N-linked and one O-linked glycosylation site are evident. The O-linked carbohydrate moiety apears to play no

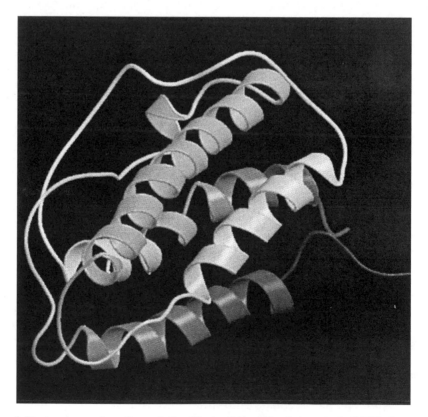

Figure 6.4. 3-D structure of erythropoietin. Photo from Cheetham *et al.* (1998), by courtesy of the Protein Data Bank: http://www.pdb.org/

essential role in the (*in vitro* or *in vivo*) biological activity of EPO. Interestingly, removal of the N-linked sugars, while having little effect on EPO's *in vitro* activity, destroys its *in vivo* activity. The sugar components of EPO are likely to contribute to the molecule's:

- solubility;
- cellular processing and secretion;
- *in vivo* metabolism.

Incomplete (N-linked) glycosylation prompts decreased *in vivo* activity due to more rapid hepatic clearance of the EPO molecule. Enzymatic removal of terminal sialic acid sugar residues from oligosaccharides exposes otherwise hidden galactose residues. These residues are then free to bind specific hepatic lectins, which promote EPO removal from the plasma. The reported plasma half-life ($t_{1/2}$) value for native EPO is 4–6 h. The $t_{1/2}$ for desialated EPO is 2 min. Comparison of native human EPO with its recombinant form produced in CHO cells reveal very similar glycosylation patterns.

Circular dichroism studies show that up to 50% of EPO's secondary structure is α-helical. The predicted tertiary structure is that of four anti-parallel helices formed by variable-sized loops, similar to many other haemopoietic growth factors.

Development of bioassays and radioimmunoassays, along with the later development of specific mRNA probes, allowed determination of the sites of production of EPO in the body. It has now been established that EPO in the human adult is synthesized almost exclusively by specialized kidney cells (peritubular interstitial cells of the kidney cortex and upper medulla). Minor quantities are also synthesized in the liver, which represents the primary EPO-producing organ of the fetus.

EPO is present in serum and (at very low concentrations) in urine, particularly of anaemic individuals. This cytokine/hormone was first purified in 1971 from the plasma of anaemic sheep, while small quantities of human EPO was later purified (in 1977) from over 2500 litres of urine collected from anaemic patients. Large-scale purification from native sources was thus impractical. The isolation (in 1985) of the human EPO gene from a genomic DNA library, facilitated its transfection into Chinese hamster ovary (CHO) cells. This now facilitates large-scale commercial production of the recombinant human product (rhEPO), which has found widespread medical application.

EPO stimulates erythropoiesis by:

- increasing the number of committed cells capable of differentiating into erythrocytes;
- accelerating the rate of differentiation of such precursors;
- increasing the rate of haemoglobin synthesis in developing cells.

An overview of the best-characterized stages in the process of erythropoiesis is given in Figure 6.5.

The erythroid precursor cells, BFU-E (burst forming unit-erythroid), display EPO receptors on their surface. The growth and differentiation of these cells into CFU-Es (colony forming unit-erythroid), require the presence not only of EPO but also of IL-3 and/or GM-CSF. CFU-E cells display the greatest density of EPO cell surface receptors. These cells, not surprisingly, also display the greatest biological response to EPO. Progressively more mature erythrocyte precursors display progressively fewer EPO receptors on their cell surfaces. Erythrocytes themselves are devoid of EPO receptors. EPO binding to its receptor on CFU-E cells promotes their differentiation into pro-erythroblasts and the rate at which this differentiation occurs

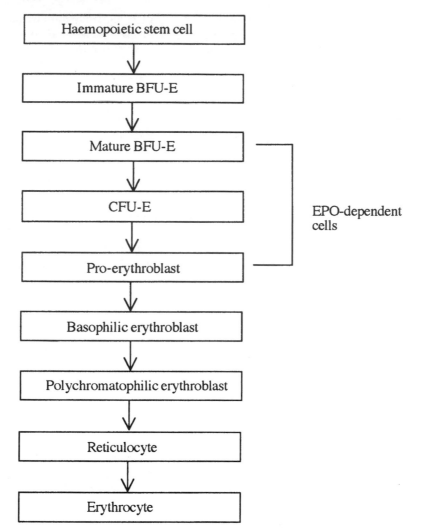

Figure 6.5. Stages in the differentiation of haemopoietic stem cells, yielding mature erythrocytes. The EPO-sensitive cells are indicated. Each cell undergoes proliferation as well as differentiation, thus greater numbers of the more highly differentiated daughter cells are produced. The proliferation phase ends at the reticulocyte stage; each reticulocyte matures over a 2 day period, yielding a single mature erythrocyte

appears to determine the rate of erythropoiesis. CFU-E cells are also responsive to insulin-like growth factor 1 (IGF-1).

Although the major physiological role of EPO is certainly to promote red blood cell production, EPO mRNA has also been detected in bone marrow macrophages, as well as some multipotential haemopoietic stem cells. Although the physiological relevance is unclear, it is possible that EPO produced by such sources may play a localized paracrine (or autocrine) role in promoting erythroid differentiation.

The EPO receptor and signal transduction

The availability of biologically active ^{125}I-labelled EPO facilitated the detection and study of cell surface receptors. In addition to erythroid precursors, various other cell lines were shown to express EPO receptors, at least when cultured *in vitro*. Many harboured two classes of receptors: a high-affinity and a low-affinity form. Most appeared to express between 1000 and 3000 receptors/cell. Radiotracer experiments illustrated that the EPO receptor is rapidly internalized after ligand binding and the EPO–receptor complex is subsequently degraded within lysosomes.

The human EPO receptor is encoded by a single gene on chromosome 19. The gene houses eight exons, the first five of which appear to code for the 233 amino acid extracellular receptor portion. The sixth encodes a single 23 amino acid transmembrane domain, while the remaining two exons encode the 236 amino acid cytoplasmic domain. The mature receptor displays a molecular mass of 85–100 kDa. It is heavily glycosylated through multiple O-linked (and a single N-linked) glycosylation site. High- versus low-affinity receptor variants may be generated by self-association.

The EPO receptor is a member of the haemopoietic cytokine receptor superfamily. Its intracellular domain displays no known catalytic activity but it appears to couple directly to the JAK 2 kinase (Chapter 4), which probably promotes the early events of EPO signal transduction. Other studies have implicated additional possible signalling mechanisms, including the involvement of G proteins, protein kinase C and Ca^{2+}. The exact molecular events underlining EPO signal transduction remain to be elucidated in detail.

Binding of EPO to its receptor stimulates the proliferation of BFU-E cells and triggers CFU-Es to undergo terminal differentiation. As well as such stimulatory roles, EPO may play a permissive role, in that it also appears to inhibit apoptosis (programmed cell death) of these cells. With this scenario, 'normal' serum EPO levels permit survival of a specific fraction of BFU-E and CFU-Es, which dictates the observed rate of haemopoiesis. Increased serum EPO concentrations permit survival of a greater fraction of these progenitor cells, thus increasing the number of red blood cells ultimately produced. The relative physiological importance of EPO stimulatory versus permissive activities has yet to be determined.

Regulation of EPO production

The level of EPO production in the kidneys (or liver) is primarily regulated by the oxygen demand of the producer cells, relative to their oxygen supply. Under normal conditions, when the producer cells are supplied with adequate oxygen via the blood, EPO (or EPO mRNA) levels are barely detectable. However, the onset of hypoxia (a deficiency of oxygen in the tissues) results in a very rapid increase of EPO mRNA in producer cells. This is followed within 2 h by an increase in serum EPO levels. This process is prevented by inhibitors of RNA and protein synthesis, indicating that EPO is not stored in producer cells, but synthesized *de novo* when required.

Interestingly, hypoxia prompts increased renal and hepatic EPO synthesis in different ways. In the kidney, the quantity of EPO produced by an individual cell remains constant, while an increase in the number of EPO-producing cells is evident. In the liver, the quantity of EPO produced by individual cells appears to simply increase in response to the hypoxic stimulus.

A range of conditions capable of inducing hypoxia stimulate enhanced production of EPO, thus stimulating erythropoiesis. These conditions include:

- moving to a higher altitude;
- blood loss;
- increased renal sodium transport;
- decreased renal blood flow;
- increased haemoglobin oxygen affinity;
- chronic pulmonary disease;
- some forms of heart disease.

On the other hand, hyperoxic conditions (excess tissue oxygen levels) promote a decrease in EPO production.

The exact mechanism by which hypoxia stimulates EPO production remains to be elucidated. This process has been studied *in vitro* using an EPO-producing cancerous liver (hepatoma) cell line as a model system. These studies suggest the existence of a haem protein (probably membrane-bound), which effectively acts as an oxygen sensor (Figure 6.6). Adequate ambient oxygen concentration retains the haem group in an oxygenated state. Hypoxia, however, promotes a deoxy-configuration, which alters the haem conformation. The deoxy- form of haem is postulated to be capable of generating an active transcription factor which, upon migration to the nucleus, enhances transcription of the EPO gene. Evidence cited to support such a theory includes the fact that cobalt promotes erythropoiesis (cobalt can substitute for the iron atom in the haem porphyrin ring; Cobalt–haem, however, remains in the deoxy-conformation, even in the presence of a high oxygen tension). In addition to oxygen levels, a number of other regulatory factors can stimulate EPO synthesis, either on their own or in synergy with hypoxia (Table 6.6).

Therapeutic applications of EPO

A number of clinical circumstances have been identified which are characterized by an often profoundly depressed rate of erythropoiesis (Table 6.7). Many, if not all, such conditions could be/are responsive to administration of exogenous EPO. The prevalence of anaemia, and the medical complications which ensue, prompts tremendous therapeutic interest in this haemopoietic growth factor. EPO has been approved for use to treat various forms of anaemia (Table 6.8). It was the first therapeutic protein produced by genetic engineering, whose annual sales value topped $1 billion. Its current annual sales value is now close to $2 billion. EPO used therapeutically is produced by recombinant means in CHO cells.

Neorecormon is one such product. Produced in an engineered CHO cell line constitutively expressing the EPO gene, the product displays an amino acid sequence identical to the native human molecule. An overview of its manufacturing process is presented in Figure 6.7. The final freeze-dried product contains urea, sodium chloride, polysorbate, phosphate buffer and several amino acids as excipients. It displays a shelf-life of 3 years when stored at 2–8 °C. A pre-filled syrine form of the product (in solution) is also available, which is assigned a 2 year shelf-life at 2–8 °C.

EPO can be administered intravenously or, more commonly, by subcutaneous (s.c.) injection. Peak serum concentrations are witnessed 8–24 h after s.c. administration. Although they are lower than the values achieved by i.v. administration, the effect is more prolonged, lasting for several hours. In healthy individuals, less than 10% of administered EPO is excreted intact in the urine. This suggests that the kidneys play, at best, a minor role in the excretion of this hormone.

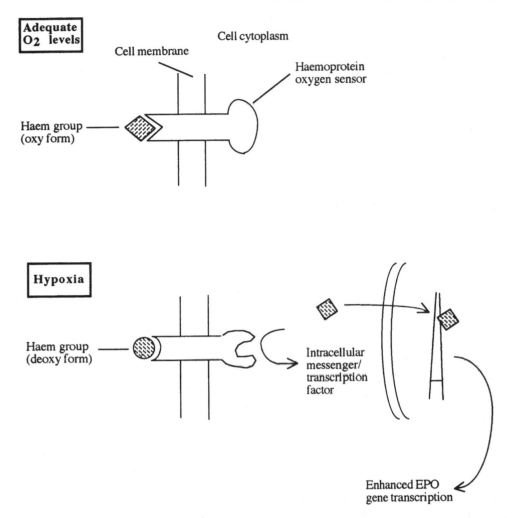

Figure 6.6. Proposed mechanism by which hypoxic conditions stimulate enhanced EPO synthesis (see text for details)

Table 6.6. Some additional regulatory factors that can promote increased EPO production. Other regulatory factors, including IL-3 and CSFs, which also influence the rate of erythropoiesis, are omitted as they have been discussed previously

---

Growth hormone
Thyroxine
Adrenocorticotrophic hormone
Adrenaline
Angiotensin II
Androgens and anabolic steroids

Table 6.7. Diseases (and other medical conditions) for which anaemia is one frequently observed symptom

Renal failure
Rheumatoid arthritis
Cancer
AIDS
Infections
Bone marrow transplantation

Table 6.8. EPO preparations that have gained regulatory approval or are undergoing clinical trials

Product	Status	Company
Epogen (rhEPO)	Approved	Amgen
Procrit (rhEPO)	Approved	Ortho Biotech
Neorecormon (rhEPO)	Approved	Boehringer–Mannheim
Aranesp (rEPO analogue)	Approved	Amgen
Nespo (rEPO analogue)	Approved	Dompé Biotec
rEPO	In clinical trials	Aventis

More recently, an engineered form of EPO has gained marketing approval. Darbepoetin-α is its international non-proprietary name and it is marketed under the tradenames Aranesp (Amgen) and Nespo (Dompé Biotec, Italy). The 165 amino acid protein is altered in amino acid sequence when compared to the native human product. The alteration entails introducing two new N-glycosylation sites, so that the recombinant product, produced in an engineered CHO cell line, displays five glycosylation sites as opposed to the normal three. The presence of two additional carbohydrate chains confers a prolonged serum half-life on the molecule (up to 21 h as compared to 4–6 h for the native molecule).

EPO was first used therapeutically in 1989 for the treatment of anaemia associated with chronic kidney failure. This anaemia is largely caused by insufficient endogenous EPO production by the diseased kidneys. Prior to EPO approval, this condition could only be treated by direct blood transfusion. It responds well, and in a dose-dependent manner, to the administration of recombinant human EPO (rhEPO). The administration of EPO is effective in the case of both patients receiving dialysis and those who have not yet received this treatment.

Administration of doses of 50–150 IU EPO/kg three times weekly is normally sufficient to elevate the patient's haematocrit values to a desired 32–35% (haematocrit refers to 'packed cell volume', i.e. the percentage of the total volume of whole blood that is composed of erythrocytes). Plasma EPO concentrations generally vary between 5 and 25 IU/l in healthy individuals. One IU (international unit) of EPO activity is defined as the activity which promotes the same level of stimulation of erythropoiesis as 5 mmol cobalt.

In addition to enhancing erythropoiesis, EPO treatment also improves tolerance to exercise, as well as patients' sense of well-being. Furthermore, reducing/eliminating the necessity for blood transfusions also reduces/eliminates the associated risk of accidental transmission of blood-borne infectious agents, as well as the risk of precipitating adverse transfusion reactions

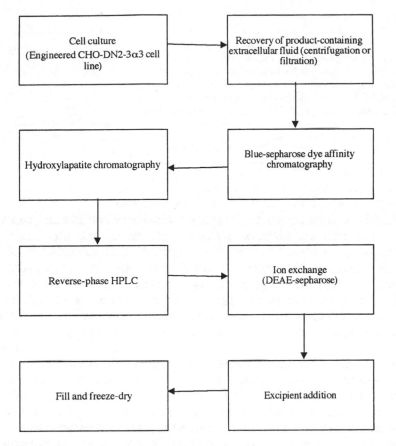

Figure 6.7. Schematic overview of the production of the erythropoietin-based product Neorecormon. Refer to text for further details

in recipients. An American study calculated the average cost of rhEPO therapy to be of the order of $6000/patient/annum, compared to approx. $4600 for transfusion therapy. However, due to the additional benefits described, the cost:benefit ratio appears to favour EPO therapy. The therapeutic spotlight upon EPO has now shifted to additional (non-renal) applications (Table 6.9).

Chronic disease and cancer chemotherapy

Anaemia often becomes a characteristic feature of several chronic diseases, such as rheumatoid arthritis. In most instances this can be linked to lower than normal endogenous serum EPO levels (although in some cases, a deficiency of iron or folic acid can also represent a contributory factor). Several small clinical trials have confirmed that administration of EPO increases haematocrit and serum haemoglobin levels in patients suffering from rheumatoid arthritis. A satisfactory response in some patients, however, required high-dose therapy, which could render this therapeutic approach unattractive from a cost:benefit perspective.

Table 6.9. Some non-renal applications of EPO (refer to text for details)

Treatment of anaemia associated with chronic disease
Treatment of anaemia associated with cancer/chemotherapy
Treatment of anaemia associated with prematurity
To facilitate autologous blood donations before surgery
To reduce transfusion requirements after surgery
To prevent anaemia after bone marrow transplantation

Severe, and in particular chronic, infection can also sometimes induce anaemia — which is often made worse by drugs used to combat the infection, e.g. anaemia is evident in 8% of patients with asymptomatic HIV infection. This incidence increases to 20% for those with AIDS-related complex and is greater than 60% for patients who have developed Kaposi's sarcoma. Up to one-third of AIDS patients treated with zidovudine also develop anaemia. Again, several trials have confirmed that EPO treatment of AIDS sufferers (be they receiving zidovudine or not) can increase haematocrit values and decrease transfusion requirements.

Various malignancies can also induce an anaemic state. This is often associated with decreased serum EPO levels, although iron deficiency, blood loss or tumour infiltration of the bone marrow can be complicating factors. In addition, chemotherapeutic agents administered to this patient group often adversely affect stem cell populations, thus rendering the anaemia even more severe.

Administration of EPO to patients suffering from various cancers/receiving various chemotherapeutic agents yielded encouraging results, with significant improvements in haematocrit levels being recorded in approximately 50% of cases. In one large US study (2000 patients, most receiving chemotherapy) s.c. administration of an average of 150 IU EPO/kg, three times weekly, for 4 months, reduced the number of patients requiring blood transfusions from 22% to 10%. Improvement in the sense of well-being and overall quality of life was also noted. The success rate of EPO in alleviating cancer-associated anaemia has varied in different trials, ranging from 32% to 85%.

The EPO receptor is expressed not only by specific erythrocyte precursor cells but also by endothelial, neural and myeloma cells. Concern has been expressed that EPO, therefore, might actually stimulate growth of some tumour types, particularly those derived from such cells. To date, no evidence (*in vitro* or *in vivo*) has been obtained to support this hypothesis.

Additional non-renal applications

Babies, especially babies born prematurely, often exhibit anaemia, which is characterized by a steadily decreasing serum haemoglobin level during the first 8 weeks of life. While multiple factors contribute to development of anaemia of prematurity, a lower than normal serum EPO level is a characteristic trait. *In vitro* studies indicate that BFU-E and CFU-E cells from such babies are responsive to EPO, and several pilot clinical trials have been initiated. Administration of 300–600 IU EPO/kg/week generally was found to enhance erythropoiesis and reduced the number of transfusions required by up to 30%.

Patients who have received an allogeneic bone marrow transplant characteristically display depressed serum EPO levels for up to 6 months post-transplantation. Administration of EPO thus seems a logical approach to counteract this effect. Several clinical studies have validated this approach, observing accelerated erythropoiesis, resulting in attainment of satisfactory haematocrit levels within a shorter period post-transplant.

Tolerability

In general, rhEPO is well tolerated. The most pronounced adverse effects appear to be associated with its long-term administration to patients with end-stage renal failure. Particularly noteworthy is an increase in blood pressure levels in some patients and the increased risk of thromboembolic events (a thromboembolic event, i.e. a thromboembolism, describes the circumstance where a blood clot forms at one point in the circulation but detaches, only to become lodged at another point; Chapter 9).

Most short-term applications of EPO are non-renal related, and generally display very few side-effects; i.v. administration can sometimes prompt a transient flu-like syndrome, while s.c. administration can render the site of injection painful. This latter effect appears, however, to be due to excipients present in the EOP preparations, most notably the citrate buffer. EPO administration can also cause bone pain, although this rarely limits its clinical use.

Overall, therefore, rhEPO has proved both effective and safe in the treatment of a variety of clinical conditions and its range of therapeutic applications is likely to increase over the coming years.

THROMBOPOIETIN

Thrombopoietin (TPO) is the haemopoietic growth factor now shown to be the primary physiological regulator of platelet production. Although its existence had been inferred for several decades, its purification from blood proved an almost impossible task, due to its low production levels and the availability of only an extremely cumbersome TPO bioassay. Its existence was finally proved in the mid-1990s when thrombopoietin cDNA was cloned. This molecule is likely to represent an important future therapeutic agent in combating depressed plasma platelet levels, although this remains to be proved by clinical trials.

Platelets (thrombocytes) carry out several functions in the body, all of which relate to the arrest of bleeding. They are disc-shaped structures $1-2\,\mu m$ in diameter, and are present in the blood of healthy individuals at levels of approximately $250\times10^9/l$. They are formed by a lineage-specific stem cell differentiation process, as depicted in Figure 6.8. The terminal stages of this process entails the maturation of large progenitor cells termed 'megakaryocytes'. Platelets represent small vesicles which bud off from the megakaryocyte cell surface and enter the circulation.

A number of disorders have been identified that are primarily caused by the presence of abnormal platelet levels in the blood. Thrombocythaemia is a disease characterized by abnormal megakaryocyte proliferation, leading to elevated blood platelet levels. In many instances, this results in an elevated risk of spontaneous clot formation within blood vessels. In other instances, the platelets produced are defective, which can increase the risk of spontaneous or prolonged bleeding events.

Thrombocytopenia, on the other hand, is a condition characterized by reduced blood platelet levels. Spontaneous bruising, bleeding into the skin (purpura) and prolonged bleeding after injury represent typical symptoms. Thrombocytopenia is induced by a number of clinical conditions, including:

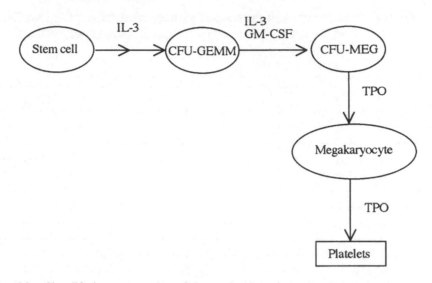

Figure 6.8.   Simplified representation of the production of platelets from stem cells. CFU-megakaryocytes and in particular, mature megakaryocytes, are most sensitive to the stimulatory actions of TPO. These two cell types also display a limited response to IL-6, IL-11 and LIF

- bone marrow failure;
- chemotherapy (or radiotherapy);
- various viral infections.

TPO should alleviate thrombocytopenia in most instances by encouraging platelet production. Currently, the standard therapy for the condition entails administration of 5 units of platelets to the sufferer (1 unit equals the quantity of platelets derived in one sitting from a single blood donor). TPO therapy is a particularly attractive potential alternative because:

- it eliminates the possibility of accidental transmission of disease via transfusions;
- platelets harvested from blood donations have a short shelf-life (5 days), and must be stored during that time at 22°C on mechanical shakers;
- platelets exhibit surface antigens, and can thus promote antibody production. Repeat administrations may thus be less effective, due to the potential presence of neutralizing antibodies.

The most likely initial TPO therapeutic target is thrombocytopenia induced by cancer chemo- or radiotherapy. This indication generally accounts for up to 80% of all platelet transfusions undertaken. In the USA alone, close to 2 million people receive platelet transfusions annually. Human TPO is a 332 amino acid, 60 kDa glycoprotein, containing six potential N-linked glycosylation sites. These are all localized towards the C-terminus of the molecule. The N-terminal half exhibits a high degree of amino acid homology with EPO and represents the biologically active domain of the molecule.

Sources of TPO include kidney and skeletal muscle cells but it is primarily produced by the liver, from where it is excreted constantly into the blood. This regulatory factor supports the proliferation, differentiation and maturation of megakaryocytes and their progenitors and promotes the production of platelets from megakaryocytes (Figure 6.8). It also appears to modulate the growth/differentiation of progenitor cells, which eventually give rise to both erythrocytes and macrophages.

TPO induces its characteristic effects by binding to a specific TPO receptor present on the surface of sensitive cells. The receptor, also known as c-mpl, is a single chain, 610 amino acid transmembrane glycoprotein. The mechanism of signal transduction triggered upon TPO-binding remains to be elucidated.

Currently, at least two recombinant TPO-based products are being assessed in clinical trials. One product is a recombinant glycosylated form produced in a mammalian cell line, the other is a non-glycosylated variant, expressed in *E. coli*. The latter molecule, also known as megakaryocyte growth and development factor (MGDF), is PEGylated subsequent to its purification. PEGylation, as already described in the context of several other protein-based therapeutics, extends the molecule's plasma half-life.

Additional cytokines (IL-3, IL-6, IL-11 and LIF) also promote a proliferative response in megakaryocytes. Although these exhibit some ability to increase platelet levels, the physiological significance of this remains unclear. TPO, on the other hand, induces a far swifter, greater and more specific response. In one study, its administration to mice over a period of 6 days resulted in a four-fold increase in platelet count (although some other studies reported a less pronounced effect). Furthermore, TPO administration to animals whose platelet production had been severely compromised by radio- or chemotherapy accelerated subsequent recovery of platelet numbers to normal values. The future clinical outlook for this haemopoietic growth factor looks bright.

FURTHER READING

Books

Dallman, M. (2000). *Haemapoietic and Lymphoid Cell Culture*. Cambridge University Press, Cambridge.
Kuter, D. *et al.* (Eds) (1997). *Thrombopoiesis and Thrombopoietins*. Humana, Totowa, NJ, USA.
Medkalf, D. (1995) *Haemopoietic Colony-stimulating Factors: From Biology to Clinical Applications*. Cambridge University Press, Cambridge.
Morstyn, G. (1998). *Filgrastim in Clinical Practice*. Marcel Dekker, New York.
Orlic, D. (1999). *Haematopoietic Stem Cells*. New York Academy of Science, New York.

Articles

Erythropoietin and thrombopoietin

Basser, R. (2002). The impact of thrombopoietin on clinical practice. *Curr. Pharmaceut. Design* **8**(5), 369–377.
Bottomley, A. *et al.* (2002). Human recombinant erythropoietin and quality of life: a wonder drug or something to wonder about? *Lancet Oncol.* **3**(3), 145–153.
Buemi, M. *et al.* (2002). Recombinant human erythropoietin: more than just the correction of uremic anemia. *J. Nephrol.* **15**(2), 97–103.
Fried, W. (1995). Erythropoietin. *Ann. Rev. Nutrit.* **15**, 353–377.
Geddis, A. *et al.* (2002). Thrombopoietin: a pan-hematopoietic cytokine. *Cytokine Growth Factor Rev.* **13**(1), 61–73.
Kaushansky, K. (1995). Thrombopoietin: the primary regulator of platelet production. *Blood* **86**(2), 419–431.
Kaushansky, K. (1997). Thrombopoietin — understanding and manipulating platelet production. *Annu. Rev. Med.* **48**, 1–11.
Kaushansky, K. & Drachman, J. (2002). The molecular and cellular biology of thrombopoietin: the primary regulator of platelet production. *Oncogene* **21**(21), 3359–3367.
Kendall, R. (2001). Erythropoietin. *Clin. Lab. Haematol.* **23**(2), 71–80.
Lok, S. *et al.* (1994). Cloning and expression of murine thrombopoietin cDNA and stimulation of platelet production *in vivo*. *Nature* **369**, 565–568.

Markham, A. & Bryson, H. (1995). Epoetin Alfa, a review of its pharmacodynamic and pharmacokinetic properties and therapeutic use in non-renal applications. *Drugs* **49**(2), 232–254.

Metcalf, D. (1994). Thrombopoietin—at last. *Nature* **369**, 519–520.

Miyazaki, H. & Kato, T. (1999). Thrombopoietin: biology and clinical potential. *Int. J. Haematol.* **70**(4), 216–225.

Ogden, J. (1994). Thrombopoietin—the erythropoietin of platelets? *Trends Biotechnol.* **12**, 389–390.

Roberts, D. & Smith, D. (1994). Erythropoietin: induction of synthesis to signal transduction. *J. Mol. Endocrinol.* **12**, 131–148.

Spivak, J. (1994). Recombinant human erythropoietin and the anaemia of cancer. *Blood* **84**(4), 997–1004.

CSFs

Cheetham, J.C., Smith, D.M., Aoki, K.H. *et al.* (1998). NMR structure of human erythropoietin and a comparison with its receptor-bound conformation. *Nature Struct. Biol.* **5**, 861.

Dranoff, G. *et al.* (1994). Involvement of granulocyte-macrophage colony-stimulating factor in pulmonary homeostasis. *Science* **264**, 713–715.

Duarte, R. & Frank, D. (2002). The synergy between stem cell factor (SCF) and granulocyte colony stimulating factor (G-CSF): molecular basis and clinical relevance. *Leukaemia Lymphoma* **43**(6), 1179–1187.

Frampton, J. *et al.* (1994). Filgrastim, a review of its pharmacological properties and therapeutic efficacy in neutropenia. *Drugs* **48**(5), 731–760.

Frampton, J. *et al.* (1995). Lenograstim, a review of its pharmacological properties and therapeutic efficacy in neutropenia and related clinical settings. *Drugs* **49**(5), 767–793.

Hamilton, J. (1997). CSF-1 signal transduction. *J. Leukocyte Biol.* **62**(2), 145–155.

Harousseau, J. (1997). The role of colony-stimulating factors in the treatment of acute leukaemia. *Biodrugs* **7**(6), 448–460.

Spangrude, G. (1994). Biological and clinical aspects of haematopoietic stem cells. *Ann. Rev. Med.* **45**, 93–104.

Tabbara, I. *et al.* (1996). The clinical applications of granulocyte-colony-stimulating factor in haematopoietic stem cell transplantation—a review. *Anticancer Res.* **16**(6B), 3901–3905.

Walter, M.R., Cook, W.J., Ealick, S.E. *et al.* (1992). Three-dimensional structure of recombinant human granulocyte-macrophage colony-stimulating factor. *J. Mol. Ecol.* **224**, 1075.

Watowich, F. *et al.* (1996). Cytokine receptor signal transduction and the control of haematopoietic cell development. *Ann. Rev. Cell Dev. Biol.* **12**, 91–128.

Chapter 7
Growth factors

The growth of eukaryotic cells is modulated by various influences, of which growth factors are amongst the most important for many cell types. A wide range of polypeptide growth factors have been identified (Table 7.1) and more undoubtedly remain to be characterized. Factors that inhibit cell growth also exist, e.g. interferons (IFNs) and tumour necrosis factor (TNF) inhibit proliferation of various cell types.

Some growth factors may be classified as cytokines, e.g. ILs, transforming growth factor-β (TGF-β) and colony stimulating factors (CSFs). Others, e.g. insulin-like growth factors (IGFs) are not members of this family. Each growth factor has a mitogenic (promotes cell division) effect on a characteristic range of cells. While some such factors affect only a few cell types, most stimulate the growth of a wide range of cells. The range of growth factors considered in this chapter is limited to those that have not received attention in previous chapters.

The ability of such factors to promote accelerated cellular growth and division has predictably attracted the attention of the pharmaceutical industry. The clinical potential of a range of such factors, e.g. to accelerate the wound-healing process, is currently being assessed in various clinical trials (Table 7.2).

GROWTH FACTORS AND WOUND HEALING

The wound-healing process is complex and as yet not fully understood. The area of tissue damage becomes the focus of various events, often beginning with immunological and inflammatory reactions. The various cells involved in such processes, as well as additional cells at the site of the wound, also secrete various growth factors. These mitogens stimulate the growth and activation of various cell types, including fibroblasts (which produce collagen and elastin precursors, and ground substance), epithelial cells (e.g. skin cells) and vascular endothelial cells. Such cells advance healing by promoting processes such as granulation (growth of connective tissue and small blood vessels at the healing surface) and subsequent epithelialization. The growth factors that appear most significant to this process include fibroblast growth factors (FGFs), transforming growth factors (TGFs), platelet-derived growth factor (PDGF), insulin-like growth factor 1 (IGF-1) and epidermal growth factor (EGF).

Wounds can be categorized as acute (healing quickly on their own) or chronic (healing slowly, and often requiring medication). Chronic wounds, such as ulcers (Table 7.3), occur if some

Biopharmaceuticals: Biochemistry and Biotechnology, Second Edition by Gary Walsh
John Wiley & Sons Ltd: ISBN 0 470 84326 8 (ppc), ISBN 0 470 84327 6 (pbk)

Table 7.1. Overview of some polypeptide growth factors. Many can be grouped into families on the basis of amino acid sequence homology, or the cell types affected. Most growth factors are produced by more than one cell type and display endocrine, paracrine or autocrine effects on target cells by interacting with specific cell surface receptors

Growth factor	Major target cells
Interleukins	Various, mainly cells mediating immunity and inflammation
Interferon-γ	Mainly lymphocytes and additional cells mediating immunity (and inflammation)
Colony stimulating factors	Mainly haemopoietic cells
Erythropoietin	Erythroid precursor cells
Thrombopoietin	Mainly megakaryocytes
Neurotrophic factors	Several, but mainly neuronal cell populations
Insulin	Various
Insulin-like growth factors	A very wide range of cells found in various tissue types
Epidermal growth factor	Various, including epithelial and endothelial cells and fibroblasts
Platelet-derived growth factor	Various, including fibroblasts, glial cells and smooth muscle cells
Fibroblast growth factors	Various, including fibroblasts, osteoblasts and vascular endothelial cells
Transforming growth factors-α	Various
Leukaemia inhibitory factor	Mainly various haemopoietic cells

Table 7.2. Some growth factors which may have significant future therapeutic application, and the conditions they aim to treat

Growth factor	Possible medical indication
Insulin-like growth factor-1 (IGF-1)	Certain forms of dwarfism, type II diabetes, kidney disease, growth hormone insensitivity, cachexia, amyotrophic lateral sclerosis, peripheral neuropathy
Epidermal growth factor (EGF)	Wound healing, skin ulcers
Platelet-derived growth factor (PDGF)	Diabetic ulcers, wound healing
Transforming growth factor-β (TGF-β)	Bone healing, skin ulcers, detached retinas
Fibroblast growth factors (FGFs)	Soft tissue ulcers, wound healing
Neurotrophic factors (NTs)	Mainly conditions caused by/associated with neurodegeneration, including peripheral neuropathies, amyotrophic lateral sclerosis and neurodegenerative diseases of the brain

influence disrupts the normal healing process. Such influences can include diabetes, malnutrition, rheumatoid arthritis and ischaemia (inadequate flow of blood to any part of the body). Elderly people are particularly susceptible to developing chronic wounds, often resulting in the necessity for hospitalization. Ulceration (particularly of the limbs or extremities) associated with old age, diabetes, etc. remains the underlying cause of up to 50% of all amputations carried out in the USA.

The fluid exuded from a fresh or acute wound generally exhibits high levels of various growth factors (as determined by bioassay or immunoassay analysis). In contrast, the concentration of

Table 7.3. Various types of ulcers along with their underlying cause. An ulcer may simply be described as a break or cut in the skin or membrane lining the digestive tract which fails to heal. The damaged area may then become inflamed

Ulcer category	Description
Decubitus ulcer (e.g. bed sores, pressure sores)	Ulcer due to continuous pressure exerted on a particular area of skin; often associated with bed-ridden patients
Diabetic ulcers	Ulcers (e.g. 'diabetic leg') caused by complications of diabetes
Varicose ulcers	Due to defective circulation, sometimes associated with varicose veins
Rodent ulcers	An ulcerous cancer (basal cell carcinoma), usually affecting the face
Peptic ulcers	Ulcer of the digestive tract, caused by digestion of the mucosa by acid and pepsin; may occur in e.g. the duodenum (duodenal ulcer), or the stomach (gastric ulcer)

such mitogens present in chronic wounds is usually several-fold lower. Direct (topical) application of exogenous growth factors results in accelerated wound healing in animals. While some encouraging results have been observed in human trials, the overall results obtained thus far have been disappointing. Having said this, one such factor (rPDGF) has been approved for topical administration on diabetic ulcers, as described later. Future studies may well also focus on application of a cocktail of growth factors instead of a single such factor to a wound surface.

A greater understanding of wound physiology and biochemistry may also facilitate greater success in future trials. It has been established, for example, that the fluid exuded from chronic wounds harbours high levels of proteolytic activity (almost 200-fold higher than associated with acute wounds). Failure of mitogens to stimulate wound healing thus may be due, in part, to their rapid proteolytic degradation (and/or the degradation of growth factor receptors present on the surface of susceptible cells). Identification of suitable protease inhibitors, and their application in conjunction with exogenous growth factor therapy, may improve clinical results recorded in the future.

INSULIN-LIKE GROWTH FACTORS (IGFs)

The insulin-like growth factors (also termed 'somatomedins'), constitute a family of two closely related (small) polypeptides: insulin-like growth factor 1 (IGF-1) and insulin-like growth factor 2 (IGF-2). As the names suggest, these growth factors bear a strong structural resemblance to insulin (or, more accurately, proinsulin). Infusion of IGF-1 decreases circulating levels of insulin and glucagon, increases tissue glucose uptake and inhibits hepatic glucose export. IGFs display pluripotent activities, regulating the growth, activation, differentiation (and maintenance of the differentiated state) of a wide variety of cell and tissue types (discussed later). The full complexity and variety of their biological activities are only now beginning to be appreciated.

The liver represents the major site of synthesis of the IGFs, from where they enter the blood stream, thereby acting in a classical endocrine fashion. A wide variety of body cells express IGF receptors, of which there are two types. Furthermore, IGFs are also synthesized in smaller quantities at numerous sites in the body and function in an autocrine or paracrine manner at these specific locations. IGF activity is also modulated by a family of IGF binding proteins (IGFBPs), of which there are at least six.

IGF biochemistry

IGF-1 and -2 were first isolated from adult human plasma, although recombinant versions of both are now available. The human IGF-1 gene is present on chromosome 12 and contains six exons. The IGF-2 gene is located on chromosome 11, adjacent to the insulin gene. It consists of nine exons. Organization and regulation of both genes is complex, with transcription potentially regulated by one of several promoters (which may facilitate tissue-specific control of expression). Differential transcripts are also observed, allowing the possible production of several species of each factor, which may differ slightly from one another. The common form of IGF-1 is a 70 amino acid polypeptide displaying three intra-chain disulphide linkages and a molecular mass of 7.6 kDa. IGF-2 (67 amino acids; 7.5 kDa) also has three disulphide linkages.

IGF-1 and -2 display identical amino acid residues at 45 positions, and exhibit in excess of 60% sequence homology. Both display A and B domains, connected by a short C domain — similar to proinsulin. However, unlike in the case of proinsulin, the IGF's C domain is not subsequently removed. The predicted tertiary structure of both IGFs closely resemble that of proinsulin. The overall amino acid homology displayed between insulin and the two IGFs is in excess of 40%.

Hepatic transcription of IGF-1, in particular, is initiated upon binding of growth hormone (GH) to its hepatic receptors and, indeed, most of the growth-promoting actions of GH are directly mediated by IGF-1.

IGF receptors

IGFs induce their characteristic effects by binding to specific receptors present on the surface of sensitive cells. At least three receptor types have been identified: the IGF-1 receptor, the IGF-2 receptor and the insulin receptor. As is evident from Table 7.4 (with one important exception), IGF-1, IGF-2 and insulin can bind the three receptor types, but with varying affinities. This renders delineation of which factor is inducing any one characteristic effect quite difficult.

The IGF-1 receptor is structurally similar to the insulin receptor, both in its primary and tertiary structure (Figure 7.1). As is the case for the insulin receptor, the IGF-1 receptor is encoded by a single large gene (displaying 22 exons) whose primary product is a 1367 amino acid receptor precursor. This is proteolytically processed, yielding mature α- and β-subunits, with the biologically active form being an $\alpha_2\beta_2$ tetramer (Figure 7.1). The intracellular tyrosine kinase domains of the human IGF and insulin receptors display 84% amino acid homology, while the extracellular cysteine-rich domains (α-subunits) exhibit 40% homology. As is the case

Table 7.4. The various IGF receptors and the ligands capable of binding to them. $\tilde{A}\tilde{A}$ denotes binding with high affinity (K_d=approximately 10^{-10} M), $\tilde{A}$=weaker binding (K_d=approximately 10^{-8}–10^{-9} M). –=failure to bind

	Ligand		
Receptor (R)	IGF-I	IGF-II	Insulin
IGF-I R	$\tilde{A}\tilde{A}$	$\tilde{A}\tilde{A}$	$\tilde{A}$
IGF-II R	$\tilde{A}$	$\tilde{A}\tilde{A}$	–
Insulin R	$\tilde{A}$	$\tilde{A}$	$\tilde{A}\tilde{A}$

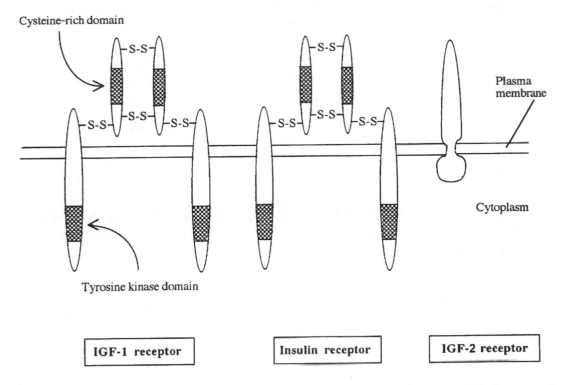

Cysteine-rich domain

Plasma membrane

Cytoplasm

Tyrosine kinase domain

| IGF-1 receptor | Insulin receptor | IGF-2 receptor |

Figure 7.1.   Comparison of the structure of the IGF-1, IGF-2 and the insulin receptors. Refer to text for specific details

for the insulin receptor, binding of ligand to the IGF-1 receptor α-subunit triggers activation of the β-subunit tyrosine kinase activity, resulting in autophosphorylation of several β-tyrosine residues. This, in turn, facilitates phosphorylation of several additional cytoplasmic polypeptide substrates. This triggers further intracellular events, culminating in an appropriate cellular response to ligand binding. This (IGF-1) receptor is expressed on virtually all cell types and is thus widely distributed throughout the body. It appears that it mediates the mitogenic effects of IGF-1, IGF-2 and insulin.

The IGF-2 receptor is structurally and functionally distinct from the IGF-1/insulin receptor family. The bulk of this 250 kDa receptor resides extracellularly (Figure 7.1), and its short cytoplasmic domain displays no known enzymatic activity. IGF-2 binds to this receptor with greatest affinity, whereas insulin fails to bind. The mechanism of signal transduction remains to be elucidated, although G proteins appear to play a prominent role. Its physiological significance is also less clear than that of the IGF-1 receptor. It is expressed at highest levels during fetal development, with receptor numbers declining rapidly after birth (this pattern is also paralleled by IGF-2 expression). Thus IGF-2 and its receptor may be most relevant during fetal tissue development.

Recent studies also point to the existence of a fourth receptor species. This appears to be a hybrid structure, composed of an insulin receptor α–β dimer crosslinked to an IGF-1 receptor α–β dimer. Although this receptor type displays a marked reduction in its affinity for insulin,

Table 7.5. The range of human IGF binding proteins (IGF BPs or 'BPs'), and an indication of their relative affinities for ligand. ÃÃ indicates a higher affinity than Ã. The approximate range of IGF BP association constants (K_a) is 1×10^{-9}–1×10^{-10} M

	IGF I	IGF II
IGF BP 1	ÃÃ	ÃÃ
IGF BP 2	Ã	ÃÃ
IGF BP 3	ÃÃ	ÃÃ
IGF BP 4	ÃÃ	ÃÃ
IGF BP 5	ÃÃ	ÃÃ
IGF BP 6	Ã	ÃÃ

physiological concentrations of IGF-1 prompts autophosphorylation of its intracellular tyrosine kinase domain. The *in vivo* importance of this hybrid receptor remains to be elucidated.

IGF-binding proteins

IGFs typically display 5–6% of the hypoglycaemic (reduction in blood glucose concentrations) potency of insulin. As IGF serum concentrations are of the order of 1000 times higher than insulin concentrations, profound IGF-associated hypoglycaemia would be expected under normal physiological conditions. This is avoided as IGFs, found in the serum or other extracellular fluids, are invariably tightly complexed to an additional protein, termed an IGF-binding protein (IGFBP). This prevents IGF interaction with its receptors, hence preventing uncontrolled IGF activity. Six different IGFBPs have been identified (Table 7.5). Individual members of this family generally exhibit in the region of 50% homology with each other, although they vary in molecular weight from 23 kDa (BP6) to 31.5 kDa (BP2). Although they display differences in their binding affinities for IGF ligands, the IGFs appear to bind them more tightly than they do their cell surface receptors.

IGFBPs are widely expressed, but high levels of BP1 and BP2 in particular are found in the liver. The bulk of serum IGF-1 and -2 is found complexed to BP3 and an acid-labile polypeptide. The remaining molecules of serum IGFs are usually found complexed to BP1, BP2 or BP4.

The IGFBPs probably fulfil several biological functions in addition to preventing hypoglycaemia. They likely protect the mitogen (e.g. from proteolysis) in the blood, and appear to significantly increase the IGF's plasma half-life. They also probably modulate IGF function locally at the surface of IGF-sensitive cells.

Biological effects

IGFs exhibit a wide range of gross physiological effects (Table 7.6), all of which are explained primarily by the ability of these growth factors to stimulate cellular growth and differentiation. Virtually all mammalian cell types display surface IGF receptors. IGFs play a major stimulatory role in promoting the cell cycle (specifically, it is the sole mitogen required to promote the G_1b phase, i.e. the progression phase. Various other phases of the cycle can be stimulated by additional growth factors). IGF activity can also contribute to sustaining the uncontrolled cell growth characteristic of cancer cells. Many transformed cells exhibit very high levels of IGF

Table 7.6. Overview of some of the effects of the IGFs

Promotes cell cycle progression in most cell types
Fetal development: promotes growth and differentiation of fetal cells and organogenesis
Promotes longitudinal body growth and increased body weight
Promotes enhanced functioning of the male and female reproductive tissue
Promotes growth and differentiation of neuronal tissue

---

receptors, and growth of these cells can be inhibited *in vitro* by the addition of antibodies capable of blocking IGF-receptor binding.

IGF and fetal development

IGFs 1 and 2, along with insulin, play an essential role in promoting fetal growth and development. IGF-2, and its receptor is expressed by the growing embryo as early as the two-cell stage (i.e. even before implantation in the womb wall). Later, the developing embryo also begins to synthesize IGF-1 and insulin. These mitogens and their receptors are expressed in virtually every fetal tissue in a coordinated manner.

IGFs and growth

Most of the growth-promoting effects of growth hormone (GH) are actually mediated by IGF-1. Direct injection of IGF-1 into hypophysectomized animals (animals whose pituitary — the source of GH — is surgically removed) stimulates longitudinal bone growth, as well as growth of several organs/glands (e.g. kidney, spleen, thymus). Bone and surrounding connective tissue represents a rich source of IGFs and various other growth factors. IGFs (particularly IGF-1) promotes bone growth largely due to its ability to stimulate osteoblast differentiation and proliferation. Osteoblasts are the cells primarily responsible for bone formation. The initial stages of bone development are marked by the deposition of a meshwork of collagen fibres in connective tissue, followed by their cementing by polysaccharides. This is then impregnated in the final stages with crystals of calcium salts.

Several experiments utilizing transgenic animals confirm the importance of IGFs in promoting longitudinal body growth and increasing body weight. Transgenic mice over-expressing IGF-1 grow faster and larger than non-transgenic controls. Furthermore, transgenic mice whose IGF-2 gene was rendered dysfunctional, grew only to 60% of their ultimate expected body weight. Such effects render IGFs likely therapeutic candidates in treating the various forms of dwarfism caused by a dysfunction in some element of the GH–IGF growth axis (Table 7.2). Initial trials show that s.c. administration of recombinant human IGF-1 over a 12 month period significantly increases the growth rate of Laron type dwarfs (LTD; a condition caused by a mutation in the GH receptor, rendering it dysfunctional; as a result, GH cannot promote any of its usual effects, including promotion of IGF synthesis). GH in turn functions as a primary regulator of IGF-1 synthesis. Unlike the pulsatile nature of GH secretion, however, serum IGF levels tend to remain relatively constant. Nutritional status also affects IGF-1 levels, which are significantly decreased during starvation, despite concurrently elevated GH levels.

In addition to promoting fetal and childhood growth, IGFs play a core role in tissue renewal and repair (e.g. wound healing) during adulthood, e.g. these growth factors play a central role in bone remodelling (i.e. reabsorption and rebuilding—which helps keep bones strong and contributes to whole body calcium homeostasis). Reabsorption of calcified bone is undertaken by osteoclasts, cells of haemopoietic origin whose formation is stimulated by IGFs. These mitogens may, therefore, influence the development of osteoporosis, a prevalent condition (especially amongst the elderly), which is characterized by brittle, uncalcified bone.

IGFs also stimulate a more generalized short- and long-term whole body anabolic effect. Studies in calorie-restricted animals and humans show that IGF administration can retard or reverse catabolic events, such as tissue degradation and catabolism of body protein. Such effects have attracted the interest of some athletes who have used it illegally as a performance-enhancing drug. Detection is rendered complex, due to the relatively wide range of IGF concentrations classified as 'normal' and the fact that exercise naturally boosts endogenous IGF-1 production. IGF effects have also prompted speculation that these growth factors might be of clinical use in retarding/preventing/reversing cachexia, the generalized wasting of body tissues associated with chronic disease and many cancer types. Many IGF metabolic effects (particularly IGF-1) exhibit similarities to several metabolic effects induced by insulin. These similarities (particularly IGF's ability to enhance cellular glucose uptake), suggests a possible role for this growth factor in the treatment of certain forms of diabetes, most notably non-insulin dependent diabetes (type II diabetes; Table 7.2). Initial studies have shown that IGF can reduce hyperglycaemia in patients unresponsive to insulin and further more detailed studies are now ongoing.

Renal and reproductive effects

IGFs (in particular IGF-1 and also IGFBP-1) are localized within various areas of the kidney. Direct infusion of IGF-1 influences (usually enhances) renal function by a number of means, including promoting:

- increased glomerular filtration rate;
- increased renal plasma flow;
- increased kidney size and weight.

These responses are obviously mediated by multiple effects on the growth and activity of several renal cell types and suggest that IGFs play a physiological role in regulating renal function. Not surprisingly, IGF-1 is currently being assessed as a potential therapeutic agent in the treatment of various forms of kidney disease.

GH deficiency often leads to delayed puberty. This condition often responds to exogenous GH administration. IGFs, as well as their receptors and binding proteins, are widespreadly expressed in the male and female reproductive tissue. Thus, IGFs are believed to affect reproductive function by both (GH-stimulated) endocrine action and via paracrine- and autocrine-based activity.

In the human female, IGF-1 is expressed by follicular theca cells, while IGF-2 is synthesized by granulosa cells (Chapter 8). The IGF-1 and -2 receptors are widely expressed in ovarian tissue, and synthesis of both growth factors and their receptors are influenced by circulating gonadotrophin levels. IGF-1 exerts a direct mitogenic effect on human granulosa cells, and promotes increased androgen and oestradiol synthesis by these cells. IGF-1 also promotes increased expression of FSH and LH receptors in ovarian tissue.

In the male, IGF-1 is synthesized by the Sertoli and Leydig cells of the testes. It also stimulates testosterone production by the Leydig cells, and promotes growth and maintenance of various additional testis cell types.

IGFs thus play an essential role in many facets of reproductive function. Traditionally, therapeutic intervention in reproductive disorders at a molecular level has relied almost exclusively upon administration of gonadotrophins or LHRH (luteinizing hormone releasing hormone; Chapter 8). Because of their widespread reproductive effects, IGFs may yet prove a valuable adjunct therapy in some instances.

Neuronal and other effects

IGF-1 is widely expressed in the CNS. IGF-2 is also present, being produced mainly by tissues at vascular interfaces with the brain. Both growth factors, along with insulin, play a number of important roles in the nervous system. They stimulate the growth and development of various neuronal populations and promote neurotrophic effects (discussed later).

IGF-1 promotes differentiation of various neuronal cells, playing a central role in fostering neurite outgrowth and synapse formation, as well as myelin formation. In addition to affecting neuronal development and maintenance, it may also stimulate regeneration of damaged peripheral neurons. This activity has prompted investigation of the therapeutic potential of IGFs (particularly IGF-1) in the treatment of some neurodegenerative conditions most notably amyotrophic lateral sclerosis (ALS), which is also called motor neuron disease (MND) in the USA (strictly speaking, these two terms are not interchangeable, owing to slight differences in their pathogenicities). ALS (and MND) are caused by a progressive degeneration of specific motor neurons stretching out from the spinal cord. This leads to wasting of the muscle cells the motor neurons normally enervate. Remission is unknown, and death is the usual outcome. Clinical application of IGFs may be tempered by side effects. High-dose administration can induce hypoglycaemia, hypotension and arrhythmias.

EPIDERMAL GROWTH FACTOR (EGF)

EGF was one of the first growth factors discovered. Its existence was initially noted in the 1960s as a factor present in saliva, which could promote premature tooth eruption and eyelid opening in neonatal mice. It was first purified from urine and named urogastrone, owing to its ability to inhibit the secretion of gastric acid. EGF has subsequently proved to exert a powerful mitogenic effect on many cell types, and its receptor is expressed by most cells. Its influence on endothelial cells, epithelial cells and fibroblasts is particularly noteworthy, and the skin appears to be its major physiological target. It stimulates growth of the epidermal layer. Along with several other growth factors, EGF plays a role in the wound-healing process. EGF is synthesized mainly by monocytes and ectodermal cells, as well as by the kidney and duodenal glands. It is found in most bodily fluids, especially milk.

The gene coding for human EGF is located on chromosome 4. It is an extensive structure, consisting of 24 exons and giving rise to a 110 kb primary transcript. After splicing, this yields a mRNA coding for a 1208 amino acid prepro-EGF. In addition to the EGF sequence, this contains seven EGF-like domains, whose biological function remains unknown. Proteolytic processing of the larger molecule releases soluble EGF, a 6 kDa, 53 amino acid unglycosylated peptide. Mature EGF is very stable. Its 3-D structure, as revealed by nuclear magnetic

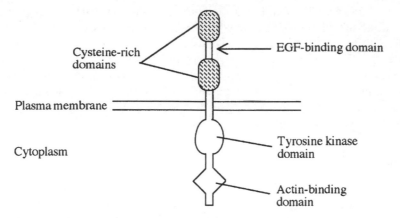

Figure 7.2. The EGF receptor. The N-terminal, extracellular region of the receptor contains 622 amino acids. It displays two cysteine-rich regions, between which the ligand binding domain is located. A 23 amino acid hydrophobic domain spans the plasma membrane. The receptor cytoplasmic region contains some 542 amino acids. It displays a tyrosine kinase domain, which includes several tyrosine autophosphorylation sites, and an actin-binding domain that may facilitate interaction with the cell cytoskeleton

resonance (NMR) studies, exhibits two stretches of anti-parallel β-sheet. It also contains three disulphide linkages, which contribute to this stability.

The EGF receptor

The cell-surface EGF receptor also serves as the receptor for the closely related TGF-α growth factor, as discussed later. The receptor gene is located on chromosome 7. The mature product is a 170 kDa glycoprotein, possessing 11 potential glycosylation sites (Figure 7.2).

Binding of ligand appears to induce receptor dimerization, which in turn prompts receptor activation. A variety of intracellular events are then triggered, which combine to yield the characteristic growth-promoting response. These events include:

(a) Activation of the receptor's endogenous tyrosine kinase activity, which promotes autophosphorylation of several of its tyrosine residues. The phosphorylated residues represent docking sites for several cytoplasmic proteins, including a phospholipase C. Docking activates the phospholipase C, which in turn catalyses degradation of the membrane lipid phosphoinositol bisphosphate (PIP2). This yields two well known cellular second messengers:
   - Inositol triphosphate (IP3), which raises intracellular Ca^{2+} concentrations by inducing its release from intracellular stores. This Ca^{2+}, in turn, activates a cytoplasmic serine/threonine protein kinase.
   - Diacylglycerol (DG), which subsequently activates protein kinase C.
(b) Activation of the Ras pathway (Ras proteins are G proteins). Their activation, upon binding of GTP, results in triggering intracellular mitogenic events.
(c) The EGF-receptor complex also appears to be capable of translocating to the nucleus. The significance of this remains to be determined.

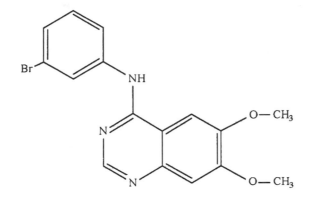

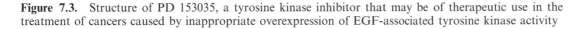

Figure 7.3. Structure of PD 153035, a tyrosine kinase inhibitor that may be of therapeutic use in the treatment of cancers caused by inappropriate overexpression of EGF-associated tyrosine kinase activity

Several cancer cell types are characterized by expressing a truncated EGF receptor. The related viral oncogene, V-*erb*B, also encodes a truncated receptor which lacks most of the extracellular domain (the EGF receptor is also known as C-erbB). Mutant receptors that display inappropriate constitutive activity can lead to cellular transformation, due to the continuous generation of mitogenic signal.

Overexpression of the EGF receptor (or any of its ligands), can also induce cancer in both cell lines and transgenic animal models. Monoclonal antibodies capable of blocking receptor activity can promote tumour regression in mice suffering from various carcinomas. A direct correlation also exists between elevated EGF receptor numbers and a shorter patient survival span in the case of several forms of breast, oesophageal, bladder and squamous cell carcinomas.

Tyrosine kinase inhibitors may represent effective chemotherapeutic agents for such cancers. Potentially attractive candidates include the inhibitor known as PD 153035 (Figure 7.3) which, even at picomolar (pM) concentrations, inhibits EGF-associated tyrosine kinase activity. While PD 153035 also inhibits additional cellular tyrosine kinases, it does so only at concentrations in the micromolar (μM) range.

EGF may also find a novel agricultural application in the defleecing of sheep. Administration of EGF to sheep has a transient effect on the wool follicle bulb cell, which results in a weakening of the root that holds the wool in place. While novel, this approach to defleecing is unlikely to be economically attractive.

PLATELET-DERIVED GROWTH FACTOR (PDGF)

Platelet-derived growth factor (PDGF) is a polypeptide growth factor which is sometimes termed 'osteosarcoma-derived growth factor' (ODGF) or 'glioma-derived growth factor' (GDGF). It was first identified over 20 years ago as being the major growth factor synthesized by platelets. It is also produced by a variety of cell types. PDGF exhibits a mitogenic effect on fibroblasts, smooth muscle cells and glial cells, and exerts various additional biological activities (Table 7.7).

PDGF plays an important role in the wound healing process. It is released at the site of damage by activated platelets, and acts as a mitogen/chemoattractant for many of the cells

Table 7.7. Range of cells producing PDGF and its major biological activities

Synthesized by	Platelets	Macrophages
	Fibroblasts	Endothelial cells
	Astrocytes	Megakaryocytes
	Myoblasts	Kidney epithelial cells
	Vascular smooth muscle cells	Many transformed cell types
Biological activities		
Mitogen for	Fibroblasts	Variety of transformed cells
	Smooth muscle cells	Glial cells
Chemoattractant for	Fibroblasts	Monocytes
	Neutrophils	Smooth muscle cells

responsible for initiation of tissue repair. It thus tends to act primarily in a paracrine manner. It also represents an autocrine/paracrine growth factor for a variety of malignant cells.

Active PDGF is a dimer. Two constituent polypeptides, A and B, have been identified and three active PDGF isoforms are possible: AA, BB and AB. Two slightly different isoforms of the human PDGF A polypeptide (generated by differential mRNA splicing) have been identified. The short A form contains 110 amino acids, while the long form contains 125 amino acids. Both exhibit one potential glycosylation site and 3 intra-chain disulphide bonds. The B-chain closely resembles the p28^{sic} protein, the transforming protein of the simian sarcoma virus. It is a 16 kDa, 109 amino acid polypeptide, which also exhibits three intra-chain disulphide linkages. Mature dimeric PDGF contains two additional inter-chain disulphide linkages. PDGF A- and B-chains are products of distinct genes, although they do display a high degree of homology. Transcription of the two genes are subject to different regulatory mechanisms, resulting in the production of the A- and B-chains in different ratios in different cells. Dimerization thus yields a range of different isomers (PDGF of platelets consist approximately of 70% AB, 20% BB and 10% AA species). Unlike AA/AB, which is generally secreted, a large proportion of the BB homodimer remains attached to the plasma membrane, mainly via electrostatic interactions.

The PDGF receptor and signal transduction

Two PDGF receptor subunits have been identified. Both are transmembrane glycoproteins whose cytoplasmic domains display tyrosine kinase activity upon activation. The mature α-receptor contains 1066 amino acids and exhibits a molecular mass of 170 kDa. The β-receptor is slightly larger (1074 amino acid residues).

Binding of ligand promotes receptor dimerization and hence activation. Three isoforms of the receptor exist: $\alpha\alpha$, $\alpha\beta$ and $\beta\beta$. The particular dimeric form of ligand that binds dictates the

Table 7.8. The range of human PDGF receptor dimers which may form upon binding of different PDGF isoforms

PDGF ligand	Receptor species formed
AA	$\alpha\alpha$
BB	$\alpha\alpha$, $\alpha\beta$, $\beta\beta$
AB	$\alpha\alpha$, $\alpha\beta$

possible combination of dimers present in the corresponding receptor (Table 7.8). Ligand-induced dimerization triggers a variety of intracellular events, including receptor auto-phosphorylation, with subsequent activation of phospholipase C.

PDGF and wound healing

In vitro and *in vivo* studies support the thesis that PDGF is of value in wound management — particularly with regard to chronic wounds. All three isoforms of PDGF are available from a range of recombinant systems. *In vitro* studies, using various cell lines, suggest that PDGF AB or BB dimeric isoforms are most potent.

Normal skin appears to be devoid of PDGF receptors. Animal studies illustrate that rapid expression of both α- and β-receptor subunits is induced upon generation of an experimental wound (e.g. a surgical incision). Receptor expression is again switched off following re-epithelialization and complete healing of the wound.

Initial human trials have found that daily topical application of PDGF (BB isoform) stimulated higher healing rates of chronic pressure wounds, although the improvement recorded fell just short of being statistically significant. A second trial found that daily topical application of PDGF (BB) did promote statistically significant accelerated healing rates of chronic diabetic ulcers.

The product (tradename Regranex) was approved for general medical use in the late 1990s. Its active ingredient is manufactured by Chiron Corporation, in an engineered strain of *Saccharomyces cerevisiae* harbouring the PDGF B-chain gene. Regranex is notable in that it is formulated as a non-sterile (low bioburden) gel, destined for topical administration. The final formulation contains methylparaben, propylparaben and *m*-cresol as preservatives. In addition, as is the case with EGF, PDGF antagonists may also prove valuable in the treatment of some cancer types in which inappropriately high generation of PDGF-like mitogenic signals leads to the transformed state.

FIBROBLAST GROWTH FACTORS (FGFs)

Fibroblast growth factors (FGFs) constitute a family of about 20 proteins (numbered consecutively FGF-1 to FGF-20). Typically, they display a molecular mass in the region of 18–28 kDa and induce a range of mitogenic, chemotactic and angiogenic responses. Classification as an FGF is based upon structural similarity. All display a 140 amino acid central core which is highly homologous between all family members. All FGFs also tightly bind heparin and heparin-like glycosaminoglycans found in the extracellular matrix. This property has been used to purify several such FGFs via heparin affinity chromatography. Subsequent to binding to the immobilized heparin, FGF can be eluted by inclusion of high NaCl concentrations in the eluting buffer. Although many of the original members of this family stimulate the growth/development of fibroblasts (hence the name), several newer members have little or no effect upon fibroblasts.

The means by which FGFs are secreted from their producer cells remains to be fully elucidated. Several (e.g. FGF-1 and FGF-2, also known as acidic-FGF and basic-FGF, respectively; Figure 7.4) do not contain a classical signal sequence for secretion (i.e. a short N-terminus stretch of hydrophobic amino acid residues which direct newly synthesized polypeptides to the endoplasmic reticulum and hence ultimately facilitates their extracellular release). Interestingly, several such FGFs display a nucleas localization motif and have been found in association with the nucleas. In this way, they may induce selected biological responses independent of the extracellular route.

FGFs induce the majority of their characteristic responses via binding to high-affinity cell surface receptors. Four such receptors, which show 55–72% homology at the amino acid level, have been identified to date. The receptors are multi-domain, consisting of three extracellular immunoglobulin-like domains (Ig domains), a highly hydrophobic transmembrane domain and two intracellular tyrosine kinase domains. Different receptors are found on different cell types and each receptor is either strongly, moderately, poorly or not activated by its own characteristic range of FGFs. This signalling complexity underscores the complexity of biological responses induced by FGFs.

Ligand (FGF) binding typically triggers receptor dimerization with associated transphosphorylation of critical tyrosine residues. Once phosphorylated, various cytoplasmic proteins dock at/are activated by the FGF receptor. Docking is most likely mediated by a characteristic interaction between Src-homology 2 (SH2) domains of the cytoplasmic proteins and the phosphotyrosine residues on the activated receptor. The next stages of signal transduction are characterized only in part. Studies with FGFR-1 implicate at least four signalling pathways (Figure 7.5).

Phospholipase C-γ (PLC-γ) activation promotes the cleavage of phosphatidyl inositol 4,5 bisphosphate, generating inositol triphosphate and diacylglycerol, which, in turn, trigger an increase in intracellular calcium ion concentration and activation of protein kinase C. Interaction with FGFR-1 also appears to activate Src, a non-receptor tyrosine kinase. This, in turn, influences cytoskeletal structure. CrK is an additional 'adaptor' protein which may link the FGFR to the intracellular signalling molecules Shc, C3G and Cas, all of which could propagate mitogenic signals. Finally, the activated FGF-1 is known to phosphorylate (activate) the protein SNT-1 (i.e. FRS2). This protein, in turn, is important in the Ras/MAPK signalling pathway, known to mediate growth factor-induced cell cycle progression.

Whatever the mode of signal transduction, FGFs display a wide range of biological activities. They function as growth factors for a range of cell types and are known to promote wound repair. Some FGFs are known to promote repair to damaged myocardial tissue in animal models. Although no FGF-based product has thus far been approved for general medical use, such biological activities render them attractive candidates for clinical appraisal. In addition, FGFs play a central role in embryonic development and inappropriate FGF-like signalling has been linked to various tumour types. Autocrine over-stimulation linked to overexpression of FGFs is a characteristic feature of most human gliomas. Overexpression of/the presence of constitutively activated FGF receptor mutants is observed in various cancers of the brain, breast, prostrate, thyroid and skin. As such, downregulation of FGF signal transduction activity could be of benefit in the future treatment of various cancer types.

TRANSFORMING GROWTH FACTORS (TGFs)

Transforming growth factors (TGFs) represent yet another family of polypeptide mitogens. The members of this family include TGF-α, as well as several species of TGF-β.

TGF-α

TGF-α is initially synthesized as an integral membrane protein. Proteolytic cleavage releases the soluble growth factor, which is a 50 amino acid polypeptide. This growth factor exhibits a high

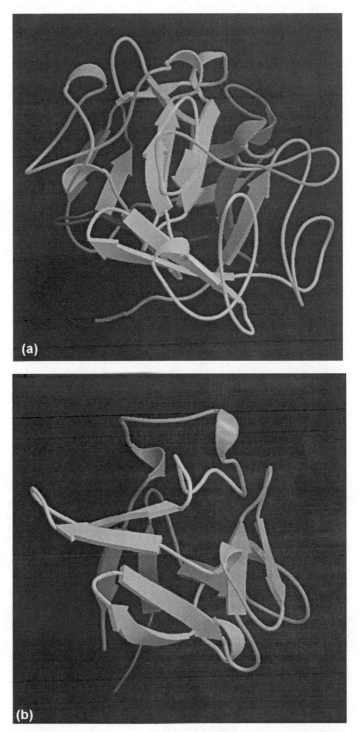

Figure 7.4.   3-D of acidic (a) and basic (b) fibroblast growth factor. Photos from Zhu *et al.* (1991), by courtesy of the Protein Data Bank: http://www.rcsb.org/pdb/

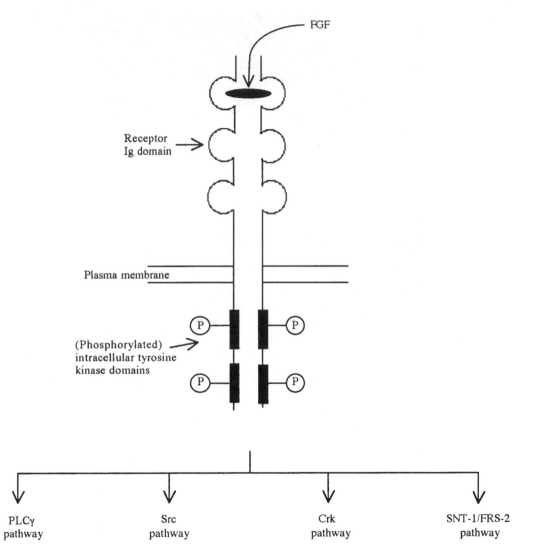

Figure 7.5. Binding of FGF to an FGF receptor, and the possible intracellular events triggered upon binding. Refer to the text for specific details

amino acid homology with EGF, and it induces its biological effects by binding to the EGF receptor. It is synthesized by various body tissues, as well as by monocytes and keratinocytes. It is also manufactured by many tumour cell types, for which it can act as an autocrine growth factor.

TGF-β

TGF-β was first described as a growth factor capable of inducing transformation of several fibroblast cell lines (hence the name, transforming growth factors). It is now recognized that

'TGF-β' actually consists of three separate growth factors: TGF-β1, -β2 and -β3. Although the product of distinct genes, all exhibit close homology. In the mature form, they exist as homodimers, with each subunit containing 112 amino acid residues. Most body cells synthesize TGF-β, singly or in combination.

TGF-βs are pleiotrophic cytokines. They are capable of inhibiting the cell cycle and hence growth of several cell types, most notably epithelial and haemopoietic cells. These factors, however, stimulate the growth of other cell types, most notably cells that give rise to connective tissue, cartilage and bone. They induce the synthesis of extracellular matrix proteins, and modulate the expression of matrix proteases. They also serve as a powerful chemoattractant for monocytes and fibroblasts. Given such activities, it is not surprising that the major physiological impact of TGF-βs appear to relate to:

- tissue remodelling;
- wound repair;
- haemopoiesis.

Such activities render them potentially useful therapeutic agents and several are being assessed medically (Table 7.2). The effect of TGF-β on haemopoietic cells has recently received increasing attention. Along with TNF-α and IFN-γ, TGF-β is a physiologically relevant negative regulator of haemopoiesis. TGF-β also inhibits the growth of various human leukaemia cell lines *in vitro*, rendering it of potential interest as a putative anti-cancer agent.

The TGF-βs exert their biological actions by binding to specific receptors, of which there are three types (I, II and III). All are transmembrane glycoproteins. All three TGF-βs bind to all three receptor types, although they bind with higher affinity to types I and II receptors (53 kDa and 65 kDa, respectively). The intracellular domains of the type I and II receptors display endogenous serine/threonine protein kinase activity.

The larger (829 amino acid) type III receptor is a proteoglycan (a class of very highly glycosylated acidic glycoprotein). Also known as β-glycan, it is characterized by a short cytoplasmic domain and displays no capability of transducing signals. The type III receptor (which is less widely distributed than the others) may function to concentrate ligand and present it to type I and II receptors. The exact molecular events underlining TGF signal transduction remain to be elucidated, although co-expression of type I and II receptors appears to be a necessary prerequisite. This has led to speculation that active signal transduction requires ligand-induced formation of a hetromeric complex containing both type I and II receptor units. A family of cytoplasmic proteins, Smad proteins, are also known to transiently associate with activated TGF-β receptors. Interaction results in the activation via phosphorylation of the Smads, which then translocate to the nucleas. Here they function as transcriptional activators of various genes.

NEUROTROPHIC FACTORS

Neurotrophic factors constitute a group of cytokines that regulate the development, maintenance and survival of neurons in both the central and peripheral nervous systems (Table 7.9). While the first member of this family (nerve growth factor, NGF) was discovered more than 50 years ago, it is only in the last decade that the other members have been identified and characterized. The major sub-family of neurotrophic factors are the neurotrophins.

The original understanding of the term 'neurotrophic factor' was that of a soluble agent found in limiting quantities in the environment of sensitive neurons, and being generally

Table 7.9. Molecules displaying neurotrophic activity *in vivo* and/ or with neurons in culture

---

Nerve growth factor (NGF)
Brain-derived neurotrophic factor (BDNF)
Neurotrophin 3 (NT-3)
Neurotrophin 4/5 (NT-4/5)
Neurotrophin 6 (NT-6)
Ciliary neurotrophic factor (CNTF)
Glial cell-line-derived neurotrophic factor (GDNF)
Fibroblast growth factors (FGFs)
Platelet-derived growth factor (PDGF)
Insulin-like growth factors 1 and 2 (IGFs 1 and 2)
Transforming growth factor $\beta1$ (TGF-$\beta1$)
Granulocyte-macrophage colony-stimulating factor (GM-CSF)
Erythropoietin (EPO)
Leukaemia inhibitory factor (LIF)

---

manufactured by the neuronal target cells. It specifically promoted the growth and maintenance of those neurons (see also Box 7.1). This description is now considered to be oversimplistic. Many neurotrophic factors are also synthesized by non-nerve target cells and influence cells other than neurons (e.g. NGF is synthesized by mast cells and influences various cells of the immune system). Furthermore, various cytokines (including several growth factors; Table 7.9), discovered because of their ability to stimulate the growth of non-neuronal cells, are now also known to influence neuronal cells.

Each neurotrophic factor influences the growth and development of a specific group of neuronal types, with some cells being sensitive to several such factors. Many sustain specific neuronal populations whose death underlines various neurodegenerative diseases. This raises the possibility that these regulatory molecules may be of benefit in treating such diseases. Results from early clinical trials have been mixed, but many remain optimistic that neurotrophic factors may provide future effective treatments for some currently incurable neurodegenerative conditions.

The neurotrophins

The neurotrophins are a group of neurotrophic factors which all belong to the same gene family. They include NGF, as well as brain-derived neurotrophic factor (BDNF), neurotrophin-3 (NT-3), neurotrophin 4/5 (NT-4/5) and neurotrophin-6 (NT-6). All are small, basic proteins sharing approximately 50% amino acid homology. They exist mainly as homodimers and promote signal transduction by binding to a member of the Trk family of tyrosine kinase receptors (Table 7.10).

NGF is the prototypic neurotrophin. The mature NGF polypeptide contains 120 amino acids, exhibits a molecular mass of 26 kDa and a pI of approximately 10. It contains three intra-chain disulphide linkages, which are essential for activity. NGF is synthesized and released from target tissues of sympathetic neurons and cholinergic basal forebrain neurons. It is also synthesized by non-neuronal tissue, including salivary glands, the prostate and mast cells. It functions to

Box 7.1. The nervous system revisited

Neurons constitute the communicative element of the nervous sytem, which consists of the central nervous system (CNS; the brain and spinal cord) and the peripheral nervous system (PNS; additional neuronal elements). Sensory neurons are those leading from a stimulus-detecting receptor cell, while motor neurons are those that normally carry on nerve impulses to an effector cell, often a muscle cell. Neurons, although varying in shape and size, consist of the nucleus-containing cell body (perikaryon), from which various elongated extensions (processes) emerge — the dendrites, which normally carry nerve impulses towards the perikaryon and the axon, the terminal branches of which form the junction (synapse) with the cell to which the nerve impulse will be transmitted.

The neuronal cytoskeleton provides the axon with mechanical support and is directly involved in the transport of materials from the cell body towards the synapse (anterograde transport) and in the opposite direction (retrograde transport). Axons are generally covered (insulated) with a myelin sheath, which is formed by oligodendrocytes (in the CNS) or Schwann cells (PNS).

During their initial development, immature neurons sprout outgrowths (neurites) representing axons or dendrites. At the tip of the neurite is the star-like growth cone, which helps guide the growing neurite towards its target tissue. The direction of growth of the developing axon seems to be directed (a) by guidance molecules resident on the surface of surrounding cells (cell adhesion molecules, CAMs) and (b) by soluble chemoattractants released from the target cell. Receptors for both of these types of guiding molecules are present on the growth cone surface. Failure of a developing axon to innervate the target tissue results in neuronal death.

Neurotrophic factors play a central role in development and maintenance of neuronal cells. After release from the target cells, they bind specific receptors on the nerve termini, are internalized and carried up the axon to the perikaryon by retrograde transport. This process helps guide the direction of neurite growth (i.e. a chemoattractant activity) during neuronal development, and also serves to 'nourish' the developing cell. Once established, the process of retrograde transport must continue if the cell is to survive and remain differentiated.

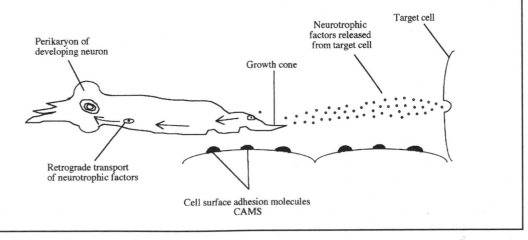

Table 7.10. Biochemical characteristic of the neurotrophin family of neurotrophic factors. Except for NT-6, the molecular masses quoted are those of the homodimeric structure, which represents their biologically active forms. See text for further details

Neurotrophin	Molecular mass (kDa)	pI	Receptor type
NGF	26	10	Trk A
BDNF	27	10	Trk B
NT-3	27	9.5	Trk A, B, C
NT-4/5	28	10.8	Trk B
NT-6	15.9	10.8	?

promote survival and stimulate growth of sensitive neurons, and accelerates neurotransmitter biosynthesis in most such cells. It also appears to stimulate growth and differentiation of B and T lymphocytes, thus potentially promoting cross-talk between the nervous and immune systems.

The restricted neuronal specificity of NGF suggested the existence of additional neurotrophic factors capable of influencing non-NGF-sensitive neuronal populations. Research efforts in the early 1980s led to the discovery of BDNF, a 119 amino acid (13.5 kDa) basic protein. In contrast to NGF, BDNF is predominantly localized within the CNS. Predictably, most BDNF-responsive neurons are located in (or project into) the CNS.

Studies (mainly *in vitro*) illustrate that BDNF promotes the survival of embryonic retina ganglion cells, dopaminergic neurons, as well as cholinergic neurons of the basal forebrain, embryonic spinal motor neurons and cortical neurons.

The synthesis of oligonucleotide primers, based upon conserved sequences between the NGF and BDNF genes, allowed researchers to fish for additional members of the neurotrophin family by PCR analysis. In 1991 this led to the discovery of neurotrophin 3 (NT-3), which is expressed early in — and throughout — embryogenesis. It supports the development of various neuronal populations in culture, although its role *in vivo* is less well understood.

Two additional neurotrophins, originally cloned from *Xenopus* and mammals, respectively, turned out to be counterparts, and this neurotrophin is now termed, NT-4/5. Mammalian NT-4/5 is quite similar to the other neurotrophins but exhibits its own unique neuronal target cell specificities. It is synthesized mainly in the prostate but also in skeletal muscle, placenta and the thymus.

More recently, an additional member of this family (NT-6) has been discovered in the fish *Xiphophorus*. The activities of this neurotrophin remain to be characterized in detail, but the spectrum of sensitive neurons appear to be similar to that of NGF. NT-6 is different from the other neurotrophins in that it appears that the mature molecule is not released from the producing cell; instead, it remains associated with the cell surface (or with the extracellular matrix).

Neurotrophin receptors

Most neurotrophin-sensitive cells express two receptor types on their surface: a high-affinity receptor, which appears to mediate most/all of the biological actions of the neurotrophins, and a low-affinity receptor. The high-affinity receptors are all members of a family of tyrosine kinases (the Trks). They are similar to the receptors of many other growth factors, but are expressed almost exclusively on neuronal tissue.

Three Trks have been identified, Trk A, B and C. Ligand-binding induces Trk receptor homodimerization. This activates the intrinsic cytoplasmic tyrosine kinase activity, resulting in receptor autophosphorylation and initiation of an intracellular response. A characteristic feature of the Trk family of receptors is the presence of a leucine-rich region near the N-terminal (extracellular) end of the molecule.

Trk A functions as the high-affinity receptor for NGF ($K_d = 10^{-11}$ M), and mediates all of its neurotrophic activities. It is expressed on the surface of sensory and sympathetic neurons, as well as the neuron-associated Schwann cells (Box 7.1). It is also expressed on the surface of mast cells, monocytes and lymphocytes. The mature Trk A receptor is a transmembrane glycoprotein of molecular mass, 140 kDa. It also functions as a receptor for NT-3 (Table 7.10).

The closely related Trk B serves as a receptor for BDNF. Two variants of this glycoprotein have been characterized: a larger (145 kDa) form and a truncated (95 kDa) form. While exhibiting identical extracellular domains, the 95 kDa protein has a short (23 amino acid) cytoplasmic region, whereas the 145 kDa form displays a larger (tyrosine kinase) cytoplasmic domain. Trk B also serves as a functional receptor for NT-3 and NT-4/5 and is expressed widely throughout the central and peripheral nervous system.

Trk C (along with Trk A and B) represents the functional receptor for NT-3. This 145 kDa glycoprotein is expressed by various neuronal cell populations, both in the brain (particularly the hippocampus and cerebellum) and the peripheral nervous system.

The neurotrophin low-affinity receptor

All the neurotrophins are also capable of binding to a low-affinity receptor known as LNGFR, or P75. P75 is a 75 kDa cell surface glycoprotein. It exhibits no known enzymatic activity. It is widely expressed, both on neuronal and non-neuronal cell populations. p75's exact physiological role remains to be defined, but its presence on non-neuronal cells suggests that it may serve to bind neurotrophic factors and present them to developing axons bearing high-affinity receptors. This could direct axonal growth towards its neurotrophin-synthesizing target cell during development (Box 7.1). It may also function to regulate apoptosis, as it belongs to a superfamily of TNF receptors, some of which mediate such activities *in vivo*.

Ciliary neurotrophic factor and glial cell line-derived neurotrophic factor

Ciliary neurotrophic factor (CNTF) and glial cell line-derived neurotrophic factor (GDNF) represent the most recently discovered members of the neurotrophic factor family. These, however, display no homology to the neurotrophins previously discussed.

CNTF, originally characterized as a survival factor for chick ciliary neurons, is now known to influence a much broader range of neuronal cells, including spinal motor neurons. Studies detailing CNTF's regional distribution and developmental expression, together with the fact that it is a cytoplasmic protein, suggests that this molecule is not a target-derived neurotrophic factor. It may well exert a neurotrophic activity upon release from damaged cells. CNTF is a 200 amino acid (22 kDa) polypeptide. It induces a biological response by binding to a specific CNTF receptor on the surface of susceptible cells. The CNTF receptor is unusual in that it is not a transmembrane protein, but is anchored to the membrane by a glycosyl-phosphatidylinositol linkage. The receptor is unrelated to the Trk family of neurotrophin receptors but displays homology with the IL-6 receptor. Ligand-binding appears to induce CNTF interaction with additional membrane proteins, notably the LIF receptor and a protein termed gp130. This, in turn, promotes phosphorylation of these latter two molecules. The CNTF receptor is expressed mainly within the nervous system and on skeletal muscle. It is also expressed (at lower densities) on skin, liver and kidney cells.

GDNF is a 34 kDa homodimeric glycosylated protein, which is a member of the TGF-β family. It influences a wide range of neuronal populations, including spinal sensory and motor neurons. It also stimulates dopaminergic neurons and is the most potent known survival factor for motor neurons *in vitro*. Because of the range of neuronal cells sensitive to this factor, it may well prove to be amongst the most clinically useful of all neurotrophic factors.

NEUROTROPHIC FACTORS AND NEURODEGENERATIVE DISEASE

Neurodegenerative diseases are generally characterized by the death of specific neuronal populations. Many such neurons are responsive, *in vitro* at least, to one or more neurotrophic factor. This infers a potential therapeutic role for these molecules in the treatment of such conditions (Table 7.11). Lack of current effective therapies for the treatment of any neurodegenerative disease renders this avenue of investigation even more attractive. Target diseases include amyotrophic lateral sclerosis and peripheral neuropathies, as well as various neurodegenerative diseases of the brain, including Alzheimer's and Parkinson's.

Disappointing initial clinical trials serve, however, to underline the fact that data from *in vitro* investigations or animal studies do not necessarily equate to a physiologically significant response in humans.

Amyotrophic lateral sclerosis (ALS) and peripheral neuropathy

ALS, as already discussed, is a condition characterized by degeneration of the spinal and brainstem motor neurons, resulting in muscle wasting and eventually death. It affects approximately 70 000 people worldwide. Several neurotrophic factors known to positively influence motor neurons *in vitro* and/or *in vivo* (Table 7.11) have or are being assessed in clinical trials as therapeutic agents for ALS.

Pre-clinical trials (as well as phase I and II clinical trials) utilizing CNTF yielded promising results, but the neurotrophic factor then failed phase III clinical trials on the basis of insufficient efficacy. However, myotrophin (IGF-1, produced by Cephalon Inc.) has proved more successful. A 266 patient phase III clinical study found that IGF-1 administration to ALS sufferers resulted in reduced severity of symptoms, and slower disease progression, although this or no related product has yet been approved for medical use. The potential world market for an ALS therapeutic agent approaches $1 billion.

Peripheral neuropathy (degeneration of peripheral sensory and/or motor neurons) represents another target for neurotrophic intervention. It often occurs as a complication of diabetes or in cancer patients receiving chemotherapy. In severe cases, amputation of limbs affected by neuronal loss is warranted. Pre-clinical studies have clearly shown that sensory and sympathetic neurons depleted in peripheral neuropathy respond to NGF. Indeed, NGF, along with IGF-1, can prevent the occurrence of drug-induced peripheral neuropathy in animals. Human clinical trials continue.

Neurotrophic factors and neurodegenerative diseases of the brain

Unlike the neurodegenerative conditions discussed above, diseases such as Alzheimer's and Parkinson's are underlined by the death of CNS neurons. Many of these cells respond to specific

Table 7.11. Some neurodegenerative diseases for which no current effective therapy exists, and neurotrophic factors known to stimulate growth of neuronal populations affected by these conditions

Disease	Neurons mainly affected	Neurotrophic factors to which cell may respond
Peripheral neuropathies	Sensory/motor neurons	NGF, IGF-1, NT-3, CNTF
Amyotrophic lateral sclerosis	Spinal motor neurons	BDNF, IGF-1, CNTF, GDNF, NT-4/5
Alzheimer's disease	Forebrain cholinergic neurons	NGF, BDNF, NT-4/5
Parkinson's disease	Nigral dopamine neurons	GDNF, BDNF, NT-3, NT-4/5
Huntington's disease	Striatal GABA neurons	BDNF, NT-4/5

neurotrophic factors, which therefore may constitute effective therapies in the treatment of these incurable conditions. The existence of the blood–brain barrier represents a complication, as it precludes delivery of the drug to the brain via intravenous injection. A number of approaches have been adopted to circumvent this problem, including:

- direct injection of neurotrophic factor into the brain;
- use of cranial infusion pumps;
- intraventricular transplantation of recombinant polymer-encapsulated cells which secrete neurotrophic factors.

While such approaches may be technically feasible, the associated risks render unlikely their widespread clinical application. An alternative approach that may prove more acceptable involves conjugating the neurotrophic factor to monoclonal antibodies raised against the transferrin receptor. This normally transports iron across the blood–brain barrier; i.v. administration of NGF–anti-transferrin antibody conjugate results in its translocation across the blood–brain barrier. Upon entry into the brain, the conjugate was found to promote survival of NGF-sensitive neurons. Amongst these are cholinergic striatal interneurons, which degenerate in Huntington's disease.

Loss of cholinergic neurons of the basal forebrain is a characteristic feature of Alzheimer's disease. These neurons enervate the hippocampus (the brain's memory centre). They respond to NGF, BDNF and NT-4/5, e.g. NGF can rescue such cells in rodents after damage induced by cutting their axons.

Degeneration of these same neurons is also associated with an age-dependent decrease in learning and memory ability. Infusion of NGF and NT-4/5 to aged rats appears to improve their spatial memory ability. Further studies in rodents have shown that physical exercise increased BDNF expression, which may explain why exercise is often a predictor of high mental function during ageing.

Dopaminergic neurons of the substantia nigra represent the major neural population degenerating in patients suffering from Parkinson's disease. Several neurotrophic factors, including NT-4/5, BDNF and GDNF, sustain these cells *in vitro* and, hence, may be useful in treating this disease. Pre-clinical studies show that direct injection of GDNF to sites adjacent to the substantia nigra prevents degeneration of these neurons when they are experimentally damaged by cutting their axons.

Likewise, GDNF prevents dopaminergic loss (in animals) subsequent to the administration of the neurotoxin, MPTP, which induces parkinsonian symptoms in man. Even more encouragingly, administration of GDNF subsequent to MPTP-induced dopaminergic damage in mice promoted significant restoration of the nigrostriatal dopamine system. This observation leaves open the tantalizing possibility that GDNF might play a therapeutic role in halting, or even reversing, the clinical progression of Parkinson's. This can only be assessed by actual human clinical trials.

The use of a combination of neurotrophic factors in the treatment of neurodegenerative disease may well prove an avenue worthy of consideration. For example, pre-clinical studies reveal that administration of a combination of CNTF and BDNF to Wobbler mice (an animal model of motor neuron disease), prevented progression of motor neuron dysfuction, whereas administration of either factor on its own only slowed progression of the disease.

Such an approach could be underpinned by the development of engineered proteins displaying multiple neurotrophic activities. Pan-neurotrophin-1, for example, is an engineered chimaeric neurotrophin, containing the active domains of NGF, BDNF and NT-3. This hybrid molecule can bind the neurotrophin receptors Trk A, B and C, as well as P75.

Limited clinical success keeps optimism alive that neurotrophic factors will find application in the treatment of some neurodegenerative disease. However, no member of this family of regulatory proteins have been approved for medical use, despite all the clinical investigations undertaken over the last decade and a half.

FURTHER READING

Books

Evrard, P. (2002). *The Newborn Brain*. Cambridge University Press, Cambridge.
McKay, I. (1998). *Growth Factors and Receptors*. Oxford University Press, Oxford.
Nilsen, H. (1994). *Growth Factors and Signal Transduction in Development*. Wiley-Liss, New York.
Thomson, A. (1998). *Cytokine Handbook*. Academic Press, London.

Articles

Insulin-like growth factors

Bach, L. (1999). The insulin-like growth factor system: basic and clinical aspects. *Aust. N. Z. J. Med.* **29**(3), 355–361.
Cohick, W. & Clemmons, D. (1993). The insulin-like growth factors. *Ann. Rev. Physiol.* **55**, 131–153.
Dercole, A. *et al.* (1996). The role of insulin-like growth factors in the central nervous system. *Mol. Neurobiol.* **13**(3), 227–255.
Furstenberger, G. & Senn, H. (2002). Insulin-like growth factors and cancer. *Lancet Oncol.* **3**(5), 298–302.
Kostecka, Z. & Blahovec, J. (2002). Animal insulin-like growth factor binding proteins and their biological functions. *Vet. Med.* **47**(2–3), 75–84.
Leroith, D. *et al.* (1997). Insulin-like growth factors. *N. Engl. J. Med.* **336**(9), 633–640.
Schmid, C. (1995). Insulin-like growth factors. *Cell Biol. Int.* **19**(5), 445–457.
Zumkeller, W. (2002). The insulin-like growth factor system in hematopoietic cells. *Leukaemia Lymphoma* **43**(3), 487–491.

EGF and PDGF

Adjej, A. (2001). Epidermal growth factor receptor tyrosine kinase inhibitors in cancer therapy. *Drugs Future* **26**(11), 1087–1092.
Boonstra, J. *et al.* (1995). The epidermal growth factor. *Cell Biol. Int.* **19**(5), 413–430.
Claesson-Welsh, L. (1994). Platelet-derived growth factor receptor signals. *J. Biol. Chem.* **269**(51), 32023–32026.
Downward, J. *et al.* (1984). Close similarity of EGF receptor and V-erb-B oncogene protein sequences. *Nature* **307**, 521–527.
Johnstone P. (2002). The epidermal growth factor receptor: a new target for anticancer therapy—introduction. *Curr. Probl. Cancer* **26**(3), 114–164.
Leserer, M. *et al.* (2000). Epidermal growth factor receptor signal transactivation. *IUBMB Life* **49**(5), 405–430.

Meyer-Ingold, W. & Eichner, W. (1995). Platelet-derived growth factor. *Cell Biol. Int.* **19**(5), 389–398.
Wakeling, A. (2002). Epidermal growth factor receptor tyrosine kinase inhibitors. *Curr. Opin. Pharmacol.* **2**(4), 382–387.

FGF/TGF

Dennler, S. *et al.* (2002). Transforming growth factor-β signal transduction. *J. Leukocyte Biol.* **71**(5), 731–740.
Derynck, R. (1994). TGF-β-receptor-mediated signalling. *Trends Biochem. Sci.* **19**, 548–553.
Hu, X. & Zuckerman, K. (2001). Transforming growth factor: signal transduction pathways, cell cycle mediation, and effects on hematopoiesis. *J. Hematother. Stem Cell Res.* **10**(1), 67–74.
Powers, C. *et. al.* (2000). Fibroblast growth factors, their receptors and signalling. *Endocr. Rel. Cancer* **7**(3), 165–197.
Souchelnytskyi, S. (2002). Transforming growth factor-β signalling and its role in cancer. *Exp. Oncol.* **24**(1), 3–12.
Zhu, X., Komiya, A., Chirino, S. *et al.* (1991). Three-dimensional structures of acidic and basic fibroblast growth factors. *Science* **251**, 90.

Wound-healing and growth factors

Deuel, T. *et al.* (1991). Growth factors and wound healing: platelet-derived growth factor as a model cytokine. *Ann. Rev. Med.* **42**, 567–584.
Martin, P. (1997). Wound healing—aiming for perfect skin regeneration. *Science* **276**(5309), 75–81.
Meyer-Ingold, W. (1993). Wound therapy: growth factors as agents to promote healing. *Trends Biotechnol.* **11**, 387–392.
Mustoe, T. *et al.* (1987). Accelerated healing of incisional wounds in rats induced by transforming growth factor type β. *Science* **347**, 1333–1336.
Pierce, G. & Mustoe, T. (1995). Pharmacologic enhancement of wound healing. *Ann. Rev. Med.* **46**, 467–481.

Neurotrophic and related factors

Butte, M. (2001). Neurotrophic factor structure reveals clues to evolution, binding, specificity and receptor activation. *Cell. Mol. Life Sci.* **58**(8), 1003–1013.
Ebadi, M. *et al.* (1997). Neurotrophins and their receptors in nerve injury and repair. *Neurochem. Int.* **30**, 347–374.
Fu, S. & Gordon, T. (1997). The cellular and molecular basis of peripheral nerve regeneration. *Mol. Neurobiol.* **14**, 67–116.
Haque, N. *et al.* (1997). Therapeutic strategies for Huntington's disease, based on a molecular understanding of the disorder. *Mol. Med. Today* **3**(4), 175–183.
Hefti, F. (1997). Pharmacology of neurotrophic factors. *Ann. Rev. Pharmacol. Toxicol.* **37**, 239–267.
J. Neurobiol. (1994) **25**(11), special issue devoted exclusively to neurotrophic factors.
Kwon, Y. (2002). Effect of neurotrophic factors on neuronal stem cell death. *J. Biochem. Mol. Biol.* **35**(1), 87–93.
Raffioni, S. *et al.* (1993). The receptor for nerve growth factor and other neurotrophins. *Ann. Rev. Biochem.* **62**, 823–850.
Sofroniew, M. *et al.* (2001). Nerve growth factor signalling, neuroprotection and neural repair. *Ann. Rev. Neurosci.* **24**, 1217–1281.
Streppel, M. *et al.* (2002). Focal application of neutralizing antibodies to soluble neurotrophic factors reduces collateral axonal branching after peripheral nerve lesion. *Eur. J. Neurosci.* **15**(8), 1327–1342.
Tatagiba, M. *et al.* (1997). Regeneration of injured axons in the adult mammalian central nervous system. *Neurosurgery* **40**(3), 541–546.
Thorne, R. & Frey, W. (2001). Delivery of neurotrophic factors to the central nervous system—pharmacokinetic considerations. *Clin. Pharmacokinet.* **40**(12), 907–946.
Walsh, G. (1995). Nervous excitement over neurotrophic factors. *Bio/Technology* **13**, 1167–1171.
Yamada, K. *et al.* (2002). Role for brain derived neurotrophic factor in learning and memory. *Life Sci.* **70**(7), 735–744.
Yamada, M. *et al.* (1997). The neurotrophic action and signalling of epidermal growth factor. *Progr. Neurobiol.* **51**(1), 19–37.

Chapter 8

Hormones of therapeutic interest

Hormones are amongst the most important group of regulatory molecules produced by the body. Originally, the term 'hormone' was defined as a substance synthesized and released from a specific gland in the body which, by interacting with a receptor present in or on a distant sensitive cell, brought about a change in that target cell. Hormones travel to the target cell via the circulatory system. This describes what is now termed a 'true endocrine hormone'.

At its loosest definition, some now consider a hormone to be any regulatory substance that carries a signal to generate some alteration at a cellular level. This embraces the concept of paracrine regulators (i.e. produced in the immediate vicinity of their target cells) and autocrine regulators (i.e. producer cell is also the target cell). Under such a broad definition, all cytokines, for example, could be considered hormones. The delineation between a cytokine and a hormone is already quite fuzzy using any definition.

True endocrine hormones, however, remain a fairly well-defined group. Virtually all of the hormones used therapeutically (discussed below) fit into this grouping. Examples include insulin, glucagon, growth hormone and the gonadotrophins.

INSULIN

Insulin is a polypeptide hormone produced by the β cells of the pancreatic islets of Langerhans. It plays a central role in regulating blood glucose levels, generally keeping it within narrow defined limits (3.5–8.0 mmol/l), irrespective of the nutritional status of the animal. It also has a profound effect on the metabolism of proteins and lipids and displays some mitogenic activity. The latter is particularly evident in *in vitro* studies and at high insulin concentrations. Some of these mitogenic effects are likely mediated via the insulin-like growth factor 1 (1GF-1) receptor and their physiological relevance is questionable.

Although many cells in the body express the insulin receptor, its most important targets are skeletal muscle fibres, hepatocytes and adipocytes, where it often antagonizes the effects of glucagon (Table 8.1). The most potent known stimulus of pancreatic insulin release is an increase in blood glucose levels, often occurring after meal times. Insulin orchestrates a suitable metabolic response to the absorption of glucose and other nutrients in a number of ways:

Biopharmaceuticals: Biochemistry and Biotechnology, Second Edition by Gary Walsh
John Wiley & Sons Ltd: ISBN 0 470 84326 8 (ppc), ISBN 0 470 84327 6 (pbk)

Table 8.1. Some metabolic effects of insulin. These effects are generally countered by other hormones (glucagon and, in some cases, adrenaline). Hence, the overall effect noted often reflects the relative rates of these hormones present in the plasma

Metabolic pathway	Target tissue	Effect of insulin	Effect of glucagon
Glycogen synthesis	Liver	↑	↓
Glycogen degradation	Liver	↓	↑
Gluconeogenesis	Liver	↓	↑
Glycogen synthesis	Muscle	↑	–
Glycogen degradation	Muscle	–	–
Fatty acid synthesis	Adipose	↑	↓
Fatty acid degradation	Adipose	↓	↑

- it stimulates glucose transport (and transport of amino acids, K^+ ions and other nutrients) into cells, thus reducing their blood concentration;
- it stimulates (or helps to stimulate) intracellular biosynthetic (anabolic) pathways, such as glycogen synthesis (Table 8.1), which helps to convert the nutrients into a storage form in the cells;
- it inhibits (or helps to inhibit) catabolic pathways, such as glycogenolysis;
- it stimulates protein and DNA synthesis (which underlies insulin's growth-promoting activity).

In general, insulin achieves such metabolic control by inducing the dephosphorylation of several key regulatory enzymes in mainline catabolic or anabolic pathways. This inhibits the former and stimulates the latter pathway types. These effects are often opposed by other hormones, notably glucagon and adrenaline. Thus, when blood glucose concentrations decrease (e.g. during fasting), insulin levels decrease and the (largely catabolic) effects of glucagon become more prominent. Insulin also induces its characteristic effects by altering the level of transcription of various genes, many of which code for metabolic enzymes. Another gene upregulated by insulin is that of the integral membrane glucose transporter.

Diabetes mellitus

Failure of the body to synthesize sufficient insulin results in the development of insulin dependent diabetes mellitus (IDDM). This is also known as type 1 diabetes or juvenile-onset diabetes (Box 8.1).

IDDM is caused by T cell-mediated autoimmune destruction of the insulin-producing β-pancreatic islet cells in genetically predisposed individuals. This is probably due to the expression of a 'super antigen' on the surface of the β cells in such individuals, although the molecular detail of what extent factors trigger onset of the β cell destruction remain to be elucidated. IDDM may, however, be controlled by parenteral administration of exogenous insulin preparations, usually by regular s.c. injection.

The insulin molecule

Insulin was first identified as an anti-diabetic factor in 1921 (Box 8.1), and was introduced clinically the following year. Its complete amino acid sequence was determined in 1951. Although mature insulin is a dimeric structure, it is synthesized as a single polypeptide

Box 8.1.   Diabetes and the discovery of insulin

The symptoms of diabetes have been recognized and recorded for thousands of years. They generally consist of excessive thirst and urination, loss of weight and, until recently, certain death.

Diabetes mellitus, the most common form of diabetes, is caused by the partial or complete absence of insulin-triggered biological responses. Two forms of diabetes mellitus exist: insulin dependent diabetes mellitus (IDDM) and non-insulin dependent diabetes mellitus (NIDDM).

IDDM, also known as type I diabetes, normally occurs during childhood or teens. It is caused by an autoimmune-mediated destruction of the insulin-producing pancreatic B cells. It is thus characterized by the absence or near-absence of insulin in the blood, even at elevated blood glucose levels.

In the case of NIDDM (maturity onset or type II diabetes mellitus), insulin is present in the blood at normal (or even elevated) levels, but fails to promote any of its characteristic effects. A number of factors can contribute to such insulin resistance, including:

- reduced numbers of insulin receptors on sensitive cells;
- reduced receptor affinity for insulin;
- total/partial failure of insulin binding to initiate an intracellular response.

Diabetes mellitus is currently the fourth leading cause of death in most developed countries. The worldwide incidence of diabetes is increasing. In 1995, some 135 million people were affected. This figure is projected to increase to 300 million by 2025. The increasing incidence is due to a number of factors, including increasing world population, population ageing, unhealthy diets, sedentary lifestyles and obesity.

A second form of diabetes is also recognized: diabetes insipidus, which is caused by a deficiency of the pituitary hormone, vasopressin. Vasopressin promotes water reabsorption from the kidney, hence a deficiency also induces symptoms of excessive urination and thirst. A key diagnostic difference between the common diabetes mellitus and the rare diabetes insipidus, is the absence of glucose in the urine in the latter case. Until a few decades ago, a popular way to differentiate between the two diseases was to taste the patient's urine to see if it was sweet.

The first proof that diabetes mellitus was caused by a factor produced by the pancreas was obtained in 1889, when two Strasburg doctors removed a dog's pancreas and found that the dog promptly developed diabetes. By the early 1900s, doctors in the USA had illustrated that the islets of Langerhans of diabetics were completely/almost completely destroyed. In the Spring of 1921, two researchers at the University of Toronto (Frederick Banting and Charles Best) showed that injection of an extract from the islets of Langerhans could revive diabetic dogs who were close to death. The researchers then decided to try out their discovery on humans, initially checking its safety by injecting each other (they were lucky to have used low doses).

The first diabetic patient to receive insulin was a 14-year-old boy, Leonard Thompson. His recovery from near-death was speedy and he was discharged from hospital within a few weeks — although dependent on regular insulin injections.

Toxicity problems (due to impurities) associated with prolonged repeat insulin administration soon put this treatment in jeopardy. However, a biochemist, James Collip, devised an improved purification scheme entailing insulin crystallization, which overcame such toxicity.

The work culminated in Banting and John MacLeod (his Professor) receiving the Nobel prize, although many felt that the contribution of Best and Collip also deserved Nobel recognition.

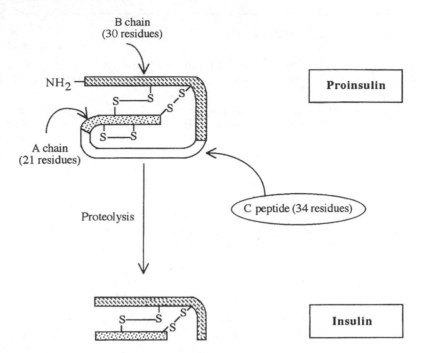

B chain
(30 residues)

NH₂

Proinsulin

A chain
(21 residues)

Proteolysis

C peptide (34 residues)

Insulin

Figure 8.1. Proteolytic processing of proinsulin, yielding mature insulin, as occurs within the coated secretory granules

precursor, preproinsulin. This 108 amino acid polypeptide contains a 23 amino acid signal sequence at its amino terminal end. This guides it through the endoplasmic reticulum membrane, where the signal sequence is removed by a specific peptidase.

Proinsulin-containing vesicles bud off from the endoplasmic reticulum and fuse with the Golgi apparatus. Subsequently, proinsulin-containing vesicles (clathrin-coated secretory vesicles), in turn, bud off from the Golgi. As they move away from the Golgi, they lose their clathrin coat, becoming non-coated secretory vesicles. These vesicles serve as a storage form of insulin in the β cell. Elevated levels of blood glucose, or other appropriate signals, cause the vesicles to fuse with the plasma membrane, thereby releasing their contents into the blood via the process of exocytosis.

Proinsulin is proteolytically processed in the coated secretory granules, yielding mature insulin and a 34 amino acid connecting peptide (C peptide, Figure 8.1). The C peptide is further proteolytically modified by removal of a dipeptide from each of its ends. The secretory granules thus contain low levels of proinsulin, C peptide and proteases, in addition to insulin itself. The insulin is stored in the form of a characteristic zinc–insulin hexamer, consisting of six molecules of insulin stabilized by two zinc atoms.

Mature insulin consists of two polypeptide chains connected by two interchain disulphide linkages. The A-chain contains 21 amino acids, whereas the larger B-chain is composed of 30 residues. Insulins from various species conforms to this basic structure, while varying slightly in their amino acid sequence. Porcine insulin (5777 Da) varies from the human form (5807 Da) by a single amino acid, whereas bovine insulin (5733 Da) differs by three residues.

Although a high degree of homology is evident between insulins from various species, the same is not true for proinsulins, as the C peptide sequence can vary considerably. This has therapeutic implications, as the presence of proinsulin in animal-derived insulin preparations can potentially elicit an immune response in humans.

The insulin receptor and signal transduction

The insulin receptor is a tetrameric integral membrane glycoprotein consisting of two 735 amino acid α-chains and two 620 amino acid β-chains. These are held together by disulphide linkages (Figure 8.2). The α-chain resides entirely on the extracellular side of the plasma membrane and contains the cysteine-rich insulin-binding domain.

Each β-subunit is composed of three regions; the extracellular domain, the transmembrane domain and a large cytoplasmic domain that displays tyrosine kinase activity. In the absence of insulin, tyrosine kinase activity is very weak. Proteolytic digestion of the α-subunit results in activation of this kinase activity. It is believed that the intact α-subunit exerts a negative influence on the endogenous kinase of the β-subunit and that binding of insulin, by causing a conformational shift in α-subunits, relieves this negative influence.

The cytoplasmic domain of the β-subunit displays three distinct sub-domains: (a) the 'juxtamembrane domain', implicated in recognition/binding of intracellular substrate molecules; (b) the tyrosine kinase domain, which (upon receptor activation) displays tyrosine kinase activity; and (c) the C-terminal domain, whose exact function is less clear although site-directed mutagenesis studies implicate it promoting insulin's mitogenic effects.

The molecular mechanisms central to insulin signal transduction are complex and have yet to be fully elucidated. However, considerable progress in this regard has been made over the last decade. Binding of insulin to its receptor promotes the autophosphorylation of three specific tyrosine residues in the tyrosine kinase domain (Figure 8.2(b)). This in turn promotes an alteration in the conformational state of the entire β-subunit, unmasking ATP (the phosphate donor) binding sites as well as substrate docking sites and activating its tyrosine kinase activity. Depending upon which specific intracellular substrates are then phosphorylated, at least two different signal transduction pathways are initiated (Figure 8.2(c)). Activation of the 'MAP kinase' pathway is ultimately responsible for triggering insulin's mitogenic effects, whereas activation of the PI-3 kinase pathway apparently mediates the majority of insulin's metabolic effects. Many of these effects, particularly the mitogenic effects, are promoted via transcriptional regulation of insulin-sensitive genes, of which there are probably in excess of 100 (Table 8.2).

Insulin production

Insulin preparations used initially were little more than crude pancreatic extracts. The therapeutic value of such products was marginal, as severe adverse reactions were commonplace (due to the presence of impurities). This was made worse by the frequency of injections required. The introduction of an acid–alcohol precipitation step yielded insulin preparations of moderate purity, thus partially overcoming the range and severity of side effects noted.

Although insulin was first crystallized in 1926, the factors promoting crystal growth were poorly understood and yielded inconsistent results. It was almost 10 years later when researchers discovered that the addition of zinc to a crude extract promoted reproducible crystallization (zinc addition yields a characteristic rhombohedral crystal, the basic crystal unit being the insulin hexamer, stabilized by the two zinc atoms).

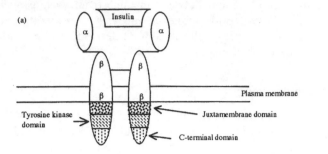

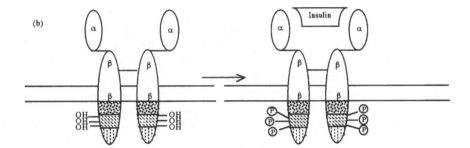

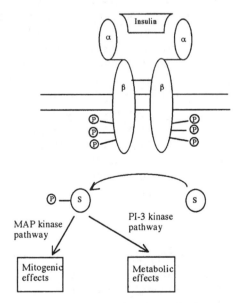

Figure 8.2. Structure of the insulin receptor (a). Binding of insulin promotes autophosphorylation of the β-subunits, where each β-subunit phosphorylates the other β-subunit. Phosphate groups are attached to three specific tyrosine residues (1158, 1162 and 1163), as indicated in (b). Activation of the β-subunit's tyrosine kinase activity in turn results in the phosphorylation of various intracellular (protein) substrates which trigger the MAP kinase and/or the IP-3 kinase pathway, responsible for inducing insulin's mitogenic and metabolic effects. The underlying molecular events occurring in these pathways are complex (see e.g. Combettes-Souverain and Issad, 1998)

Table 8.2. Selected genes whose rate of transcription is altered by binding of insulin to its receptor. In virtually all instances, the ultimate effect is to promote anabolic events characteristic of insulin action. Two-dimensional gel electrophoresis has also pinpointed dozens of proteins of unknown function whose cellular level is altered by insulin

Protein class	Gene product	Insulin effect (↑ or ↓ in transcription rate)
Integral membrane proteins	Insulin receptor	↑↓
	Growth hormone receptor	↑
	Glucose transporters	↑
Enzymes	Fatty acid synthetase	↑
	Glutamine synthetase	↑↓
	Pyruvate kinase	↑
	Fructose 1,6 bis-phosphatase	↓
	Phosphoenolpyruvate carboxykinase	↓
	Glucokinase	↑
Hormones	IGF-1	↑
	Glucagon	↓
	GH	↓
Transcription factors	C-Myc	↑
	C-Fos	↑
	egr-1	↑

By the mid-1930s, commercial insulin was being prepared by crystallization from crude porcine or bovine extracts. The crystallized preparation was generally subjected to a recrystallization step in order to further increase the product's purity. Such preparations are termed 'conventional insulins' (Box 8.2).

Chromatographic or electrophoretic analysis of conventional insulins generally yields three major fractions or bands (a, b and c). Fraction a contains high molecular mass material which can be removed from the product by additional recrystallization steps. The major components of fraction b are proinsulin and insulin dimers, while insulin, as well as slightly modified forms of insulin (e.g. arginine-insulin and desamido-insulin), are found in fraction c.

Additional impurities, such as glucagon, somatostatin, pancreatic polypeptide and vasoactive intestinal polypeptide, are present in most conventional insulin preparations at lower levels. The presence of such contaminants can impact upon product safety and efficacy in a number of ways.

Many of the contaminants are immunogenic in man. This is particularly significant in the case of insulin as, unlike most other biopharmaceuticals, it usually must be administered daily for life. The frequency of administration will ultimately trigger a strong immunological response, even against weak immunogens. Porcine insulin, differing from human insulin by only a single amino acid (residue 30 of the B-chain; threonine in humans, alanine in pigs), is essentially non-immunogenic in man. However, many of the porcine insulin contaminants (including porcine proinsulin) are immunogenic.

Bovine insulin, differing from the human form by three amino acids, does elicit an immunological response in humans. This can trigger long-term complications, including insulin resistance (as anti-insulin antibodies neutralize some of the administered product). The presence of these antibodies can also affect the pharmacokinetic profile of the drug, as antibody-bound insulin molecules are largely resistant to the normal insulin degradative process. (Pharmacokinetics is the study of how a drug interacts with the body in terms of its absorption, distribution, metabolism and excretion; Chapter 2.)

Box 8.2.   Insulin products: a glossary of terms

Conventional insulins: bovine or porcine insulin purified only by crystallization

Single peak insulins: bovine or porcine insulin that have undergone a further gel filtration purification step

Highly purified insulins: insulin purified by gel filtration and ion-exchange chromatography

Human insulin (emp):   insulin of human sequence manufactured by enzymatic modification of porcine insulin

Human insulin (crb):   recombinant human insulin in which A- and B-chains are expressed separately in bacteria

Human insulin (prb):   recombinant human insulin in which proinsulin is expressed in bacteria

Human insulin (pyr):   recombinant human insulin produced in yeast

Insulin B.P./Eur.P./USP: insulin of bovine or porcine origin

Human insulin B.P./Eur.P.:   insulin of human sequence produced either by enzymatic modification of porcine insulin or by recombinant DNA technology

Insulin human USP: insulin of human sequence produced either by enzymatic modification of porcine insulin or by recombinant DNA technology

Soluble insulin=regular insulin=unmodified insulin: any insulin solution from any source which is not formulated/changed in any way in order to prolong its duration of action

Protamine zinc insulin: insulin complexed to excess protamine in order to prolong its duration of action

Isophane insulin: preparations containing equimolar quantities of insulin and protamine in order to prolong its duration of action

Insulin–zinc suspension: suspension of insulin, generated by crystallization with zinc, formulated in this way in order to prolong its duration of action

Biphasic insulin: mixture of insulin preparations that provide for immediate and prolonged action

The higher molecular mass contaminants in conventional insulin preparations include various proteases. Such preparations are generally maintained in solution at acidic pH values (often as low as pH 2.5–3.5). This minimizes the risk of proteolytic degradation of the insulin molecules, as contaminant proteases are inactive at such pH values.

Modern animal-derived insulin preparations are subjected to one or more chromatographic steps in order to further reduce the content of product impurities. Recrystallized insulins subjected to a gel filtration step are termed 'single peak' insulins. Process-scale gel filtration chromatographic systems (usually using Sephadex G-50 chromatography media), with bed volumes of up to 100 litres, are routinely used in this regard. Depending upon the system, a single column run takes 5–8 h and can yield up to 50 g of purified insulin.

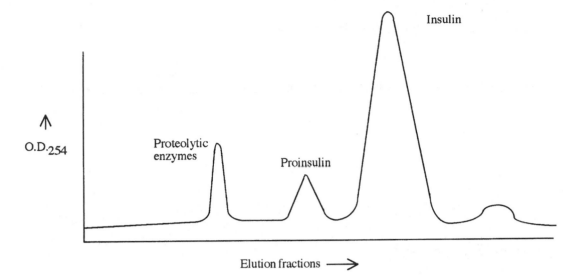

Figure 8.3. Chromatographic purification of recrystallized insulin on a Sephadex G-50 gel filtration column. Separation of high molecular mass proteolytic enzymes, as well as proinsulin and some very low molecular mass material, is obvious. Insulin elutes from the column as a single peak, hence the term 'single peak insulin'

Gel filtration separates the high molecular mass (mainly proteolytic) fraction, as well as proinsulin and insulin dimers, from the insulin product. It fails to remove slightly modified forms of the insulin molecule itself (e.g. desamido-insulin), which are of limited clinical significance in any case (Figure 8.3). A variety of additional pancreatic polypeptides of similar molecular mass to insulin also co-elute with it. Thus, while being substantially purified, single peak insulins are nowhere near to being homogeneous preparations. However, removal of proteolytic enzymes facilitates formulation of the insulin in buffers at neutral pH. This is important, as such insulin products are 'fast-acting', as discussed later.

An additional ion-exchange step substantially improves the electrophoretic purity of single-peak insulins, removing not only most pancreatic polypeptides of similar size, but also modified insulins. Importantly, it also achieves separation of much of the proinsulin contaminant, often bringing its level to below 10 ppm. A combination of gel filtration and ion-exchange chromatography is used to generate product known as 'purified insulin' in the USA or 'highly purified insulin' in the UK (Box 8.2).

Enzymatic conversion of porcine insulin

As previously described, porcine insulin differs from human insulin by only one amino acid (the B30 residue). In the early 1970s, a method was developed by which porcine insulin could be converted into a preparation of identical amino acid sequence to that of human insulin (Figure 8.4). This method utilizes a combination of enzymatic and chemical treatment of the porcine product.

The porcine insulin is first subjected to digestion with chymotrypsin-free trypsin at pH 7.5 for in excess of 45 min. This results in the selective cleavage of the peptide bond linking arginine 22

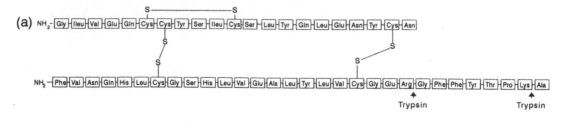

Figure 8.4. Amino acid sequence of porcine insulin is depicted in (a). Trypsin cleavage sites are also indicated. Trypsin therefore effectively removes the insulin carboxy-terminus B chain octapeptide. The amino acid sequence of human insulin differs from that of porcine insulin by only one amino acid residue. Porcine insulin contains an alanine residue at position 30 of the B-chain, whereas human insulin contains a threonine residue at that position. Insulin exhibiting a human amino acid sequence may thus be synthesized from porcine insulin by treating the latter with trypsin, removal of the C terminus fragments, generated and replacement of this with the synthetic octapeptide shown in (b). Reproduced by permission of John Wiley & Sons Ltd from Walsh & Headon (1994)

and glycine 23 in the insulin B-chain. The reaction products are a shortened insulin molecule and the B-chain terminal octapeptide (which can be further proteolysed by trypsin; Figure 8.4). The tryptic digest is then applied to a Sephadex G-75 gel filtration column in order to separate the reaction products.

An octapeptide, corresponding in sequence to the C-terminal octapeptide found in the human insulin B-chain, is prepared by chemical synthesis. This octapeptide is then coupled to the shortened insulin using a well-established chemical method, thus yielding a semi-synthetic human insulin product ('human insulin *emp*'; Box 8.2).

Typically, 7.0 g of human insulin can be prepared from 10 g of purified porcine insulin. The process allows large-scale production of human insulin simply and inexpensively. The complete *de novo* synthesis of human insulin, while technically possible, is economically unattractive.

Production of human insulin by recombinant DNA technology

Human insulin produced by recombinant DNA technology was first approved for general medical use in 1982, initially in the USA, West Germany, the UK and The Netherlands. As such, it was the first product of recombinant DNA technology to be approved for therapeutic use in humans. Production of insulin by recombinant means displays several advantages, including,

- reliability of supply;
- elimination of the risk of accidental transmission of disease, due to the presence of pathogens in animal pancreatic tissue;
- economically attractive (once initial capital investment has been made).

The quantity of purified insulin obtained from the pancreas of one pig satisfies the requirements of one diabetic for 3 days. The supply of pancreatic tissue is dependent upon the demand for meat, which does not necessarily correlate with the increasing worldwide incidence of diabetes. Recombinant DNA technology provides an obvious way to ensure future adequate supply of insulin.

The initial approach taken (by scientists at Genentech) entailed inserting the nucleotide sequence coding for the insulin A- and B-chains into two different *E. coli* cells (both strain K12). These cells were then cultured separately in large-scale fermentation vessels, with subsequent chromatographic purification of the insulin chains produced. The A- and B-chains are then incubated together under appropriate oxidizing conditions in order to promote interchain disulphide bond formation, forming human insulin *crb* (Box 8.2).

An alternative method (developed in the Eli Lilly research laboratories) entails inserting a nucleotide sequence coding for human proinsulin into recombinant *E. coli*. This is followed by purification of the expressed proinsulin and subsequent proteolytic excision of the C peptide *in vitro*. This approach has become more popular, largely due to the requirement for a single fermentation and subsequent purification scheme. Such preparations have been termed human insulin *prb*.

A number of studies have shown conclusively that the recombinant insulins are chemically and functionally identical to native human insulin. Sequencing data confirms the expected amino acid sequence. HPLC analysis also yields identical chromatograms (Figure 8.5). Circular dichromism studies, which evaluate tertiary structure, also yield identical patterns, as does X-ray crystallographic analysis. Radioreceptor- and radioimmuno-assays yield identical results, as does the traditional bioassay for insulin (measure of the hormone's ability to induce a hypoglycaemic response in rabbits). Prior to its approval for medical use, human clinical trials also found the recombinant insulin to be as effective as previously available products in terms of controlling hyperglycaemia. Recombinant human insulins are now routinely produced in 10 000 gallon fermentation vessels and several such products have gained marketing approval (Table 8.3).

While the recombinant product is identical to native insulin, any impurities present will be *E. coli*-derived and, hence, potentially highly immunogenic. Stringent purification of the recombinant product must thus be undertaken. This entails several chromatographic steps (often gel filtration and ion-exchange, along with additional steps which exploit differences in molecular hydrophobicity, e.g. hydrophobic interaction chromatography or reverse-phase chromatography) (Figure 8.6).

A 'clean-up' process-scale reverse-phase HPLC (RP-HPLC) step has been introduced into production of human insulin *prb*. The C8 or C18 RP-HPLC column used displays an internal volume of 80 l or more, and up to 1200 g of insulin may be loaded during a single purification run (Figure 8.7). Separation is achieved using an acidic (often acetic acid-based) mobile phase (i.e. set at a pH value sufficiently below the insulin pI value of 5.3 in order to keep it fully in solution). The insulin is usually loaded in the water-rich acidic mobile phase, followed by gradient elution using acetonitrile (insulin typically elutes at 15–30% acetonitrile).

(a)

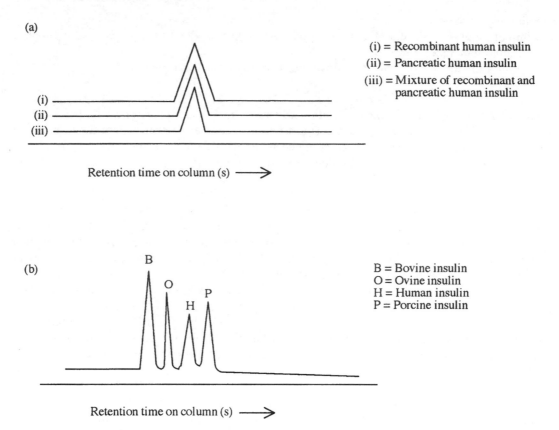

(i) = Recombinant human insulin
(ii) = Pancreatic human insulin
(iii) = Mixture of recombinant and
pancreatic human insulin

(i)
(ii)
(iii)

Retention time on column (s) ——→

(b)

B = Bovine insulin
O = Ovine insulin
H = Human insulin
P = Porcine insulin

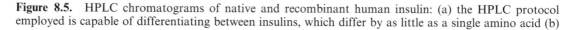

Retention time on column (s) ——→

Figure 8.5. HPLC chromatograms of native and recombinant human insulin: (a) the HPLC protocol employed is capable of differentiating between insulins, which differ by as little as a single amino acid (b)

While the starting material loaded onto the column is fairly pure (~92%), this step yields a final product of approximately 99% purity. Over 95% of the insulin activity loaded onto the column can be recovered. A single column run takes in the order of 1 h.

The RP-HPLC 'polishing' step not only removes *E. coli*-derived impurities, but also effectively separates modified insulin derivatives from the native insulin product. The resultant extremely low levels of impurities remaining in these insulin preparations fail to elicit any significant immunological response in diabetic recipients.

Formulation of insulin products

Insulin, whatever its source, may be formulated in a number of ways. This directly affects its activity profile upon administration to diabetic patients. Fast (short)-acting insulins are those preparations that yield an elevated blood insulin concentration relatively quickly after their administration, which is usually by s.c. or, less commonly, by i.m. injection. Slow-acting insulins, on the other hand, enter the circulation much more slowly from the depot (injection) site. This is characterized by a slower onset of action, but one of longer duration (Table 8.4).

Table 8.3. Native and engineered human insulin preparations that have gained approval for general medical use. Refer to text for further detail. rh=recombinant human

Product	Company
Humulin (rh-insulin)	Eli Lilly
Novolin (rh-insulin)	Novo Nordisk
Humalog (Insulin Lispro, an insulin analogue)	Eli Lilly
Insuman (rh-insulin)	Hoechst AG
Liprolog (Bio Lysprol, a short-acting insulin)	Eli Lilly
NovoRapid (Insulin Aspart, short-acting rh-insulin analogue)	Novo Nordisk
Novomix 30 (contains Insulin Aspart, short-acting rh-insulin analogue (see NovoRapid) as one ingredient	Novo Nordisk
Novolog (Insulin Aspart, short acting rh-insulin; see also NovoRapid entry above)	Novo Nordisk
Novolog mix 70/30 (contains Insulin Aspart, short acting rh-insulin analogue as one ingredient; see also Novomix 30 entry above)	Novo Nordisk
Actrapid/Velosulin/Monotard/Insulatard/Protaphane/Mixtard/Actraphane/ Ultratard (all contain rh-insulin produced in *S. cerevisiae*, formulated as short/intermediate/long-acting products)	Novo Nordisk
Lantus (insulin glargine, long acting rh-insulin)	Aventis Pharmaceuticals
Optisulin (insulin glargine, long-acting rh-insulin analogue, see Lantus)	Aventis Pharma

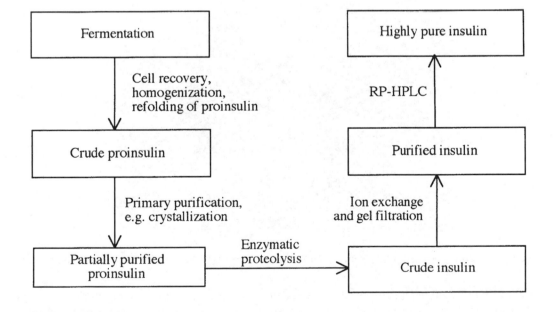

Figure 8.6. A likely purification scheme for human insulin prb. A final RP–HPLC polishing step yields a highly pure product. Refer to text for details

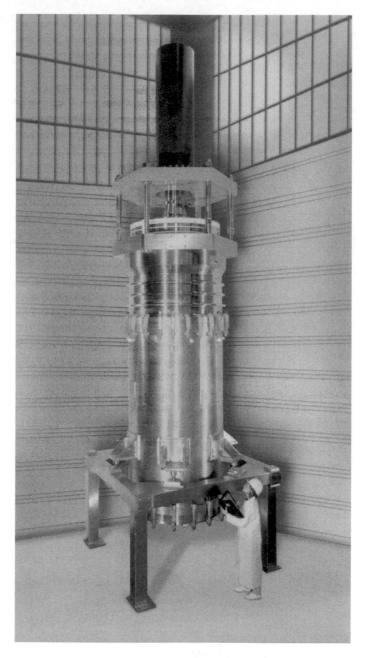

Figure 8.7.   Process-scale HPLC column. Photo courtesy of NovaSep Ltd: http://www.novasep.com

In healthy individuals, insulin is typically secreted continuously into the bloodstream at low basal levels, with rapid increases evident in response to elevated blood sugar levels. Insulin secretion usually peaks approximately 1 h after a meal, falling off to base levels once again within the following 2 h.

Table 8.4. Some pharmacokinetic characteristics of short, intermediate and long-acting insulin preparations

Category	Onset (hours after administration)	Peak activity (hours after administration)	Duration (hours)
Short-acting	1/2–1	2–5	6–8
Intermediate-acting	2	4–12	Up to 24
Long-acting	4	10–20	Up to 36

The blood insulin level is continuously up- or downregulated as appropriate for the blood glucose levels at any given instant. Conventional insulin therapy does not accurately reproduce such precise endogenous control. Therapy consists of injections of slow- and fast-acting insulins, as appropriate, or a mixture of both. No slow-acting insulin preparation, however, accurately reproduces normal serum insulin baseline levels. An injection of fast-acting insulin will not produce a plasma hormone peak for 1.5–2 h post-injection, and levels then remain elevated for up to 5 h. Hence, if fast-acting insulin is administered at meal time, diabetics will still experience hyperglycaemia for the first hour, and hypoglycaemia after 4–5 h. Such traditional animal or human insulin preparations must thus be administered 1 h before eating — and the patient must not subsequently alter his/her planned mealtime.

Insulin, at typical normal plasma concentrations (approximately 1×10^{-9} M) exists in true solution as a monomer. Any insulin injected directly into the bloodstream exhibits a half-life of only a few minutes.

The concentration of insulin present in soluble insulin preparations (i.e. fast-acting insulins), is much higher (approximately 1×10^{-3} M). At this concentration, the soluble insulin exists as a mixture of monomer, dimer, tetramer and zinc–insulin hexamer. These insulin complexes have to dissociate in order to be absorbed from the injection site into the blood, which slows down the onset of hormone action.

In order to prolong the duration of insulin action, soluble insulin may be formulated to generate insulin suspensions. This is generally achieved in one of two ways:

1. Addition of zinc in order to promote zinc–insulin crystal growth (which take longer to disassociate and, hence, longer to leak into the blood stream from the injection depot site).
2. Addition of a protein to which the insulin will complex, and from which the insulin will only be slowly released. The proteins normally used are protamines, basic polypeptides naturally found in association with nucleic acid in the sperm of several species of fish. Depending on the relative molar ratios of insulin:protamine used, the resulting long-acting insulins generated are termed protamine–Zn–insulin or isophane insulin (Box 8.2). Biphasic insulins include mixtures of short- and long-acting insulins, which attempt to mimic normal insulin rhythms in the body.

Engineered insulins

Recombinant DNA technology facilitates not only production of human insulin in microbial systems, but also facilitates generation of insulins of modified amino acid sequences. The major aims of generating such engineered insulin analogues include:

- identification of insulins with altered pharmacokinetic properties, such as faster-acting or slower-acting insulins;
- identification of super-potent insulin forms (insulins with higher receptor affinities). This is due to commercial considerations, namely the economic benefits which would accrue from utilizing smaller quantities of insulin per therapeutic dose.

The insulin amino acid residues which interact with the insulin receptor have been identified (A1, A5, A19, A21, B10, B16, B23–25), and a number of analogues containing amino acid substitutions at several of these points have been manufactured, e.g. conversion of histidine to glutamate at the B10 position yields an analogue displaying five-fold higher activity *in vitro*. Other substitutions have generated analogues with even higher specific activities. However, increased *in vitro* activity does not always translate to increased *in vivo* activity.

Attempts to generate faster-acting insulins have centred upon developing analogues which do not dimerize or form higher polymers at therapeutic dose concentrations. The contact points between individual insulin molecules in insulin dimers/oligomers include amino acids at positions B8, B9, B12–13, B16 and B23–28. Thus, analogues with various substitutions at these positions have been generated. The approach adopted generally entails insertion of charged or bulky amino acids, in order to promote charge repulsion or steric hindrance between individual insulin monomers. Several are absorbed from the site of injection into the bloodstream far more quickly than native soluble (fast-acting) insulin. Such modified insulins could thus be injected at mealtimes, rather than 1 h before, and several such fast-acting engineered insulins have now been approved for medical use (Table 8.3). Insulin Lispro was the first such engineered short-acting insulin to come to market (Box 8.3 and Figure 8.8).

Insulin Aspart is a second fast-acting engineered human insulin analogue now approved for general medical use. It differs from native human insulin in that the proline^{B28} residue has been replaced by aspartic acid. This single amino acid substitution also decreases the propensity of individual molecules to self-associate, ensuring that they begin to enter the bloodstream from the site of injection immediately upon administration.

A number of studies have also focused upon the generation of longer-acting insulin analogues. The currently used Zn–insulin suspensions, or protamine–Zn–insulin suspensions, generally display a plasma half-life of 20–25 h. Selected amino acid substitutions have generated insulins which, even in soluble form, exhibit plasma half-lives of up to 35 h.

Optisulin or Lantus are the trade names given to one such analogue that gained general marketing approval in 2000 (Table 8.3). The international non-proprietary name (inn) for this engineered molecule is 'insulin glargine'. It differs from native human insulin in that the C-terminal asparagine residue of the α-chain has been replaced by a glycine residue and the β-chain has been elongated (again from its C-terminus) by two arginine residues. The overall effect is to increase the molecule's isoelectric point (pI, the pH at which the molecule displays a net overall zero charge and consequently is least soluble) from 5.4 to a value approaching 7.0. The engineered insulin is expressed in a recombinant *E. coli* K12 host strain and is produced via the 'proinsulin route', as previously described. The purified product is formulated at pH 4.0, a pH value at which it is fully soluble.

Upon s.c. injection, the insulin experiences an increase in pH towards more neutral values and, consequently, appears to precipitate in the subcutaneous tissue. It resolubilizes very slowly and hence a greatly prolonged duration of release into the bloodstream is noted. Consequently, a single daily injection supports the maintenance of acceptable basal blood insulin levels, and insulin molecules are still detected at the site of injection more than 24 h after administration.

Box 8.3. Insulin Lispro

Insulin Lispro was the first recombinant fast-acting insulin analogue to gain marketing approval (Table 8.3). It displays an amino acid sequence identical to native human insulin, with one alteration—an inversion of the natural proline–lysine sequence found at positions 28 and 29 of the insulin β-chain. This simple alteration significantly decreased the propensity of individual insulin molecules to self-associate when stored at therapeutic dose concentrations. The dimerization constant for Insulin Lispro is 300 times lower than that exhibited by unmodified human insulin. Structurally, this appears to occur as the change in sequence disrupts the formation of inter-chain hydrophobic interactions critical to self-association.

Insulin Lispro was developed by scientists at Eli Lilly (which, along with Novo Nordisk, are the world's largest producers of therapeutic insulins). The rationale underlying the sequence alteration was rooted in studies, not of insulin, but of insulin-like growth factor-1 (IGF-1; Chapter 7). The latter displays a strong structural resemblance to proinsulin, with up to 50% of amino acid residues within the IGF-1 A- and B-domains being identical to those found in comparable positions in the insulin A- and B-chains. When compared to insulin, IGF-1 molecules display a significantly decreased propensity to self-associate. Sequencing studies earlier revealed that the Proline^{B28}–Lysine^{B29} sequence characteristic of insulin is reversed in IGF-1. It was suggested that, if this sequence difference was responsible for the differences in self-association propensity, then inversion of the Proline^{B28}–Lysine^{B29} sequence in insulin would result in its decreased self-association. Direct experimentation proved this hypothesis accurate.

Insulin Lispro is manufactured commercially in a manner quite similar to the 'proinsulin' route used to manufacture native recombinant human insulin. A synthetic gene coding for Lys^{B28}–Pro^{B29} proinsulin is expressed in *E. coli*. Following fermentation and recovery, the proinsulin is treated with trypsin and carboxypeptidase B, resulting in the proteolytic excision of the engineered insulin molecule. It is then purified to homogeneity by a number of high-resolution chromatographic steps. The final product formulation also contains *m*-cresol (preservative and stabilizer), zinc oxide (stabilizer), glycerol (tonicity modifier) and a phosphate-based buffer. The commercial product has a shelf-life of 2 years when stored at 2–8°C.

The generation of engineered insulin analogues raises several important issues relating to product safety and efficacy. As mentioned in a general context in Chapter 3, alteration of a native protein's amino acid sequence could render the engineered product immunogenic. Such an effect would be particularly significant in the case of insulin, as the product is generally administered daily for life. In addition, alteration in structure could have unintended (in addition to intended) influences upon pharmacokinetic and/or pharmacodynamic characteristics of the drug. Preclinical and, in particular, clinical evaluations undertaken upon the analogues thus far approved, however, have confirmed their safety as well as efficacy. The sequence changes introduced are relatively minor and do not seem to elicit an immunological response. Fortuitously, neither have the alterations made affected the ability of the insulin molecule to interact with the insulin receptor and trigger the resultant characteristic biological responses.

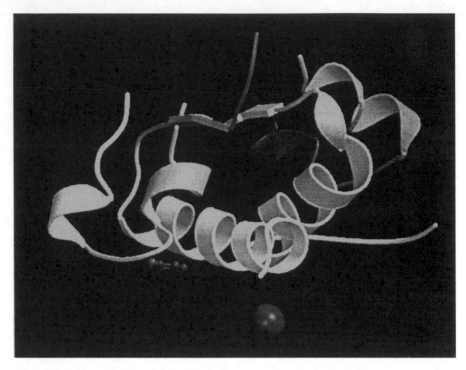

Figure 8.8.   3-D structure of the engineered fast-acting insulin, 'Insulin Lispro'. Photo from Ciszak *et al.* (1995), by courtesy of the Protein Data Bank: http://www.rcsb.org.pdb/

Additional means of insulin administration

Chapter 2 details recent progress in developing insulin formulations for delivery via the oral or pulmonary route. An additional approach, which may mimic more closely the normal changes in blood insulin levels, entails the use of infusion systems which constantly deliver insulin to the patient. The simplest design in this regard is termed an 'open loop system'. This consists of an infusion pump which automatically infuses soluble insulin subcutaneously, via a catheter. Blood glucose levels are monitored manually and the infusion rate is programmed accordingly.

While the potential of such systems is obvious, they have not become popular in practice, mainly due to complications which can potentially arise, including:

- abscess formation or development of cellulitis at the site of injection;
- possible pump malfunction;
- catheter obstruction;
- hypersensitivity reactions to components of the system;
- requirement for manual blood glucose monitoring.

The closed-loop system (often termed the 'artificial pancreas') is essentially a more sophisticated version of the system described above. It consists not only of a pump and infusion device, but also an integral glucose sensor and computer, which analyses the blood glucose data obtained and adjusts the flow-rate accordingly. The true potential of such systems remains to be assessed.

Treating diabetics with insulin-producing cells

While infusion pumps can go some way towards mimicking normal control of blood insulin levels, transplantation of insulin-producing pancreatic cells should effectively 'cure' the diabetic patient. This approach has been adopted thus far with almost 200 patients, with encouraging results.

Initial experiments in the 1970s using inbred strains of rats illustrated the feasibility of this approach. Insulin-producing pancreatic islet cells 'donated' by one set of rats were transplanted into other rats of the same strain, first made diabetic by injection with drugs such as streptozotocin, which destroy the pancreatic B cells.

Such islet grafts permanently returned blood glucose levels in the diabetic animals to normal values. Even more encouraging, this treatment prevented development of diabetic-associated complications of kidney and eye function (which, in human diabetics, can lead to kidney failure and partial blindness).

The technique simply entails injecting the insulin-producing islets into the portal vein. These cells subsequently lodge in smaller vessels branching from the vein. Here, they can constantly monitor blood glucose levels and secrete insulin accordingly. About 400 000–800 000 islet B cells are usually transplanted. In most instances, these function for up to 3 years, although they often fail to control blood glucose levels fully, i.e. supplemental insulin injections are sometimes required.

The islet cells transplanted into humans are obtained from pancreatic tissue of deceased human donors (Figure 8.9). Implantation of these cells in recipients displaying a competent immune system would, at best, be of transient therapeutic benefit. The ensuing immune response would quickly destroy the foreign cells. Studies conducted thus far in humans have utilized diabetic patients who have received kidney transplants, as these are already subject to immunosuppressive therapy. However, a major stumbling block to the widespread adoption of this therapeutic approach is, predictably, the requirement to induce concurrent immune suppression.

GLUCAGON

Glucagon is a single-chain polypeptide of 29 amino acid residues and a molecular mass of 3500 Da. It is synthesized by the A cells of the Islets of Langerhans, and also by related cells found in the digestive tract. Like insulin, it is synthesized as a high molecular mass polypeptide from which the mature hormone is released by selective proteolysis.

The major biological actions of glucagon tend to oppose those of insulin, particularly with regard to regulation of metabolism. Glucagon has an overall catabolic effect, stimulating the breakdown of glycogen, lipid and protein. A prominent metabolic effect is to increase blood glucose levels (i.e. it is a hyperglycaemic hormone). Indeed, the major physiological function of glucagon is to prevent hypoglycaemia. The hormone is stored in secretory vesicles, after synthesis in the pancreatic A cells, and released by exocytosis upon experiencing a drop in blood glucose concentration.

Glucagon initiates its metabolic (and other) effects by binding to a specific cell surface receptor, thus activating a membrane-bound adenylate kinase. This in turn, promotes activation of a cAMP-dependent protein kinase (Figure 8.10). The kinase phosphorylates key regulatory enzymes in carbohydrate metabolism, thereby modulating their activity. Hepatic glycogen phosphorylase, for example, is activated via phosphorylation, while glycogen synthetase is

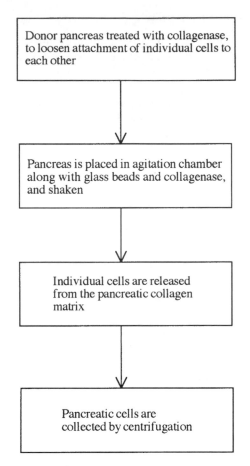

Figure 8.9. Overview of the extraction of pancreatic cells from a human donor pancreas. Typically, a pancreas will house approximately 1 million such cells, of which around 40% are recovered by this procedure

inactivated, thus promoting glycogen breakdown. The rate of gluconeogenesis is also stimulated by the inactivation of pyruvate kinase and simultaneous activation of fructose 1,6 bisphosphatase.

Hypoglycaemia remains the most frequent complication of insulin administration to diabetics. It usually occurs due to (a) administration of an excessive amount of insulin; (b) administration of insulin prior to a mealtime, but with subsequent omission of the meal; or (c) due to increased physical activity. In severe cases, this can lead to loss of consciousness and even death. Although it may be treated by oral or i.v. administration of glucose, insulin-induced hypoglycaemia is sometimes treated by administration of glucagon.

Glucagon is also used medically as a diagnostic aid during certain radiological examinations of the stomach, small and large intestine where decreased intestinal motility is advantageous (the hormone has an inhibitory effect on the motility of the smooth muscle lining the walls of the gastrointestinal tract).

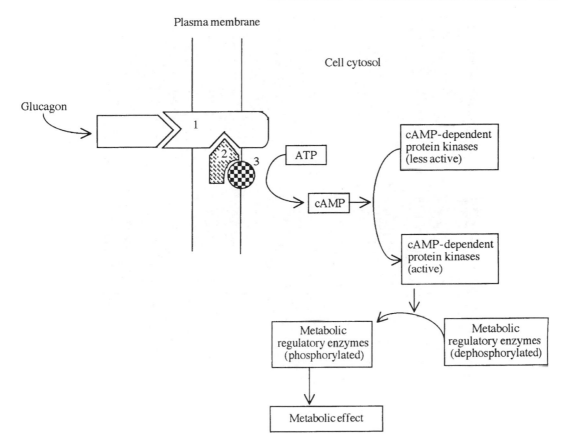

Figure 8.10. Initiation of a metabolic response to the binding of glucagon to its receptor. (1)=glucagon cell surface receptor; (2)=G protein; (3)=adenylate cyclase (see text for further detail)

Traditionally, glucagon preparations utilized therapeutically are chromatographically purified from bovine or porcine pancreatic tissue (the structure of bovine, porcine and human glucagon is identical, thus eliminating the possibility of direct immunological complications). Such commercial preparations are generally formulated with lactose and sodium chloride and sold in freeze-dried form; 0.5–1.0 units of glucagon (approximately 0.5–1.0 mg freeze-dried hormone) are administered to the patient by s.c. or i.m. injection.

More recently, glucagon preparations produced via recombinant means have also become available. 'GlucaGen' is the trade name given to one such product, produced by Novo Nordisk using an engineered *Saccharomyces cerevisiae* strain. Upstream processing (aerobic batch-fed fermentation) is followed by an upward adjustment of media pH in order to dissolve precipitated product (glucagon is insoluble in aqueous-based media between pH 3–9.5). This facilitates subsequent removal of the yeast by centrifugation. Glucagon is then recovered and purified from the media by a series of further precipitation as well as high-resolution

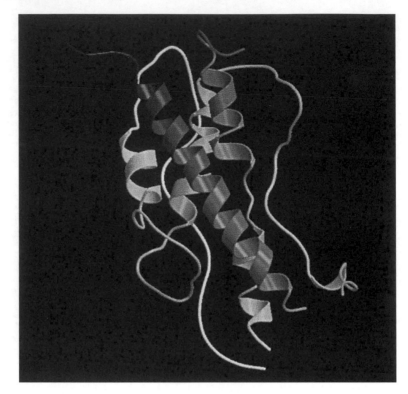

Figure 8.11.   3-D structure of human growth hormone. Photo from Chantalat *et al.* (1995), by courtesy of the Protein Data Bank: http://www.rcsb.org/pdb/

chromatographic steps. Eli Lilly also produces a recombinant glucagon product using an engineered *E. coli* strain.

HUMAN GROWTH HORMONE (hGH)

Human growth hormone (hGH, somatotrophin; Figure 8.11) is a polypeptide hormone synthesized in the anterior pituitary. It promotes normal body growth and lactation and influences various aspects of cellular metabolism.

Mature hGH contains 191 amino acid residues and displays a molecular mass of 22 kDa. It also contains two characteristic intra-chain disulphide linkages. hGH mRNA can also undergo alternate splicing, yielding a shortened GH molecule (20 kDa), which appears to display biological activities indistinguishable from the 22 kDa species.

hGH displays significant, although not absolute, species specificity. GHs isolated from other primates are the only preparations biologically active in humans (this precluded the earlier use of bovine/porcine preparations for medical use in humans).

Growth hormone synthesis and release from the pituitary is regulated by two hypothalamic factors: growth hormone releasing hormone (GHRH, also known as growth hormone releasing factor, GHRF, or somatorelin) and growth hormone release inhibiting hormone (GHRIH) or

Table 8.5. Some factors known to affect the rate of secretion of GH. Most of these factors influence GH release indirectly by affecting the rate and level of secretion of GHRH and/or GHRIH

Factors promoting increased GH secretion	Factors promoting decreased GH secretion
Starvation	Obesity
Sleep	Elevated blood glucose
Stress	β-Adrenergic antagonists
Exercise	β-Adrenergic agonists
Low blood glucose	
Several amino acids	
Glucagon	
Vasopressin	
α-Adrenergic agonists	
β-Adrenergic antagonists	

somatostatin (Table 8.5). Furthermore, while GH directly mediates some of its biological actions, its major influence on body growth is mediated indirectly via IGF-1, as discussed below. GHRH, GHRIH, GH and IGF-1 thus form a hormonal axis, as depicted in Figure 8.12.

Growth hormone releasing factor (GHRF) and inhibitory factor (GHRIF)

GHRF and GHRIF are peptides secreted by hypothalamic neurons termed 'neuroendocrine transducers' (the name is apt, as these interface between the nervous and endocrine systems). The factors that regulate their secretion are poorly understood but probably involve both nerve impulses originating from within the brain and feedback mechanisms, possibly involving pituitary hormones.

37, 40 and 44 amino acid GHRF variants have been identified. All can promote GH release from the pituitary, an activity which apparently resides in the first 29 amino acid residues of these molecules. Administration of GHRH to GH-deficient individuals generally promotes modest increases in GH secretion, thereby increasing growth rate.

Hypothalamic GHRIF is a cyclic 14 amino-acid peptide, although a 28 amino acid form is also found in some other tissues. GHRIF inhibits the release not only of GH but also of tyrotrophin and corticotrophin from the pituitary, and insulin and glucagon from the pancreas. It can also regulate the level of duodenal secretions.

The GH receptor

GH induces its characteristic biological effects by binding to a specific cell surface receptor. The human receptor is a single chain 620 amino acid transmembrane polypeptide. Sequence analysis indicates it is a member of the haemopoietic receptor superfamily (which includes receptors for several ILs, GM-CSF and EPO). X-ray crystallographic analysis shows that GH binds simultaneously to the extracellular domains of two receptor molecules, effectively promoting receptor dimerization (Figure 8.13). The exact molecular detail of the subsequent signal transduction events remain to be determined. However, ligand binding does induce receptor autophosphorylation, as well as phosphorylation of additional cellular substances and protein kinase C activation.

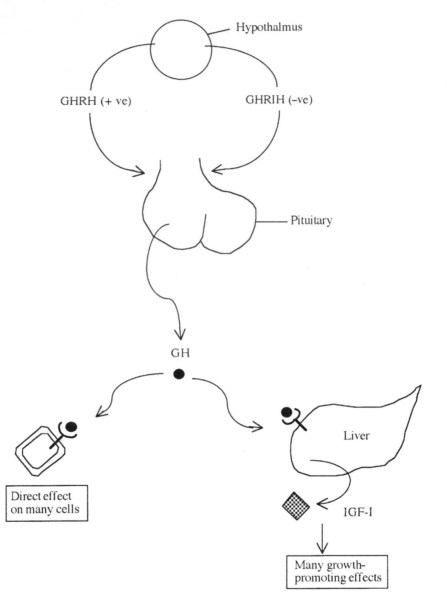

Figure 8.12. Overview of the mechanisms by which GH induces its biological effects and how its secretion from the pituitary is regulated

Soluble GH-binding proteins (GHBPs) are also found in the circulation. In humans, these GHBPs are generated by enzymatic cleavage of the integral membrane receptor, releasing the GH-binding extracellular domain. In rodents, however, the GHBPs are derived from alternatively cleaved GH-receptor mRNA. The exact physiological role of these binding proteins remains to be elucidated. In serum, GH binds to two such GHBPs, an action which prolongs the hormone's plasma half-life.

GH bound to GH binding proteins

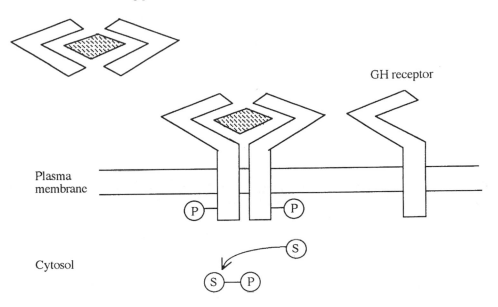

Figure 8.13. Growth hormone found in the circulation is generally bound to GH-binding proteins. Binding to the cell surface receptor promotes receptor dimerization and phosphorylation and hence activation. This leads to the phosphorylation of various cystolic protein substrates, which mediate intracellular effects of the hormone

Biological effects of GH

GH primarily displays an anabolic activity. It partially stimulates the growth of bone, muscle and cartilage cells directly. Binding of GH to its hepatic receptor results in the synthesis and release of insulin-like growth factor (IGF-1), which mediates most of GH's growth-promoting activity on, for example, bone and skeletal muscle (Chapter 7). The major effects mediated by hGH are summarized in Table 8.6.

A deficiency in the secretion of hGH during the years of active body growth results in pituitary dwarfism (a condition responsive to exogenous hGH administration). On the other hand, overproduction of hGH during active body growth results in gigantism. hGH overproduction after primary body growth has occurred results in acromegaly, a condition characterized by enlarged hands and feet, as well as coarse features.

Table 8.6. Some of the major biological effects promoted by growth hormone. While many of these are direct, other effects are mediated via IGF-1 (Chapter 7)

Increased body growth (particularly bone and skeletal muscle)
Stimulation of protein synthesis in many tissues
Mobilization of depot lipids from adipose tissue (lipolytic effect)
Elevation of blood glucose levels (anti-insulin effect)
Increase of muscle and cardiac glycogen stores
Increased kidney size and enhanced renal function
Reticulocytosis (increased reticulocyte production in the bone marrow)

Table 8.7. Some actual or likely therapeutic uses for hGH. Refer to text for details

---

Treatment of short stature caused by GH deficiency
Treatment of defective growth caused by various diseases/medical conditions
Induction of lactation
Counteracting ageing
Treatment of obesity
Body building
Induction of ovulation

Therapeutic uses of GH

GH has a potentially wide range of therapeutic uses (Table 8.7). To date, however, its major application has been for the treatment of short stature. hGH extracted from human pituitary glands was first used to treat pituitary dwarfism (i.e. caused by sub-optimal pituitary GH secretion), in 1958. It has subsequently proved effective in the treatment of short stature caused by a variety of other conditions, including:

- Turner's syndrome;
- idiopathic short stature;
- chronic renal failure.

The use of hGH extracted from the pituitaries of deceased human donors came to an abrupt end in 1985, when a link between treatment and Creutzfeldt–Jakob disease (CJD, a rare, but fatal, neurological disorder) was discovered. In this year, a young man who had received hGH therapy some 15 years previously died from CJD, which, investigators concluded, he had contracted from infected pituitary extract (CJD appears to be caused by a prion). At least an additional 12 CJD cases suspected of being caused in the same way have subsequently been documented. Fortunately, several recombinant hGH (rhGH) preparations were coming on-stream at that time (Table 8.8), and now all hGH preparations used clinically are derived from recombinant sources. Currently, in excess of 20 000 people are in receipt of rhGH therapy.

rhGH was first produced in *E. coli* in the early 1980s. The initial recombinant preparations differed from the native human hormone only in that they contained an extra methionine residue (due to the AUG start codon inserted at the beginning of the gene). Subsequently, a different cloning strategy allowed production in *E. coli* of products devoid of this terminal methionine.

In vitro analysis, including tryptic peptide mapping, amino acid analysis and comparative immunoassays, show the native and recombinant form of the molecule to be identical. Clinical trials in humans have also confirmed that the recombinant version promotes identical biological responses to the native hormone. rhGH was first purified (on a lab scale) by Genentech scientists using the strategy outlined in Figure 8.14. A somewhat similar strategy is likely used in its process-scale purification.

Recombinant hGH (rhGH) and pituitary dwarfism

Various studies have confirmed that rhGH promotes increased linear growth rates in children suffering from pituitary dwarfism (classical growth hormone deficiency). Dosages are generally

Table 8.8. Recombinant human growth hormone (rhGH) preparations approved for general medical use

Product (trade name)	Company	Indication
Humatrope	Eli Lilly	hGH deficiency in children
Nutropin	Genentech	hGH deficiency in children
Nutropin AQ	Schwartz Pharma AG	Growth failure, Turner's syndrome
BioTropin	Biotechnology General	hGH deficiency in children
Genotropin	Pharmacia and Upjohn	hGH deficiency in children
Saizen	Serono Laboratories	hGH deficiency in children
Serostim	Serono Laboratories	Treatment of AIDS-associated catabolism/wasting
Norditropin	Novo Nordisk	Treatment of growth failure in children due to inadequate growth hormone secretion

administered on a weekly basis by i.m. or s.c. injection. Duration of treatment typically varies from 6 months to 2 years, although on occasion administration has continued for up to 4 years.

Increased growth rates are generally observed, although the extent varies with, for example, the recipient's age at onset of treatment, sex and baseline growth rates. rhGH-induced growth

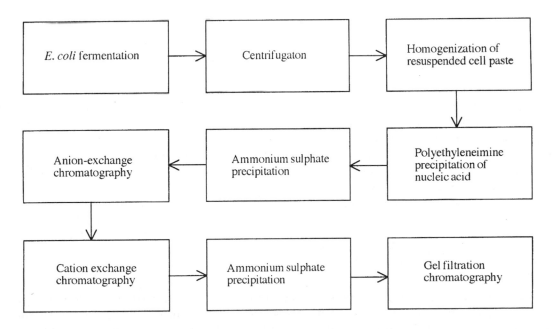

Figure 8.14. Production of recombinant human growth hormone (rhGH) in *E. coli* (as an intracellular protein). Subsequent to fermentation, the cells are collected by centrifugation or filtration. After homogenization, nucleic acids and some membrane constituents are precipitated by the addition of polyethyleneimine. Ammonium sulphate precipitation of the supernatant concentrates the crude rhGH preparation. Chromatographic purification follows, as illustrated

acceleration is most notable during the initial stages of treatment, with relative effect decreasing with time. In most cases, growth hormone treatment ensures a final body height several centimetres greater than would otherwise be attained in recipients.

Idiopathic short stature and Turner's syndrome

In many cases, a root cause for slower than normal growth rate in children of short stature is not immediately obvious (idiopathic short stature). Endogenous GH levels are often considered to be within a normal range (although there may be changes in its pusatile secretion patterns). A host of clinical trials have shown, however, that rhGH administration can increase the growth rate of many children with idiopathic short stature. Several trials lasting up to 3 years showed that, although the response was most dramatic during the first year, even during year three, mean growth rates were over 3 cm/year greater than expected.

Turner's syndrome is a genetic defect that affects females (sufferers carry only one of the usual two X chromosomes). These individuals are infertile, often show developmental defects, mental retardation and short stature. Virtually all clinical trials involving Turner's syndrome patients confirm that administration of GH significantly increases growth velocity, indicating its therapeutic usefulness in these cases.

Metabolic effects of hGH

The twin metabolic effects of hGH in promoting increased body protein synthesis and increased lipolytic activity suggest a role for the hormone in influencing body lean mass/fat composition. Attention in this regard has focused upon treating obesity and burns, as well as counteracting some of the effects of old age. Clinical studies in dieting obese people suggest that GH treatment (typically for 3–12 weeks) did not promote reduction of body fat levels any faster than in persons' dieting, but without treatment. A lipolytic effect was, however, observed in obese people who were not subject to caloric restriction during rhGH treatment. A future role for this hormone in treating obesity is, therefore, far from certain.

Clinical trials have also revealed a role for rhGH in the treatment of severe burns, particularly in children. The fear and emotional trauma (as well as physical damage) associated with receiving a severe burn triggers a neurological and immune-mediated response termed the stress response. This is characterized by:

- protein catabolism;
- loss of lean body mass;
- increased metabolic rate;
- futile substrate cycling and lipolysis;
- elevated body temperature.

rhGH treatment is aimed largely at slowing/preventing elevated protein catabolism. Initial trials in burn patients showed that GH administration reduced protein loss by 50% compared to (untreated) controls. Subsequent GH studies in children with massive burning (over 50% of total body surface), revealed accelerated wound healing, particularly at the skin graft donor site. This, in turn, facilitated further skin grafting within shorter time periods, thus reducing the time to close the burn wound. On the basis of such results, GH may well play a future expanding role in burn care management.

The production of GH is age-modulated. The highest production levels are recorded immediately after birth, with a second increase noted at puberty. GH secretion decreases steadily after age 40, and this decline is likely linked to age-associated decreased muscle, bone and skin mass, all of which contribute to age-associated frailty.

In recent years, several pilot clinical trials, assessing the effects of GH administration to ageing adults, have been carried out. Typically, trial duration is 4–6 months. A 7% increase in lean body mass and skin thickness, along with a 14% drop in body fat, was observed in one trial, although results recorded in other trials were less striking. More detailed clinical trials and cost:benefit analysis must be carried out in order to fully assess the potential of GH to counteract some of the effects of ageing in the elderly population.

GH, lactation and ovulation

Recombinant bovine GH (bovine somatotrophin, BST), has been used for a number of years to boost milk yield in dairy cattle (by up to 20%). More recent studies in monkeys showed that GH administration increased milk yields as well as promoting a slight increase in milk fat levels. This suggested that GH might be beneficial in the treatment of human lactation failure. Treatment of a small group of breast-feeding women with rhGH for 1 week has been shown to increase milk production (although it had no effect on the milk's nutritional composition, including fat levels).

GH also appears to impact upon ovarian physiology, mainly although not exclusively through IGF-1. IGF-1 stimulates replication of cultured mammalian granulosa cells (see gonadotrophin section) and potentiates FSH action on the ovary. While GH appears not to play an essential role in ovulation or fertility, it seems to act synergistically with gonadotrophins and other reproductive hormones. One clinical trial, involving women subfertile due to the lack of endogenous FSH secretion, showed that co-treatment with rhGH decreased the quantity of exogenous FSH required to induce ovulation.

The range of potential applications of rhGH in clinical medicine continues to grow. The use of GH is also facilitated by the absence of any serious side effects in most instances. Although its efficacy in promoting growth in persons of short stature is beyond doubt, more convincing clinical evidence is required before its approved clinical applications are expanded further.

THE GONADOTROPHINS

The gonadotrophins are a family of hormones for which the gonads represent their primary target (Table 8.9). They directly and indirectly regulate reproductive function and, in some cases, the development of secondary sexual characteristics. Insufficient endogenous production of any member of this family will adversely affect reproductive function, which can be treated by administration of an exogenous preparation of the hormone in question. Most gonadotrophins are synthesized by the pituitary, although some are made by reproductive and associated tissues.

Follicle stimulating hormone (FSH), luteinizing hormone (LH) and human chorionic gonadotrophin (hCG)

Follicle stimulating hormone (FSH) and luteinizing hormone (LH) play critical roles in the development and maintenance of male and particularly female reproductive function (Box 8.4). Human chorionic gonadotrophin (hCG), produced by pregnant women, plays a central role in maintaining support systems for the developing embryo during early pregnancy. All three are

Table 8.9. The gonadotrophins, their site of synthesis and their major biological effects

Gonadotrophin	Site of synthesis	Major effects
Follicle stimulating hormone (FSH)	Pituitary	Stimulates folicular growth (female), enhanced spermatogenesis (male)
Luteinizing hormone (LH)	Pituitary	Induction of ovulation (female), synthesis of testosterone (male)
Chorionic gonadotrophin (CG)		Maintenance of the corpus luteum in pregnant females
Pregnant mare serum gonadotrophin (PMSG, horses only)	Endometrial cups	Maintenance of pregnancy in equids
Inhibin	Gonads	Inhibition of FSH synthesis, probably tumour repressor
Activin	Gonads	Stimulation of FSH synthesis

heterodimeric hormones, containing an identical α-polypeptide subunit and a unique β-polypeptide subunit which confers biological specificity to each gonadotrophin. In each case, both subunits of the mature proteins are glycosylated. Human FSH displays four N-linked (asparagine or Asn-linked) glycosylation sites, located at positions Asn 52 and 78 of the α-subunit and Asn 7 and 24 of the β-subunit. Some 30% of the hormone's overall molecular mass is accounted for by its carbohydrate component. Structurally, the attached oligosaccharides are heterogenous in nature, varying in particular in terms of the content of sialic acid residues and sulphate groups present. This represents the structural basis of the charge heterogeneity characteristic of this (and other) gonadotrophins.

The oligosaccharide components play a direct and central role in the biosynthesis, secretion, serum half-life and potency of the gonadotrophins. The sugar components attached to the α-subunits play an important role in dimer assembly and stability, as well as hormone secretion and possibly signal transduction. The sugars associated with the β-subunit, while contributing to dimer assembly and secretion, appear to play a more prominent role in clearance of the hormone from circulation.

The functional effects of glycosylation take on added significance in the context of producing gonadotrophins by recombinant means. As subsequently discussed, several are now produced for clinical application in recombinant (animal cell line) systems. While the glycosylation patterns observed on the recombinant molecules can vary somewhat in composition from those associated with the native hormone, these slight differences bear no negative influence upon their clinical applicability.

The synthesis and release of both FSH and LH from the pituitary is stimulated by a hypothalmic peptide, gonadotrophin-releasing hormone (GnRH, also known as gonadorelin, luteinizing hormone-releasing hormone (LHRH), or LH/FSH-releasing factor).

FSH exhibits a molecular mass of 34 kDa. The α-subunit gene (containing four exons) is present on chromosome 6, while the β gene (three exons) is found on chromosome 11. mRNA coding for both sununits is translated separately on the rough endoplasmic recticulum, followed by removal of their signal peptides upon entry into the endoplasmic recticulum. N-linked glycosylation also takes place, as does intra-chain disulphide bond formation. The α- and β-subunits combine non-covalently and appear to be stored in secretory vesicles, separately to those containing LH. While free α-subunits are also found

Box 8.4.   An overview of the female reproductive cycle

The human female reproductive (ovarian) cycle is initiated and regulated by gonado-trophic hormones. Day 1 of the cycle is characterized by commencement of menstruation — the discharge of fragments of the endometrium (wall of the womb) from the body — signifying that fertilization has not occurred in the last cycle. At this stage, plasma levels of FSH and LH are low, but these begin to increase slowly over the subsequent 10–14 days.

During the first phase of the cycle, a group of follicles (each of which houses an egg) begins to develop and grow, largely under the influence of FSH. Shortly thereafter, a single dominant follicle normally emerges, and the remainder regress. The growing follicle begins to synthesize oestrogens, which in turn trigger a surge in LH secretion at the cycle mid-point (day 14). A combination of elevated FSH and LH levels (along with additional factors such as prostaglandin F_{2a}) promotes follicular rupture. This releases the egg cell (ovulation) and converts the follicle into the progesterone-secreting follicular reminant, the corpus luteum (CL). Release of the egg marks the end of the first half (follicular phase) of the cycle and the commencement of the second (luteal) phase.

In the absence of fertilization subsequent to ovulation, the maximum life span of the corpus luteum is 14 days, during which time it steadily regresses. This, in turn, promotes slowly decreasing levels of CL hormones — oestrogen and progesterone. Progesterone normally serves to prepare (thicken) the lining of the womb for implantation of an embryo, should fertilization occur. Withdrawal of hormonal support as the CL regresses results in the shedding of the endometrial tissue, which marks commencement of the next cycle. However, if ovulation is followed by fertilization, the CL does not regress but is maintained by hCG, synthesized in the placenta of pregnant females.

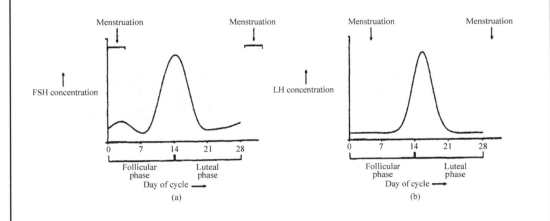

Changes in plasma FSH (a) and LH (b) levels during the reproductive cycle of a healthy human female. Reproduced by permission of John Wiley & Sons Ltd from Walsh & Headon (1994)

within the pituitary, few β-subunits are present in unassociated form. Such free β-subunits are rapidly degraded.

The major FSH target in the male are the Sertoli cells, found in the walls of the seminiferous tubules of the testis. They function to anchor and nourish the spermatids, which are subsequently transformed into spermatozoa during the process of spermatogenesis. Sertoli cells also produce inhibin (discussed later), which functions as a negative feedback regulator of FSH. The major physiological effect of FSH in the male is thus sperm cell production.

Box 8.5.   Female follicular structure

The major female reproductive organs are a pair of ovaries, situated in the lower abdomen. At birth, each ovary houses approximately 1 million immature follicles. Each follicle is composed of an egg cell (ovum) surrounded by two layers of cells; an inner layer of granulosa cells and an outer layer of theca cells. During the follicular phase of the female reproductive cycle (Box 8.3), a group of follicles (ca. 20), approximately 5 mm in diameter, are recruited by FSH (i.e. they begin to grow). FSH targets the granulosa cells, prompting them to synthesize oestrogen. The dominant follicle continues to grow to a diameter of 20–25 mm. At this stage, it contains a fluid-filled cavity with the ovum attached to one side. Ovulation is characterized by bursting of the follicle and release of the ovum.

Typically, 400 follicles will mature and fully ovulate during an average woman's reproductive lifetime. The remaining 99.98% of her follicles begin to develop but regress due to inadequate FSH stimulation. The molecular detail of how FSH (and LH) promote follicular growth is described in the main body of the text.

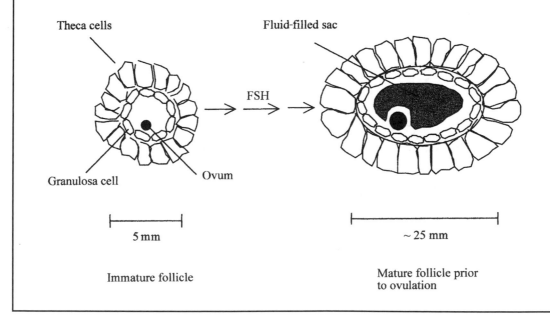

Immature follicle   Mature follicle prior
                                     to ovulation

In the female, FSH mainly targets the granulosa cells of the ovarian follicle (Box 8.5). FSH exhibits a mitogenic effect upon these cells, stimulating their division and, hence, follicular growth and development. This activity is enhanced by the paracrine action of locally-produced growth factors. FSH also triggers enzymatic production of glycosaminoglycans (GAGs), as well as expression of aromatase and other enzymes involved in oestrogen synthesis. GAGs form an essential component of the follicular fluid, while granulosa cell-derived oestrogens play multiple roles in sustaining and regulating female reproductive function.

Prior to puberty, serum FSH levels are insufficient to promote follicular recruitment and development. Subsequent to puberty, as a group of follicles begin to develop at the beginning of a cycle, the one that is most responsive to FSH (i.e. displays the lowest FSH threshold) becomes the first to secrete oestrogen. As one effect of oestrogen is to suppress FSH release from the pituitary, blood FSH levels then plateau or decline slightly. This slightly lower FSH concentration is insufficient to sustain growth of follicles of higher FSH thresholds, so they die, leaving only the single oestrogen-producing dominant follicle (Boxes 8.4 and 8.5) to mature and ovulate.

FSH exerts its molecular effects via a specific receptor on the surface of sensitive cells. This receptor contains a characteristic seven transmembrane-spanning regions and is functionally coupled (via membrane-associated G proteins) to adenylate cyclase. This generates the second messenger cAMP. FSH itself can promote increased expression of its own receptor in the short term, although longer-term exposure to elevated FSH levels downregulates receptor numbers. Cloning and analysis of gonadotrophin receptors from several species indicate a high level of homology between the FSH, LH and CG receptors.

LH exhibits a molecular mass of 28.5 kDa. The gene coding for the β-subunit of this glycoprotein hormone is present on human chromosome 19. This subunit exhibits significant amino acid homology to placental CG. Both promote identical biological effects and act via the same 93 kDa cell surface receptor. The LH receptor is present on testicular Leydig cells in males and on female ovarian theca, granulosa, luteal and interstitial cells.

LH promotes synthesis of testosterone, the major male androgen (Box 8.6) by the testicular Leydig cells. FSH sensitizes these cells to the activities of LH, probably by increasing LH receptor numbers on the cell surface. Leydig cells have a limited storage capacity for testosterone ($\sim 25\,\mu g$), but secrete 5–10 mg of the hormone into the bloodstream daily in young healthy males.

The primary cellular targets of LH in the females are the follicular theca cells, which constitutively express the LH receptor. Under the influence of LH, these cells produce androgens. The androgens (principally testosterone) are then taken up by granulosa cells and converted into oestrogens (Box 8.6) by the already-mentioned aromatase complex. Thus, the follicle represents the major female gonadal endocrine unit, in which granulosa and theca cells cooperate in the synthesis of oestrogens. Physiologically, LH in the female plays a major role in maturation of the dominant follicle and appears central to triggering ovulation.

Pregnant mare serum gonadotrophin (PMSG)

Pregnant mare serum gonadotrophin (PMSG) is a unique member of the gonadotrophin family of hormones. It is synthesized only by pregnant mares (i.e. is not found in other species). Furthermore, it displays both FSH-like and LH-like biological activities.

This glycoprotein hormone is a heterodimer, composed of an α- and β-subunit, and approximately 45% of its molecular mass is carbohydrate. Reported molecular masses range from 52 kDa to 68 kDa, a reflection of the potential variability of the hormone's carbohydrate content.

PMSG is secreted by cup-shaped outgrowths found in the horn of the uterus of pregnant horses. These equine-specific endometrial cups are of fetal rather than maternal origin. They first become visible around day 40 of gestation, and reach maximum size at about day 70, after which they steadily regress. They synthesize high levels of PMSG and secrete it into the blood, where it is detectable between days 40 and 130 of gestation.

Box 8.6.   The androgens and oestrogens

The androgens and oestrogens represent the major male and female sex hormones, respectively. The testicular Leydig cells represent the primary source of androgens in the male, of which testosterone is the major one. Testosterone, in turn, serves as a precursor for two additional steroids: dihydrotestosterone and the oestrogen. These mediate many of its biological effects.

Females, too, produce androgens, principally in the follicular theca cells. Androgens are also produced in the adrenals in both male and females.

The biological activities of androgens (only some of which are specific to males) may be summarized as:

- promoting and regulating development of the male phenotype during embryonic development;
- promoting sperm cell synthesis;
- promoting development and maintenance of male secondary sexual characteristics at and after puberty;
- general growth-promoting effects;
- behavioural effects (e.g. male aggressiveness, etc.);
- regulation of serum gonadotrophin levels.

The follicular granulosa cells are the major site of synthesis of female steroid sex hormones: the oestrogens. β-Oestradiol represents the principal female follicular oestrogen. Oestriol is producted by the placenta of pregnant females. Oestriol as well as oestrone are also produced in small quantities as products of β-oestradiol metabolism.

Testosterone represents the immediate precursor of the oestrogens, the conversion being catalysed by the aromatase complex, a microsomal enzyme system. The biological actions of oestrogens may be summarized as:

- growth and maturation of the female reproductive system;
- maintenance of reproductive capacity;
- development and maintenance of female secondary sexual characteristics;
- female behavioural effects;
- complex effects upon lipid metabolism and distribution of body fat;
- regulation of bone metabolism (oestrogen deficiency promotes bone decalcification, as seen in post-menopausal osteoporosis).

Box 8.6. *Continued*

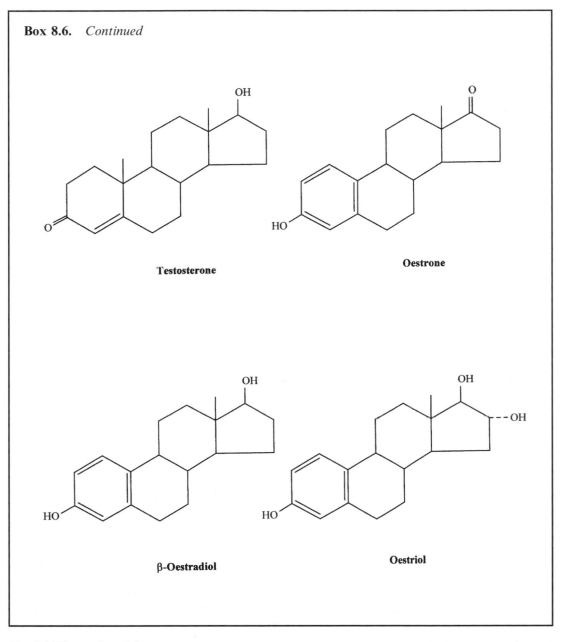

Testosterone

Oestrone

β-Oestradiol

Oestriol

The inhibins and activins

The inhibins and activins are a family of dimeric growth factors synthesized in the gonads. They exert direct effects both on gonadal and extra-gonadal tissue, and are members of the transforming growth factor-β (TGF-β) family of proteins. The inhibins are heterodimers consisting of α- and β-polypeptide subunits. Activins are $\beta\beta$ dimers. The mature form of the α-subunit is termed α_c, and it consists of 134 amino acid residues. Two closely related (but structurally distinct) β-subunit forms have been characterized: β_A and β_B. These exhibit in excess of 70% amino acid homology, and differ in size by only a single amino acid. The naming and polypeptide composition of the inhibin/activin family may be summarized as follows:

- Inhibin A $= \alpha_c \beta_A$
- Inhibin B $= \alpha_c \beta_B$
- Activin A $= \beta_A \beta_A$
- Activin AB $= \beta_A \beta_B$
- Activin B $= \beta_B \beta_B$

Inhibins and activins were initially identified as gonadal-derived proteins capable of inhibiting (inhibin) or stimulating (activin) pituitary FSH production (Figure 8.15). The major gonadal sites of inhibin synthesis are the Sertoli cells (male) and granulosa cells (female). In addition to targeting the pituitary, the inhibins/activins probably play a direct (mutually antagonistic) role as paracrine/autocrine regulators of gonadal function.

They also likely induce responses in tissues other than the pituitary and gonads, e.g. in adults inhibin is also synthesized by the adrenal glands, spleen and nervous system. Recent studies involving inhibin-deficient transgenic mice reveal a novel role for inhibin as a gonadal-specific tumour suppressor. These mice, in which the α-inhibin gene was missing, all developed normally, but all ultimately developed gonadal stromal tumours.

LHRH and regulation of gonadotrophin production

Gonadotrophin-releasing hormone (GnRH, LHRH), as previously mentioned, is a hypothalmic decapeptide amide which stimulates synthesis and release of pituitary FSH and LH. A variety of neurological influences alter hypothalmic secretion of LHRH, which tends to be pulsatile and higher during sleep. Synthesis of this regulatory peptide predictably increases at puberty. Its effects on the pituitary are mediated via a specific cell membrane receptor, which displays a typical seven transmembrane domain structure, with extracellular (ligand binding) domains and an intracellular domain that generates second messengers.

Several second messengers have been implicated in mediating GnRH's biological effects, including: calcium mobilization, diacylglycerate production (responsible for gonadotrophin release) and protein kinase C activation (which promotes transcription of the LH β-subunit). A number of factors appear to regulate levels of pituitary GnRH receptors, modulating its activity in this way. GnRH can up- or downregulate its own receptor numbers. Oestradiol increases receptor numbers, while inhibin can downregulate them.

Although GnRH promotes increased FSH and LH synthesis, it can do so differentially, at least under certain circumstances. After an injection of GnRH, the ratio of maximal to basal LH is higher than the ratio of maximal to basal FSH. This can only be partially explained on the basis that LH is cleared more slowly from circulation than FSH. Furthermore, during the normal female reproductive cycle, alterations in serum levels of LH and FSH do not always occur exactly in parallel. The exact molecular basis underlining the differential regulation of synthesis and secretion of LH and FSH is not understood at the moment. The root lies in a lack of understanding of the different intracellular pathways that trigger LH versus FSH β-subunit synthesis.

In addition to GnRH, several other effector molecules modulate secretion of gonadotrophins. These include not only inhibins and activins, but also gonadal steroids. All of these combine via complex feedback loops to modulate gonadotrophin production and, hence, reproductive function (Figure 8.15).

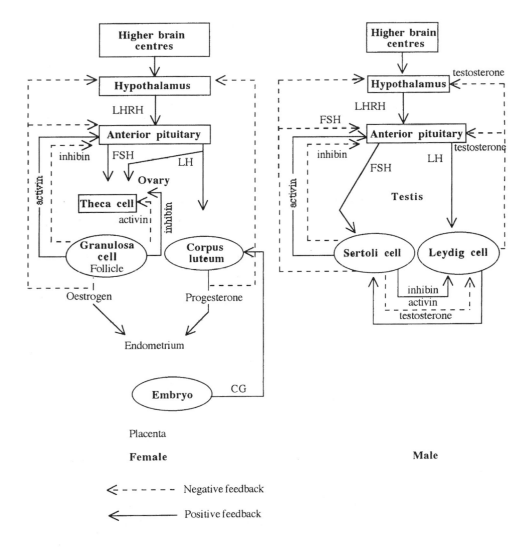

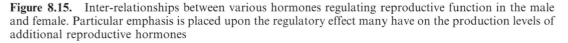

Figure 8.15. Inter-relationships between various hormones regulating reproductive function in the male and female. Particular emphasis is placed upon the regulatory effect many have on the production levels of additional reproductive hormones

Medical and veterinary applications of gonadotrophins

Because of their central role in maintaining reproductive function, the therapeutic potential of gonadotrophins in treating subfertility and some forms of infertility was obvious (Table 8.10). Gonadotrophins are also used to induce a superovulatory response in various animal species, as outlined later. The market for these hormones, while modest by pharmaceutical standards, is,

Table 8.10. Overview of gonadotrophin and related preparations used (or of potential use) in human and veterinary medicine. See text for details of each

Hormonal preparation	Source	Description/activity
Menotrophin	Urine of post-menopausal women	Contains FSH with some LH activity. Used to induce human follicular growth
P-FSH	Porcine pituitary extract	Enriched FSH extract. Contains lower levels of LH and other pituitary proteins. Used to induce superovulatory response in animals
r-FSH	Mainly recombinant mammalian production systems, notably CHO cell lines	Purified FSH (human or animal) used to treat human sub-fertility or induction of superovulation in animals
P-LH	Porcine pituitary extract	Used to induce ovulation in super-ovulated animals
r-LH	Mammalian cell production systems, e.g. CHO cell lines	Used to induce ovulation in super-ovulated animals
hCG	Urine of pregnant females	Enriched hCG preparations, used instead of LH in human medicine
PMSG	Serum of pregnant mares	Exhibits both FSH- and LH-like biological activities — used to superovulate animals
Inhibins	Produced by gonads. rDNA technology only source of large quantities	Inhibits FSH secretion. Tumour suppressor
Activins	Produced by gonads. rDNA technology only source of large quantities	Stimulates FSH secretion
GnRH	Produced by hypothalmus. Therapeutic product, manufactured by direct chemical synthesis	Stimulates synthesis and secretion of FSH and LH

none the less substantial. By the late 1990s the annual human market stood at about $250 million, of which the USA accounted for ~$110 million, Europe ~$90 million and Japan $50 million.

Sources and medical uses of FSH, LH and hCG

While the human pituitary is the obvious source of human gonadotrophins, it also constitutes an impractical source of medically useful quantities of these hormones. However, the urine of post-menopausal women does contain both FSH and LH activity. Up until relatively recently this has served as the major source, particularly of FSH, used medically.

Menotrophin (human menopausal gonadotrophin, HMG) is the name given to FSH-enriched extracts from human urine. Such preparations contain variable levels of LH activity, as well as various other proteins normally present in urine. As much as 2.5 l of urine may be required to produce one dose (75 IU, ~7.5 mg) of human FSH (hFSH).

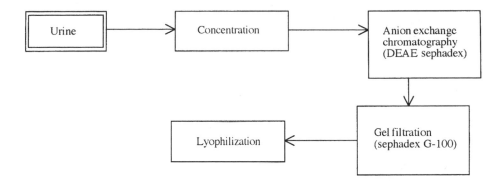

Figure 8.16. Overview of the procedure by which hCG may be purified from the urine of pregnant females at laboratory scale. Production-scale systems would be at least partially based upon such a purification strategy. Although initial concentration steps could involve precipitation, the use of ultrafiltration would now be more common

As previously mentioned, hCG exhibits similar biological activities to hLH and is excreted in the urine of pregnant women. Traditionally, hCG from this source has found medical application in humans (as an alternative to hLH; Figure 8.16).

In females, menotrophins and hCG are used for the treatment of anovulatory infertility. This condition is due to insufficient endogenous gonadotrophin production. Menotrophin is administered to stimulate follicular maturation, with subsequent administration of hCG to promote ovulation and corpus luteum formation. Mating at this point should lead to fertilization.

Dosage regimes attempt to mimic as closely as possible normal serum gonadotrophin profiles as they occur during the reproductive cycle of fertile females. This is achieved by monitoring the resultant oestrogen production, or by using ultrasonic equipment to monitor follicular response. Depending upon the basal hormonal status of the female, calculation of the optimal dosage levels can be tricky (treatments are tailored to meet the physiological requirements of individual patients). Over-dosage can, and does, result in multiple follicular development, with consequent risk of multiple pregnancy.

Treatment typically entails daily i.m. administration of gonadotrophin, often for 12 days or more, followed by a single dose of hCG. Alternatively, three equal larger doses of menotrophin may be administered on alternate days, followed by hCG administration 1–2 days after the final menotrophin dose.

Gonadotrophins are also used in assisted reproduction procedures. Here the aim is to administer therapeutic doses of FSH that exceed individual follicular FSH threshold requirements, thus stimulating multiple follicular growth. This, in turn, facilitates harvest of multiple eggs, which are then available for *in vitro* fertilization (IVF). This technique is often employed when a woman has a blocked fallopian tube, or some other impediment to normal fertilization of the egg by a sperm cell. After treatment, the resultant eggs are collected, incubated *in vitro* with her partner's sperm, incubated in culture media until the embryonic blastocyst is formed, and then implanted into the mother's uterus.

FSH and hCG also find application in the treatment of male subfertility or related conditions. Both are administered to males exhibiting hypogonadotrophic hypogonadism to stimulate

Table 8.11. Some notable non-gonadal tissues that express functional LH/hCG receptors

Pregnancy/fertility-related tissue	Other tissue
Uterus	Skin
Cervix	Blood vessels
Placenta	Adrenal cortex
Oviduct	Brain tissue
Fetal membranes	Prostate gland
Seminal vesicles	Bladder
Sperm cells	Monocytes
Breast	Macrophages

sperm synthesis and normal sexual function. hCG has found limited application in the treatment of pre-pubertal cryptorchidism (a condition characterized by failure of the testes to descend fully into the scrotum from the abdomen). The ability of this hormone to stimulate testosterone production also caught the attention of some athletes and, as a result, the International Olympic Committee has banned its use.

The LH/hCG cell surface receptor is found in a number of non-gonadal tissues, indicating that these hormones may exert physiologically relevant non-gonadal functions (Table 8.11). In addition, while liver, kidney and muscle cells are devoid of such a receptor, it is expressed by a number of these tissues before birth, hinting at a potential developmental role. Receptor levels in non-gonadal tissues are generally much lower than in gonadal tissue.

Research indicates that hCG probably has a number of pregnancy/non-pregnancy-related non-gonadal functions that may give rise to future additional clinical applications. It appears to promote effects such as increased uterine blood flow and immunosuppression at the maternal–fetal interface. As such, hCG may prove potentially useful in preventing some types of pregnancy loss. Research has also indicated that infusion of hCG into the uterus can counteract prostaglandin-induced uterine contractions. As such, it may prove useful in preventing the onset of premature labour. hCG also exhibits anti-breast cancer activity. Studies in rodents, for example, illustrate that it prevents mammary tumour formation/growth when administered prior or subsequent to various chemical carcinogens.

Recombinant gonadotrophins

Gonadotrophins are now also produced by recombinant DNA technology. The genes or cDNAs coding for gonadotrophins from several species have been identified and expressed in various recombinant host systems, particularly mammalian cell lines. rhFSH produced in CHO cells has proved clinically effective. While exhibiting an amino acid sequence identical to the human molecule, its carbohydrate composition differs slightly. When administered to humans, the preparation is well tolerated and yields no unexpected side effects. It does not elicit an immunological response, and its plasma half-life is similar to the native hormone. rhFSH has proved efficacious in stimulating follicular growth in females suffering from hypogonadotrophic hypogonadism and is effective in the treatment of males suffering from similar conditions. rhFSH was amongst the first biopharmaceutical substances to be approved for general medical

Table 8.12. Recombinant gonadotrophins now approved for general medical use in the EU and/or the USA. rh = recombinant human

Product trade name	Company	Indication
Gonal F (rhFSH)	Serono	Anovulation and superovulation
Puregon (rhFSH)	N.V. Organon	Anovulation and superovulation
Follistim (rhFSH)	Organon	Some forms of infertility
Luveris (rhLH)	Ares-Serono	Some forms of infertility
Ovitrelle (rhCG)	Serono	Used in selected assisted reproductive techniques

use in Europe by the EMEA via the centralized application procedure (Chapter 2). Recombinant gonadotrophins approved for general medical use are listed in Table 8.12.

Two of the more recent such approvals are that of Ovitrelle and Luveris. Ovitrelle is the trade name given by Serono to its recombinant hCG-based product. The producer is an engineered CHO cell line that has been co-transfected with the genes coding for both the hCG α- and β-subunits. Downstream processing entails a combination of several chromatographic and ultrafiltration steps and the final product is presented in freeze-dried form. Each vial of product contains 285 μg of active substance (hCG) and the product has been assigned a 2 year shelf-life. It is reconstituted with water for injections (WFI) immediately before use.

Luveris is a recombinant (human) luteinizing hormone (rLH) used in conjunction with FSH to stimulate follicular development in women displaying severe LH and FSH deficiency. As in the case of Ovitrelle, the producing source is an engineered CHO cell line, co-transfected in this case with the genes coding for the LH α- and β-subunits. After an initial ultrafiltration (concentration) step, the hormone is purified using a combination of several chromatographic steps. After a final ultrafiltration step (viral removal safety step), the product is filled into glass vials and freeze-dried. In addition to the active substance, the product contains a phosphate buffer, sucrose and polysorbate 20 as excipients.

Recombinant DNA technology also facilitates genetic modification of native gonadotrophins in the hope of generating variants displaying some enhanced functional characteristic (e.g. extended shelf-life, longer plasma half-life, greater potency, etc.), e.g. a carboxyl terminal peptide of the hCG β-subunit has been fused to the carboxyl terminus of the FSH β-subunit. The resulting hybrid structure displays identical biological activity to that of FSH, but with an extended plasma half-life.

The recombinant production of FSH and LH also obviously facilitates the generation of a pure preparation of any one gonadotrophin, without contamination by a second gonadotrophin. Such preparations continue to facilitate a greater understanding of the precise role each gonadotrophin plays in reproductive function.

Recombinant inhibins and activins have also been produced. This allows detailed study of the role the various members of this family play in the reproductive axis and facilitates assessment of their therapeutic potential.

Immunization of various animal species with recombinant inhibin promotes increased ovulation rates, presumably due to ensuing immunoneutralization of endogenous inhibin. While such a strategy might be useful, e.g. in producing super-fertile animals, the recent discovery of inhibins' role as a tumour suppressor may militate against such an approach.

Direct administration of recombinant inhibin inhibits ovulation in females (via inhibition of FSH secretion). It also inhibits spermatogenesis when administered to males. This last effect initially prompted interest in the use of inhibin as a potential male contraceptive, although no significant data on the safety or efficacy of such a treatment has yet been published.

Veterinary uses of gonadotrophins

Gonadotrophins may be utilized to treat subfertility in animals and are routinely used to induce a superovulatory response in valuable animals, most notably valuable horses and cattle.

The theory and practice of superovulation is quite similar to the use of gonadotrophins to assist *in vitro* fertilization procedures in humans. Exogenous FSH is administered to the animal such that multiple follicles develop simultaneously. After administration of LH to help promote ovulation, the animal is mated, thus fertilizing the released egg cells. Depending upon the specific animal and the superovulatory regime employed, anything between 0 and 50 viable embryos may be produced, although more typically the number is between 4 and 10. The embryos are then recovered from the animal (either surgically or, more usually, non-surgically) and are often maintained in cell culture for a short period of time. A single embryo is then usually re-implanted into the donor female, while remaining embryos are implanted into other recipient animals, who act as surrogate mothers, carrying the offspring to term.

This technology is most often applied to valuable animals (e.g. prize-winning horses, or high milk-yield dairy cattle) in order to boost their effective reproductive capacity several-fold. Each of the offspring will inherit its genetic complement from the biological mother (and father), irrespective of which recipient animal carries it to term.

Gonadotrophins are usually utilized to induce a superovulatory response, and include porcine FSH (p-FSH), porcine LH (p-LH) and PMSG. P-FSH is extracted from the pituitary glands of slaughterhouse pigs. The crude pituitary extract is usually subject to a precipitation step, using either ethanol or salts. The FSH-containing precipitate is normally subjected to at least one subsequent chromatographic step. The final product often contains some LH as well as low levels of additional pituitary-derived proteins.

p-LH is obtained, again, by its partial purification from the pituitary glands of slaughterhouse pigs. In both cases, a porcine source is utilized, as the target recipients are almost always cattle or horses. The use of a product derived from a species other than the intended recipient species is encouraged, as it helps minimize the danger of accidental transmission of disease via infected source material (many pathogens are species-specific).

Most superovulatory regimes utilizing p-FSH entails its administration to the recipient animal twice daily for 4–5 days. Regular injections are required, due to the relatively short half-life of FSH in serum; s.c. administration helps prolong the duration of effectiveness of each injection. The 4 or 5 days of treatment with FSH is followed by a single dose of LH, promoting final follicular maturation and ovulation.

The causes of variability of superovulatory responses are complex, and not fully understood. The general health of the animal, as well as its characteristic reproductive physiology, is important. The exact composition of the gonadotrophin preparations administered and the exact administration protocol also influences the outcome. The variability of FSH:LH ratios in many p-FSH preparations can affect the results obtained, with the most consistent super-ovulatory responses being observed when FSH preparations exhibiting low LH activity are used. The availability of recombinant FSH and LH will overcome these difficulties at least.

An alternative superovulatory regime entails administration of PMSG which, as described earlier, exhibits both FSH and LH activity. The major rationale for utilizing PMSG is its relatively long circulatory half-life. In cattle, clearance of PMSG may take up to 5 days. The

Table 8.13. GnRH and some of its analogues, along with their amino acid sequence

Analogue	Amino acid sequence
Buserelin acetate	C$_2$H$_5$-NH-Pro-Arg-Leu-Ser-Tyr-Ser-Trp-His-5oxo pro | butyl
Goserelin acetate	NH$_2$CO(NH)$_2$-Pro-Arg-Leu-Ser-Tyr-Ser-Trp-His-5oxo pro | butyl
Leuprorelin acetate	C$_2$H$_5$-NH-Pro-Arg-Leu-D-Leu-Tyr-Ser-Trp-His-5oxo pro
Nafarelin acetate	NH$_2$-Gly-Pro-Arg-Leu-D-Ala-Tyr-Ser-Try-His-5oxo pro | naphthyl
GnRH	NH$_2$-Gly-Pro-Arg-Leu-Gly-Tyr-Ser-Trp-His-5oxo pro

slow clearance rate appears to be due to the molecule's high content of N-acetyl-neuramic acid. This extended serum half-life means that a single dose of PMSG is sufficient to induce a superovulatory response. Paradoxically, however, its extended half-life limits its use in practice. Post-ovulatory stimulation of follicular growth can occur, resulting in the recovery of a reduced number of viable embryos. Attempts to negate this biological effect have centred around administration of anti-PMSG antibodies several days after PMSG administration. However, this gonadotrophin is still not widely used.

Gonadotrophin releasing hormone (GnRH)

GnRH is also used (in both human and veterinary medicine) to improve conception rates by enhancing basal hypothalamic–pituitary function. The preparations utilized clinically are manufactured by direct chemical synthesis and are usually administered by s.c. injection or, sometimes, by i.v. injection. Occasionally it has also been administered intranasally. Frequent injection is often required, particularly if administration is via the i.v. route, as the peptide's plasma half-life is of the order of a few minutes (it is hydrolysed in the plasma and excreted in the urine).

Direct chemical synthesis facilitates the manufacture of GnRH analogues of altered amino acid sequence. Several such analogues display useful clinical properties (such as extended half-life). Analogues used medically (Table 8.13) have activities similar to those of GnRH, and are used not only in the treatment of reproductive complications but also for the treatment of malignant neoplasms of the prostate and breast. Gonadal steroids can promote growth of many such tumours and a single s.c. injection of some analogues can suppress testosterone and oestradiol synthesis for up to 4 weeks. Interestingly, GnRH analogues have been reported to relieve pre-menstrual tension.

Additional recombinant hormones now approved

Two additional recombinant hormones have recently gained marketing approval: thyroid-stimulating hormone and calcitonin.

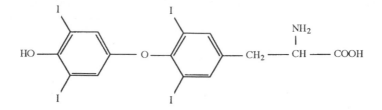

Thyroxine (T$_4$)

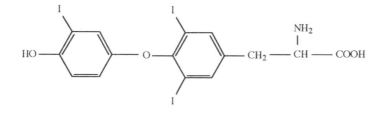

Triiodothyronine (T$_3$)

Figure 8.17. Structure of the iodine-containing amino acid-based thyroid hormones—thyroxine and triiodothyronine

Structurally, thyroid-stimulating hormone (TSH or thyrotrophin) is classified as a member of the gonadotrophin family, although functionally it targets the thyroid gland as opposed to the gonads. As with other gonadotrophins, it is a heterodimeric glycoprotein displaying a common α-subunit and a unique β-subunit. The β-subunit shows less homology to that of other members of the group. It consists of 118 amino acids, is particularly rich in cysteine residues and contains one N-linked glycosylation site (Asn 23).

TSH is synthesized by a distinct pituitary cell type; the thyrotroph. Its synthesis and release is promoted by thyrotrophin releasing hormone (TRH, a hypothalamic tripeptide hormone). TSH exerts its characteristic effects by binding specific receptors found primarily, but not exclusively, on the surface of thyroid gland cells. Binding to the receptor activates adenylate cyclase, leading to increased intracellular cAMP levels. Ultimately, this triggers TSH's characteristic effects on thyroid function, including promoting iodine uptake from the blood, synthesis of the iodine-containing thyroid hormones, thyroxine (T$_4$) and triiodothyronine (T$_3$) (Figure 8.17) and release of these hormones into the blood, from where they regulate many aspects of general tissue metabolic activity. Elevated plasma levels of T$_4$ and T$_3$ also promote decreased TSH synthesis and release by a negative feedback mechanism.

TSH is approved for medical use as a diagnostic aid in the detection of thyroid cancer/thyroid remnants in post-thyroidectomy patients. Thyroid cancer is relatively rare, exhibiting the highest incidence in adults, particularly females. First-line treatment is surgical removal of all or most of the thyroid gland (thyroidectomy). This is followed by thyroid hormone suppression therapy, which entails administration of T$_3$ or T$_4$ at levels sufficient to maintain low seum TSH levels through the negative feedback mechanism mentioned earlier. TSH suppression is required in order to prevent the TSH-mediated stimulation of remnant thyroid cancer cells. The recurrence of active thyroid cancer can be detected by administration of TSH along with radioactive iodine. TSH promotes uptake of radioactivity, which can then be detected by appropriate radio-imaging techniques.

The commercial recombinant TSH product (trade name, Thyrogen; international non-proprietary name; thyrotrophin-α) is produced in a CHO cell line co-transfected with plasmids harbouring the DNA sequences coding for the α- and β-TSH subunits. The cells are grown in batch harvest animal cell culture bioreactors. Following recovery and concentration (ultrafiltration), the TSH is chromatographically purified and formulated to a concentration of 0.9 mg/ml in phosphate buffer containing mannitol and sodium chloride as excipients. After sterile filtration and aseptic filling into glass vials, the product is freeze-dried. Finished product has been assigned a shelf-life of 3 years when stored at 2–8°C.

Calcitonin is a polypeptide hormone which (along with parathyroid hormone and the vitamin D derivative, 1,25-dihydroxycholecalciferol) plays a central role in regulating serum ionized calcium (Ca^{2+}) and inorganic phosphate (P_i) levels. The adult human body contains up to 2 kg of calcium, of which 98% is present in the skeleton (i.e. bone). Up to 85% of the 1 kg of phosphorus present in the body is also found in the skeleton (the so-called mineral fraction of bone is largely composed of $Ca_3 (PO_4)_2$ which acts as a body reservoir for both calcium and phosphorus). Calcium concentrations in human serum approximate to 0.1 mg/ml and are regulated very tightly (serum phosphate levels are more variable).

Calcitonin lowers serum Ca^{2+} and P_i levels, primarily by inhibiting the process of bone resorption, but also by decreasing resorption of P_i and Ca^{2+} in the kidney. Calcitonin receptors are predictably found primarily on bone cells (osteoclasts) and renal cells, and generation of cAMP via adenylate cyclase activation plays a prominent role in hormone signal transduction.

Calcitonin is used clinically to treat hypercalcaemia associated with some forms of malignancy and Paget's disease. The latter condition is a chronic disorder of the skeleton in which bone grows abnormally in some regions. It is characterized by substantially increased bone turnover rates which reflects over-stimulation of both osteoclasts (promote bone resorption, i.e. degradation of old bone) and osteoblasts (promotes synthesis of new bone).

In most mammals, calcitonin is synthesized by specialized parafollicular cells in the thyroid. In sub-mammalian species, it is synthesized by specialized anatomical structures known as ultimobranchial bodies.

Calcitonin produced by virtually all species is a single-chain, 32 amino acid residue polypeptide, displaying a molecular mass in the region of 3500 Da. Salmon calcitonin differs in sequence from the human hormone by nine amino acid residues. It is noteworthy, however, as it is approximately 100-fold more potent than the native hormone in humans. The higher potency appears due to both a greater affinity for the receptor and greater resistance to degradation *in vivo*. As such, salmon, as opposed to human calcitonin, is used clinically. Traditional clinical preparations were manufactured by direct chemical synthesis, although a recombinant form of the molecule has now gained marketing approval. The recombinant calcitonin is produced in an engineered *E. coli* strain. Structurally, salmon calcitonin displays C-terminal amidation. A C-terminal amide group ($-CONH_2$) replacing the usual carboxyl group is a characteristic feature of many polypeptide hormones. If present, it is usually required for full biological activity/stability. As *E. coli* cannot carry out post-translational modifications, the amidation of the recombinant calcitonin is carried out *in vitro* using an α-amidating enzyme which is itself produced by recombinant means in an engineered CHO cell line. The purified, amidated finished product is formulated in an acetate buffer and filled into glass ampoules. The (liquid) product exhibits a shelf-life of 2 years when stored at 2–8°C.

CONCLUSIONS

Several hormone preparations have a long history of use as therapeutic agents. In virtually all instances they are administered simply to compensate for lower than normal endogenous production of the hormone in question. Since it first became medically available, insulin has saved or prolonged the lives of millions of diabetics. Gonadotrophins have allowed tens, if not hundreds, of thousands of sub-fertile individuals to conceive. Growth hormone has improved the quality of life of thousands of people of short stature. Most such hormones were in medical use prior to the advent of genetic engineering. Recombinant hormonal preparations are now however gaining greater favour, mainly on safety grounds. Hormone therapy will remain a central therapeutic tool for clinicians for many years to come.

FURTHER READING

Books

Bercu, B. (1998). *Growth Hormone Secretagogues in Clinical Practice*. Marcel Dekker, New York.
Fauser, B. (1997). *FSH Action and Intraovarian Regulation*. Parthenon, Carnforth, UK.
Hakin, N. (2002). *Pancreas and Islet Transplantation*. Oxford University Press, Oxford.
Juul, A. (2000). *Growth Hormone in Adults*. Cambridge University Press, Cambridge.
Mac Hadley, E. (1999). *Endocrinology*. Prentice-Hall, Hemel Hempstead, UK.
Norman, A. (1997). *Hormones*. Academic Press, London.
O'Malley, B. (1997). *Hormones and Signalling*. Academic Press, London.
Walsh, G. & Headon, D. (1994). *Protein Biotechnology*. Wiley, Chichester.

Articles

Insulin and diabetes

Atkinson, M. & McClaren, N. (1990). What causes diabetes? *Sci. Am.* **July**, 42–46.
Blundell, T. *et al.* (1972). Insulin: the structure in the crystal and its reflection in chemistry and biology. *Adv. Protein Chem.* **26**, 279–402.
Bristow, A. (1993). Recombinant DNA derived insulin analogues as potentially useful therapeutic agents. *Trends Biotechnol.* **11**, 301–305.
Brunetti, P. & Bolli, G. (1997). Pharmacokinetics and pharmacodynamics of insulin relevance to the therapy of diabetes mellitus. *Diabet. Nutrit. Metab.* **10**(1), 24–34.
Cao, Y. & Lam, L. (2002). Projections for insulin treatment for diabetics. *Drugs Today* **38**(6), 419–427.
Ciszak, E., Beals, J. M., Frank, H. *et al.* (1995). Role of C-terminal B-chain residues in insulin assembly: the structure of hexameric LysB28 ProB29-human insulin. *Structure* **3**, 615.
Combettes-Souverain, M. & Issad, T. (1998). Molecular basis of insulin action. *Diabet. Metab.* **24**, 477–489.
Conrad, B. *et al.* (1994). Evidence for superantigen involvement in insulin-dependent diabetes mellitus aetiology. *Nature* **371**, 351–354.
Docherty, K. (1997). Gene therapy for diabetes mellitus. *Clin. Sci.* **92**(4), 321–330.
Drucker, D. (2002). Biological actions and therapeutic potential of the glucagon-like peptides. *Gastroenterology* **122**(2), 531–544.
Goa, L. *et al.* (1997). Lisinopril—a review of its pharmacology and use in the management of the complications of diabetes mellitus. *Drugs* **53**(6), 1081–1105.
Greenbaum, C. (2002). Insulin resistance in type 1 diabetes. *Diabet. Metab. Res. Rev.* **18**(3), 192–200.
Hinds, K. & Kim, S. (2002). Effects of PEG conjugation on insulin properties. *Adv. Drug Delivery Rev.* **54**(4), 505–530.
Ikegami, H. & Ogihara, T. (1996). Genetics of insulin-dependent diabetes mellitus. *Endocr. J.* **43**(6), 605–613.
Johnson, I. (1983). Human insulin from recombinant DNA technology. *Science* **219**, 632–637.
Kroeff, E. *et al.* (1989). Production scale purification of biosynthetic human insulin by reverse phase high performance liquid chromatography. *J. Chromatogr.* **461**, 45–61.

Lacy, P. (1995). Treating diabetes with transplanted cells. *Sci. Am.* **July**, 40–45.

Maassen, J. & Ouwens, D. (1997). Mechanism of insulin action. *Frontiers Hormone Res.* **22**, 201–221.

Patton, J. *et al.* (1999). Inhaled insulin. *Adv. Drug Delivery Rev.* **35**, 235–247.

Rhodes, C. & White, M. (2002). Molecular insights into insulin action and secretion. *Eur. J. Clin. Invest.* **32**, 3–13.

Secchi, A. *et al.* (1997). Pancreas and Islet transplantation—current progress, problems and perspectives. *Hormone Metab. Res.* **29**(1), 1–8.

Selam, J. (1997). Management of diabetes with glucose sensors and implantable insulin pumps—from the dream of the 60s to the realities of the 90s. *ASAIO J.* **43**(3), 137–142.

Smith, R. *et al.* (1997). Insulin internalization and other signalling pathways in the pleiotropic effects of insulin. *Int. Rev. Cytol. Surv. Cell Biol.* **173**, 243–280.

Stralfors, P. (1997). Insulin 2nd messengers. *Bioessays* **19**(4), 327–335.

Vajo, Z. *et al.* (2001). Recombinant DNA technology in the treatment of diabetes: insulin analogues. *Endocr. Rev.* **22**(5), 706–717.

Growth hormone

Artini, P. *et al.* (1996). Growth hormone co-treatment with gonadotrophins in ovulation induction. *J. Endocrinol. Invest.* **19**(11), 763–779.

Carter, C. *et al.* (2002). A critical analysis of the role of growth hormone and IGF-1 in aging and lifespan. *Trends Genet.* **18**(6), 295–301.

Chantalat, L., Jones, N. D., Korber, F. *et al.* (1995). The crystal structure of wild-type growth hormone at 2.5 Å resolution. *Protein Peptide Lett.* **2**, 333.

De Vos, A. *et al.* (1992). Human growth hormone and extracellular domain of its receptor; crystal structure of the complex. *Science* **255**, 306–312.

Gibson, F. & Hinds, C. (1997). Growth hormone and insulin-like growth factors in critical illness. *Intens. Care Med.* **23**(4), 369–378.

Hathaway, D. (2002). Growth hormone: challenges and opportunities for the biotechnology sector. *J. Anti-aging Med.* **5**(1), 57–62.

Neely, E. (1994). Use and abuse of human growth hormone. *Ann. Review Med.* **45**, 407–420.

Piwien-Pilipuk, G. *et al.* (2002). Growth hormone signal transduction. *J. Pediat. Endocrinol. Metab.* **15**(6), 771–786.

Sharara, F. & Giudice, K. (1997). Role of growth hormone in ovarian physiology and onset of puberty. *J. Soc. Gynaecol. Invest.* **4**(1), 2–7.

Simpson, H. *et al.* (2002). Growth hormone replacement therapy for adults: into the new millennium. *Growth Hormone IGF Res.* **12**(1), 1–33.

Gonadotrophins and TSH

Barbieri, R. (1992). Clinical applications of GnRH and its analogues. *Trends Endocrinol. Metab.* **3**(1), 30–34.

Bernard, D. *et al.* (2002). Minireview: inhibin binding protein, β-glycan and the continuing search for the inhibin receptor. *Mol. Endocrinol.* **16**(2), 207–212.

Cho, B. (2002). Clinical applications of TSH receptor antibodies in thyroid diseases. *J. Korean Med. Sci.* **17**(3), 293–301.

Conn, P. & Crowley, W. (1994). Gonadotropin-releasing hormone and its analogues. *Ann. Rev. Med.* **45**, 391–405.

Dardenne, M. & Savino, W. (1996). Interdependence of the endocrine and immune systems. *Adv. Neuroimmunol.* **6**(4), 297–307.

De Jong, F. (1988). Inhibin. *Physiol. Rev.* **68**, 555–595.

De Koning, W. *et al.* (1994). Recombinant reproduction. *Bio/Technology* **12**, 988–992.

Depaolo, L. (1997). Inhibins, activins and follistatins—the saga continues. *Proc. Soc. Exp. Biol. Med.* **214**(4), 328–339.

Fauser, B. & Vanheusden, A. (1997). Manipulation of human ovarian function—physiological concepts and clinical consequences. *Endocr. Rev.* **18**(1), 71–106.

Gore, A. & Roberts, J. (1997). Regulation of gonadotrophin-releasing hormone gene expression *in vivo* and *in vitro*. *Frontiers Neuroendocrinol.* **18**(2), 209–245.

Greenberg, N. *et al.* (1991). Expression of biologically active heterodimeric bovine follicle-stimulating hormone in milk of transgenic mice. *Proc. Natl Acad. Sci. USA* **88**, 8327–8331.

Hayden, C. et. al. (1999). Recombinant gonadotrophins. *Br. J. Obstet. Gynaecol.* **106**(3), 188–196.

Hillier, S. (1994). Current concepts of the role of follicle stimulating hormone and luteinizing hormone in folliculogenesis. *Hum. Reprod.* **9**(2), 188–191.

Jones, R. *et al.* (2002). Potential roles for endometrial inhibins, activins and follistatin during human embryo implantation and early pregnancy. *Trends Endocrinol. Metab.* **13**(4), 144–150.

Macklon, N. & Fauser, B. (2001). Follicle stimulating hormone and advanced follicle development in the human. *Arch. Med. Res.* **32**(6), 595–600.

Matzuk, M. *et al.* (1992). α-Inhibin is a tumor-suppressor gene with gonadal specificity in mice. *Nature* **360**, 313–319.

McCann, S. *et al.* (2001). Control of gonadotrophin secretion by follicule stimulating hormone-releasing factor, luteinizing hormone-releasing hormone and leptin. *Arch. Med. Res.* **32**(6), 476–485.

Rao, C. & Sanfilippo, J. (1997). New understanding in the biochemistry of implantation — potential direct roles of luteinizing hormone and human chorionic gonadotropin. *Endocrinologist* **7**(2), 107–111.

Risbridger, G. *et al.* (2001). Activins and inhibins in endocrine and other tumors. *Endocr. Rev.* **22**(6), 836–858.

Schwartz, N. (1995). The 1994 Stevenson Award lecture. Follicle-stimulating hormone and luteinizing hormone: a tale of two gonadotrophins. *Can. J. Physiol. Pharmacol.* **73**, 675–684.

Siarim, M. & Krishnamurthy, H. (2001). The role of follicle stimulating hormone in spermatogenesis: lessons from knockout animal models. *Arch. Med. Res.* **32**(6), 601–608.

Stewart, E. (2001). Gonadotrophins and the uterus: is there a gonad-independent pathway? *J. Soc. Gynaecol. Invest.* **8**(6), 319–326.

Sturgeon, C. & McAllister, E. (1998). Analysis of hCG: clinical applications and assay requirements. *Ann. Clin. Biochem.* **35**, 460–491.

Themmen, A. *et al.* (1997). Gonadotropin receptor mutations. *J. Endocrinol.* **153**(2), 179–183.

Ullao-Aguirre, A. *et al.* (1999). Role of glycosylation in function of follicle stimulating hormone. *Endocrine* **11**(3), 205–215.

Wonerow, P. *et al.* (2001). Thyrotropin receptor mutations as a tool to understand thyrotropin receptor action. *J. Mol. Med.* **79**(12), 707–721.

Calcitonin

Yallampalli, C. *et al.* (2002). Calcitonin gene regulated peptide in pregnancy and its emerging receptor heterogeneity. *Trends Endocrinol. Metab.* **13**(6), 263–269.

Chapter 9

Blood products and therapeutic enzymes

Blood and blood products constitute a major group of traditional biologics. The main components of blood are the red and white blood cells, along with platelets and the plasma in which these cellular elements are suspended. Whole blood remains in routine therapeutic use, as do red blood cell and platelet concentrates. A variety of therapeutically important blood proteins also continue to be purified from plasma. These include various clotting factors and immunoglobulins (immunoglobulins will be considered in the next chapter). Such blood products are summarized in Table 9.1.

DISEASE TRANSMISSION

Associated with the administration of blood or blood products is the risk of accidental transmission of infectious agents. Transmission of hepatitis, as well as AIDS, has generated prominent attention in this regard, but several bacterial and parasitic diseases may also be transmitted via infected blood products (Table 9.2).

Rigorous application of good manufacturing practice (GMP) with regard to the manufacture of blood products is required to minimize the risk of pathogen transmission. Most GMP or related guidelines contain sections that address issues particularly relevant to the production of blood products. The prevention of accidental pathogen transmission relies upon:

- careful screening of all blood donors/donations;
- introduction of methods of pathogen removal or inactivation during the processing steps;
- careful screening of all finished products.

The identity of each blood donor should be recorded, and all donor blood bags must be labelled carefully. Traceability of individual blood donors/donations is essential, in case the donor or product is subsequently found to harbour blood-borne pathogens. The risk of contamination of blood during collection/processing is minimized by using closed systems and strict aseptic technique.

Biopharmaceuticals: Biochemistry and Biotechnology, Second Edition by Gary Walsh
John Wiley & Sons Ltd: ISBN 0 470 84326 8 (ppc), ISBN 0 470 84327 6 (pbk)

Table 9.1. Major blood products that find therapeutic application. While all of these products are still sourced from human blood donations, a number of the protein-based products are now also produced by genetic engineering. Antibody preparations are considered in the next chapter

Whole blood
Red blood cells
Platelet concentrate
Plasma and plasma protein fraction
Albumin
Clotting factors (particularly factors VII_a, VIII, IX and XIII)
Haemoglobin

Table 9.2. Some of the infectious agents that have been transmitted via administration of infected blood or blood products. Transmission of viruses, particularly hepatitis A and B virus and HIV, are most common

Infectious agent	Ensuing medical condition
Hepatitis B virus	Infectious hepatitis
Hepatitis C virus	Infectious hepatitis
Human immunodeficiency virus (HIV)	AIDS
Human T-cell lymphocytotrophic viruses I and II	Possible causative agents of lymphomas
Cytomegalovirus (CMV)	Causes cold-like symptoms in healthy individuals, but more severe effects in immunocompromised persons. Causes congenital handicap in infants whose mothers contracted CMV during pregnancy
Treponema pallidum	Bacterial causative agent of syphilis
Protozoa of the genus *Plasmodium*	Malaria
Trypanosoma cruzi	Protozoal causative agent of Chagas' disease

Before any blood donation is released for issue/processing, it must be tested for the presence of various pathogens particularly likely to be present in blood. In most countries, these tests include immunoassays capable of detecting:

- hepatitis B surface antigen (HBsAg);
- antibodies to HIV;
- antibodies to hepatitis C virus (HCV);
- syphilis antibodies.

However, no immunoassay is 100% accurate and all will report a low number of false negatives (and false positives). It is believed that in the order of 1 in every 42 000 blood units reported to be HIV antibody-negative actually harbours the virus.

In general, processes capable of inactivating viral or other pathogens (e.g. heat or chemical treatment) may not be applied to whole blood or most blood-derived products. Thus, for whole blood at least, effective screening of donations is exclusively relied upon to prevent pathogen transmission. Many of the processing techniques used to derive blood products from whole blood (e.g. precipitation, but especially chromatographic purification) can be effective in separating viral or other pathogens from the final product (see also Chapter 3). Fractionated products, therefore, are less likely to harbour undetected pathogens.

WHOLE BLOOD

Whole blood is blood that has been aseptically withdrawn from humans. A suitable anticoagulant is added (often heparin or a citrate–dextrose-based substance), although no preservative is present. The blood is usually stored at temperatures in the range 1–8°C, and has a short shelf-life (48 h after collection if heparin is used as the anticoagulant; or up to 35 days if citrate–phosphate–dextrose with adenine is employed). In addition to being screened for likely pathogens, the ABO blood group and the Rh group is also determined. In the USA alone, in the region of 35 transfusion-related deaths occur annually due to errors in blood group typing or the presence of bacteria in the product.

The blood is generally warmed to 37°C immediately prior to transfusion. Whole blood is often used to replace blood lost due to injury or surgery. The number of Units (1 Unit $\simeq 510$ ml) administered depends upon the health and age of the recipient, along with the therapeutic indication. Administration of whole blood may also be undertaken to supply a recipient with a particular blood constituent (e.g. a clotting factor, immunoglobulin, platelets or red blood cells). However, this practice is minimized in favour of direct administration of the specific blood constituent needed.

PLATELETS AND RED BLOOD CELLS

Platelets play a central role in the blood clotting process. They are often administered prophylactically or therapeutically in order to prevent/minimize blood loss due to haemorrhage in persons suffering from thrombocytopenia (low blood platelet levels; see Chapter 6).

Platelet concentrate consists of platelets obtained from whole blood. The platelets obtained from a unit of blood are usually resuspended in 20–50 ml of the original plasma and contain not less than 5.5×10^{10} platelets/unit (for blood preparations, a 'unit' refers to the amount of that product purified from a single Unit of whole blood). Like whole blood, platelets have a short shelf-life and must be used within 72 h of blood collection.

Concentrated red blood cells are prepared from the whole blood of a single donor, from which the anticoagulant and some of the plasma have been removed. According to the *British Pharmacopoeia* (Chapter 3), the preparation must have a packed cell volume greater than 70% (plasma-reduced blood is similar, except that its packed cell volume must be between 60–65%).

Red blood cell preparations are usually stored at 2–8°C (although the United States Pharmacopeia includes frozen storage below −65°C). If stored unfrozen, its useful shelf-life must not exceed the shelf-life of the whole blood from which it was derived. If stored frozen, the shelf-life is extended to 3 years (although the product must subsequently be used within 24 h after thawing).

Red blood cell fractions are administered to patients suffering from severe anaemia, including patients with sickle cell anaemia and new born babies suffering from haemolytic disease.

BLOOD SUBSTITUTES

Blood substitutes, as defined here, refers to any substance which can:

- replace or maintain blood volume; or
- ensure oxygen delivery to body tissues.

Table 9.3. Some colloidal plasma volume expanders currently in therapeutic use. In addition to these, albumin and plasma protein fraction may also be used

Dextran 1
Dextran 40
Dextran 60
Dextran 70
Dextran 110
Gelatin
Starch derivatives

The majority of blood substitutes currently in use function only as plasma expanders. These maintain blood pressure by providing vascular fluid volume after haemorrhage, burns, sepsis or shock. While standard electrolyte solutions, such as physiological saline, may be administered, their effect is transitory as they subsequently diffuse back out of the vascular system.

Alternatively, colloidal plasma expanders (Table 9.3) are used. When administered at appropriate concentrations, they exert an osmotic pressure similar to that of plasma protein, hence vascular volume and blood pressure are maintained. The major disadvantages of colloidal therapy include its relatively high cost, and the risk of prompting a hypersensitivity reaction. Determined efforts to develop blood substitutes were initiated in 1985 by the US military, concerned about the issue of blood supply to future battlefields.

Dextrans

Dextrans (polysaccharides; Figure 9.1) of various molecular masses, usually 1, 40, 60, 70 or 110 kDa, are often used as plasma expanders. These polysaccharides are produced naturally by

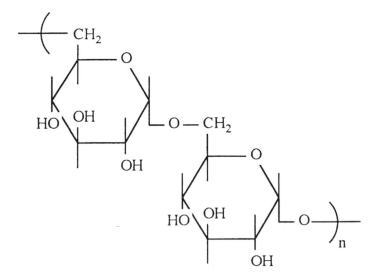

Figure 9.1. Dextran is a homopolysaccharide composed exclusively of D-glucose monomers linked predominantly by 1–6 glycosidic bonds (as in the fragment of dextran backbone shown above). Different dextran preparations vary only in molecular mass and their degree of branching

various microorganisms, although commercial production is undertaken almost exclusively using Lactobacteriaceae (usually *Leuconostoc mesenteroides*, grown on sucrose as carbon source). Native dextrans usually display a high molecular mass, and those used clinically are usually prepared by depolymerization of the native molecule, or sometimes by direct synthesis.

Higher molecular mass dextrans (particularly dextran 70, 75 and 110) are used to promote short-term expansion of plasma volume thus preventing/treating shock due to blood loss. A 6% w/v solution of these dextrans exerts an osmotic pressure similar to that of plasma proteins. Generally, an initial dose of 500 ml–1 litre is administered by i.v. infusion. Dextrans also inhibit the aggregation of red blood cells. Thus, they are often used to prevent/treat post-operative thrombo-embolic disorders (see later in this chapter) and to improve blood flow.

The lower molecular mass dextran 40 (40 kDa) exhibits similar therapeutic effects to the higher molecular mass dextrans, although it must be used at slightly higher concentrations (10%, w/v) in order to achieve the same osmotic pressure.

Dextrans may also promote a number of negative effects. Dextrans 40 and 70 have been associated with acute renal failure, although the mechanism by which this is induced is unclear. Infusion of dextrans can also prompt severe anaphylactic shock. Many patients exhibit anti-dextran antibodies, including some who have not been previously administered dextran (antibodies may be generated in response to dextran-like dietary or bacterial polysaccharides to which the patient has previously been exposed).

To prevent severe anaphylactic responses, administration of a small volume (10–20 ml) of low molecular mass dextran (Dextran 1) is often undertaken immediately prior to infusion of the higher molecular mass product. Circulatory anti-dextran antibodies will be 'mopped up' by binding to the lower molecular mass dextran. This prevents formation of high molecular mass dextran-immune complexes/precipitates which often underscore the severe anaphylactic response.

ALBUMIN

Human serum albumin (HSA) is the single most abundant protein in blood (Table 9.4). Its normal concentration is approximately 42 g/litre, representing 60% of total plasma protein. The vascular system of an average adult thus contains in the region of 150 g of albumin. HSA is responsible for over 80% of the colloidal osmotic pressure of human blood. More than any other plasma constituent, HSA is thus responsible for retaining sufficient fluid within blood vessels. It has been aptly described as the protein that makes blood thicker than water.

Albumin molecules also temporarily leave the circulation, entering the lymphatic system, which harbours a large pool of this protein (up to 230 g in an adult). Lower quantities of albumin are also present in the skin.

In addition to its osmoregulatory function, HSA serves a transport function. Various metabolites travel throughout the vascular system predominantly bound to HSA. These include fatty acids, amino acids, steroid hormones and heavy metals (e.g. copper and zinc), as well as many drugs.

HSA is a 585 amino acid, 65.5 kDa polypeptide. It is one of the few plasma proteins that is unglycosylated. A prominent feature is the presence of 17 disulphide bonds, which helps stabilize the molecule's 3-D structure. HSA is synthesized and secreted from the liver, and its gene is present on human chromosome 4.

HSA is used therapeutically as an aqueous solution, and is available in concentrated form (15–25% protein) or as an isotonic solution (4–5% protein). In both cases, in excess of 95% of

Table 9.4. The major plasma proteins of known function found in human blood

Protein	Normal plasma concentration (g/l)	Molecular mass (kDa)	Function
Albumin	35–45	66.5	Osmoregulation transport
Retinol-binding protein	0.03–0.06	21	Retinol transport
Thyroxine binding globulin	0.01–0.02	58	Binds/transports thyroxine
Transcortin	0.03–0.04	52	Cortisol and corticosterone transport
Caeruloplasmin	0.1–0.6	151	Copper transport
Haptoglobin			
Type 1-1	1.0–2.2	100	Binds and helps conserve
Type 2-1	1.6–3.0	200	haemoglobin
Type 2-2	1.2–2.6	400	
Transferrin	2.0–3.2	76.5	Iron transport
Haemopexin	0.5–1.0	57	Binds haem destined for disposal
β_2-microglobulin	0.002	11.8	Associated with HLA histocompatibility antigen
γ-Globulins	7.0–15.0	150	Antibodies
Transthyretin	0.1–0.4	55	Binds thyroxine

the protein present is albumin. It can be prepared by fractionation from normal plasma or serum, or purified from placentas. The source material must first be screened for the presence of indicator pathogens. After purification, a suitable stabilizer (often sodium caprylate) is added, but no preservative. The solution is then sterilized by filtration and aseptically filled into final sterile containers. The relative heat stability of HSA allows a measure of subsequent heat treatment, which further reduces the risk of accidental transmission of viable pathogens (particularly viruses). This treatment normally entails heating the product to 60°C for 10 h. It is then normally incubated at 30–32°C for a further 14 days and subsequently examined for any signs of microbial growth.

HSA is used as a plasma expander in the treatment of haemorrhage, shock, burns and oedema, as well as being administered to some patients after surgery. For adults, an initial infusion containing at least 25 g of albumin is used. The annual world demand for HSA exceeds 300 tonnes, representing a market value of the order of $1 billion.

Despite screening of raw material and heat treatment of final product, HSA derived from native blood will sometimes (although rarely) harbour pathogens. rDNA technology provides a way of overcoming such concerns and the HSA gene and cDNA have been expressed in a wide variety of microbial systems, including *E. coli*, *Bacillus subtilis*, *Saccharomyces cerevisiae*, *Pichia pastoris* and *Aspergillus niger* (its lack of glycosylation renders possible production of native HSA in prokaryotic as well as eukaryotic systems). However, HSA's relatively large size, as well as the presence of so many disulphide bonds, can complicate recombinant production of high levels of correctly folded products in some production systems. The main stumbling block in replacing native HSA with a recombinant version, however, is an economic one. Unlike most biopharmaceuticals, HSA can be produced in large quantities and inexpensively by direct extraction from its native source. Native HSA currently sells at $2–3/g. Although it can be guaranteed blood pathogen-free, recombinant HSA products will find it difficult to compete with this price.

Gelatin

Gelatin is produced by partial acid or partial alkaline hydrolysis of animal collagen. It has a wide variety of therapeutic and pharmaceutical uses. It is often used in the manufacture of hard and soft capsule shells, suppositories and tablets, and is sometimes used as a 'sponge' during surgical procedures, as it can absorb many times its own weight of blood.

A 4% solution of gelatin (often modified, i.e. succinylated gelatin) is also used as a plasma expander. For this application, 500 ml–1 l of the sterile solution is infused slowly. In rare occurrences, infusion (particularly rapid infusion) of the gelatin solution has been known to initiate hypersensitivity reactions. After its infusion, gelatin is excreted relatively quickly and mostly via the urine.

Oxygen-carrying blood substitutes

Thus far, the only molecules that have found even a limited clinical application as an oxygen-carrying blood substitute are the fluorocarbons and haemoglobin.

Fluosol is a fluorocarbon emulsion of perfluorodecalin and perfluorotripropylamine. Such fluorocarbon emulsions can absorb, transport and release both oxygen and carbon dioxide. Although fluosol failed to show efficacy in the treatment of life-threatening anaemia, it is used as an effective oxygen carrier during coronary angioplasty procedures. A 20% emulsion is normally used, and can be administered regardless of blood type. It also will be free of any blood-borne pathogens, and is stable for years when stored at room temperature.

Haemoglobin displays the property of reversible oxygenation and, hence, is being investigated as a blood substitute. Human haemoglobin is a tetramer of molecular mass 64 kDa. It consists of two α-chains (141 amino acids) and two β-chains (146 amino acids), with each subunit displaying an associated haem prosthetic group. The interaction of the oxygen-binding haem moiety and the globulin constituent is important, as free haem is toxic and the apoglobin is insoluble.

Because of its structural characteristics, haemoglobin displays a non-linear oxygen saturation curve, with maximal oxygen saturation occurring in arterial blood. At tissue sites, the oxygen partial pressure is lower and much of the haemoglobin-bound oxygen is released. This process is aided *in vivo* by the effector molecule 2,3-diphosphoglycerate (2,3-DPG), which binds to deoxyhaemoglobin (in the presence of 2,3-DPG and at normal tissue oxygen partial pressures, over 20% of the bound oxygen is released from haemoglobin; in the absence of 2,3-DPG, this value falls to 2–4%). Native haemoglobin, when extracted from erythrocytes, is less attractive as a tissue oxygen delivery system, as free haemoglobin no longer binds 2,3-DPG. Furthermore, outside the erythrocyte (in which haemoglobin is present at very high concentrations), haemoglobin tends to disassociate into dimers. Attempts have been made to stabilize free haemoglobin and to modify it in order to reduce its oxygen affinity.

Pyridoxal 5′-phosphate (a derivative of pyridoxal; vitamin B$_6$) is similar in size and charge to 2,3-DPG. Covalent attachment of pyridoxal 5′-phosphate reduces the oxygen affinity of the haemoglobin molecule. Covalent attachment of benzene isothiocyanates to the amino termini of the four haemoglobin polypeptide chains, also yields derivatives which display lower oxygen affinity. These may prove worthy of clinical investigation.

In addition to altered oxygen-binding characteristics, free haemoglobin in plasma disassociates rapidly into $\alpha\beta$ dimers, which are in turn rapidly oxidized and cleared by the kidneys. Indeed, high plasma concentrations can result in kidney toxicity. Development of a clinically useful modified haemoglobin would have to circumvent this, probably by polymerization or micro-encapsulation of the molecules prior to their administration.

Haemoglobin conjugated to additional high molecular mass substances, such as dextrin and polyethylene glycol, are also generating clinical interest. When compared to native haemoglobin, such high molecular mass derivatives often display prolonged vascular retention (i.e. prolonged useful half-life), reduced antigenicity (if animal haemoglobin is used) and potent plasma volume expansion properties.

Polymerized haemoglobins (usually formed by crosslinking with gluteraldehyde) have also been generated. The aim again is to prolong product half-life by preventing disassociation into dimers or monomers. Additionally, such products often display increased thermal stability, facilitating a subsequent viral-inactivation heat step.

In addition to chemical crosslinking, recombinant DNA technology has been used to generate stable intact haemoglobin variants. 'Dialpha' haemoglobin, for example, is an engineered molecule in which two α-chains are fused together, head to tail. Co-expression in *E. coli* along with the *β*-gene results in the formation of a working, stable haemoglobin analogue. Haemoglobin molecules can be obtained from whole blood/red cell concentrates. Human haemoglobin α and β genes have been expressed in a wide variety of prokaryotic and eukaryotic systems, including transgenic plants and animals.

Although research continues in an effort to develop an effective haemoglobin-based red blood cell substitute, no suitable candidate has yet been developed that has gained widespread clinical acceptance.

HAEMOSTASIS

Blood plays various vital roles within the body and it is not surprising that a number of processes have evolved capable of effectively maintaining haemostasis — the rapid arrest of blood loss upon vascular damage, in order to maintain a relatively constant blood volume. In humans, three main mechanisms underline the haemostatic process:

- The congregation and clumping of blood platelets at the site of vascular injury, thus effectively plugging the site of blood leakage.
- Localized constriction of the blood vessel, which minimizes further blood flow through the area.
- Induction of the blood coagulation cascade. This culminates in the conversion of a soluble serum protein, fibrinogen, into insoluble fibrin. Fibrin monomers then aggregate at the site of damage, thus forming a clot (thrombus), which seals it off. These mechanisms are effective in dealing with small vessel injuries, e.g. in capillaries and arterioles, although they are ineffective when the damage relates to large veins/arteries.

The coagulation pathway

The process of blood coagulation is dependent on a large number of blood clotting factors, which act in a sequential manner. At least 12 distinct factors participate in the coagulation cascade, along with several macromolecular co-factors. The clotting factors are all designated by Roman numerals (Table 9.5) and, with the exception of factor IV, all are proteins. Most factors are proteolytic zymogens, which become sequentially activated. An activated factor is indicated by inclusion of a subscript 'a' (e.g. factor XII$_a$ = activated factor XII).

Table 9.5. The coagulation factors which promote the blood clotting process. Note that the factor originally designated as VI was later shown to be factor V_a

Factor number	Common name	Pathway in which it functions	Function
I	Fibrinogen	Both	Forms structural basis of clot after its conversion to fibrin
II	Prothrombin	Both	Precursor of thrombin, which activates factors I, V, VII, VIII and XIII
III	Tissue factor (thromboplastin)	Extrinsic	Accessory tissue protein which initiates extrinsic pathway
IV	Calcium ions	Both	Required for activation of factor XIII and stabilizes some factors
V	Proaccelerin	Both	Accessory protein, enhances rate of activation of X
VII	Proconvertin	Extrinsic	Precursor of convertin (VII_a) which activates X (extrinsic system)
VIII	Anti-haemophilic factor	Intrinsic	Accessory protein, enhances activation of X (intrinsic system)
IX	Christmas factor	Intrinsic	Activated IX directly activates X (intrinsic system)
X	Stuart factor	Both	Activated form (X_a) converts prothrombin to thrombin
XI	Plasma thromboplastin antecedent	Intrinsic	Activated form (XIa) serves to activate IX
XII	Hageman factor	Intrinsic	Activated by surface contact or the kallikrenin system. XIIa helps initiate intrinsic system
XIII	Fibrin-stabilizing factor	Both	Activated form cross-links fibrin, forming a hard clot

Although the final steps of the blood clotting cascade are identical, the initial steps can occur via two distinct pathways: the extrinsic and intrinsic pathways. Both pathways are initiated when specific clotting proteins make contact with specific surface molecules exposed only upon damage to a blood vessel. Clotting occurs much more rapidly when initiated via the extrinsic pathway.

Two coagulation factors function uniquely in the extrinsic pathway: factor III (tissue factor) and factor VII. Tissue factor is an integral membrane protein present in a wide variety of tissue types (particularly lung and brain). This protein is exposed to blood constituents only upon rupture of a blood vessel, and it initiates the extrinsic coagulation cascade at the site of damage as described below.

Factor VII contains a number of γ-carboxyglutamate residues (as do factors II, IX and X), which play an essential role in facilitating their binding of Ca^{2+} ions. The initial events initiating the extrinsic pathway entail the interaction of factor VII with Ca^{2+} and tissue factor. In this associated form, factor VII becomes proteolytically active. It displays both binding affinity for, and catalytic activity against, factor X. It thus activates factor X by proteolytic processing, and factor X_a, which initiates the terminal stages of clot formation, remains attached to the tissue factor–Ca^{2+} complex at the site of damage. This ensures that clot formation only occurs at the point where it is needed (Figure 9.2).

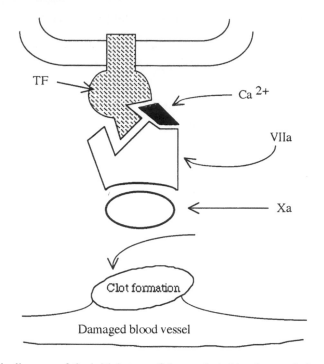

Figure 9.2. Schematic diagram of the initial steps of the extrinsic blood coagulation pathway. See text for details. TF = tissue factor

The initial steps of the intrinsic pathway are somewhat more complicated. This system requires the presence of clotting factors VIII, IX, XI and XII, all of which, except for factor VIII, are endo-acting proteases. As in the case of the extrinsic pathway, the intrinsic pathway is triggered upon exposure of the clotting factors to proteins present on the surface of body tissue exposed by vascular injury. These protein binding/activation sites probably include collagen.

Additional protein constituents of the intrinsic cascade include prekallikrein, an 88 kDa protein zymogen of the protease kallikrein, and high molecular mass kininogen (HMK), a 150 kDa plasma glycoprotein that serves as an accessory factor.

The intrinsic pathway appears to be initiated when factor XII is activated by contact with surface proteins exposed at the site of damage. High molecular mass kininogen also appears to form part of this initial activating complex (Figure 9.3).

Factor XII_a can proteolytically cleave and hence activate two substrates:

- prekallikrein, yielding kallikrein (which, in turn, can directly activate more XII to XII_a);
- factor XI, forming XI_a.

Factor XI_a, in turn, activates factor IX. Factor IX_a then promotes the activation of factor X, but only when it (i.e. IX_a) is associated with factor VIII_a. Factor VIII_a is formed by the direct action of thrombin on factor VIII. The thrombin will be present at this stage because of prior activation of the intrinsic pathway.

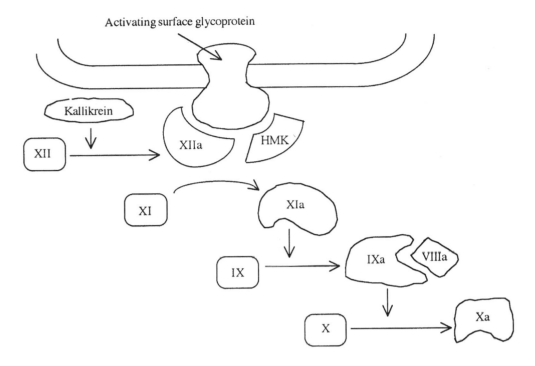

Figure 9.3. The steps unique to the intrinsic coagulation pathway. Factor XIIa can also convert prekallikrein to kallikrein by proteolysis, but this is omitted from the above diagram for the sake of clarity. Full details are given in the main text. The final steps of the coagulation cascade, which are shared by both extrinsic and intrinsic pathways, are outlined in Figure 9.4

Terminal steps of coagulation pathway

Both intrinsic and extrinsic pathways generate activated factor X. This protease, in turn, catalyses the proteolytic conversion of prothrombin (factor II) into thrombin (II_a). Thrombin, in turn, catalyses the proteolytic conversion of fibrinogen (I) into fibrin (I_a). Individual fibrin molecules aggregate forming a soft clot. Factor XIII_a catalyses the formation of covalent crosslinks between individual fibrin molecules, forming a hard clot (Figures 9.4 and 9.5).

Prothrombin (factor II) is a 582 amino acid, 72.5 kDa glycoprotein, which represents the circulating zymogen of thrombin (II_a). It contains up to six γ-carboxyglutamate residues towards its N-terminal end, via which it binds several Ca^{2+} ions. Binding of Ca^{2+} facilitates prothrombin binding to factor X_a at the site of vascular injury. The factor X_a complex then proteolytically cleaves prothrombin at two sites (arg^{274}–thr^{275} and arg^{323}–ile^{324}), yielding active thrombin and an inactive polypeptide fragment, as depicted in Figure 9.6.

Fibrinogen (factor I) is a large (340 kDa) glycoprotein consisting of two identical tri-peptide units, α,β and γ. Its overall structural composition may thus be represented as $(\alpha\,\beta\,\gamma)_2$. Interchain disulphide bonds hold together not only the $\alpha\beta$- and $\beta\gamma$-chains, but also the two tri-peptide subunits. Slight heterogeneity of plasma fibrinogen molecules have been observed. This is apparently not only caused by variation in its carbohydrate content, but also slight proteolytic degradation at its carboxyl and amino termini. The overall molecule, which exhibits a pI in the

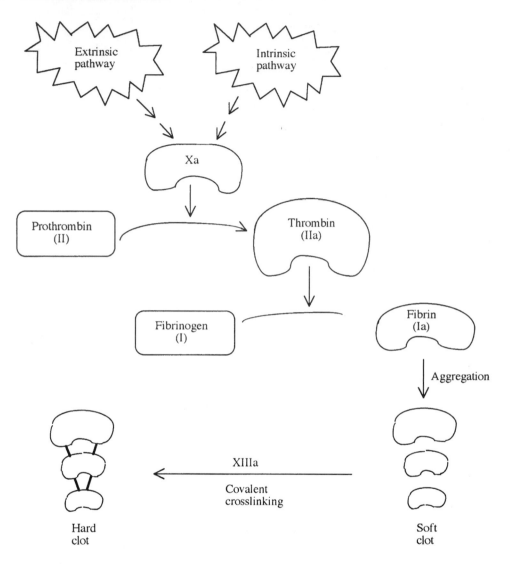

Figure 9.4. Overview of the blood coagulation cascade, with emphasis upon the molecular detail of its terminal stages. Refer to text for specific detail

region of 5.5, displays an α-helical content of approximately 33%. Its quaternary structure is characterized by three compact domain-like regions (one at either end and one in the middle), separated by two extended stretches (Figure 9.7).

The N-terminal region of the α- and β-fibrinogen chains are rich in charged amino acids, which, via charge repulsion, play an important role in preventing the aggregation of individual fibrinogen molecules. Thrombin, which catalyses the proteolytic activation of fibrinogen, hydrolyses these N-terminal peptides. This renders individual fibrin molecules more conducive

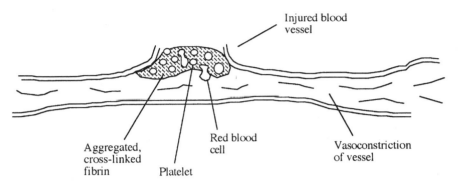

Figure 9.5. Section through a blood clot (haemostatic plug). Crosslinked fibrin molecules bind together platelets and red blood cells congregated at the site of damage, thus preventing loss of any more blood

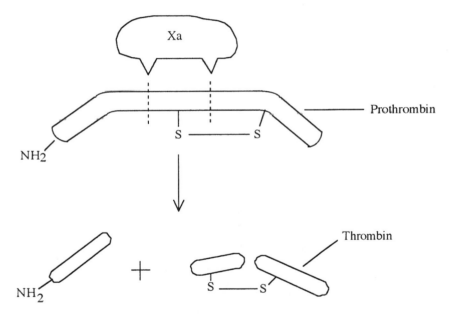

Figure 9.6. Proteolytic cleavage of prothrombin by factor Xa, yielding active thrombin. While prothrombin is a single-chain glycoprotein, thrombin consists of two polypeptides linked by what was originally the prothrombin intra-chain disulphide bond. The smaller thrombin polypeptide fragment consists of 49 amino acid residues, while the large polypeptide chain contains 259 amino acids. The N-terminal fragment released from prothrombin contains 274 amino acid residues. Activation of prothrombin by Xa does not occur in free solution but at the site of vascular damage

to aggregation, therefore promoting soft clot formation (Figure 9.7). The soft clot is stabilized by the introduction of covalent crosslinkages between individual participating fibrin molecules. This reaction is catalysed by factor XIII_a, as shown in Figure 9.8.

Factor XIII is present in both plasma and platelets. Plasma factor XIII is a 320 kDa tetramer, composed of two (70 kDa) α-chains, and two (90 kDa) β-chains. The platelet form of factor XIII

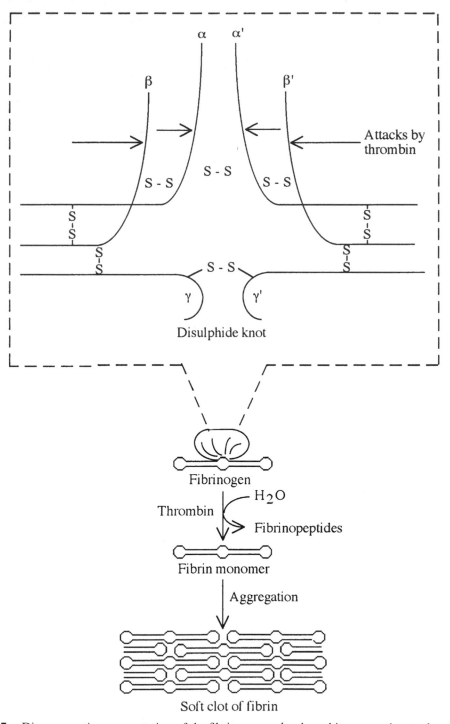

Figure 9.7. Diagrammatic representation of the fibrinogen molecule and its conversion to the soft clot of fibrin. Reproduced (in modified form) by permission from *Textbook of Biochemistry with Clinical Correlations* (3rd Ed.) Devlin (1992). This material is used by permission of John Wiley & Sons, Inc.

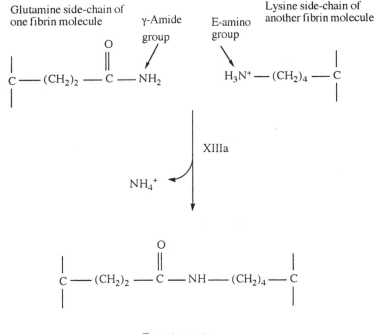

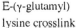

E-(γ-glutamyl)
lysine crosslink

Figure 9.8. Formation of a hard clot via the action of factor XIIIa. This activated factor displays a transglutaminase activity, which catalyses direct formation of a covalent linkage between a glutamine side-chain of one fibrin molecule and a lysine side-chain of a second fibrin molecule. The resultant highly crosslinked hard clot is both tough and insoluble

is composed solely of the two α-chains (i.e. a 140 kDa α-dimer). Both forms of factor XIII are activated upon proteolytic cleavage by thrombin (factor II_a), which hydrolyses a single arg–gly bond in the NH_2 terminal region of the α-chains. This generates a 73 amino acid peptide and a modified α-chain (α').

In the case of platelet-derived factor XIII, the resultant product $(\alpha')_2$, is the activated form. Thrombin action on plasma-derived factor XIII generates an $\alpha'_2\beta_2$ dimer, which is devoid of transglutaminase activity. However, in the presence of Ca^{2+}, the $\alpha'\beta$ chains dissociate, yielding the biologically active α'_2.

Clotting disorders

Genetic defects characterized by (a) lack of expression, or (b) an altered amino acid sequence of any clotting factor can have serious clinical consequences. In order to promote effective clotting, both intrinsic and extrinsic coagulation pathways must be functional, and the inhibition of even one of these pathways will result in severely retarded coagulation ability. The result is usually occurrence of spontaneous bruising and prolonged haemorrhage, which can be fatal. With the exception of tissue factor and Ca^{2+}, defects in all other clotting factors have been characterized.

Table 9.6. Recombinant blood coagulation factors which have been approved for the management of coagulation disorders

Product (trade name)	Company	Indication
Bioclate (rhFactor VIII)	Centeon	Haemophilia A
Benefix (rhFactor IX)	Genetics Institute	Haemophilia B
Kogenate (rhFactor VIII)	Bayer	Haemophilia A
Helixate NexGen (rhFactor VIII)	Bayer	Haemophilia A
NovoSeven (rhFactor VIIa)	Novo-Nordisk	Some forms of haemophilia
Recombinate (rhFactor VIII)	Baxter Healthcare/Genetics Institute	Haemophilia A
ReFacto (B-domain deleted rhFactor VIII)	Genetics Institute	Haemophilia A

Up to 90% of these, however, relate to a deficiency in factor VIII, while much of the remainder is due to a deficiency in factor IX.

Such clotting disorders are generally treated by ongoing administration of whole blood or, more usually, concentrates of the relevant coagulation factor purified from whole blood. This entails significant risk of accidental transmission of blood-borne disease, particularly hepatitis and AIDS. In turn, this has hastened the development of blood coagulation factors produced by genetic engineering, several of which are now approved for general medical use (Table 9.6).

Factor VIII and haemophilia

Haemophilia A (classical haemophilia, often simply termed haemophilia) is an X-linked recessive disorder which is caused by a deficiency of factor VIII. Von Willebrand's disease is a related disorder, also caused by a defect in the factor VIII complex, as discussed below.

Intact factor VIII, as usually purified from the blood, consists of two distinct gene products: factor VIII and (multiple copies of) von Willebrand's factor (vWF; Figure 9.9). This complex displays a molecular mass of 1–2 million Da, of which up to 15% is carbohydrate. The fully intact factor VIII complex is required to enhance the rate of activation of factor IX of the intrinsic system.

The factor VIII polypeptide portion of the factor VIII complex is coded for by an unusually long gene (289 kb). Transcription and processing of the mRNA generates a shorter, mature mRNA which codes for a 300 kDa protein. Upon its synthesis, this polypeptide precursor is subsequently proteolytically processed, with removal of a significant portion of its mid-region. This yields two fragments: an amino terminal 90 kDa polypeptide and an 80 kDa carboxyl terminal polypeptide. These associate non-covalently (a process requiring Ca^{2+} ions) to produce mature factor VIII (sometimes called factor VIII_c). This mature factor VIII is then released into the plasma, where it associates with multiple copies of vWF, forming the biologically active factor VIII complex. vWF stabilizes factor VIII in plasma (particularly against proteolytic degradation). It also can associate with platelets at the site of vascular damage and, hence, presumably plays a role in docking the factor VIII complex in an appropriate position where it can participate in the coagulation cascade.

Persons suffering from haemophilia A exhibit markedly reduced levels of (or the complete absence of) factor VIII complex in their blood. This is due to the lack of production of factor VIII_c. Persons suffering from (the rarer) von Willebrand's disease lack both components of

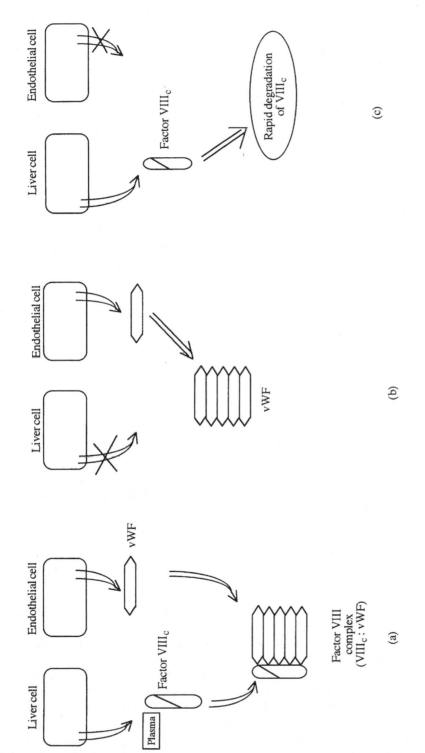

Figure 9.9. Synthesis of factor VIII complex as occurs in healthy individuals, as illustrated in (a). In the case of persons suffering from haemophilia A, synthesis of factor VIII:C is blocked (b), preventing constitution of an active factor VIII complex in plasma. Persons suffering from von Willebrand's disease fail to synthesize vWF(c). Although they can synthesize VIII:C, this is rapidly degraded upon entering the blood due to lack of its vWF stabilizing factor

mature factor VIII complex (Figure 9.9). The severity of the resultant disease is somewhat dependent upon the level of intact factor VIII complex produced. Persons completely devoid of it (or expressing levels below 1% of normal values), will experience frequent, severe and often spontaneous bouts of bleeding.

Persons expressing 5% or above of the normal complex levels, experience less severe clinical symptoms. Treatment normally entails administration of factor VIII complex purified from donated blood. More recently, recombinant forms of the product have also become available. Therapeutic regimens can require product administration on a weekly basis, for life. About 1 in 10 000 males are born with a defect in the factor VIII complex and there are approximately 25 000 haemophiliacs currently resident in the USA.

Production of factor VIII

Native factor VIII is traditionally purified from blood donations first screened for evidence of the presence of viruses such as hepatitis B and HIV. A variety of fractionation procedures (initially mainly precipitation procedures) have been used to produce a factor VIII product. The final product is filter-sterilized and filled into its finished product containers. The product is then freeze-dried and the containers are subsequently sealed under vacuum, or are flushed with an inert gas (e.g. N_2) before sealing. No preservative is added. The freeze-dried product is then stored below 8°C until shortly before its use.

Although earlier factor VIII preparations were relatively crude (i.e. contained lower levels of various other plasma proteins), many of the modern preparations are chromatographically purified to a high degree. The use of immunoaffinity chromatography has become widespread in this regard since 1988 (Figure 9.10). The extreme bioselectivity of this method can yield a single-step purification factor of several thousand-fold.

The use of monoclonal antibodies to purify factor VIII (or any other serum/therapeutic protein) exhibits a number of associated advantages, the most important of which are:

- high degree of purity obtained by a single chromatographic step;
- viral particles and other potential pathogens are rarely retained on an immuno-affinity column along with the product being purified; this provides added insurance with regard to removal of undetected pathogens from the product stream during downstream processing.

However, a number of potential disadvantages are also associated with this approach, including:

- possibility of contamination of the product stream with monoclonal antibody;
- conditions used to elute the protein off the immunoaffinity column can be harsh and, therefore, can cause limited protein denaturation.

Immobilized ligands (in this case, monoclonal antibody) may be attached to support beads by a variety of chemical means. Slow leakage of immobilized ligand characterize many affinity systems, although this has been minimized by newer immobilization coupling techniques. The potential clinical implications of leakage are unclear. Many would, however, feel that product contamination, with even very low levels of the monoclonal antibody, would be inappropriate, due to the regularity with which the product is normally administered. However, to date no significant clinical complications associated with ligand leakage have been noted in practice.

The binding between antibody and antigen is generally quite tight; thus, relatively harsh conditions are normally required to subsequently elute antigen off immuno-affinity columns. Several standard approaches may be adopted in this regard. Elution, using a buffer of low pH, is

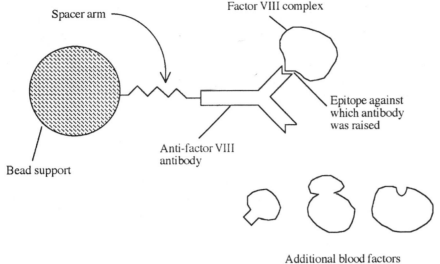

Figure 9.10. Purification of factor VIII complex using immunoaffinity chromatography. The immobilized anti-factor VIII antibody is of mouse origin. Antibodies raised against specific epitopes on both the VIII:C and vWF components have both been successfully used. Industrial-scale columns would often exhibit a bed volume of several litres. Note that the different elements in this diagram are not drawn to the correct scale relative to each other

often attempted, followed by rapid neutralization of the eluate to pH 7–8. Elution, using buffers of high pH, can also sometimes be successfully employed. In many instances, even harsher elution conditions may be required. These can include the use of chaotropic agents or detergents. Such conditions can obviously partially/completely denature the protein being eluted. Although many clotting factors are very stable when exposed to various denaturing influences, factor VIII is quite labile. Thus, the use of a monoclonal antibody with high, but not extreme, avidity for factor VIII would likely yield the most successful results.

Although fractionation can reduce very significantly the likelihood of pathogen transmission, it cannot entirely eliminate this possibility. Blood-derived factor VIII products, including those prepared by immunoaffinity chromatography, generally undergo further processing steps designed to remove/inactivate any virus present. The raw material is often heated for up to 10 h at 60°C or treated with solvent or dilute detergent prior to chromatography. Recombinant factor VIII is also often treated with dilute detergent in an effort to inactivate any viral particles potentially present.

Production of recombinant factor VIII (Table 9.6) has ended dependence on blood as the only source of this product and eliminated the possibility of transmitting blood-borne diseases specifically derived from infected blood. In the past, over 60% of haemophiliacs were likely to be accidently infected via contaminated products at some stage of their lives.

Several companies have expressed the cDNA coding for human factor VIII:C in a variety of eukaryotic production systems (human VIII:C contains 25 potential glycosylation sites).

Chinese hamster ovary (CHO) cells and baby hamster kidney (BHK) cell lines have been most commonly used, in addition to other cell lines, such as various mouse carcinoma cell lines. The recombinant factor VIII product generally contains only VIII:C (i.e. is devoid of vWF). However, both clinical and pre-clinical studies have shown that administration of this product to patients suffering from haemophilia A is equally as effective as administering blood-derived factor VIII complex. The recombinant VIII:C product appears to bind plasma vWF with equal affinity to native VIII:C, upon its injection into the patient's circulatory system. Animal and human pharmacokinetic data reveal no significant difference between the properties of recombinant and native products.

Slight variation in the glycosylation patterns of native and recombinant product were to be expected, due to the differing production systems. While this has turned out to be the case, thus far it has not proved to be of any clinical significance. Significant differences could have made the recombinant product immunogenic. Bearing in mind that most recipients would receive several thousand injections of the product over their lifetime, even a mildly immunogenic product would promote a significant immunological response.

Some patients, particularly those suffering from severe haemophilia A (i.e. those naturally producing little or no VIII:C) will mount an immune response against injected factor VIII:C, whatever its source.

The production of anti-factor VIII:C antibodies renders necessary administration of higher therapeutic doses of the product. In severe cases, the product may even become ineffective. Several approaches may be adopted in order to circumvent this problem. These include:

- Exchange transfusion of whole blood. This will transiently decrease circulating anti-factor VIII:C antibodies.
- Direct administration of factor X_a, thus bypassing the non-functional step in the coagulation cascade (Figures 9.3 and 9.4).
- Administration of high levels of a mixture of clotting factors II, VII, IX and X, which works effectively in 50% of treated patients.
- Administration of factor VII_a, as discussed subsequently.
- Administration of porcine factor VIII, which may or may not cross-react with the antibodies raised against human factor VIII_a (however, the immune system will soon begin to produce antibodies against the porcine clotting factor).
- Administration of factor VIII, with concurrent administration of immunosuppressive agents.

Due to the frequency of product administration, the purification procedure for recombinant factor VIII:C must be particularly stringent. Unlike the situation pertaining when the product is purified from human blood, any contaminant present in the final product will be non-human and hence immunogenic. Sources of such contaminants would include:

- host cell proteins;
- animal cell culture medium;
- antibody leaked from the immunoaffinity column.

Emphasis is placed not only upon ensuring the absence of contaminant proteins, but also other potential contaminants, particularly DNA (host cell line-derived DNA could harbour oncogenes; Chapter 3).

Recombinant factor VIII is gaining an increasing market share of the factor VIII market. Researchers are also attempting to develop modified forms of VIII:C (by site-directed mutagenesis) which display additional desirable characteristics. Particularly attractive in this regard would be the development of a product exhibiting an extended circulatory half-life. This could reduce the frequency of injections required by haemophilia A sufferers. However, any alteration of the primary sequence of the molecule carries with it the strong possibility of rendering the resultant mutant immunogenic.

Factors IX, VII$_a$ and XIII

Individuals who display a deficiency of factor IX develop haemophilia B, also known as Christmas disease. Although its clinical consequences are very similar to that of a deficiency of factor VIII, its general incidence in the population is far lower. Persons suffering from haemophilia B are treated by i.v. administration of a concentrate of factor IX. This was traditionally obtained by fractionation of human blood. Recombinant factor IX is now also produced in genetically engineered CHO cells.

Factor IX obtained from blood donations is normally only partially pure. In addition to factor IX, the product contains lower levels of factors II, VII and X, and has also been used to treat bleeding disorders caused by a lack of these factors.

Factor IX may also be purified by immuno-affinity chromatography, using immobilized anti-IX murine monoclonals. Purification to homogeneity is particularly important in the case of recombinant products. At least one monoclonal antibody has been raised that specifically binds only to factor IX, which contains pre-bound Ca^{2+} (i.e. the Ca^{2+}-dependent conformation of factor IX). Immobilization of this antibody allowed the development of an immuno-affinity system in which factor IX binds to the column in the presence of a Ca^{2+}-containing buffer. Subsequent elution is promoted simply by inclusion of a chelating agent (e.g. EDTA) in the elution buffer.

5–25% of individuals suffering from haemophilia A develop anti-factor VIII antibodies, while 3–6% of haemophilia B sufferers develop anti-factor IX antibodies. This complicates treatment of these conditions and, as mentioned previously, one approach to their treatment is direct administration of factor VII$_a$. The therapeutic rationale is that factor VII$_a$ could directly activate the final common steps of the coagulation cascade, independantly of either factor VIII or IX (Figure 9.2). Factor VII$_a$ forms a complex with tissue factor which, in the presence of phospholipids and Ca^{2+}, activates factor X.

A recombinant form of factor VII$_a$ (called 'NovoSeven' or 'Eptacog α-activated') is marketed by Novo-Nordisk. The recombinant molecule is produced in a BHK cell line, and the final product differs only slightly (in its glycosylation pattern only) from the native molecule.

Purification entails use of an immunoaffinity column containing immobilized murine anti-factor VII antibody. It is initially produced as an unactivated, single chain 406 amino acid polypeptide, which is subsequently proteolytically converted into the two-chain active factor VII$_a$ complex. After sterilization by filtration, the final product is aseptically filled into its final product containers and freeze-dried. The excipients present in the product include sodium chloride, calcium chloride, polysorbate 80, mannitol and glycylglycine. When freeze-dried in the presence of these stabilizing substances and stored under refrigerated conditions, the product displays a shelf-life of at least 2 years. It has proved effective in the treatment of serious bleeding events in patients displaying anti-factor VIII or IX antibodies.

A (very rare) genetic deficiency in the production of factor XIII also results in impaired clotting efficacy in affected persons. In this case, covalent links which normally characterize transformation of a soft clot into a hard clot are not formed. Factor XIII preparations, partially purified from human blood, are used to treat individuals with this condition.

Table 9.7. Anticoagulants which are used therapeutically or display therapeutic potential. Dicoumarol and related molecules are generally used over prolonged periods, while heparin is used over shorter periods. Hirudin has recently been approved for general medical use, while ancrod remains under clinical investigation

Anticoagulant	Structure	Source	Molecular mass (Da)
Heparin	Glycosaminoglycan	Beef lung, pig gastric mucosa	3000–40 000
Dicoumarol	Coumarin-based	Chemical manufacture	336.3
Warfarin	Coumarin-based	Chemical manufacture	308.4
Hirudin	Polypeptide	Leech saliva, genetic engineering	7000
Ancrod	Polypeptide	Snake venom, genetic engineering	35 000
Protein C	Glycoprotein	Human plasma	62 000

Anticoagulants

Although blood clot formation is essential to maintaining haemostasis, inappropriate clotting can give rise to serious, if not fatal, medical conditions. The formation of a blood clot (a thrombus) often occurs inappropriately within diseased blood vessels. This partially or completely obstructs the flow of blood (and hence oxygen) to the tissues normally served by that blood vessel.

Thrombus formation in a coronary artery (the arteries that supply the heart muscle itself with oxygen and nutrients) is termed coronary thrombosis. This results in a heart attack, characterized by the death (infarction) of oxygen-deprived heart muscle—hence the term 'myocardial infarction'. The development of a thrombus in a vessel supplying blood to the brain can result in development of a stroke. In addition, a thrombus (or part thereof) which has formed at a particular site in the vascular system may become detached. After travelling through the blood, this may lodge in another blood vessel, obstructing blood flow at that point. This process, which can also give rise to heart attacks or strokes, is termed embolism.

Anticoagulants are substances which can prevent blood from clotting and, hence, are of therapeutic use in cases where a high risk of coagulation is diagnosed. They are often administered to patients with coronary heart disease and to patients who have experienced a heart attack or stroke, in an effort to prevent recurrent episodes. The major anticoagulants used for therapeutic purposes are listed in Table 9.7.

Heparin

Proteoglycans are widely distributed throughout the body, being most abundant in connective tissue, where they may contribute up to 30% of that tissue's dry weight. They consist of a polypeptide backbone to which heteropolysaccharide chains are attached. However, unlike glycoproteins, proteolycans consist of up to, or in excess of, 95% carbohydrate and their properties resemble those of polysaccharides more than those of proteins.

Proteolytic digestion of proteoglycans liberates the carbohydrate side-chains, which are known as glycosaminoglycans (also known as mucopolysaccharides). All the glycosaminoglycans contain derivatives of glucosamine or galactosamine. Six major groups are known, one of which is heparin.

Heparin (Figure 9.11) is associated with many tissues but is found mainly stored intracellularly as granules in mast cells which line the endothelium of blood vessels. Upon

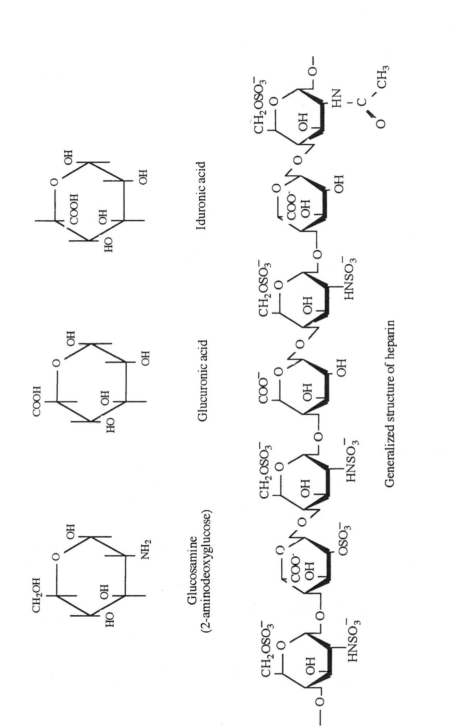

Figure 9.11. Structure of heparin. Heparin preparations, as isolated from natural sources, are a heterogeneous mixture of variably sulphated polysaccharides. The basic repeat structure consists of a D-glucosamine residue linked to a uronic acid, normally L-iduronic acid, less often D-glucuronic acid. Most of the amino groups of the glucosamine residues are modified with N-sulphate groups, while a small proportion are modified with N-acetyl groups. Many of the hydroxyl groups present at positions 2 and 6 of the iduronic ring also carry a sulphate substituent group. Molecular masses of individual molecules can vary considerably, often between 3 and 40 kDa. Individual hydrogens present on the sugar structures above have been omitted for clarity of presentation

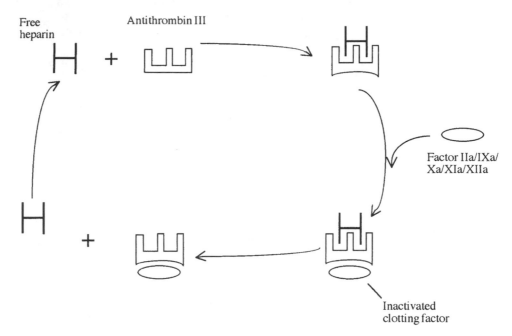

Figure 9.12. Diagramatic illustration of the mechanism by which heparin inhibits the clotting process. See text for specific details

release into the bloodstream heparin binds to, and activates, an additional plasma protein, antithrombin.

Antithrombin displays a heparin-binding site, as well as a binding site for a number of activated proteolytic clotting factors, including II_a, IX_a, X_a, XI_a and XII_a. Binding of heparin to antithrombin activates the latter, facilitating complex formation between the heparin–antithrombin and the activated clotting factor. This binding, which is of very high affinity, inactivates the clotting factor. Moreover, the heparin now disassociates from the complex and combines with another antithrombin molecule, thereby initiating another turn of this cycle (Figure 9.12).

Heparin represents one of the few carbohydrate-based biomolecules to find therapeutic application. It was originally extracted from liver (hence its name), but commercial preparations are now obtained by extraction from beef lung or porcine gastric mucosa.

While the product has proved to be an effective (and relatively inexpensive) anticoagulant, it does suffer from a number of clinical disadvantages (Table 9.8). Its requirement for a co-factor

Table 9.8. Some clinical disadvantages exhibited by the anticoagulant, heparin

Need for a co-factor (antithrombin III)
Poorly predictable dose response
Failure to effectively inhibit fibrin-bound thrombin sometimes induces serious bleeding episodes
Narrow benefit:risk ratio

(i.e. antithrombin) can lead to unpredictable clinical responses. Activated platelets also secrete at least two factors (platelet factor 4 and histidine-rich glycoprotein) that can bind and neutralize heparin. However, perhaps this molecule's most serious clinical limitation is its inability to inhibit thrombin bound to fibrin (i.e. thrombin functioning on the surface of a newly developing clot). Despite such disadvantages, however, heparin still enjoys widespread clinical use.

Vitamin K antimetabolites

Dicoumarol and warfarin are related, coumarin-based anticoagulants which, unlike heparin, may be administered orally (Figure 9.13). These compounds induce their anti-coagulant effect by preventing the vitamin K-dependent γ-carboxylation of certain blood factors, specifically factors II, VII, IX and X. Upon initial hepatic synthesis of these coagulation factors, a specific carboxylase catalyses the γ carboxylation of several of their glutamate residues (e.g. 10 of the first 33 residues present in prothrombin are γ-carboxyglutamate). This post-translational modification is required in order to allow these factors to bind Ca^{2+} ions — a prerequisite to their effective functioning. Vitamin K is an essential co-factor for the carboxylase enzyme, and its replacement with the antimetabolite, dicoumarol, renders this enzyme inactive. As a consequence, defective blood factors are produced which hinder effective functioning of the coagulation cascade.

The only major side-effect of these oral anticoagulants is prolonged bleeding, thus the dosage levels are chosen with care. Dicoumarol was first isolated from spoiled sweet clover hay, as the agent which promoted haemorrhage disease in cattle. Both dicoumarol and warfarin have also been utilized (at high doses) as rat poisons.

Hirudin

Hirudin is a leech-derived anticoagulant which functions by directly inhibiting thrombin. A range of blood-sucking animals contain substances in their saliva which specifically inhibit some element of the blood coagulation system (Table 9.9).

A bite from any such parasite is characterized by prolonged host bleeding. This property led to the documented use of leeches as an aid to blood-letting as far back as several hundred years BC. The method was particularly fashionable in Europe at the beginning of the ninteenth century. Many doctors at that time still believed that most illnesses were related in some way to blood composition and blood letting was a common, if uneffective, therapy. The Napoleonic Army surgeons, for example, used leeches to withdraw blood from soldiers suffering from conditions as diverse as infections and mental disease.

With the advent of modern medical principles, the medical usage of leeches waned somewhat. In more recent years, however, they did stage a limited comeback. They were occasionally used to drain blood from inflamed tissue, and in procedures associated with plastic surgery.

The presence of an anticoagulant in the saliva of the leech *Hirudo medicinalis* was first described in 1884. However, it was not until 1957 that the major anticoagulant activity present was purified and named hirudin. Hirudin is a short (65 amino acid) polypeptide, of molecular weight 7000 Da. The tyrosine residue at position 63 is unusual in that it contains a sulphate group. The molecule appears to have two domains; the globular N-terminal domain is stablized by three disulphide linkages, while the C-terminal domain is more elongated and exhibits a high content of acidic amino acids.

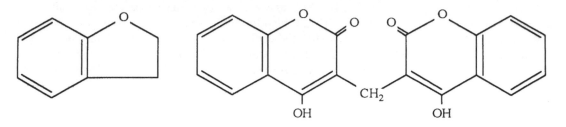

Coumaran   **Dicoumarol**

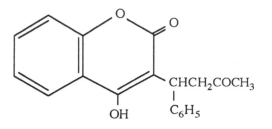

Warfarin

(a)

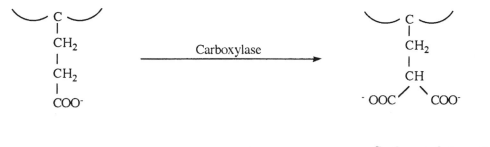

Glutamate   **γ-Carboxy-glutamate**

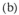

Figure 9.13. (a) Structure of coumarin, dicoumarol and warfarin. (b) Reaction catalysed by the vitamin K-dependent carboxylase. See text for details

Table 9.9. Some substances isolated from bloodsucking parasites which inhibit their host's haemostatic mechanisms. All are polypeptides of relatively low molecular mass

Polypeptide	Molecular mass (Da)	Producer	Haemostatic effect disrupted
Hirudin	7000	*Hirudo medicinalis*	Binds to and inhibits thrombin
Rhodniin	11 100	*Rhodnius prolixus*	Binds to and inhibits thrombin
Antistatin	15 000	*Haementeria officinalis*	Inhibits factor Xa
Tick anticoagulant peptide (TAP)	6800	*Ornithodoros moubata*	Inhibits factor Xa
Calin	55 000	*Hirudo medicinalis*	Inhibits platelet adhesion
Decorsin	4400	*Macrobdella decora*	Inhibits platelet adhesion

Hirudin exhibits its anticoagulant effect by tightly binding thrombin, thus inactivating it. In addition to its critical role in the production of a fibrin clot, thrombin displays several other (non-enzymatic) biological activities important in sustaining haemostasis. These include:

- it is a potent inducer of platelet activation and aggregation;
- it functions as a chemoattractant for monocytes and neutrophils;
- it stimulates endothelial transport.

One molecule of hirudin binds a single molecule of thrombin with very high affinity ($K_d \sim 10^{-12}$ M). Binding and inactivation occurs as a two-step mechanism. The C-terminal region of hirudin first binds along a groove on the surface of thrombin, resulting in a small conformational change of the enzyme. This then facilitates binding of the N-terminal region to the active site area (Figure 9.14). Binding of hirudin inhibits all the major functions of thrombin. Fragments of hirudin can also bind thrombin, but will generally only inhibit some of thrombin's range of activities, e.g. binding of an N-terminal hirudin fragment to thrombin inhibits only the thrombin catalytic activity.

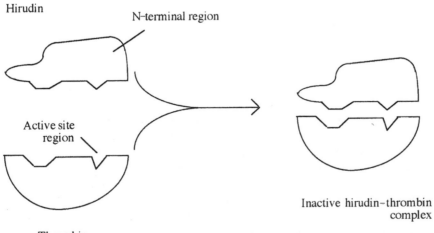

Figure 9.14. Binding of hirudin to thrombin, thus inactivating this activated coagulation factor

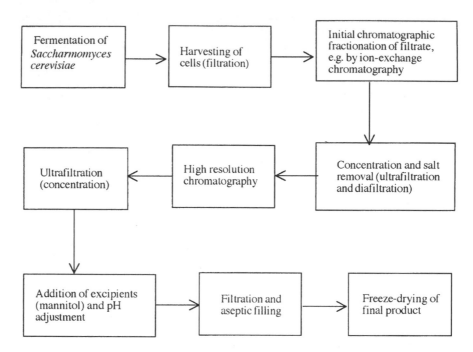

Figure 9.15. Overview of the production of Refludan (recombinant hirudin). The exact details of many steps remain confidential for obvious commercial reasons. A number of quality control checks are carried out on the final product to confirm the product's structure. These include amino acid composition, HPLC analysis and peptide mapping

Hirudin displays several potential therapeutic advantages as an anticoagulant:

- it acts directly upon thrombin;
- it does not require a co-factor;
- it is less likely than many other anticoagulants to induce unintentional haemorrhage;
- it is a weak immunogen.

Although the therapeutic potential of hirudin was appreciated for many years, insufficient material could be purified from the native source to support clinical trials, never mind its widespread medical application. The hirudin gene was cloned in the 1980s, and it has subsequently been expressed in a number of recombinant systems, including *E. coli*, *B. subtilis* and *S. cerevisiae*. A recombinant hirudin (trade name Refludan) was first approved for general medical use in 1997. The recombinant production system was constructed by insertion (via a plasmid) of a synthetic hirudin gene into a strain of *S. cerevisiae*. The yeast cells secrete the product which is then purified by various fractionation techniques (Figure 9.15). The recombinant molecule displays a slightly altered amino acid sequence when compared to the native product. Its first two amino acids, leucine and threonine, replace two valines of native hirudin. It is also devoid of the sulphate group normally present on tyrosine residue No. 63. Clinical trials, however, have proved this slightly altered product to be both safe and effective. The final product is presented in freeze-dried form with the sugar, mannitol, representing the major added excipient. The product, which displays a useful shelf-life of 2-years when stored at room temperature, is reconstituted with saline or water for injections immediately prior to its i.v. administration. A second recombinant product (trade name Revasc, also produced in *S. cerevisiae*) has also been approved.

Antithrombin

Antithrombin, already mentioned in the context of heparin, is the most abundantly occurring natural inhibitor of coagulation. It is a single-chain 432 amino acid glycoprotein displaying four oligosaccharide side-chains and an approximate molecular mass of 58 kDa. It is present in plasma at concentrations of 150 μg/ml and is a potent inhibitor of thrombin (factor IIa) as well as factors IXa and Xa. It inhibits thrombin by binding directly to it in a 1:1 stoichiometric complex.

Plasma-derived anti-thrombin (AT) concentrates have been used medically since the 1980s for the treatment of hereditary and acquired AT deficiency. Hereditary (genetic) deficiency is characterized by the presence of little/no native antithrombin activity in plasma and results in an increased risk of inappropriate blood clot/embolus formation. Acquired AT deficiency can be induced by drugs (e.g. heparin and oestrogens), liver disease (which causes decreased AT synthesis) or various other medical conditions. Recombinant AT has been successfully expressed in engineered CHO cells. Commercial production via this route, however, is rendered unattractive due to high relative production costs and, to a lesser extent, by the scale of production needed to satisfy market demand. Recombinant AT has been produced more economically in the milk of transgenic goats (Chapter 3) and this product is currently undergoing clinical trials (Figure 9.16). The recombinant product displays an identical amino acid sequence to that of native human AT, although its oligosaccharide composition does vary somewhat from the native protein.

Ceprotin (human protein C concentrate) is an additional protein-based anticoagulant now approved for general medical use. Protein C is a 62 kDa glycoprotein synthesized in the liver but

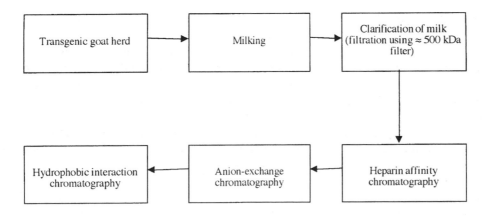

Figure 9.16. Outline of the production and purification of antithrombin (AT) from the milk of transgenic goats. Purification achieves an overall product yield in excess of 50%, with a purity greater than 99%

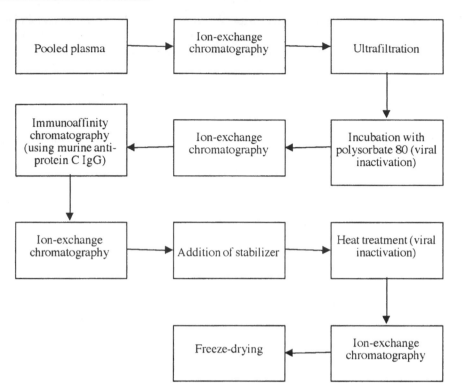

Figure 9.17. Overview of the manufacture of Ceprotin. As the active ingredient is derived directly from pooled human plasma, particular emphasis is placed upon ensuring that the finished product is pathogen-free. Precautions entail the incorporation of two independent viral inactivation steps and high-resolution chromatographic purification. Additionally, extensive screening of plasma pool source material for blood-borne pathogens is undertaken. Viral screening is undertaken using a combination of immunoassay and PCR analysis for the presence of viral nucleic acid

released into the blood as a circulating inactive zymogen. It is activated by thrombin in conjunction with another protein, thrombomodulin, and the activated form displays anti-coagulant activity. *In vivo* protein C plays an important role in controlling coagulation by preventing excessive clot formation. A range of genetic congenital deficiencies adversely affecting serum levels of functional protein C have been characterized. Sufferers generally display an increased risk of inappropriate venous thrombosis and Ceprotin has been approved for the treatment of such individuals. An overview of its method of manufacture is provided in Figure 9.17. As the protein is sourced directly from pooled human plasma, it is more properly described as a product of pharmaceutical biotechnology, as opposed to a true biopharmaceutical (Chapter 1).

Thrombolytic agents

The natural process of thrombosis functions to plug a damaged blood vessel, thus maintaining haemostasis until the damaged vessel can be repaired. Subsequent to this repair, the clot is removed via an enzymatic degradative process known as fibrinolysis. Fibrinolysis normally

Table 9.10. Thrombolytic agents approved for general medical use (r = recombinant, rh = recombinant human)

Product	Company
Activase (rh-tPA)	Genentech
Ecokinase (rtPA; differs from human tPA in that three of its five domains have been deleted)	Galenus Mannheim
Retavase (rtPA; see Ecokinase)	Boehringer-Mannheim/Centocor
Rapilysin (rtPA; see Ecokinase)	Boehringer-Mannheim
Tenecteplase (also marketed as Metalyse) (TNK-tPA, modified rtPA)	Boehringer-Ingelheim
TNKase (Tenecteplase; modified rtPA; see Tenecteplase)	Genentech
Streptokinase (produced by *Streptokinase haemolyticus*)	Various
Urokinase (extracted from human urine)	Various
Staphylokinase (extracted from *Staphylococcus aureus* and produced in various recombinant systems)	Various

depends upon the serine protease plasmin, which is capable of degrading the fibrin strands present in the clot.

In situations where inappropriate clot formation results in the blockage of a blood vessel, the tissue damage that ensues depends, to a point, upon how long the clot blocks blood flow. Rapid removal of the clot can often minimize the severity of tissue damage. Thus, several thrombolytic (clot-degrading) agents have found medical application (Table 9.10). The market for an effective thrombolytic agent is substantial. In the USA alone, it is estimated that 1.5 million people suffer acute myocardial infarction each year, while another 0.5 million suffer strokes.

Tissue plasminogen activator (tPA)

The natural thrombolytic process is illustrated in Figure 9.18. Plasmin is a protease which catalyses the proteolytic degradation of fibrin present in clots, thus effectively dissolving the clot. Plasmin is derived from plasminogen, its circulating zymogen. Plasminogen is synthesized in, and released from, the kidneys. It is a single-chain 90 kDa glycoprotein, which is stabilized by several disulphide linkages.

Tissue plasminogen activator (tPA, also known as fibrinokinase) represents the most important physiological activator of plasminogen. tPA is a 527 amino acid serine protease. It is synthesized predominantly in vascular endothelial cells (cells lining the inside of blood vessels) and displays five structural domains, each of which has a specific function (Table 9.11). tPA displays four potential glycosylation sites, three of which are normally glycosylated (residues 117, 184 and 448). The carbohydrate moieties play an important role in mediating hepatic uptake of tPA and hence its clearance from plasma. It is normally found in the blood in two forms; a single-chain polypeptide (type I tPA) and a two-chain structure (type II) proteolytically derived from the single chain structure. The two-chain form is the one predominantly associated with clots undergoing lysis, but both forms display fibrinolytic activity.

Fibrin contains binding sites for both plasminogen and tPA, thus bringing these into close proximity. This facilitates direct activation of the plasminogen at the clot surface (Figure 9.18). This activation process is potentiated by the fact that binding of tPA to fibrin (a) enhances the subsequent binding of plasminogen and (b) increases tPA's activity towards plasminogen by up to 600-fold.

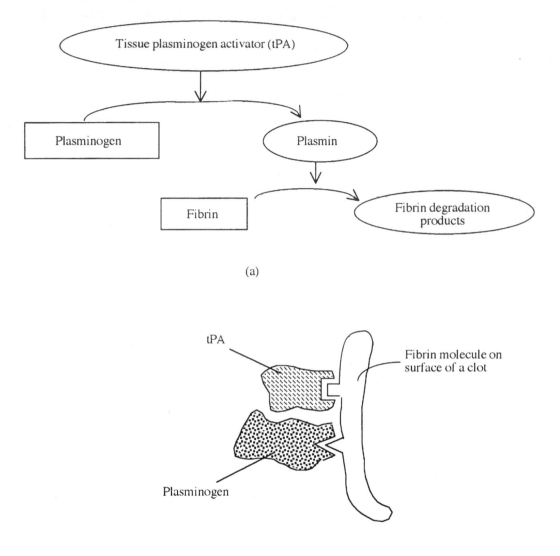

(a)

(b)

Figure 9.18. (a) The fibrinolytic system, in which tissue plasminogen activator (tPA) proteolytically converts the zymogen plasminogen into active plasmin, which in turn degrades the fibrin strands, thus dissolving the clot. tPA and plasminogen both bind to the surface of fibrin strands (b), thus ensuring rapid and efficient activation of the thrombolytic process

Overall, therefore, activation of the thrombolytic cascade occurs exactly where it is needed — on the surface of the clot. This is important as the substrate specificity of plasmin is poor, and circulating plasmin displays the catalytic potential to proteolyse fibrinogen, factor V and factor VIII. Although soluble serum tPA displays a much reduced activity towards plasminogen, some free circulating plasmin is produced by this reaction. If uncontrolled, this could increase the risk of subsequent haemorrhage. This scenario is usually averted, as circulating plasmin is rapidly

Table 9.11. The five domains that constitute human tPA and the biological function of each domain

tPA domain	Function
Finger domain (F domain)	Promotes tPA binding to fibrin with high affinity
Protease domain (P domain)	Displays plasminogen-specific proteolytic activity
Epidermal growth factor domain (EGF domain)	Binds hepatic receptors thereby mediating hepatic clearance of tPA from blood
Kringle-1 domain (K_1 domain)	Associated with binding to the hepatic receptor
Kringle-2 domain (K_2 domain)	Facilitates stimulation of tPA's proteolytic activity by fibrin

neutralized by another plasma protein, α_2-antiplasmin (α_2-antiplasmin, a 70 kDa, single-chain glycoprotein, binds plasmin very tightly in a 1:1 complex). In contrast to free plasmin, plasmin present on a clot surface is very slowly inactivated by α_1-antiplasmin. The thrombolytic system has thus evolved in a self-regulating fashion, which facilitates efficient clot degradation with minimal potential disruption to other elements of the haemostatic mechanism.

First-generation tPA. Although tPA was first studied in the late 1940s, its extensive characterization was hampered by the low levels at which it is normally synthesized. Detailed studies were facilitated in the 1980s after the discovery that the Bowes melanoma cell line produces and secretes large quantities of this protein. This also facilitated its initial clinical appraisal. The tPA gene was cloned from the melanoma cell line in 1983, and this facilitated subsequent large-scale production in CHO cell lines by recombinant DNA technology. The tPA cDNA contains 2530 nucleotides and encodes a mature protein of 527 amino acids. The glycosylation pattern was similar, although not identical, to the native human molecule. A marketing licence for the product was first issued in the USA to Genentech in 1987 (under the trade name Activase). The therapeutic indication was for the treatment of acute myocardial infarction. The production process entails an initial (10 000 litre) fermentation step, during which the cultured CHO cells produce and secrete tPA into the fermentation medium. After removal of the cells by sub-micron filtration and initial concentration, the product is purified by a combination of several chromatographic steps. The final product has been shown to be greater than 99% pure by several analytical techniques, including HPLC, SDS–PAGE, tryptic mapping and N-terminal sequencing.

Activase has proved effective in the early treatment of patients with acute myocardial infarction (i.e. those treated within 12 h after the first symptoms occur). Significantly increased rates of patient survival (as measured 1 day and 30 days after the initial event), are noted when tPA is administered in favour of streptokinase, a standard therapy (see later). tPA has thus established itself as a first-line option in the management of acute myocardial infarction. A therapeutic dose of 90–100 mg (often administered by infusion over 90 min), results in a steady-state Activase concentration of 3–4 mg/l during that period. The product is, however, cleared rapidly by the liver, displaying a serum half-life of approximately 3 min. As is the case for most thrombolytic agents, the most significant risk associated with tPA administration is the possible induction of severe haemorrhage.

Engineered tPA. Modified forms of tPA have also been generated in an effort to develop a product with an improved therapeutic profile (e.g. faster-acting or exhibiting a prolonged

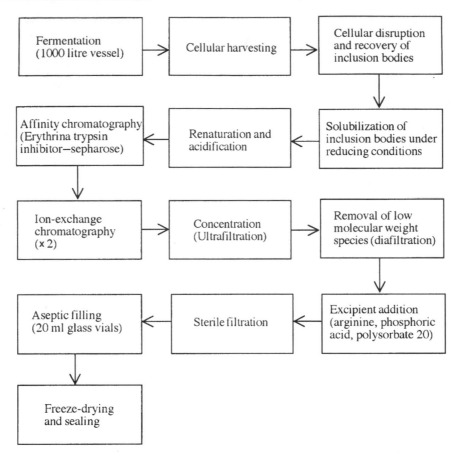

Figure 9.19. Production of Ecokinase, a modified tPA molecule which gained regulatory approval in Europe in 1996. The production cell line is recombinant *E. coli* K12, which harbours a nucleotide sequence coding for the shortened tPA molecule. The product accumulates intracellularly in the form of inclusion bodies

plasma half-life). Reteplase is the international non-proprietary name given to one such modified human tPA produced in recombinant *E. coli* cells and is sold under the tradenames Ecokinase, Retavase and Rapilysin (Table 9.10). This product's development was based upon the generation of a synthetic nucleotide sequence encoding a shortened (355 amino acid) tPA molecule. This analogue contained only the tPA domains responsible for fibrin selectivity and catalytic activity. The nucleotide sequence was integrated into an expression vector subsequently introduced into *E. coli* (strain K12) by treatment with calcium chloride. The protein is expressed intracellularly where it accumulates in the form of an inclusion body. Due to the prokaryotic production system, the product is non-glycosylated. The final sterile freeze-dried product exhibits a 2 year shelf-life when stored at temperatures below 25°C. An overview of the production process is presented in Figure 9.19.

The lack of glycosylation as well as the absence of the EGF and K_1 domains (Table 9.11) confers an extended serum half-life upon the engineered molecule. Reteplase-based products display a serum half-life of up to 20 min, facilitating its administration as a single bolus injection as opposed to continuous infusion. Absence of the molecule's F_1 domain also reduces the product's fibrin-binding affinity. It is theorized that this may further enhance clot degradation, as it facilitates more extensive diffusion of the thrombolytic agent into the interior of the clot. Tenecteplase (also marketed under the tradename, Metalyse) is yet an additional engineered tPA now on the market. Produced in a CHO cell line, this glycosylated variant differs in sequence to native tPA by six amino acids (Thr 103 converted to Asn; Asn 117 converted to Gln and the Lys–His–Arg–Arg sequence at position 296–299 converted to Ala–Ala–Ala–Ala). Collectively, these modifications result in a prolonged plasma half-life (to 15–19 min), as well as an increased resistance to PAI-1 (plasminogen activator inhibitor-1, a natural tPA inhibitor).

Streptokinase

Streptokinase is an extracellular bacterial protein produced by several strains of *Streptococcus haemolyticus* group C. It displays a molecular mass in the region of 48 kDa and an isoelectric point of 4.7. Its ability to induce lysis of blood clots was first demonstrated in 1933. Early therapeutic preparations administered to patients often caused immunological and other complications, usually prompted by impurities present in these products. Chromatographic purification (particularly using gel filtration and ion-exchange columns), overcame many of these initial difficulties. Modern chromatographically pure streptokinase preparations are usually supplied in freeze-dried form. These preparations often contain albumin as an excipient. The albumin prevents flocculation of the active ingredient upon its reconstitution.

Streptokinase is a widespreadly employed thrombolytic agent. It is administered to treat a variety of thrombo-embolic disorders, including:

- pulmonary embolism (blockage of the pulmonary artery by an embolism), which can cause acute heart failure and sudden death (the pulmonary artery carries blood from the heart to the lungs for oxygenation);
- deep-vein thrombosis (thrombus formation in deep veins, usually in the legs);
- arterial occlusions (obstruction of an artery);
- acute myocardial infarction.

Streptokinase induces its thrombolytic effect by binding specifically and tightly to plasminogen. This induces a conformational change in the plasminogen molecule, which renders it proteolytically active. In this way, the streptokinase–plasminogen complex catalyses the proteolytic conversion of plasminogen to active plasmin.

As a bacterial protein, streptokinase is viewed by the human immune system as an antigenic substance. In some cases, its administration has elicited allergic responses, ranging from mild rashes to more serious anaphylactic shock (anaphylactic shock represents an extreme and generalized allergic response, characterized by swelling, constriction of the bronchioles, circulatory collapse and heart failure).

Another disadvantage of streptokinase administration is the associated increased risk of haemorrhage. Streptokinase-activated plasminogen is capable of lysing not only clot-associated fibrin, but also free plasma fibrinogen. This can result in low serum fibrinogen levels and hence compromise haemostatic ability. It should not, for example, be administered to patients suffering from coagulation disorders or bleeding conditions such as ulcers. Despite such potenital clinical complications, careful administration of streptokinase has saved countless thousands of lives.

Urokinase

The ability of some components of human urine to dissolve fibrin clots was first noted in 1885, but it was not until the 1950s that the active substance was isolated and named 'urokinase'.

Urokinase is a serine protease produced by the kidney and is found in both the plasma and urine. It is capable of proteolytically converting plasminogen into plasmin. Two variants of the enzyme have been isolated: a 54 kDa species and a lower molecular mass (33 kDa) variant. The lower molecular mass form appears to be derived from the higher molecular mass moiety by proteolytic processing. Both forms exhibit enzymatic activity against plasminogen.

Urokinase is used clinically under the same circumstances as streptokinase and, because of its human origin, adverse immunological responses are less likely. Following acute medical events such as pulmonary embolism, the product is normally administered to the patient at initial high doses (by infusion) for several minutes. This is followed by hourly i.v. injections for up to 12 h.

Urokinase utilized medically is generally purified directly from human urine. It binds to a range of adsorbants, such as silica gel and, especially, kaolin (hydrated aluminium silicate), which can be used to initially concentrate and partially purify the product. It may also be concentrated and partially purified by precipitation using sodium chloride, ammonium sulphate or ethanol as precipitants.

Various chromatographic techniques may be utilized to further purify urokinase. Commonly employed methods include anion (DEAE-based) exchange chromatography, gel filtration on Sephadex G-100 and chromatography on hydroxyapatite columns. Urokinase is a relatively stable molecule. It remains active subsequent to incubation at 60°C for several hours, or brief incubation at pHs as low as 1.0 or as high as 10.0.

After its purification, sterile filtration and aseptic filling, human urokinase is normally freeze-dried. Because of its heat stability, the final product may also be heated to 60°C for up to 10 h in an effort to inactivate any undetected viral particles present. The product utilized clinically contains both molecular mass forms, with the higher molecular mass moiety predominating. Urokinase can also be produced by techniques of animal cell culture utilizing human kidney cells or by recombinant DNA technology.

Staphylokinase

Staphylokinase is a protein produced by a number of strains of *Staphylococcus aureus*, which also displays therapeutic potenital as a thrombolytic agent. The protein has been purified from its natural source by a combination of ammonium sulphate precipitation and cation-exchange chromatography on CM cellulose. Affinity chromatography using plasmin or plasminogen immobilized to sepharose beads has also been used. The pure product is a 136 amino acid polypeptide displaying a molecular mass in the region of 16.5 kDa. Lower molecular mass derivatives lacking the first six or 10 NH_2-terminal amino acids have also been characterized. All three appear to display similar thrombolytic activity *in vitro* at least.

The staphylokinase gene has been cloned in *E. coli*, as well as various other recombinant systems. The protein is expressed intracellularly in *E. coli* at high levels, representing 10–15% of total cellular protein. It can be purified directly from the clarified cellular homogenate by a combination of ion-exchange and hydrophobic interaction chromatography.

Although staphylokinase shows no significant homology with streptokinase, it induces a thrombolytic effect by a somewhat similar mechanism — it also forms a 1:1 stoichiometric complex with plasminogen. The proposed mechanism by which staphylokinase induces

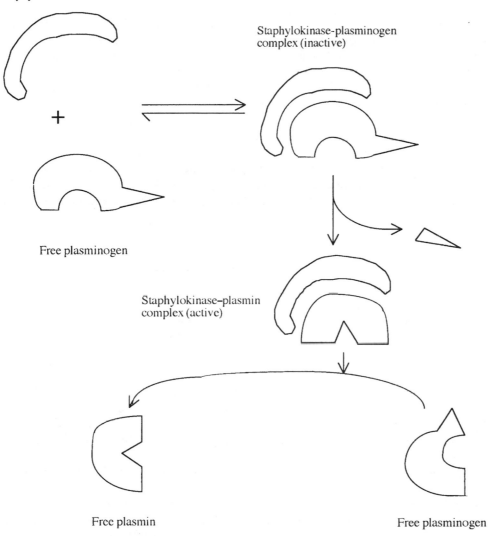

Figure 9.20. Schematic representation of the mechanism by which staphylokinase appears to activate the thrombolytic process via the generation of plasmin. See text for details

plasminogen activation is outlined in Figure 9.20. Binding of the staphylokinase to plasminogen appears to initially yield an inactive staphylokinase–plasminogen complex. However, complex formation somehow induces subsequent proteolytic cleavage of the bound plasminogen, forming plasmin, which remains complexed to the staphylokinase. This complex (via the plasmin) then appears to catalyse the conversion of free plasminogen to plasmin, and may even accelerate the process of conversion of other staphylokinase–plasminogen complexes into staphylokinase–plasmin complexes. The net effect is generation of active plasmin, which displays a direct thrombolytic effect by degrading clot-based fibrin, as described previously (Figure 9.18).

The serum protein α_2-antiplasmin can inhibit the activated plasmin–staphylokinase complex. It appears that the α_2-antiplasmin can interact with the active plasmin moiety of the complex, resulting in dissociation of staphylokinase, and consequent formation of an inactive plasmin–α_2–antiplasmin complex.

The thrombolytic ability of (recombinant) staphylokinase has been evaluated in initial clinical trials, with encouraging results; 80% of patients suffering from acute myocardial infarction who received staphylokinase responded positively (10 mg staphylokinase was administered by infusion over 30 min). The native molecule displays a relatively short serum half-life (6.3 min), although covalent attachment of polyethylene glycol (PEG) reduces the rate of serum clearance, hence effectively increasing the molecule's half-life significantly. As with streptokinase, patients administered staphylokinase develop neutralizing antibodies. A number of engineered (domain-deleted) variants have been generated, which display significantly reduced immunogenicity.

α_1-Antitrypsin

The respiratory tract is protected by a number of defence mechanisms which include:

- particle removal in the nostril/nasopharynx;
- particle expulsion (e.g. by coughing);
- upward removal of substances via mucociliary transport;
- presence in the lungs of immune cells, such as alveolar macrophages;
- production/presence of soluble protective factors, including α_1-antitrypsin, lysozyme, lactoferrin and interferon.

Failure/ineffective functioning of one or more of these mechanisms can impair normal respiratory function, e.g. emphysema is a condition in which the alveoli of the lungs are damaged, which compromises the lung's capacity to exchange gases, and breathlessness often results. This condition is often promoted by smoking, respiratory infections or a deficiency in the production of serum α_1-antitrypsin.

α_1-Antitrypsin is a 394 amino acid, 52 kDa serum glycoprotein. It is synthesized in the liver and secreted into the blood, where it is normally present at concentrations of 2–4 g/l. It constitutes in excess of 90% of the α_1-globulin fraction of blood.

The α_1-antitrypsin gene is located on chromosome 14. A number of α_1-antitrypsin gene variants have been described. Their gene products can be distinguished by their differential mobility upon gel electrophoresis. The normal form is termed M, while point mutations in the gene have generated two major additional forms, S and Z. These mutations results in a greatly reduced level of synthesis and secretion into the blood of the mature α_1-antitrypsin. Persons inheriting two copies of the Z gene, in particular, display greatly reduced levels of serum α_1-antitrypsin activity. This is often associated with the development of emphysema (particularly in smokers). The condition may be treated by the administration of purified α_1-antitrypsin. This protein constitutes the major serine protease inhibitor present in blood. It is a potent inhibitor of the protease elastase, and serves to protect the lung from proteolytic damage by inhibiting neutrophil elastase. The product is administered on an ongoing basis to sufferers, who receive up to 200 g of the inhibitor each year. It is normally prepared by limited fractionation of whole human blood, although the large quantities required by patients heightens the risk of accidental transmission of blood-borne pathogens. The α_1-antitrypsin gene has been expressed in a number

Table 9.12. Enzymes used therapeutically

Enzyme	Application
Tissue plasminogen activator	Thrombolytic agent
Urokinase	Thrombolytic agent
Ancrod	Anticoagulant
Factor IXa	Haemophilia B
Asparaginase	Anti-cancer agent
Nuclease (DNase)	Cystic fibrosis
Glucocerebrosidase	Gaucher's disease
α-Galactosidase	Fabry's disease
Urate oxidase	Hyperuricaemia
Superoxide dismutase	Oxygen toxicity
Trypsin/papain/collagenase	Debriding/anti-inflammatory agents
Lactase/pepsin/papain/pancrelipase	Digestive aids

of recombinant systems, including in the milk of transgenic sheep. While use of the recombinant product would all but preclude blood pathogen transmission, it appears significantly more costly to produce.

Enzymes of therapeutic value

Enzymes are used for a variety of therapeutic purposes, the most significant of which are listed in Table 9.12. A number of specific examples have already been discussed in detail within this chapter, including tPA, urokinase and factor IXa. The additional therapeutic enzymes now become the focus of the remainder of the chapter.

Although a limited number of polymer-degrading enzymes, (used as digestive aids), are given orally, most enzymes are administered intravenously. Such enzymes will often elicit an immunological response upon their injection into the body. Although a long-term consequence can be a decrease in therapeutic efficacy due to antibody formation, enzymes, like any other proteins, can also potentially induce an immediate allergic/anaphylactic response in some patients. In addition, most enzymes administered intravenously are removed from the blood stream and rapidly degraded.

Attempts to overcome antigenicity and short plasma half-lives have centred around protecting the enzyme by encapsulation or covalent modification. Encapsulation of the enzyme in microspheres physically protects it from elements of the immune system and generally increases its circulatory half-life. It is important that the microsphere itself be constructed from a non-antigenic substance. The semi-permeable membrane of the microsphere should display a pore size too small to allow enzymes to leak out, but large enough to facilitate free inward diffusion of substrate and free outward diffusion of product (Figure 9.21). The microsphere can be made of natural polymers, such as albumin, or from synthetic materials such as nylon, polyacrylamide or cellulose nitrate. Enzymes can also be entrapped in erythrocyte ghosts or in liposomes.

Liposomes, in particular, may offer the future possibility of delivering enzymes (and other drugs) to specific body tissues. This could be attained by incorporating target molecules (e.g. specific receptors, glycoproteins or antibodies) in the liposome membrane, which selectively

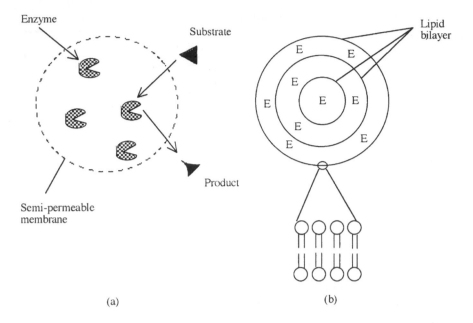

Figure 9.21. (a) Microencapsulation of enzyme molecules within a semipermeable membrane. Substrate molecules can diffuse inwards from the surrounding fluid (e.g. blood), to be catalytically converted by the enzyme. The resultant product molecules can diffuse back out of the microsphere. (b) Typical structure of a liposome. The simplest structure would consist of a single lipid bilayer (thus somewhat resembling a cell membrane). By controlling the synthesis process, liposomes containing different numbers of lipid bilayers can be generated. The compartments between the individual bilayers are aqueous-based and thus can be used to house enzymes (E above)

interact with ligands present on the surface of the specific target tissue. Fusion of the liposome membrane with the cell in question would facilitate entry of the liposome contents into that cell.

Chemical modification, particularly succinylation, or coupling to polyglycols, can also increase the plasma half-life of enzymes. Conjugation with polyethylene glycol [PEG; $H(OCH_2CH_2)_nOH$] has successfully been employed to stabilize and protect several therapeutic enzymes. Such modification, for example, increases the plasma half-life of superoxide dismutase from 5 h to over 30 h. PEG-coupled asparaginase was approved for general medical use by the FDA in 1994.

Asparaginase

Asparaginase is an enzyme capable of catalysing the hydrolysis of L-asparagine, yielding aspartic acid and ammonia (Figure 9.22). In the late 1970s, researchers illustrated that serum transferred from healthy guinea pigs into mice suffering from leukaemia, contained some agent capable of inhibiting the proliferation of the leukaemic cells. A search revealed the agent to be asparaginase.

Most healthy (untransformed) mammalian cells are capable of directly synthesizing asparagine from glutamine (Figure 9.22). Hence, asparagine is generally classified as a non-essential amino acid (i.e. we do not require it as an essential component of our diet). However,

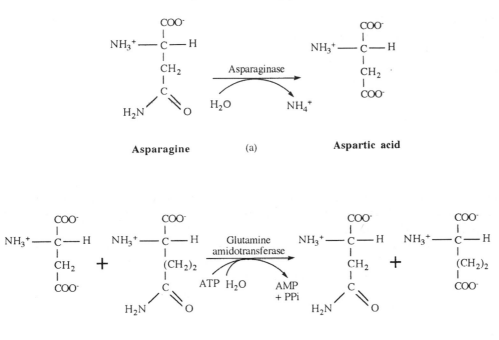

Figure 9.22. (a) Hydrolytic reaction catalysed by L-asparaginase. (b) Reaction by which asparagine is synthesized in most mammalian cells

many transformed cells lose the ability to synthesize asparagine themselves. For these, asparagine becomes an essential amino acid. In the case of leukaemic mice, guinea-pig asparaginase deprived the transformed cells of this amino acid by hydrolysing plasma asparaginase. This approach has been successfully applied to treating some forms of human leukaemia, e.g. the PEG–L-asparaginase previously mentioned was approved for the treatment of refractory childhood acute lymphoblastic leukaemia.

Generally, the plasma concentration of asparagine is quite low ($\sim 40 \, \mu M$). Therefore, therapeutically useful asparaginases must display a high substrate affinity (i.e. low K_m values). Asparaginase from *E. coli* and *Erwinia*, as well as *Pseudomonas* and *Acinetobacter* have been studied in greatest detail. All have proved effective in inhibiting growth of various leukaemias and other transformed cell lines. PEG-coupled enzymes are often preferred, as they display an extended plasma half-life.

Although asparaginase therapy has proved effective, a number of side-effects have been associated with initiation of therapy. These have included severe nausea, vomiting and diarrhoea, as well as compromised liver and kidney function. Side-effects are probably due to a transient asparaginase deficiency in various tissues. Under normal circumstances, dietary-derived plasma asparagine levels are sufficient to meet normal tissue demands, and the cellular asparagine biosynthetic pathway remains repressed. Reduced plasma asparagine levels result in the induction of cellular asparagine synthesis. High-dose asparaginase administration will immediately reduce plasma asparagine levels. However, the ensuing initiation of cellular asparagine synthesis may not occur for several hours. Thus, a more suitable therapeutic regimen may entail initial low-dose asparaginase administration, followed by stepwise increasing dosage levels.

DNase

Recombinant DNase preparations have been used in the treatment of cystic fibrosis (CF) since the end of 1993. This genetic disorder is common, particularly in ethnic groups of northern European extraction, where the frequency of occurrence can be as high as 1 in 2500 live births. A higher than average incidence has also been recorded in southern Europe, as well as in some Jewish populations and American blacks.

A number of clinical symptoms characterize cystic fibrosis. Predominant among these is the presence of excess sodium chloride in CF patients' sweat. Indeed, measurement of chloride levels in sweat remains the major diagnostic indicator of this disease. Another characteristic is the production of an extremely viscous, custard-like mucus in various body glands/organs, which severely compromise their function. Particularly affected are:

- the lungs, in which mucus compromises respiratory function;
- the pancreas, in which the mucus blocks its ducts in 85% of CF patients, causing pancreatic insufficiency; this is chiefly characterized by secretion of greatly reduced levels of digestive enzymes into the small intestine;
- the reproductive tract, in which changes can render males, in particular, sub-fertile or infertile;
- the liver, in which bile ducts can become clogged;
- the small intestine, which can become obstructed by mucus mixed with digesta.

These clinical features are dominated by those associated with the respiratory tract. The physiological changes induced in the lung of cystic fibrosis sufferers renders this tissue susceptible to frequent and recurrent microbial infection, particularly by *Pseudomonas* species. The presence of microorganisms in the lung attracts immune elements, particularly phagocytic neutrophils. These begin to ingest the microorganisms and large quantities of DNA are released from damaged microbes and neutrophils at the site of infection. High molecular mass DNA is itself extremely viscous and substantially increases the viscosity of the respiratory mucus.

The genetic basis of this disease was underlined by the finding of a putative CF gene in 1989. Specific mutations in this gene, which resides on human chromosome 7, were linked to the development of cystic fibrosis, and the gene is expressed largely by cells present in sweat glands, the lung, pancreas, intestine and reproductive tract.

70% of all CF patients exhibit a specific three-base pair deletion in the gene, which results in the loss of a single amino acid (phenylalanine 508) from its final polypeptide product. Other CF patients display various other mutations in the same gene.

The gene product is termed CFTR (cystic fibrosis transmembrane conductance regulator), and it codes for a chloride ion channel. It may also carry out additional (as yet undetermined) functions.

Although therapeutic approaches based upon gene therapy (Chapter 11) may well one day cure cystic fibrosis, current therapeutic intervention focuses upon alleviating CF symptoms, particularly those relating to respiratory function. Improved patient care has increased the life expectancy of CF patients to well into their 30s. The major elements of CF management include:

- chest percussion (physically pounding on the chest) in order to help dislodge respiratory tract mucus, rendering the patient better able to expel it;
- antibiotic administration, to control respiratory and other infections;
- pancreatic enzyme replacement;
- attention to nutritional status.

A relatively recent innovation in CF therapy is the use of DNase to reduce the viscosity of respiratory mucus. Scientists had been aware since the 1950s that free DNA concentrations in the lung of cystic fibrosis sufferers were extremely high (3–14 mg/ml). They realized that this could contribute to the mucus viscosity. Pioneering experiments were undertaken, entailing inhalation of DNase-enriched extracts of bovine pancreas, but both product safety and efficacy were called into question. The observed toxicity was probably due to trypsin or other contaminants that were damaging to the underlying lung tissue. The host immune system was also probably neutralizing much of the bovine DNase.

The advent of genetic engineering and improvements in chromatographic methodology facilitated the production of highly purified recombinant human DNase (rhDNase) prepara-tions. Initial *in vitro* studies proved encouraging—incubation of the enzyme with sputum derived from a CF patient resulted in a significant reduction of the sputum's viscosity. Clinical trials also showed the product to be safe and effective, and Genentech received marketing authorization for the product in December, 1993 under the trade name 'Pulmozyme'. The annual cost of treatment varies, but is often $10 000–$15 000.

Pulmozyme is produced in an engineered CHO cell line harbouring a nucleotide sequence coding for native human DNase. Subsequent to upstream processing, the protein is purified by tangential flow filtration followed by a combination of chromatographic steps. The purified 260 amino acid glycoprotein displays a molecular mass of 37 kDa. It is formulated as an aqueous solution at a concentration of 1.0 mg/ml, with the addition of calcium chloride and sodium chloride as excipients. The solution, which contains no preservative, displays a final pH of 6.3. It is administered directly into the lungs by inhalation of an aerosol mist generated by a compressed air-based nebulizer system.

Glucocerebrosidase

Glucocerebrosidase preparations are administered to relieve the symptoms of Gaucher's disease, which affects some 5000 people worldwide. This is a lysosomal storage disease affecting lipid metabolism, specifically the degradation of glucocerebrosides. Glucocerebrosides are a specific class of lipid, consisting of a molecule of sphingosine, a fatty acid and a glucose molecule (Figure 9.23). They are found in many body tissues, particularly in the brain and other neural tissue, in which they are often associated with the myelin sheath of nerves. Glucocerebrosides, however, are not abundant structural components of membranes, but are mostly formed as intermediates in the synthesis and degradation of more complex glycosphingolipids. Their degradation is undertaken by specific lysosomal enzymes, particularly in cells of the reticulo-endothelial system (i.e. phagocytes, which are spread throughout the body and which function as: (a) a defence against microbial infection and, (b), removal of worn-out blood cells from the plasma. These phagocytes are particularly prevalent in the spleen, bone marrow and liver).

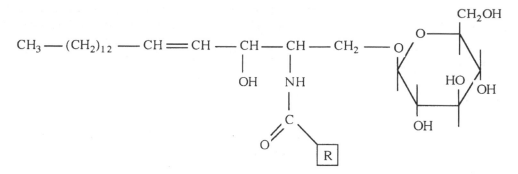

Figure 9.23. Generalized structure of a glucocerebroside

Gaucher's disease is an inborn error of metabolism characterized by lack of the enzyme glucocerebrosidase, with consequent accumulation of glucocerebrosides, particularly in tissue-based macrophages. Clinical systems include enlargement and compromised function of these macrophage-containing tissues, particularly the liver and spleen, as well as damage to long bones and, sometimes, mental retardation. Administration of exogenous glucocerebrosidase as enzyme replacement therapy, has been shown to reduce the main symptoms of this disease. The enzyme is normally administered by slow intravenous infusion (over a period of 2 h) once every 2 weeks.

Genzyme Corporation were granted marketing authorization in 1991 for a glucocerebrosidase preparation to be used for the treatment of Gaucher's disease. This Genzyme product (trade name Ceredase) was extracted from placentas (afterbirths) obtained from maternity hospital wards. The enzyme displays a molecular mass of 65 kDa and four of its five potential glycosylation sites are glycosylated. It had been estimated that 1 year's supply of enzyme for an average patient required extraction of 27 000 placentas, which renders treatment extremely expensive. Genzyme then gained regulatory approval for a recombinant version of glucocerebrosidase produced in CHO cells. This product (trade name Cerezyme) has been on the market since 1994 and the total world market for glucocerebrosidase is estimated to be in the region of $200 million.

Cerezyme is produced in a CHO cell line harbouring the cDNA coding for human β-glucocerebrosidase. The purified product is presented as a freeze-dried powder and also contains mannitol, sodium citrate, citric acid and polysorbate 80 as excipients. It exhibits a shelf-life of 2 years when stored at 2°C–8°C.

An integral part of the downstream processing process entails the modification of Cerezyme's oligosaccharide components. The native enzyme's sugar side-chains are complex and, for the most part, are capped with a terminal sialic acid or galactose residue. Animal studies indicate that in excess of 95% of injected glucocerebrosidase is removed from the circulation by the liver via binding to hepatocyte surface lectins. As such, the intact enzyme is not available for uptake by the affected cell type — the tissue macrophages. These macrophages display high levels of surface mannose receptors. Treatment of native glucocerebrosidase with exoglycosidases, by removing terminal sugar residues, can expose mannose residues present in their sugar side-chains, resulting in their binding to and uptake by the macrophages. In this way, the 'mannose-engineered' enzyme is selectively targeted to the affected cells.

α-Galactosidase and urate oxidase

Recombinant α-galactosidase and urate oxidase represent two additional biopharmaceuticals recently approved for general medical use. α-Galactosidase is approved for long-term enzyme replacement therapy in patients with Fabry's disease. Like Gaucher's disease, Fabry's disease is a genetic disease of lipid metabolism. Sufferers display little or no liposomal α-galactosidase A activity. This results in the progressive accumulation of glycosphingolipids in several body cell types. Resultant clinical manifestations are complex, affecting the nervous system, vascular endothelial cells and major organs. Although the condition is rare (500–1000 patients within the European Union), untreated sufferers usually die in their 40s or 50s.

Two recombinant α-galactosidase products are now on the market ('Fabrazyme', produced by Genzyme and 'Replagal', produced by TKT Europe). Fabrazyme is produced in an engineered CHO cell line, and downstream processing entails a combination of five chromatographic purification steps, followed by concentration and diafiltration. Excipients added include mannitol and sodium phosphate buffering agents and the final product is freeze-dried after filling into glass vials. Replagal is produced in a continuous human cell line and is also purified by a combination of five chromatographic purification steps, although it is marketed as a liquid solution.

Human α-galactosidase is a 100 kDa homodimeric glycoprotein. Each 398 amino acid monomer displays a molecular mass of 45.3 kDa (excluding the glycocomponent) and is glycosylated at three positions (asparagines 108, 161 and 184). After administration (usually every second week by a 40 min infusion), the enzyme is taken up by various body cell types and directed to the lysosomes. This cellular uptake and delivery process appears to be mediated by mannose-6-phosphate residues present in the oligosaccharide side-chains of the enzyme. Mannose-6-phosphate receptors are found on the surface of various cell types and also intracellularly, associated with the Golgi complex, which then directs the enzyme to the lysosomes.

The enzyme urate oxidase has also found medical application for the treatment of acute hyperuricaemia (elevated plasma uric acid levels), associated with various tumours, particularly during their treatment with chemotherapy.

Uric acid is the end product of purine metabolism in humans, other primates, birds and reptiles. It is produced in the liver by the oxidation of xanthine and hypoxanthine (Figure 9.24) and is excreted via the kidneys. Due to its relatively low solubility, an increase in serum uric acid levels often triggers the formation and precipitation of uric acid crystals, typically resulting in conditions such as gout or urate stones in the urinary tract. Significantly elevated serum uric acid concentrations can also be associated with rapidly proliferating cancers or, in particular, with onset of chemotherapy. In the former instance, rapid cellular turnover results in increased rates of nucleic acid catabolism and hence uric acid production. In the latter case, chemotherapy-induced cellular lysis results in the release of intracellular contents, including free purines and purine-containing nucleic acids, into the bloodstream. The increased associated purine metabolism then triggers hyperuricaemia. The elevated uric acid concentrations often trigger crystal formation in the renal tubules, and hence renal failure.

Purine metabolism in some mammals is characterized by a further oxidation of uric acid to allantoin by the enzyme, urate oxidase. Allantoin is significantly more water-soluble than uric acid and is also freely excreted via the renal route.

Administration of urate oxidase to humans suffering from hyperuricaemia results in the reduction of serum uric acid levels through its conversion to allantoin. Urate oxidase purified

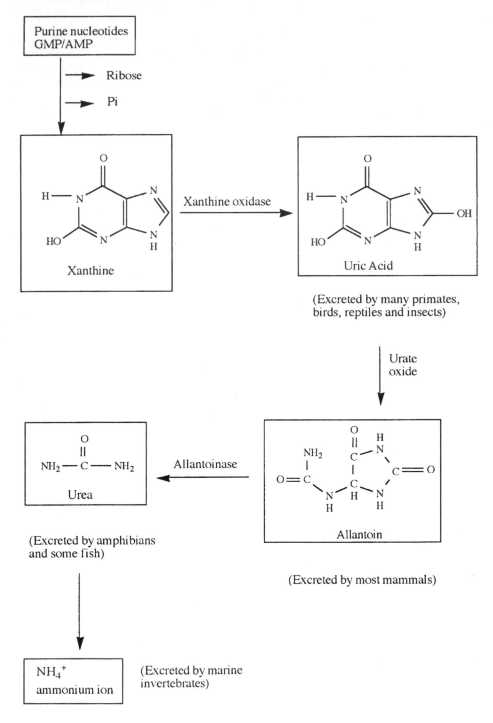

Figure 9.24.   Summary overview of purine metabolism

directly from cultures of the fungus *Aspergillus flavus* has been used to treat this condition for a number of years. More recently, a recombinant form of the fungal enzyme (trade name Fasturtec), has gained regulatory approval in the European Union. Produced in an engineered strain of *S. cerevisiae*, the enzyme is a tetramer composed of four identical polypeptide subunits. Each subunit contains 301 amino acids, displays a molecular mass of 34 kDa and is N-terminal acetylated.

Superoxide dismutase

Under normal circumstances in aerobic metabolism, oxygen is reduced by four electrons, forming H_2O. While this usually occurs uneventfully, incomplete reduction will result in the generation of oxygen radicals and other reactive species. These are: the superoxide radical, O_2^-, hydrogen peroxide (H_2O_2) and the hydroxyl radical (OH^-). The superoxide and hydroxyl radicals are particularly reactive and can attack membrane components, nucleic acids and other cellular macromolecules, leading to their destruction or modification. O_2^- and OH^- radicals, for example, are believed to be amongst the most mutagenic substances generated by ionizing radiation.

Oxygen-utilizing organisms have generally evolved specific enzyme-mediated systems that serve to protect the cell from such reactive species. These enzymes include superoxide dismutase (SOD) and catalase or glutathione peroxidase (GSH-px), which catalyse the following reactions:

$$O_2^{-\cdot} + O_2^{-\cdot} + 2H^+ \xrightarrow{\text{SOD}} H_2O_2 + O_2$$

$$H_2O_2 + H_2O_2 \xrightarrow{\text{Catalase or GSH-px}} 2H_2O + O_2$$

In general, all aerobic organisms harbour these oxygen-defence systems. At least three types of SODs have been identified: a cytosolic eukaryotic dismutase, generally a 31 kDa dimer, containing both copper and zinc; a 75 kDa mitochondrial form and a 40 kDa bacterial form, each of which contain two manganese atoms and an iron-containing form, found in some bacteria, blue-green algae and many plants. The metal ions play a direct role in the catalytic conversion, serving as transient acceptors/donors of electrons.

In humans, increased generation of O_2^- and/or reduced SOD levels have been implicated in a wide range of pathological conditions, including ageing, asthma, accelerated tumour growth, neurodegenerative diseases and inflammatory tissue necrosis. Furthermore, administration of SOD has been found to reduce tissue damage due to irradiation or other conditions that generate O_2^-. Increased SOD production in *Drosophila melanogaster* leads to increased oxygen tolerance and, interestingly, increased lifespan.

SOD isolated from bovine liver or erythrocytes has been used medically as an anti-inflammatory agent. Human SOD has also been expressed in several recombinant systems, and is currently being evaluated to assess its ability to prevent tissue damage induced by exposure to excessively oxygen-rich blood.

Debriding agents

Debridement refers to the process of cleaning a wound by removal of foreign material and dead tissue. Cleansing of the wound facilitates rapid healing and minimizes the risk of infection due to the presence of bacteria at the wound surface. The formation of a clot, followed by a scab, on a wound surface can trap bacteria, which then multiply (usually evidenced by the production of pus), slowing the healing process. Although debridement may be undertaken by physical means (e.g. cutting away dead tissue, washing/cleaning the wound), proteolytic enzymes are also often used to facilitate this process.

The value of proteases in cleansing tissue wounds have been appreciated for several hundred years. Wounds were sometimes cleansed in the past by application of protease-containing maggot saliva. Nowadays, this is usually more acceptably achieved by topical application of the enzyme to the wound surface. In some cases, the enzyme is formulated in an aqueous-based cream, while in others, it is impregnated into special bandages. Trypsin, papain, collagenase and various microbial enzymes have been used in this regard.

Trypsin is a 24 kDa proteolytic enzyme synthesized by the mammalian pancreas in an inactive zymogen form, trypsinogen. Upon its release into the small intestine, it is proteolytically converted into trypsin by an enteropeptidase. Active trypsin plays a digestive role, hydrolysing peptide bonds in which the carboxyl group has been contributed by an arginine or lysine. Trypsin used medically is generally obtained by the enzymatic activation of trypsinogen, extracted from the pancreatic tissue of slaughterhouse animals.

Papain is a cysteine protease isolated from the latex of the immature fruit and leaves of the plant, *Carica papaya*. It consists of a single 23.4 kDa, 212 amino acid polypeptide and the purified enzyme exhibits broad proteolytic activity. Although it can be used as a debriding agent, it is also used for a variety of other industrial processes, including meat tenderizing, and for the clarification of beverages.

Collagenase is a protease that can utilize collagen as a substrate. Although it can be produced by animal cell culture, certain microorganisms also produce this enzyme, most notably certain species of *Clostridium* (the ability of these pathogens to produce collagenase facilitates their rapid spread throughout the body). Collagenase used therapeutically is usually obtained from cell fermentation supernatants of *Clostridium histolyticum*. Such preparations are applied topically to promote debridement of wounds, skin ulcers and burns.

Chymotrypsin has also been utilized to promote debridement, as well as the reduction of soft tissue inflammation. It is also used in some ophthalmic procedures—particularly in facilitating cataract extraction. It is prepared by activation of its zymogen, chymotrypsinogen, which is extracted from bovine pancreatic tissue.

Yet another proteolytic preparation used for debridement of wounds and skin ulcers consists of proteolytic enzymes derived from *Bacillus subtilis*. The preparation displays broad proteolytic activity and is usually applied several times daily to the wound surface.

Digestive aids

A number of enzymes may be used as digestive aids (Table 9.13). In some instances, a single enzymatic activity is utilized, whereas other preparations contain multiple enzyme activities. These enzyme preparations may be used to supplement normal digestive activity, or to confer upon an individual a new digestive capability.

The use of enzymes as digestive aids is only applied under specific medical circumstances. Some medical conditions (e.g. cystic fibrosis) can result in compromised digestive function due to insufficient production/secretion of endogenous digestive enzymes. Digestive enzyme preparations are often formulated in powder (particularly tablet) form, and are recommended to be taken orally immediately prior to or during meals. As the product never enters the blood

Table 9.13. Enzymes that are used as digestive aids

Enzyme	Application
α-Amylase	Aids in digestion of starch
Cellulase	Promotes partial digestion of cellulose
α-Galactosidase	Promotes degradation of flatulance factors
Lactase	Counteracts lactose intolerance
Papain	
Pepsin }	Enhanced degradation of dietary protein
Bromelains	
Pancreatin	Enhanced degradation of dietary carbohydrate, fat and protein

stream, the product purity need not be as stringent as enzymes (or other proteins) administered intravenously. Most digestive enzymes are, at best, semi-pure preparations.

In some instances, there is a possibility that the efficacy of these preparations may be compromised by conditions associated with the digestive tract. Most function at pH values approaching neutrality. They would thus display activity possibly in saliva and particularly in the small intestine. However, the acidic conditions of the stomach (where the pH can be below 1.5), may denature some of these enzymes. Furthermore, the ingested enzymes would also be exposed to endogenous proteolytic activities associated with the stomach and small intestine. Some of these difficulties, however, may be at least partially overcome by formulating the product as a tablet coated with an acid-resistant film to protect the enzyme as it passes through the stomach.

Pancreatin is a pancreatic extract usually obtained from the pancrease of slaughterhouse animals. It contains a mixture of enzymes, principally amylase, protease and lipase and, thus, exhibits a broad digestive capability. It is administered orally, mainly for the treatment of pancreatic insufficiency caused by cystic fibrosis or pancreatitis. As it is sensitive to stomach acid, it must be administered in high doses or, more usually, as enteric coated granules or capsules which may be taken directly, or sprinkled upon the food prior to its ingestion. Individual digestive activities, such as papain, pepsin or bromelains (proteases), or α-amylase are sometimes used in place of pancreatin.

Cellulase is not produced in the human digestive system. Cellulolytic enzyme preparations obtained from *Aspergillus niger* or other fungal sources are available and it is thought that their ingestion may improve overall digestion, particularly in relation to high-fibre diets.

α-Galactosides are oligosaccharides present in plant matter, particularly beans. They are not normally degraded in the human digestive tract due to the absence of an appropriate endogenous digestive enzyme (i.e. an α-galactosidase). However, upon their entry into the large intestine, these oligosaccharides are degraded by microbial α1,6-galactosidases, thus stimulating microbial fermentation. The end-products of fermentation include volatile fatty acids, carbon dioxide, methane and hydrogen, which lead to flatulance. This can be avoided by minimizing dietary intake of food containing α-galactosides. Another approach entails the simultaneous ingestion of tablets containing α-galactosidase activity. If these 'flatulance factors' are degraded before or upon reaching the small intestine, the monosaccharides released will be absorbed and, hence, will subsequently be unavailable to promote undesirable microbial fermentations in the large intestine.

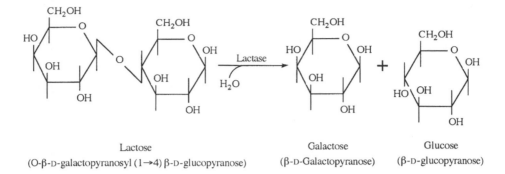

Figure 9.25.   Hydrolysis of lactose by lactase (β-galactosidase)

Lactase

Lactose, the major disaccharide present in milk, is composed of a molecule of glucose linked via a glycosidic bond to a molecule of galactose. The digestive tract of young (suckling) animals generally produces significant quantities of the enzyme β-galactosidase (lactase), which catalyses the hydrolysis of lactose, releasing the constituent monosaccharides (Figure 9.25). This is a prerequisite to their subsequent absorption.

The digestive tract of many adult human populations, however, produce little or no lactase, rendering these individuals lactose-intolerant. This is particularly common in Asia, Africa, Latin America and the Middle East. It severely curtails the ability of these peoples to drink milk without feeling ill. In the absence of sufficient endogenous digestive lactase activity, milk lactose is not absorbed and thus serves as a carbon source for intestinal microorganisms. The resultant production of lactic acid, CO_2 and other gases causes gastrointestinal irritation and diarrhoea. A number of approaches have been adopted in an effort to circumvent this problem. Most involve the application of microbial lactase enzymes. In some instances, the enzyme has been immobilized in a column format, such that passage of milk through the column results in lactose hydrolysis. Free lactase has also been added to milk immediately prior to its bottling, so that lactose hydrolysis can slowly occur prior to its eventual consumption (i.e. during transport and storage).

Fungal and other microbial lactase preparations have also been formulated into tablet form, or sold in powder form. These can be ingested immediately prior to the consumption of milk or lactose-containing milk products, or can be sprinkled over the food before eating it. Such lactose preparations are available in supermarkets in many parts of the world.

FURTHER READING

Books

Becker, R. (2000). *Thrombolytic and Antithrombolytic Therapy.* Oxford University Press, Oxford.
Devlin, T. (1992). *Textbook of Biochemistry with Clinical Correlations*, 3rd edn. Wiley-Liss, New York.
Goodnight, S. (2001). *Disorders of Hemostasis and Thrombosis.* McGraw Hill, New York.
Kirchmaier, C. (1991). *New Aspects on Hirudin.* Karger, Basel.
Lauwers, A. & Scharpe, S. (Eds) (1997). *Pharmaceutical Enzymes.* Marcel Dekker, New York.
Poller, H. (1996). *Oral Anticoagulants.* Arnold, London.

Articles

Plasma proteins, including coagulation factors

Bowen, D. (2002). Haemophilia A and haemophilia B: molecular insights. *J. Clin. Pathol. Mol. Pathol.* **55**(1), 1–18.

Chuang, V. *et al.* (2002). Pharmaceutical strategies utilizing recombinant human serum albumin. *Pharmaceut. Res.* **19**(5), 569–577.

Crevenakova, L. *et al.* (2002). Factor VIII and transmissible spongiform encephalopathy: the case for safety. *Haemophilia* **8**(2), 63–75.

Federici, A. & Mannucci, P. (2002). Advances in the genetics and treatment of von Willebrand disease. *Curr. Opin. Pediat.* **14**(1) 23–33.

Goodey, A. (1993). The production of heterologous plasma proteins. *Trends Biotechnol.* **11**, 430–433.

Kingdon, H & Lundblad, R. (2002). An adventure in biotechnology: the development of haemophilia A therapeutics— from whole blood transfusion to recombinant DNA technology to gene therapy. *Biotechnol. Appl. Biochem.* **35**, 141–148.

Klinge, J. *et al.* (2002) Hemophilia A—from basic science to clinical practice. *Semin. Thrombosis Hemostasis.* **28**(3), 309–321.

Legaz, M. *et al.* (1973). Isolation and characterization of human factor VIII (antihaemophilic factor). *J. Biol. Chem.* **248**, 3946–3955.

Nicholson, J. *et al.* (2000). The role of albumin in critical illness. *Br. J. Anaesth.* **85**(4), 599–610.

Ogden, J. (1992). Recombinant haemoglobin in the development of red blood cell substitutes. *Trends in Biotech.* **10**, 91–95.

Winslow, R. (2000). Blood substitutes: refocusing an elusive goal. *Br. J. Haematol.* **111**(2), 387–396.

Wright, G. *et al.* (1991). High level expression of active human α-1-antitrypsin in the milk of transgenic sheep. *Bio/ Technology* **9**, 830–834.

Anticoagulants and related substances

Dodt, J. (1995). Anti-coagulatory substances of bloodsucking animals: from hirudin to hirudin mimetics. *Angew. Chem. Int. Ed. Engl.* **34**, 867–880.

Eldora, A. *et al.* (1996). The role of the leech in medical therapeutics. *Blood Rev.* **10**(4), 201–209.

Fitzgerald, G. (1996). The human pharmacology of thrombin inhibition. *Coronary Artery Dis.* **7**(12), 911–918.

Markwardt, F. (1991). Hirudin and its derivatives as anticoagulant agents. *Thromb. Haemost.* **66**, 141–152.

Pineo, G. & Hull, R. (1997). Low molecular weight heparin—prophylaxis and treatment of venous thromboembolism. *Ann. Rev. Med.* **48**, 79–91.

Salzet, M. (2002). Leech thrombin inhibitors. *Curr. Pharmaceut. Design* **8**(7), 493–503.

Sawyer, R. (1991). Thrombolytics and anticoagulants from leeches. *Bio/Technology* **9**, 513–518.

Schulman, S. (1996). Anticoagulation in venous thrombosis. *J. R. Soc. Med.* **89**(11), 624–630.

Sohn, J. *et al.* (2001). Current status of the anticoagulant hirudin: its biotechnological production and clinical practice. *Appl. Microbiol. Biotechnol.* **57**(5–6), 606–613.

Tencate, H. *et al.* (1996). Developments in anti-thrombolic therapy—state of the art, anno 1996. *Pharmacy World Sci.* **18**(6), 195–203.

Walker, C & Royston, D. (2002). Thrombin generation and its inhibition: a review of the scientific basis and mechanism of action of anticoagulant therapies. *Br. J. Anaesth.* **88**(6), 848–863.

Thrombolytics

Al-Buhairi, A. & Jan, M. (2002). Recombinant tissue plasminogen activator for acute ischemic stroke. *Saudi Med. J.* **23**(1), 13–19.

Blasi, F. (1999). The urokinase receptor. A cell surface, regulated chemokine. *APMIS* **107**(1), 96–101.

Castillo, P. *et al.* (1997). Cost-effectiveness of thrombolytic therapy for acute myocardial infarction. *Ann. Pharmacother.* **31**(5), 596–603.

Collen, D. & Lijnen, H. (1994). Staphylokinase, a fibrin-specific plasminogen activator with therapeutic potential? *Blood* **84**(3), 680–686.

Collen, D. (1998). Staphylokinase: a potent, uniquely fibrin-selective thrombolytic agent. *Nature Med.* **4**(3), 279–284.

Collins, R. *et al.* (1997). Drug therapy—aspirin, heparin and fibrinolytic therapy in suspected acute myocardial infarction. *N. Engl. J. Med.* **336**(12), 847–860.

Datar, R. *et al.* (1993). Process economics of animal cell and bacterial fermentations: a case study analysis of tissue plasminogen activator. *Bio/Technology* **11**, 349–357.

Emeis, J. *et al.* (1997). Progress in clinical fibrinolysis. *Fibrinolysis Proteolysis* **11**(2), 67–84.

Gillis, J. *et al.* (1995). Alteplase. A reappraisal of its pharmacological properties and therapeutic use in acute myocardial infarction. *Drugs* **50**(1), 102–136.

Marder, V. & Stewart, D. (2002). Towards safer thrombolytic therapy. *Semin. Haematol.* **39**(3), 206–216.

Preissner, K. *et al.* (2000). Urokinase receptor: a molecular organizer in cellular communication. *Curr. Opin. Cell Biol.* **12**(5), 621–628.

Rabasseda, X. (2001). Tenecteplase (TNK tissue plasminogen activator): a new fibrinolytic for the acute treatment of myocardial infarction. *Drugs Today* **37**(11), 749–760.

Schoebel, F. *et al.* (1997). Antithrombotic treatment in stable coronary syndromes—long-term intermittent urokinase therapy in end-stage coronary-artery disease and refractory angina pectoris. *Heart* **77**(1), 13–17.

Tsirka, S. (1997). Clinical implications of the involvement of tPA in neuronal cell death. *J. Mol. Med.* **75**(5), 341–347.

Verstraete, M. *et al.* (1995). Thrombolytic agents in development. *Drugs,* **50**(1), 29–42.

Verstraete, M. (2000). Third generation thrombolyic drugs. *Am. J. Med.* **109**(1), 52–58.

Enzyme therapeutics

Barranger, J. *et al.* (1995). Molecular biology of glucocerebrosidase and the treatment of Gaucher's disease. *Cytokines Mol. Ther.* **1**(3), 149–163.

Chakrabarti, R. & Schuster, S. (1997). L-Asparaginase—perspectives on the mechanisms of action and resistance. *Int. J. Pediat. Haematol./Oncol.* **4**(6), 597–611.

Chapple, L. (1997). Reactive oxygen species and antioxidants in inflammatory diseases. *J. Clin. Periodontol.* **24**(5), 287–296.

Conway, S. & Littlewood, J. (1997). rhDNase in cystic fibrosis. *Br. J. Hosp. Med.* **57**(8), 371–372.

Conway, S. & Watson, A. (1997). Nebulized bronchodilators, corticosteroids and rhDNase in adult patients with cystic fibrosis. *Thorax* **52**(2), S64–S68.

Edgington, S. (1993). Nuclease therapeutics in the clinic. *Bio/Technology* **11**, 580–582.

James, E. (1994). Superoxide dismutase. *Parasitol. Today* **10**(12), 482–484.

Mistry, P & Cox, T. (1993). The glucocerebrosidase locus in Gaucher's disease—molecular analysis of a lysosomal enzyme. *J. Med. Genet.* **30**(11), 889–894.

Ronghe, M. *et al.* (2001). Remission induction therapy for childhood acute lymphoblastic leukaemia: clinical and cellular pharmacology of vincristine, corticosteroids, L-asparaginase and anthracyclines. *Cancer Treat. Rev.* **27**(6), 327–337.

Welsh, M. & Smith, A. (1995). Cystic fibrosis. *Sci. Am.* (December), 36–43.

Wileman, T. (1991). Properties of asparaginase–dextran conjugates. *Adv. Drug Delivery Rev.* **6**(2), 167–180.

Zhao, H & Grabowski. G. (2002). Gaucher's disease: perspectives on a prototype lysosomal disease. *Cell. Mol. Life Sci.* **59**(4), 694–707.

Chapter 10
Antibodies, vaccines and adjuvants

Few substances have had a greater positive impact upon human healthcare management than antibodies, vaccines and adjuvants. For most of this century, these immunological agents have enjoyed widespread medical application, predominantly for the treatment/prevention of infectious diseases. As a group, they are often referred to as 'biologics' (generally speaking, the term 'biologic' refers to vaccines, serum, toxins and medicinal products derived from human blood or plasma; Chapter 1).

Polyclonal antibody preparations have been used to induce passive immunity against a range of foreign (harmful) agents, while vaccines are used to efficiently and safely promote active immunization. Adjuvants are usually co-administered with the vaccine preparation, in order to enhance the immune response against the vaccine. The development of modern biotechnological methodology has had an enormous impact upon the therapeutic application of immunological agents, as discussed later. Monoclonal/engineered antibodies find a range of therapeutic uses, while many of the newer vaccine preparations are now produced by recombinant DNA technology.

POLYCLONAL ANTIBODY PREPARATIONS

Polyclonal antibody preparations have been used for several decades to induce passive immunization against infectious diseases and other harmful agents, particularly toxins. The antibody preparations are usually administered by direct i.v. injection. While this affords immediate immunological protection, its effect is transitory, usually persisting for only 2–3 weeks (i.e. until the antibodies are excreted). Passive immunization can be used prophylactically (i.e. to prevent a future medical episode) or therapeutically (i.e. to treat a medical condition that is already established). An example of the former would be prior administration of a specific anti-snake toxin antibody preparation to an individual before he/she travelled to a world region in which these snakes are commonly found. An example of the latter would be administration of the anti-venom antibody immediately after the individual has experienced a snake bite.

Antibody preparations used to induce passive immunity may be obtained from either animal or human sources. Preparations of animal origin are generally termed 'antisera', while those sourced from humans are called 'immunoglobulin preparations'. In both cases, the predominant antibody type present is immunoglobulin G (IgG).

Biopharmaceuticals: Biochemistry and Biotechnology, Second Edition by Gary Walsh
John Wiley & Sons Ltd: ISBN 0 470 84326 8 (ppc), ISBN 0 470 84327 6 (pbk)

Antisera are generally produced by immunizing healthy animals (e.g. horses) with appropriate antigen. Small samples of blood are subsequently withdrawn from the animal on a regular basis and quantitatively analysed for the presence of the desired antibodies (often using ELISA-based immunoassays). This facilitates harvesting of the blood at the most appropriate time points. Large animals, such as horses, can withstand withdrawal of 1–2 l of blood every 10–14 days and antibody levels are usually maintained by administration of repeat antigen booster injections.

The blood is collected using aseptic technique into sterile containers. It can then be allowed to clot, with subsequent recovery of the antibody-containing antisera by centrifugation. Alternatively, the blood may be collected in the presence of heparin, or another suitable anti-coagulant, with subsequent removal of the suspended cellular elements, again by centrifugation. In this case, the resultant antibody-containing solution is termed 'plasma'.

The antibody fraction is then purified from the serum (or plasma). Traditionally, this entailed precipitation steps, usually using ethanol and/or ammonium sulphate as precipitants. The precipitated antibody preparations, however, are only partially purified and modern preparations are generally subjected to additional high-resolution chromatographic fractionation (Figure 10.1). Ion-exchange chromatography is often employed, as is protein A affinity chromatography (IgG from many species binds fairly selectively to protein A).

Following high-resolution purification, the antibody titre is determined, usually using an appropriate bioassay or an immunoassay. Stabilizing agents, such as NaCl (0.9% w/v) or glycine (2–3% w/v) are often added, as are anti-microbial preservatives. Addition of preservative is particularly important if the product is subsequently filled into multi-dose containers. Phenol, at concentrations less than 0.25%, is often used. After adjustment of the potency to fall within specification, the product is sterile-filtered and aseptically filled into sterile containers. These are sealed immediately if the product is to be marketed in liquid form. Such antibody solutions are often filled under an oxygen-free nitrogen atmosphere in order to prevent oxidative degradation during subsequent storage. Such a product, if stored at 2–8°C, should exhibit a shelf-life of up to 5 years.

As is the case with all other pharmaceutical substances, all aspects of antisera production must be undertaken by means conducive to the principles of GMP. Most regulatory authorities publish guidelines which outline acceptable standards/procedures for the production of such blood-derived products. Donor animals must be healthy and screened for the presence of (particularly blood-borne) pathogens. They must be housed in appropriate animal facilities, and withdrawal of blood must be undertaken by aseptic technique. Subsequent downstream processing must be undertaken according to the principles of GMP, as laid down in Chapter 3.

While specific antisera have proved invaluable in the treatment of a variety of medical conditions (Table 10.1), they can also induce unwanted side effects. Particularly noteworthy is their ability to induce hypersensitivity reactions. While some such sensitivity reactions (e.g. 'serum sickness') are often not acute, others (e.g. anaphylaxis) can be life-threatening. Because of such risks, antibody preparations derived from human donors (i.e. immunoglobulins) are usually preferred as passive immunizing agents.

Immunoglobulins are purified from the serum (or plasma) of human donors by methods similar to those used to purify animal-derived antibodies. In most instances, the immunoglobulin preparations are enriched in antibodies capable of binding to a specific antigen (usually an infectious microorganism/virus). These may be purified from donated blood of individuals who have:

- recently been immunized against the antigen of interest;
- recently recovered from an infection caused by the antigen of interest.

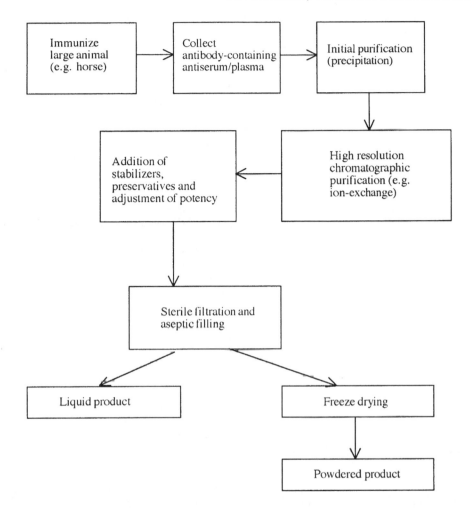

Figure 10.1. Overview of the production of antisera for therapeutic use to induce passive immunization. Refer to text for specific details

Although hypersensitivity reactions can occur upon administration of immunoglobulin preparations, the incidence of such events are far less frequent than is the case upon administration of antibody preparations of animal origin. As with all blood-derived products, the serum from which the immunoglobulins are due to be purified is first assayed for the presence of infectious agents before its use.

The major polyclonal antibody preparations used therapeutically are listed in Table 10.1. These may generally be categorized into one of several groups, on the basis of their target specificities. These groups include:

- antibodies raised against specific microbial or viral pathogens;
- antibodies raised against microbial toxins;
- antibodies raised against snake/spider venoms (anti-venins).

Table 10.1. Polyclonal antibody preparations of human or animal origin used to induce passive immunity against specific biological agents

Antibody	Source	Specificity
Anti-D immunoglobulin	Human	Specificity against rhesus D antigen
Botulism antitoxin	Horse	Specificity against toxins of type A, B or E *Clostridium botulinum*
Cytomegalovirus immunoglobulin	Human	Antibodies exhibiting specificity for cytomegalovirus
Diphtheria antitoxin	Horse	Antibodies raised against diphtheria toxoid
Diphtheria immunoglobulin	Human	Antibodies exhibiting specificity for diphtheria toxoid
Endotoxin antibodies	Horse	Antibodies raised against Gram-negative bacterial lipopolysaccharide
Gas gangrene antitoxins	Horse	Antibodies raised against α-toxin of *Clostridum novyi*, *C. perfringens* and *C. septicum*
Haemophilus influenzae immunoglobulins	Human	Antibodies raised against surface capsular polysaccharide of *Haemophilus influenzae*
Hepatitis A immunoglobulin	Human	Specificity against hepatitis A surface antigen
Hepatitis B immunoglobulin	Human	Specificity against hepatitis B surface antigen
Leptospira antisera	Animal	Antibodies raised against *Leptospira icterohaemorrhagiae* (used to treat Weil's disease)
Measles immunoglobulin	Human	Specificity against measles virus
Normal immunoglobulin	Human	Specificities against variety of infectious and other biological agents prevalent in general population
Rabies immunoglobulin	Human	Specificity against rabies virus
Scorpion venom antisera	Horse	Specificity against venom of one or more species of scorpion
Snake venom antisera	Horse	Antibodies raised against venom of various poisonous snakes
Spider antivenins	Horse	Antibodies raised against venom of various spiders
Tetanus antitoxin	Horse	Specificity against toxin of *Clostridium tetani*
Tetanus immunoglobulin	Human	Specificity against toxin of *Clostridium tetani*
Tick-borne encephalitis immunoglobulin	Human	Antibodies against tick-borne encephalitis virus
Varicella-zoster virus immunoglobulin	Human	Specificity for causative agent of chicken pox

Anti-D immunoglobulin

In addition to the major blood group antigens (i.e. A and B), a number of additional erythrocyte alloantigens (antigens that differ between individuals of the same species) are known to exist. These include the rhesus antigen (Rh-antigen), of which a number of related gene products exist. By far the most significant Rh-antigen is known as the 'D' antigen.

Due to the gene's dominant inheritance pattern, when an Rh-negative female becomes pregnant by an Rh-positive male, the fetal erythrocytes will be Rh-positive. Although small quantities of fetal blood enter the maternal circulation during pregnancy, the levels generally appear insufficient to stimulate a strong maternal immunological reaction. However, during childbirth, significant quantities of fetal blood cells do enter the maternal circulation. In the normal course of events, this effectively immunizes the mother against the Rh-antigen. This can endanger fetal health during subsequent pregnancies, as maternal anti-Rh antibodies can cross the placenta and enter the fetal circulation. Binding of anti-Rh antibodies to fetal erythrocytes can induce haemolysis. This results in medical complications, with the newborn baby often suffering from erythroblastosis fetalis (haemolytic disease of the newborn). Moreover, with each successive birth, the mother effectively receives booster shots of Rh-antigen. After several pregnancies, maternal anti-Rh antibody levels can be sufficiently high to threaten fetal viability.

This scenario can be prevented by administration of anti-Rh (usually anti-D) antibodies to Rh-negative mothers immediately upon the birth of a Rh-positive baby. The administered antibodies bind the fetal Rh-positive erythrocytes, marking them for destruction before a maternal immunological reaction is triggered. Usually a dose of 200–300 μg of antibody is administered immediately post-delivery. This would be sufficient to suppress an immune response for up to 10 ml of Rh-positive red blood cells.

The anti-D immunological preparations used are purified from the serum or plasma of Rh-negative individuals who have been immunized against Rh-D antigen. The purified antibody preparations may be marketed as a liquid (shelf-life of 2 years when stored refrigerated) or as a freeze-dried preparation, which exhibits a shelf-life of up to 5 years.

Normal immunoglobulins

Normal immunoglobulins (often termed 'immune globulins' in the USA) represent antibody preparations purified from the plasma, serum or placentas of normal, healthy donors. Blood obtained from such individuals will contain a wide range of antibody specificities. The range of specificities were produced over many years, as the individual's immune system came into contact with various antigens, either naturally (infections) or artificially (by vaccination).

Normal immunoglobulin preparations are purified from pooled material obtained from 1000 or more donors. They will generally contain antibodies against diphtheria, measles, poliomyelitis, hepatitis A, rubella and varicella. Normal immunoglobulin may, therefore, be used to provide passive immunization against these diseases.

Therapeutic antibody preparations generally contain in excess of 90% IgG, the concentration of which is usually greater than 10 times the average starting concentration in the original pooled material. The final protein concentration is generally 15–16% (w/v). Stabilizers (often glycine) may be added, as may preservatives—but only to product destined for sale as liquid preparations. Aqueous preparations retain potency for 3 years when stored refrigerated. Alternatively, the product may be freeze-dried and stored in the final product container under vacuum or an inert gas (e.g. N_2). Such preparations are generally assigned shelf-lives of 5 years.

Hepatitis B and tetanus immunoglobulin

Hepatitis B immunoglobulin is an example of an antibody preparation known to contain antibodies displaying a specificity for a specific pathogen, in this case hepatitis B virus. Hepatitis B immunoglobulins are purified from the serum or plasma of donors who exhibit high titres of anti-hepatitis B surface antigen (HBsAg) antibodies. IgG represents in excess of 80% of the total protein in the product. As in the case of other immunoglobulin preparations, it may be marketed as a liquid or freeze-dried preparation.

Hepatitis B immunoglobulins are administered to persons who have come into contact with hepatitis B, including newborn infants whose mothers have recently been infected with the virus.

Tetanus immunoglobulin is an example of an antibody preparation used to induce passive immunization against a microbial toxin. Tetanus (lockjaw) is an infectious disease caused by the bacterium, *Clostridium tetani*. Bacterial spores can commonly contaminate surface wounds and the resulting bacterial cells produce a toxin as they multiply. The toxin interferes with normal neurological function, particularly at neuromuscular junctions. The result is spasmodic contraction of muscles and, if untreated, mortality rates are high. Treatment with antibiotics and anti-toxin, however, is highly effective if administered promptly.

Tetanus antitoxin is routinely administered as part of the management of tetanus-prone wounds. The antibody preparation is purified from pooled serum/plasma of human donors who have been immunized with tetanus toxin.

Snake and spider antivenins

Polyclonal antibody preparations raised against toxins of poisonous snakes and spiders (i.e. venins), are used in the medical management of individuals who have suffered bites from these creatures. In many instances immediate administration of the appropriate antiserum can prevent almost certain death.

Venomous snakes can be largely categorized as Viperidae (Vipers), Elapidae (cobras, kraits and mambas) and Hydrophiidae (sea snakes). The venom of these snakes consists largely of complex protein mixtures, some of which display enzymatic activity. In general, snake venom antiserum is prepared by injecting healthy horses with (usually inactivated) venom, or a mixture of venoms (i.e. monovalent or polyvalent preparations). The resultant antibodies are subsequently purified by the general scheme outlined in Figure 10.1. The requirement for supplies of specific antivenins obviously varies from region to region, being dependent upon the snake species indigenous to a particular area. Some of the major antivenins available commercially are listed in Table 10.2.

In the UK, the adder (*Vipera berus*) represents the only indigenous poisonous snake and adder antivenin preparations are termed 'Zagreb antisera'. European viper venom antisera contain antibodies capable of neutralizing the venoms of one or more species of viper (*Vipera ammodytes*, *V. aspis*, *V. berus* and *V. ursinii*). In many instances, antivenin preparations are polyvalent in nature. This is particularly helpful in cases where the victims are unsure of which snake actually bit them.

Antivenins capable of neutralizing the toxins present in the venom of various poisonous spiders are also available. The major preparations available include *Latrodectus mactans* antivenin, which contains antibodies raised against the venom of the black widow spider, and

Table 10.2. Some polyclonal antibody preparations raised in horses against specific snake toxins

Antivenin preparation	Confers immunological protection (passive immunity) against
Zagreb antivenin	Adder bites
European viper venom antisera	One or more species of viper
Polyvalent Crotalidae antivenin	Any one of four species of pit viper (including Western diamond back and South American rattlesnake
Micrurus fulvius antivenin	Eastern coral snake (*Micrurus fulvius*)
Australian polyvalent antivenins	Any one or combination of: black snake, brown snake, death adder, taipan and tiger snake

antivenins that neutralize the venom of the funnel-web spider (*Atrax robustus*). Scorpion venom antisera preparations are also available. These neutralize the venom produced by one or more species of scorpion. The stings of scorpions found in Africa and the Middle East are usually not fatal. However, South and Central American scorpion stings quite often result in death.

MONOCLONAL ANTIBODIES

In the last 20 years or so, antibody-based therapeutics have mainly focused upon the medical application of monoclonal antibodies. Monoclonal antibody technology was first developed in the mid-1970s, when Kohler and Milstein successfully fused immortal myeloma cells with antibody-producing B lymphocytes. A proportion of the resultant hybrids were found to be stable, cancerous, antibody-producing cells. These 'hybridoma' cells represented an inexhaustible source of monospecific (monoclonal) antibody. Hybridoma technology facilitates the relatively straightforward production of monospecific antibodies against virtually any desired antigen.

The production process (Box 10.1) entails initial immunization of a mouse with the antigen of interest. The mouse is subsequently sacrificed and its spleen removed (the spleen is an organ enriched in B lymphocytes. Because of the immunization process, a significant proportion of these lymphocytes are likely capable of producing antibodies recognizing specific epitopes on the antigen).

Spleen-derived B lymphocytes are then incubated with mouse myeloma cells in the presence of propylene glycol. This promotes fusion of the cells. The resultant immortalized antibody-producing hybridomas are subsequently selected from unfused cells by culture in a specific

---

Box 10.1.   The basis of monoclonal antibody production by hybridoma technology

When antigen enters the body, it stimulates an immune response. A major element of this response entails activation of selected B lymphocytes to produce antibodies capable of binding the antigen (the humoral immune response). The binding of antibody can reduce/inactivate the biological activity of the antigen (especially if it is, for example, a toxin) and also marks the antigen for destruction by other elements of the immune system. Any given antibody will bind only to a specific region of the antigen called an epitope (in the example shown, the antigen contains just three epitopes). Most antigens encountered naturally (e.g. proteins, viruses, bacteria, etc.) contain hundreds, if not thousands, of different epitopes. A typical epitope region on a protein surface would comprise of 5–7 amino acid residues. Each specific antibody, which recognizes a specific epitope, is produced by a specific B lymphocyte. If one single antibody-producing cell could be isolated and cultured *in vitro*, it would be a source of monoclonal (monospecific) antibody. However, B lymphocytes die after a short time when cultured *in vitro*, and hence are an impractical source of long-term antibody production.

Monoclonal antibody technology entails isolation of such B lymphocytes, with subsequent fusion of these cells with transformed (myeloma) cells. Many of the resultant hybrid cells retain immortal characteristics, while producing large quantities of the monospecific antibody. These hybridoma cells can be cultured long term to effectively produce an inexhaustible supply of the monoclonal antibody of choice.

Box 10.1.   (*Continued*)

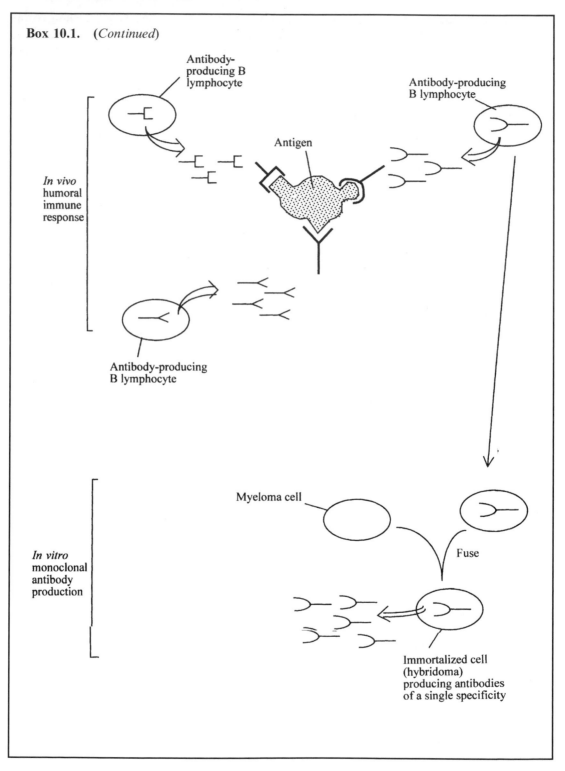

In vivo humoral immune response

Antibody-producing B lymphocyte

Antibody-producing B lymphocyte

Antigen

Antibody-producing B lymphocyte

In vitro monoclonal antibody production

Myeloma cell

Fuse

Immortalized cell (hybridoma) producing antibodies of a single specificity

selection medium. Individual hybridomas can be separated from each other by simple dilution and subsequently grown in culture, producing a clone. Individual clones can be screened to identify which ones produce murine (monoclonal) antibody, which binds the antigen of interest. Appropriate clones are then selected and grown on a larger scale in order to produce biotechnologically useful quantities of antibody.

Production of monoclonals via hybridoma technology

The culture of hybridomas, thereby producing monoclonal antibodies, may be undertaken by ascites production or by direct animal cell culture. Ascites production entails injection of the hybridoma cells into the peritoneal cavity of mice (the mice essentially serve as a live fermentation chamber). The transplanted hybridoma cells produce antibody as they grow. Ascitic fluid collects in the cavity, which contains high concentrations (up to 15 mg/ml) of the desired antibody. On average, 5 ml of this fluid can be extracted per mouse. Most of the earlier monoclonal antibody preparations were produced in this manner, e.g. OKT-3, the first monoclonal antibody to be approved for therapeutic use by the FDA (see later), is produced using this strategy.

Ascites production, however, suffers from a number of drawbacks. It is costly, and the product is contaminated by significant levels of various mouse proteins, rendering subsequent downstream processing more complex. As a result, monoclonal antibody production by standard animal cell culture techniques has become the method of choice for the production of pharmaceutical-grade monoclonal antibody preparations.

Optimal fermentation parameters have been well established and air-lift, stirred tank, and hollow fibre systems have all been used. At commercial scale, fermentation volumes in excess of 1000 litres can be used, which can yield 100 g or more of final product. While hybridoma growth is straightforward, production levels of antibody can be quite low compared with ascites-based production systems. Typically, fermentation yields antibody concentrations of 0.1–0.5 mg/ml. Removal of cells from the antibody-containing media is achieved by centrifugation or filtration. An ultrafiltration step is then normally undertaken in order to concentrate the filtrate by up to 20-fold.

The concentrated extract is next subjected to 2–4 chromatographic purification steps (Figure 10.2). These serve not only to remove contaminating proteins but also to reduce or remove additional contaminants, including nucleic acids, endotoxin and adventitious agents. Affinity chromatography on protein A agarose columns is often employed as a high-resolution initial (IgG) purification step. The selectivity of protein A for most sub-species of IgG results in a high degree of purification, while maintaining a high product yield. This step is often followed by ion-exchange chromatography. Often both anion and cation exchange steps are undertaken sequentially. In some instances, hydrophobic interaction chromatography is also employed. Gel filtration is usually used as the final polishing step, yielding an essentially pure antibody preparation.

Depending upon the intended application, the antibody may next be conjugated to specific molecular tags (e.g. a radionuclide or toxin). Finally, stabilizing agents (e.g. buffer components, glycine or sometimes human serum albumin) are added to the product. This is then aseptically filled into the final containers after sterile filtration. The product is then usually freeze-dried and sealed under an atmosphere of an inert gas.

As with all biopharmaceuticals, strict and numerous QC checks are made upon the product during all stages of manufacture. Because some issues of GMP are particularly relevant or

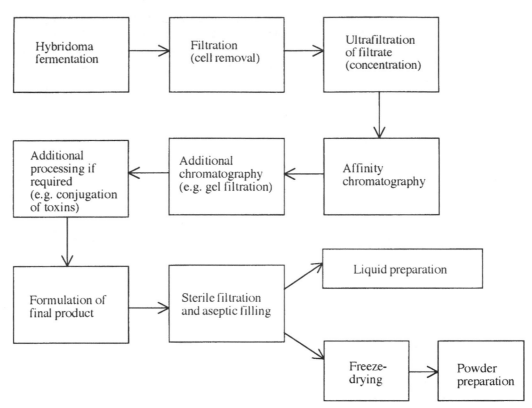

Figure 10.2. Overview of the production by hybridoma cell culture of monoclonal antibodies destined for pharmaceutical use. Refer to text for specific details

unique to monoclonal antibody production, most regulatory authorities publish specific supplemental GMP guidelines. Examples include the FDA's *Points to Consider in the Manufacture and Testing of Monoclonal Antibody Products for Human Use.*

Antibody screening: phage display technology

Phage display technology provides an extremely powerful way to generate a library of (protein) ligands and subsequently screen these ligands for their ability to bind a selected target molecule. The technique, as the name implies, employs filamentous 'phage' (bacteriophage), which replicate in *E. coli.*

The principle of phage display is presented in Figure 10.3. A library of genes (one of which codes for the protein of interest) is first generated/obtained. These genes are inserted (batch-cloned) into a phage library fused to a gene encoding one of the phage coat proteins (pIII, pIV or pVIII). The phage are then incubated with *E. coli*, which facilitates phage replication. Expression of the fusion gene product during replication and the subsequent incorporation of the fusion product into the mature phage coat results in the gene product being 'presented' on the phage surface. The entire phage library can then be screened in order to identify the one(s) coding for the protein of interest. This is usually achieved by affinity selection (biopanning).

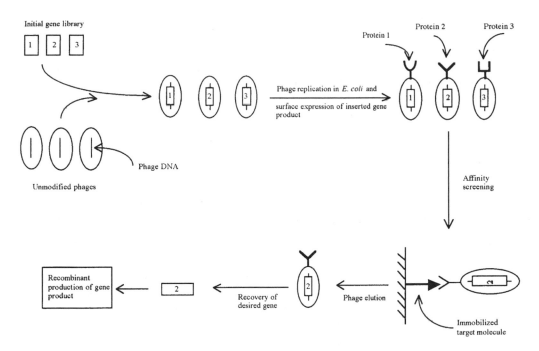

Figure 10.3. Phage display technology and the screening of a library for a protein capable of binding to a desired target molecule. In this simplified example, an initial library of three genes are inserted into three phages. One (gene 2) codes for the desired protein. In reality, libraries typically consist of hundreds of thousands/millions of different genes. Refer to text for further details

Biopanning entails passing the library over immobilized target molecules, usually in immobilized column format. Only the phage expressing the protein of desired specificity should be retained in the immobilized column. The bound phage can subsequently be eluted, e.g. by reducing the pH of the elution buffer or inclusion of a competitive ligand — usually free target molecules — in the buffer. Eluted phage can then be repassed over the affinity column in order to isolate those binding the immobilized ligand with the highest specificity/affinity. Once this is achieved, the gene coding for the protein of interest can be excised from the phage genome by standard techniques of molecular biology. It can then be incorporated into an appropriate microbial/animal cell/transgenic expression system (Chapter 3), facilitating large-scale production of the gene product. Variations of the phage display approach have been developed, some of which utilize engineered phage (phagemids), while others achieve library expression, not on the surface of phage but on the surface of bacteria.

Amongst the first and still most prominent application of phage display technology is the production and screening of antibody libraries in order to isolate/identify an antibody capable of binding to a desired target molecule. As such, this technology has now come to the fore in identifying antibodies suited to clinical application.

Genes/cDNA libraries coding for antibodies or antigen-binding antibody fragments have been obtained from human and animal (e.g. mice, rabbit and chicken) sources. Two types of library can be generated. 'Immune libraries' are obtained by cloning antibody or antibody fragment coding sequences derived from B lymphocytes (usually from spleens) of donors previously immunized with the target antigen. A high number of hits (positive clones) should be obtained from such libraries.

Non-immune libraries are produced in a similar fashion, but using B lymphocytes from non-immunized donors as a source of antibody genes. This approach becomes necessary if initial immunization with the antigen of interest is not possible (due to ethical considerations, for example). While such libraries will generate a lower number of positive clones, they can be screened against multiple antigens. Such native non-immune libraries can also be the starting point for the generation of so-called 'synthetic immune libraries'. Their generation entails initial *in vitro* engineering of the non-immune library of antibody genes in order to increase still further the level of antibody diversity generated.

Therapeutic application of monoclonal antibodies

The unrivalled specificity of monoclonal antibodies, coupled with their relatively straightforward production and their continuity of supply, renders them attractive biochemical tools. Therapeutically, they represent by far the single largest category of biopharmaceutical substances under investigation. Several hundred such preparations are currently undergoing pre-clinical and clinical trials. Throughout the 1980s the focus of attention rested upon their use as either *in vivo* imaging (i.e. diagnostic) agents or direct therapeutic agents. Initial studies centred mainly around cancer, but monoclonal antibody preparations are now used in a variety of other medical circumstances (Table 10.3).

All *in vivo* diagnostic/therapeutic applications are dependent upon the selective interaction of a monoclonal antibody with a specific target cell type in the body (e.g. a cancer cell). Therefore, a prerequisite to application of monoclonal antibody-based products in this way is the identification of a cell surface antigen unique to the target cell type (Figure 10.4). Once identified and characterized, monoclonal antibodies may be raised against that unique surface antigen (USAg). The specificity of antibody-antigen binding should ensure that, once injected into the body, the antibody will selectively congregate on the surface of only the target cells. Depending upon the specific intended therapeutic/diagnostic application, the antibodies employed may have nothing attached to them or may be conjugated to a radioisotope, drug or toxin (Figure 10.4). With the latter approaches, the antibody is used as a 'magic bullet', delivering a radioactive/drug load to specific cells in the body. All of these various strategies have been adopted in practice and specific examples will be provided in subsequent sections of this chapter.

In the context of antibody-mediated cell targeting, it is also important to appreciate that binding of an antibody to a USAg can, by itself, trigger a number of responses. In some instances, the antibody–antigen (Ab–USAg) complex is quickly internalized. In other instances, the Ab-USAg complex is shed from the cell surface, while in yet other cases binding induces neither response. The specific response triggered is generally only determined by direct experimentation. The induction of Ab–USAg shedding renders an anti-TSA antibody clinically useless.

Table 10.3.   Range of clinical applications of monoclonal antibodies

Induction of passive immunity
Diagnostic imaging (e.g. of cancer, infectious diseases, cardiovascular disease and
    deep vein thrombosis)
Therapy for cancers, transplantations and cardiovascular disease

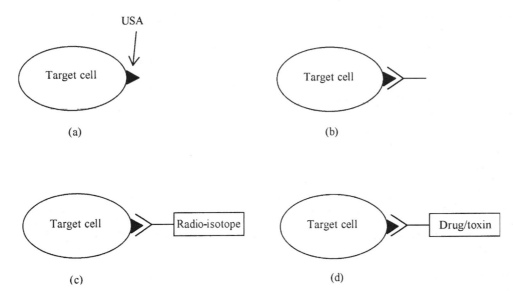

Figure 10.4. Underlying principle/approaches taken during the development and use of antibody-mediated target cell detection and destruction. A prerequisite for adoption of this strategy is the identification and characterization of a surface antigen unique to the target cell type (unique surface antigen, USA or USAg) (a). Antibodies raised against the USA should selectively interact with the target cell (b). In some instances the antibody is chemically coupled to a radioactive tag (c), a drug or a toxin (d)

By mid-2002, a total of 20 such antibody-based products had gained marketing approval in some world regions at least (Table 10.4). Over half of these aim to detect/treat various cancers and cancer represents the single most significant indication for antibody-based products currently in clinical trials. The application of antibodies in the context of cancer is overviewed in the next section. A minority of the products approved or in trials are intact antibodies produced by classical hybridoma technology. The majority are engineered antibodies ('chimaeric' or 'humanized') or antibody fragments. The generation and rationale for use of such engineered products is also discussed subsequently in this chapter.

Tumour immunology

Some elements of tumour immunology have already been discussed in the context of IL-2 and cancer treatment (Chapter 5). To recap, the transformation of a cell to the cancerous state is normally associated with increased surface expression of antigens recognized as foreign by the host immune system. These surface antigens, often termed tumour antigens or tumour surface antigens, are either not expressed at all by the untransformed cell or are expressed at such low levels that they fail to induce immunological tolerance.

The presence of tumour-specific antigens implies that the immune system should be capable of recognizing and destroying transformed cells. This concept, known as immunosurveillance, probably does function to some extent in the body. The immune system does respond to the presence of some tumours, causing their partial or complete regression. The major anti-tumour immune elements include:

Table 10.4. Monoclonal/engineered antibodies thus far approved for medical use. The sponsoring companies and therapeutic indications are also listed

Product	Company	Indication
CEA-scan (Arcitumomab, murine monoclonal antibody (Mab) fragment (Fab), directed against human carcinoembryonic antigen, CEA)	Immunomedics	Detection of recurrent/ metastatic colorectal cancer
MyoScint (Imiciromab-Pentetate, murine Mab fragment directed against human cardiac myosin)	Centocor	Myocardial infarction imaging agent
OncoScint CR/OV (Satumomab Pendetide, murine Mab directed against TAG-72, a high molecular weight tumour-associated glycoprotein)	Cytogen	Detection/staging/follow-up of colorectal and ovarian cancers
Orthoclone OKT3 (Muromomab CD3, murine Mab directed against the T lymphocyte surface antigen CD3)	Ortho Biotech	Reversal of acute kidney transplant rejection
ProstaScint (Capromab Pentetate, murine Mab directed against the tumour surface antigen PSMA)	Cytogen	Detection/staging/follow-up of prostate adeno-carcinoma
ReoPro (Abciximab, Fab fragments derived from a chimaeric Mab, directed against the platelet surface receptor $GPII_b/III_a$)	Centocor	Prevention of blood clots
Rituxan (Rituximab chimaeric Mab directed against CD20 antigen found on the surface of B lymphocytes)	Genentech/IDEC Pharmaceuticals	Non-Hodgkin's lymphoma
Verluma (Nofetumomab, murine Mab fragments (Fab) directed against carcinoma-associated antigen)	Boehringer Ingelheim/ NeoRx	Detection of small cell lung cancer
Zenapax (Daclizumab, humanized Mab directed against the α-chain of the IL-2 receptor)	Hoffman La Roche	Prevention of acute kidney transplant rejection
Simulect (Basiliximab, chimaeric Mab directed against the α-chain of the IL-2 receptor)	Novartis	Prophylaxis of acute organ rejection in allogeneic renal transplantation
Remicade (Infliximab, chimaeric Mab directed against TNF-α)	Centocor	Treatment of Crohn's disease
Synagis (Palivizumab, humanized Mab directed against an epitope on the surface of respiratory syncytial virus)	MedImmune (USA) Abbott (EU)	Prophylaxis of lower respiratory tract disease caused by respiratory syncytial virus in paediatric patients
Herceptin (Trastuzumab, humanized antibody directed against HER2, i.e. human epidermal growth factor receptor 2)	Genentech (USA) Roche Registration (EU)	Treatment of metastatic breast cancer if tumour overexpresses HER2 protein
Indimacis 125 (Igovomab, murine Mab fragment (Fab_2) directed against the tumour-associated antigen CA 125)	CIS Bio	Diagnosis of ovarian adenocarcimona
Tecnemab KI (murine Mab fragments (Fab/Fab_2 mix) directed against HMW-MAA, i.e. high molecular weight meloma-associated antigen)	Sorin	Diagnosis of cutaneous melanoma lesions
LeukoScan (Sulesomab, murine Mab fragment (Fab) directed against NCA 90, a surface granulocyte non-specific cross-reacting antigen)	Immunomedics	Diagnostic imaging for infection/inflammation in bone of patients with osteomyelitis

Table 10.4. (*Continued*)

Product	Company	Indication
Humaspect (Votumumab, human Mab directed against cytokeratin tumour-associated antigen)	Organon Teknika	Detection of carcinoma of the colon or rectum
Mabthera (Rituximab, chimaeric Mab directed against CD20 surface antigen of B lymphocytes)	Hoffmann La Roche (see also Rituxan)	Non-Hodgkin's lymphoma
Mabcampath (EU) or Campath (USA); Alemtuzumab; a humanized monoclonal antibody directed against CD52 surface antigen of B lymphocytes)	Millennium and ILEX (EU); Berlex, ILEX oncology and Millennium Pharmaceuticals (USA)	Chronic lymphocytic leukaemia
Mylotarg (Gemtuzumab zogamicin; a humanized antibody–toxic antibiotic conjugate targeted against CD33 antigen found on leukaemic blast cells)	Wyeth Ayerst	Acute myeloid leukaemia
Zevalin (Ibritumomab Tiuxetan; murine monoclonal antibody, produced in a CHO cell line, targeted against the CD20 antigen)	IDEC Pharmaceuticals	Non-Hodgkin's lymphoma

- T lymphocytes, which are capable of recognizing and lysing malignant cells.
- Natural killer (NK) cells which, like some T cells, can induce lysis of tumour cells. The tumoricidal activity of NK cells is potentiated by various cytokines (e.g. IL-2 and TNF).
- Macrophages can destroy tumour cells, largely by releasing damaging lysosomal enzymes and reactive oxygen metabolites at the tumour cell surface. Macrophages also produce TNF, which can kill tumour cells by: (a) binding to high-affinity TNF cell surface receptors, which is directly toxic to the cells; and (b) promoting synthesis of additional cytokines, which can, indirectly, lead to tumour destruction via activation of other elements of immunity.
- Antibodies which, by binding to the cell surface antigen, mark the tumour cell for destruction. NK cells and macrophages express cell surface receptors which bind to the antibody Fc region (Box 10.2). Thus, antibody bound to tumour antigens directs these immune elements directly to the tumour surface. Antibodies also activate complement, which is capable of directly lysing tumour cells.

The methods by which some transformed cells likely escape immune detection have already been outlined in detail in Chapter 5.

Antibody-based strategies for tumour detection/destruction

Clear identification of tumour-associated antigens would facilitate the production of monoclonal antibodies capable of selectively binding to tumour tissue. Such antibodies could be employed to detect and/or destroy the tumour cells (Figure 10.5).

The antibody preparations could be administered unaltered or (more commonly) after their conjugation to radioisotopes or toxins. Binding of unaltered monoclonal antibodies to a tumour surface alone should facilitate increased destruction of tumour cells (Figure 10.6). This approach, however, has yielded disappointing results, as the monoclonal antibody preparations used to date have largely been murine in origin. The Fc region of such mouse antibodies are very poor activators of human immune function. Technical advances allowing the production of human/humanized monoclonals (see later) may render this therapeutic approach more attractive in the future.

Box 10.2.   Antibody architecture

Five major classes of antibodies (immunoglobulins; Igs) have been characterized: IgM, IgG, IgA, IgD and IgE). Immunoglobulins of all classes display a similar basic four-chain structure consisting of two identical light (L) chains and two identical heavy (H) chains. The overall structure is held together by disulphide linkages and non-covalent interactions. Different heavy chain types are present in immunoglobulins of different classes. In addition, some classes can be further sub-divided into sub-classes (isotypes) based upon more subtle differences. Thus, human IgG can be sub-divided into IgG_1, IgG_2, IgG_3 and IgG_4. Murine IgG can be sub-divided into IgG_1, IgG_{2a}, IgG_{2b} and IgG_3.

In their native conformation, each immunoglobulin chain is seen to be composed of discrete domain structures, stabilized by intrachain disulphide linkages (not shown below). Each domain contains ca. 110 amino acid residues. H chains and L chains contain both variable (V) and constant (C) domains. Variable regions house the actual antigen-binding site of the antibody. Variable regions of antibodies displaying different (antigen-binding) specificities differ in amino acid sequence. Constant regions (within any one antibody class/sub-class) do not. L chains contain one variable (V_L) and one constant (C_L) domain. H chains contain one variable (V_H) and three constant (C_H1, C_H2 and C_H3) domains. In addition, H chains display a single short sequence joining C_H1 and C_H2. This is the flexible hinge (H) region, which contains several proline residues.

Treatment with certain proteolytic enzymes (e.g. papain) results in cleavage of the immunoglobulin at the hinge region, yielding two separate antigen-binding fragments ($2 \times Fab$), and a constant fragment (Fc). The Fc region mediates the various antibody effector functions. Fab fragments, while retaining their antigen-binding properties, are no longer capable of precipitating antigen *in vitro*. However, immunoglobulin incubation with other proteases, e.g. pepsin, results in antibody fragmentation immediately below the hinge region. This leaves intact two inter-chain disulphide linkages towards the C-terminus of the hinge region. This holds the two antigen binding fragments together. The products of this fragmentation are termed Fab_2 and Fc. Because of its bivalent nature, Fab_2 retains the ability to precipitate antigen *in vitro*.

Fv fragments consist of V_H and V_L domains, and can easily be produced by recombinant DNA technology (as can other antibody fragments). Two Fv domains can be stabilized by the introduction of an interchain covalent linkage (e.g. a disulphide linkage, or via direct chemical coupling). 'Single chain' Fv fragments may also be generated by the introduction of a short peptide linker sequence between the two Fv domains. Selected regions within the antibody's variable domain display greater variability in amino acid sequence (from one antibody to another) than do other variable regions. These so-called 'hypervariable' regions (complementarity-determining regions: CDRs) are brought into close proximity upon antibody folding into its native conformation, and represent the antigen-binding sites. The remaining areas of the variable domain are termed 'framework' regions.

Immunoglobulins are glycoproteins. The carbohydrate moiety is attached to the heavy chain (usually the C_H2 domain) via an N-linked glycosidic bond. Removal of the carbohydrate group has no effect upon antigen binding but does affect various antibody effector functions and alters its serum half-life.

ANTIBODIES, VACCINES AND ADJUVANTS 419

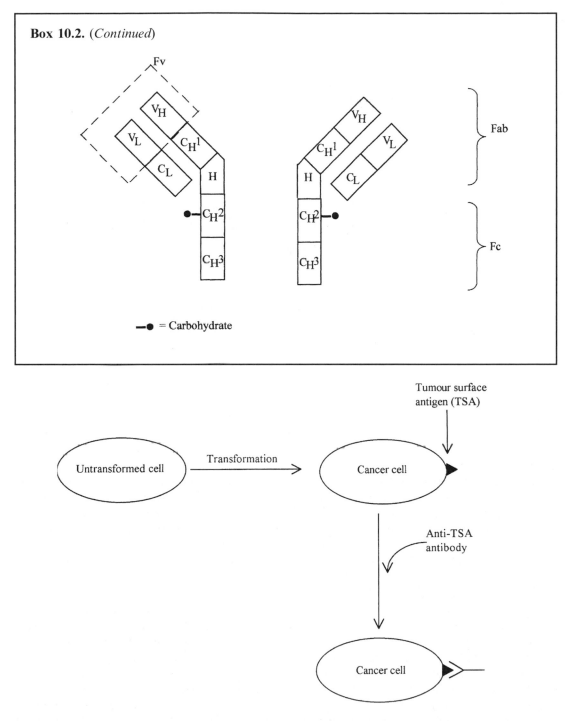

Figure 10.5. Upon transformation, cancer cells often express unique surface antigens termed 'tumour surface antigens' (TSAs). Antibodies raised against these will selectively bind the tumour cells. The antibody used may be unconjugated or conjugated to a drug, toxin or radioactive tag

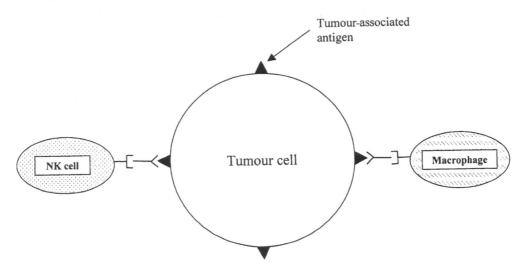

Figure 10.6.   Binding of appropriate antibody to tumour-associated antigens marks the tumour cell for destruction. This is largely due to the presence of a domain on the antibody Fc region (see also Box 10.2), which is recognized and bound by macrophages and NK cells. Congregation of such cells on the surface of the tumour is therefore encouraged. This greatly facilitates their cytocidal activity towards the transformed cells

Several clinical trials have evaluated (or continue to evaluate) monoclonal antibodies to which a radioactive tag has been conjugated. These are usually employed as potential anti-cancer agents. The rationale is selective delivery of the radioactivity directly to the tumour site. Most of the radio-isotopes being evaluated are β-emitters; these include ^{125}I and ^{131}I (iodine), ^{186}Re and ^{188}Re (rhenium) and ^{90}Y (yttrium). The medium-energy radioactivity these emit is capable of penetrating a thickness of several cells. Congregation of radioactivity at the tumour surface could thus promote irradiation of several layers of tumour cells—as well as nearby healthy cells (Figure 10.7). Higher-energy α-emitters are also being evaluated. Although their effective path length is only about one cell deep, each emission has a greater likelihood of killing all cells in its path.

An allied application of radiolabelled anti-tumour monoclonal antibodies is that of diagnostic imaging (immunoscintigraphy). In this case, the radioisotope employed must be a γ-emitter (such that the radioactivity can penetrate outward through the body for detection purposes). Although various radioisotopes of iodine have been evaluated, ^{99m}Tc (technetium) is the one most commonly employed. It has a γ-ray emission energy, which is sufficient, but a relatively short half-life of 6 h (this minimizes long-term exposure of patient to high-energy γ-rays). It can also be generated at nuclear installations relatively easily and is inexpensive. Equally important, chemical methodologies exist which facilitate its (stable) coupling to antibody molecules. Direct labelling with ^{99m}Tc generally entails initial reduction of antibody disulphide residues, forming free sulphydryl (–SH) groups. This is achieved by incubation with a suitable reducing agent, such as ascorbic acid or sodium dithionite. A source of ^{99m}Tc (e.g. Na^{99m}TcO$_4$) is then reduced separately. Subsequent mixing under nitrogen gas (to maintain reducing conditions) results in direct linkage of the radioisotope to the antibody.

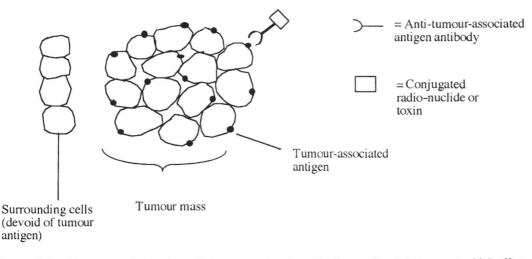

Figure 10.7. Theoretical basis for utilizing monoclonal antibodies conjugated to a cytocidal effector molecule as a cancer therapeutic agent. Binding specificity for tumour-associated antigen renders the antibody a 'magic bullet', capable of selectively binding to tumour cells

Upon administration, the anti-tumour ^{99m}Tc conjugate will congregate at the tumour site. The tumour can then be visualized using suitable γ-ray detection equipment, such as a planar γ-camera.

A number of radiolabelled monoclonal antibodies have been approved as tumour-diagnostic imaging agents (Table 10.4), e.g. CEA-SCAN is a Fab fragment of a specific murine monoclonal raised against human carcinoembryonic antigen (CEA). As discussed in detail in the section on tumour-associated antigens, CEA is expressed at high levels by some tumours. This is particularly true of tumours of the gastrointestinal tract, such as carcinomas of the colon or rectum. CEA-SCAN (non-proprietary name, arcitumomab) is used to detect these carcinomas. However, CEA is expressed naturally (albeit at much lower levels) by some non-transformed cells. Therefore, this antibody fragment is used mostly to image recurrence and/or metastases of histologically demonstrated carcinoma of the colon or rectum. It is used as an adjunct to standard imaging techniques, such as a computed tomography (CT) scan or ultrasonography. Its industrial method of production is overviewed in Figure 10.8. The product is administered by i.v. injection, and only relatively mild side effects are usually noted. These can include nausea, fever, rash and headaches.

Tecnemab-K-1 is an additional antibody fragment used for tumour imaging. Its overall method of production is quite similar to that of CEA-SCAN, except that the final product consists of a mixture of $F(ab)_2$ (ca. 70%) and Fab (ca. 30%) fragments. The Tecnemab-K-1 antibody fragment recognizes a specific antigen present on the surface of most malignant lesions of melanocyte origin (melanomas). However, as in the case of CEA, absolute tumour specificity is not recorded and the antibody cross-reacts to some extent with peripheral nerves, skin and muscle cells.

Tecnemab-K-1 is used to image the extent of/presence of metastases from confirmed cases of melanoma. Tumour visualization is via radio-immunoscintigraphy and the approach is generally used in combination with additional diagnostic procedures. In clinical trials involving several hundred patients with confirmed melanoma lesions, the antibody fragments detected

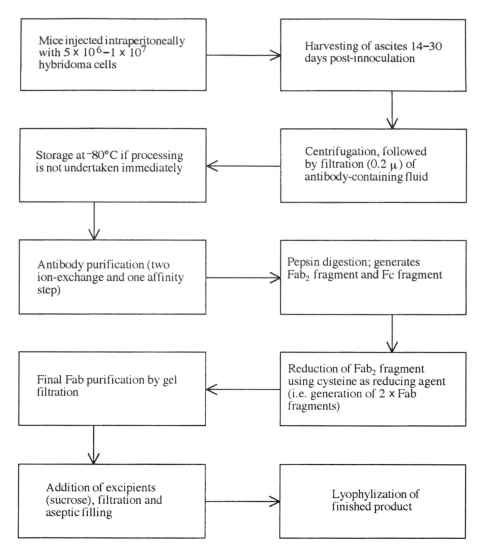

Figure 10.8.   Outline of the production strategy of CEA-SCAN. The antibody-producing hybridoma cell line was originally obtained by standard methods of hybridoma generation. Spleen-derived murine B-lymphocytes were fused with murine myeloma calls. The resulting stable hybridomas were screened for the production of anti-CEA monoclonals. The clone chosen produces an IgG anti-CEA antibody. Note that the finished product outlined above is not radio-labelled. The freeze-dried antibody preparation (which has a shelf-life of 2 years at 2–8°C) is reconstituted immediately prior to its medical use. The reconstituting solution contains ^{99m}Tc, and is formulated to facilitate direct conjugation of the radio-label to the antibody fragment

these lesions in 80% of cases (the other 20% thus being false negatives). Again, no significant side effects are generally noted upon administration of this antibody preparation.

Anti-tumour monoclonal antibodies can also be used to deliver toxins to tumour sites. Some of the toxins conjugated to therapeutic antibodies are listed in Table 10.5. After binding to the

Table 10.5. The major toxins which have been conjugated to monoclonal antibody preparations for clinical use as anti-cancer agents. Refer to text for details

Ricin	Diphtheria toxin
Pokeweed	Abrin
Gelonin	Antiviral protein
Pseudomonas endotoxin	

cell surface, the antibody–toxin conjugate is often internalized via endocytosis. It is presumed that, rather than being destroyed, the toxin is subsequently made available inside the cell, such that it can induce its toxic effects. One such antibody-based product now approved for general medical use is Mylotarg (Table 10.4). The product consists of an engineered antibody (a 'humanized' antibody, as described later), conjugated to a cytotoxic anti-tumour antibiotic, calicheamicin (Figure 10.9). The antibody binds specifically to a cell surface antigen, CD33. This is a sialic acid-dependent adhesion protein found on the surface of leukaemic cells in more than 80% of patients suffering from acute myeloid leukaemia (AML). The production process entails initial culture of the antibody-producing mammalian cell line, with subsequent purification of the antibody by a series of chromatographic steps. Downstream processing also incorporates ultrafiltration and low pH incubation steps designed to remove or inactivate any virus potentially present. The cytotoxic antibiotic is obtained separately via fermentation of its producer microrganism, *Micromonospora echinospora* ssp. *calichensis*. Direct chemical linkage of antibiotic to antibody is achieved using a bifunctional linker.

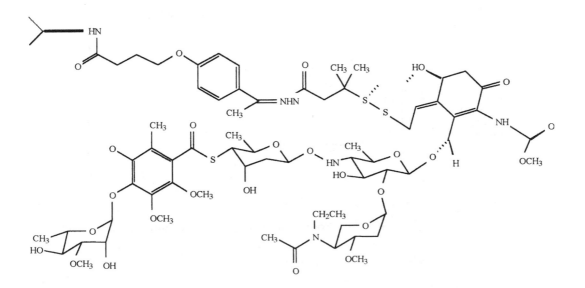

Figure 10.9. Schematic diagram of the antibody-based product Mylotarg, with emphasis upon the toxin's chemical structure. In reality, three to five molecules of toxin are attached to each antibody molecule

Mylotarg administration results in congregation of the antibody–toxin conjugate on the surface of (CD33-positive) leukaemic cells. Binding triggers internalization of the conjugate. Lysosomal degradation ensues but a significant proportion of the intact antibiotic escapes and induces its cytotoxic affect by binding DNA in its minor groove. This, in turn, induces double-strand breakage.

Mylotarg (like most other drugs) does induce some side effects, the most significant of which is immunosuppression. This is induced because certain additional (non-cancerous) white blood cell precursors also display the CD-33 antigen on their surface. The immunosuppressive effect is reversed upon termination of treatment, as pluripotent haemopoietic stem cells (Chapter 6) are unaffected by the product.

Drug-based tumour immunotherapy

In addition to tumour-selective delivery of toxins and radioisotopes, antibodies may also be used to mediate tumour-targeted drug delivery. At its simplest, this involves conjugation of a chemotherapeutic drug to a tumour-specific antibody. Therapeutic drugs used include adriamycin, aminopterin, methotrexate and vinca alkaloids. This direct approach to tumour drug delivery has met with some success, mainly in animal studies. However, a limited number of drug molecules can be conjugated to each antibody molecule, thus somewhat limiting the drug delivery load.

An alternative approach is the use of a tumour-specific antibody to which a pro-drug activating enzyme has been attached. Therapeutically inactive prodrugs could be administered by, for example, i.v. injection. This would subsequently be activated only at the tumor surface

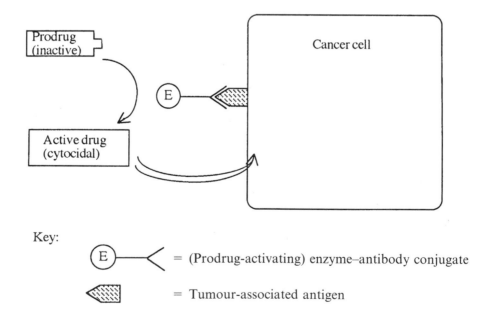

Figure 10.10. Outline of antibody-directed enzyme prodrug therapy (ADEPT). Subsequent to its enzymatic activation, the active drug is taken up by the cell, upon which it exhibits a cytocidal effect. Refer to text for specific details

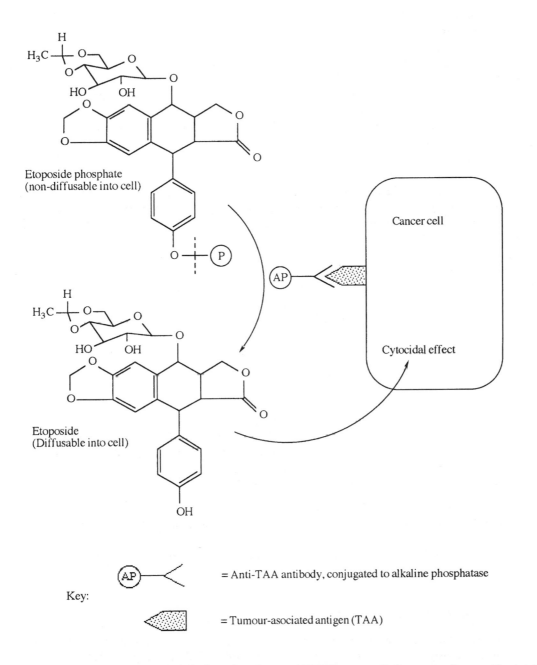

Etoposide phosphate
(non-diffusable into cell)

Cancer cell

AP

Cytocidal effect

Etoposide
(Diffusable into cell)

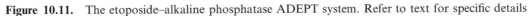

AP   = Anti-TAA antibody, conjugated to alkaline phosphatase

Key:

= Tumour-asociated antigen (TAA)

Figure 10.11.   The etoposide–alkaline phosphatase ADEPT system. Refer to text for specific details

(Figure 10.10). This approach has been termed 'antibody-directed enzyme prodrug therapy' (ADEPT) or 'antibody-directed catalysis' (ADC).

Because of its catalytic nature, a single antibody–enzyme conjugate would activate many molecules of the prodrug in question. Much of the active cytocidal agent released at the tumour surface would be taken up by the tumour cells via simple diffusion or carrier-mediated active transport. Administration of etoposide in prodrug form exemplifies this approach (Figure 10.11). Etoposide ($C_{29}H_{32}O_{13}$; molecular mass 588.6) is a semi-synthetic derivative of podophyllotoxin, produced naturally by the North American plant, *Podophyllum peltatum*. It is used as an anti-cancer agent. Its cellular uptake is diffusion-dependent and, once inside the cell, it exerts its cytocidal effect. Phosphorylated etoposide is non-diffusable and hence represents an inactive prodrug form of etoposide (attachment of a charged group to most diffusion-dependent drugs prevents their cellular uptake). Alkaline phosphatase, however, can cleave the phosphate group, releasing free cytocidal agent. Administration of a tumour-detecting antibody–alkaline phosphatase conjugate thus effectively targets the enzyme to the tumour surface. Subsequent administration of phosphorylated etoposide results in etoposide liberation at the tumour surface, which can then enter tumour cells by diffusion (Figure 10.11). Various other prodrug–enzyme combinations have now been developed, including phenoxyacetamide derivatives of doxorubicin (activated by penicillin amidase) and 5-fluorocytosine (activated by cytosine deaminase).

Prodrugs used should be inexpensive, readily available and stable to chemical/enzymatic degradation *in vivo*. The enzymes used should also be stable under physiological conditions, display a reasonable turnover number *in vivo* and not be dependent upon a co-factor for activity. Mammalian enzymes would be likely less immunogenic than microbial enzymes. However, the use of a prodrug capable of being activated by a mammalian enzyme can lead to complications if that enzyme's (human) endogenous counterpart is capable of activating the drug at sites distant from the tumour.

First-generation anti-tumour antibodies: clinical disappointment

Despite the scientific elegance of the antibody-mediated approach to tumour detection/destruction, initial clinical trials proved disappointing. A number of factors contributed to their poor therapeutic performance, particularly against solid tumours. Most such factors relate directly or indirectly to the fact that the first generation of such drugs utilized whole monoclonal antibody preparations of murine origin. These factors include:

- insufficient information exists regarding tumour antigens;
- murine monoclonals prompt an immune response when administered to humans;
- poor penetration of tumour mass by antibody;
- murine monoclonals display a relatively short half-life when administered to man;
- poor recognition of murine antibody Fc domain by human effector mechanisms.

Tumour-associated antigens

In this text, the term 'tumour-associated antigen' represents any antigen associated with any cancer cell, no matter what factor(s) originally prompted cellular transformation (in some circles, the term 'tumour-associated antigen' is often applied more specifically—to antigens associated with virally transformed cells). Identification of tumour-associated antigens forms a core requirement for effective tumour immunotherapy. Identification of such tumour-associated antigens remains a very active area of biomedical research. From the limited data generated to date, tumor-associated antigens can generally be categorized into one of three groups (Table 10.6).

Table 10.6. Characterization of tumour-associated antigens. Antigens commonly expressed by a number of different tumour types renders practical the application of tumour immunodetection/immunotherapy in those cases

Cell-transforming factors	Associated tumour antigen
Tumours induced by chemical carcinogens or irradiation	Each tumour usually displays distinct antigen specificity
Virally-induced tumours	Various tumour types display identical tumour-associated antigens (especially if tumours are induced by the same virus)
Various induction factors (often unknown)	The same oncofetal antigen can be expressed by a number of different tumour types

Many tumour types are induced by chemical and/or physical carcinogens we encounter in our living and working environments. Most of these tumours are initiated when the carcinogen induces a point mutation in a nucleotide sequence, thus perhaps altering expression levels of the gene product or altering its functional characteristics. Because such mutations are random, it is not surprising that each resulting tumour displays its own unique tumour-associated antigen(s). This renders an immunological approach to detection/therapy impractical in such instances, as the specific tumour-associated antigens unique to that case would first have to be identified.

In contrast to the above situation, cancers induced by viruses generally exhibit immunological cross-reactivity. Any specific virus will often induce expression of the same tumour antigen, no matter what cell type it transforms. Moreover, in some cases, different transforming viruses can induce production of the same tumor antigen(s). Immunodetection/immunotherapy of such cancers is thus rendered attractive. Once a tumour antigen is identified, antibodies raised against it will likely cross-react with several other tumour types.

DNA viruses, such as adenoviruses and papovaviruses (e.g. polyoma and SV40), induce cellular transformation in rodents. Other viruses have been implicated in human cancers, e.g. Epstein–Barr virus has been implicated with nasopharyngeal carcinoma, β-cell lymphomas and Hodgkin's lymphoma; human papilloma virus is linked to most cervical cancers.

Certain RNA viruses, particularly retroviruses, have also proven capable of inducing cancer. Retroviruses known to induce cancer in animals include Rous sarcoma virus, Kirsten murine sarcoma virus, avian myelocytomatosis virus, as well as various murine leukaemia viruses. Thus far, the only well-characterized human RNA transforming virus is that of human T cell lymphocytotropic virus-1 (HTLV-1), which can induce adult T cell leukaemia/lymphoma (ATL). Identification of antigens uniquely associated with various tumour types, and identification of additional cancer-causing viruses, remain areas of very active research.

Another group of antigens associated with some tumour types are oncofetal antigens. These antigens are proteins that are normally expressed during certain stages of fetal development. Subsequent repression of their structural genes, however, prevents their expression at later stages of development and/or into adulthood. Characteristic of some cancers is the re-expression of oncofetal antigens. Some such antigens remain attached to the cancer cell surface, while others are secreted in soluble form. Although these oncofetal proteins are not recognized as foreign by the host's own immune system, they do represent important potential diagnostic markers. While some such markers have been identified, efforts continue to identify additional members of this family.

Carcinoembryonic antigen (CEA) and α-fetoprotein (AFP) represent the most extensively characterized oncofetal antigens thus far. We have already encountered CEA in the guise of its use as a marker for cancers of the colon and rectum. CEA is a 180 kDa integral membrane glycoprotein. It also may be secreted into the blood in soluble form. It is expressed mainly in the gut, liver and pancreas during the first 6 months of fetal development. However, it is now known to be expressed (although at greatly reduced levels) by adult colonic mucosal cells and in the lactating breast. Elevated levels of either soluble (serum) or cell-bound CEA is normally indicative of cancers of the gastrointestinal tract.

α-Fetoprotein is a 70 kDa glycoprotein found in the circulatory system of the developing fetus. It is synthesized primarily by the yolk sac and (fetal) liver. AFP is present only in vanishing low quantities in the serum of adults (where it is replaced by serum albumin). Elevated adult serum levels of this marker are often associated with various cancers of the liver as well as germ cell tumours. It is also sometimes expressed by gastric and pancreatic cancer cells. Although a useful tumour marker, increased serum AFP levels also often accompany cirrhosis and some other non-cancerous liver diseases.

CA125 represents an oncofetal protein which is expressed by up to 90% of ovarian adenocarcinomas. Some of the protein is released from the tumour site into the general circulation. Elevated serum CA125 levels, therefore, have some diagnostic value. Imaging of the actual tumour site can also be undertaken using radio-labelled antibody coupled to immunoscintigraphy. Indimacis-125 is the trade name given to such a product approved in 1996 for use in the EU. The product is an ^{111}In-labelled F(ab)$_2$ fragment derived from a murine hybridoma cell line (In stands for indium). Although some of the product is likely absorbed by the circulatory form of the oncofetal protein, the product has proved effective in imaging relapsing ovarian adenocarcinoma.

In summary, tumour surface antigen (TSA)-based complications in the context of developing antibody-based cancer therapies include:

- Limited numbers of TSAs currently characterized.
- Some cancer types, depending upon their cause, may display unique TSAs in different patients.
- TSAs are often expressed, albeit at lower levels, by one or more additional (non-transformed) body cell types.
- In some instances, binding of antibody results in immediate shedding of Ab-TSA from the cell surface.
- TSA expression can be transient. For many tumours, only a proportion (albeit a large one) of the tumour cells express TSAs at any given timepoint.

Antigenicity of murine monoclonals

Antibody immunogenicity remains one of the inherent therapeutic limitations associated with administration of murine monoclonals to human subjects. In most instances, a single injection of the murine monoclonal will elicit an immune response in 50–80% of patients. Human anti-mouse antibodies (HAMA) will generally be detected within 14 days of antibody administration. Repeated administration of the monoclonal (usually required if the monoclonal is used for therapeutic purposes) will increase the HAMA response significantly. It will also induce a HAMA response in the majority of individuals who display no such response after the initial injection. The HAMA response will effectively and immediately destroy subsequent doses of monoclonal administered. In practice, therefore, therapeutic efficacy of murine monoclonals is limited to the first and, at most, the second dose administered.

An obvious strategy for overcoming the immunogenicity problem would be the generation and use of monoclonal antibodies of human origin. This is possible but difficult. Human antibody-producing lymphocytes can potentially be rendered immortal by:

- transformation by Epstein–Barr virus infection;
- fusion with murine monoclonals;
- fusion with human lymphoblastoid cell lines.

However, a number of technical hurdles remain which prevent routine production of human monoclonal preparations. These include:

- source of antibody-producing cell;
- reliable methods for lymphocyte immortalization;
- stability and antibody-producing capacity of the resulting immortalized cells.

Initial stages in the production of murine monoclonals entail administration of the antigen of interest to a mouse. This is followed by sacrifice of the mouse and recovery of activated B lymphocytes from the spleen. A similar approach to the production of human monoclonals would be unethical. Administration of some antigens to humans could endanger their health. Although B lymphocytes could be obtained from the peripheral circulation, the majority of these are unstimulated, and recovery of (stimulated) B lymphocytes from the spleen is impractical.

Although Epstein–Barr virus (EBV) is capable of inducing cellular transformation, few antibody-producing B lymphocytes display the viral cell surface receptor. Most, therefore, are immune to EBV infection. Even upon successful transformation, most produce low-affinity IgM antibodies, and the cells are often unstable. Having said that, one monoclonal antibody approved for medical use (Humaspect, Table 10.4) is produced by a human lymphoblastoid cell line originally transformed by EBV.

Fusion of human lymphocytes with human lymphoblastoid cell lines is a very inefficient process. Fusion of human lymphocytes with murine myeloma cells lead to very unstable hybrids. Upon fusion, preferential loss of human genetic elements is often observed. Unfortunately, particularly common is the loss of chromosomes 2, 14 and 22, which encode antibody light- and heavy-chain loci.

The production yields of human monoclonals upon immortalization of the human B lymphocyte (by whatever means) are also low. Recoveries of 10–20 μg per 10^6 transformed cells are not unusual. Such figures are approximately 10-fold lower than production levels of murine monoclonals. In addition, immortalized human B lymphocytes grow to a much lower cell density than that achievable with its murine counterpart. These latter factors render the production of human monoclonals an expensive process.

Chimaeric and humanized antibodies

Recombinant DNA technology has provided an alternative (and successful) route for reducing the innate immunity of murine monoclonals. The genes for all human immunoglobulin subtypes have been cloned and this has allowed generation of various hybrid antibody structures of reduced immunogenicity.

The first strategy entails production of 'chimaeric' antibodies, consisting of mouse variable regions and human constant regions (Figure 10.12). The chimaeric antibody would display the

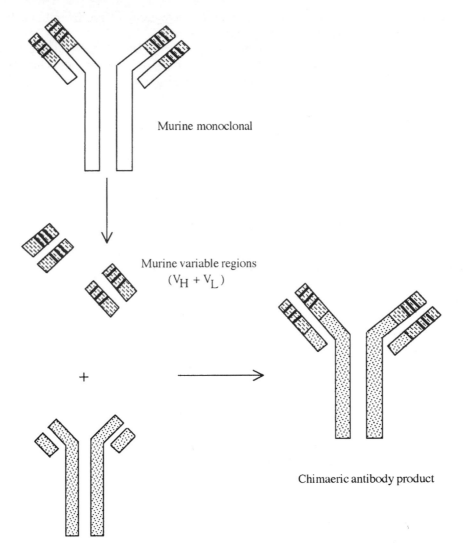

Murine monoclonal

Murine variable regions
($V_H + V_L$)

+

Chimaeric antibody product

Human antibody lacking variable region

(a)

Figure 10.12a

specificity of the original murine antibody but would be largely human in sequence. It was hoped that such chimaeric antibodies, when compared to murine antibodies, would be:

- significantly less immunogenic;
- display a prolonged serum half-life;
- allow activation of various Fc-mediated functions.

Reduced immunogenicity was expected, as only a minor proportion of chimaeric antibodies are murine in origin. Furthermore, the HAMA response is normally directed largely at epitopes

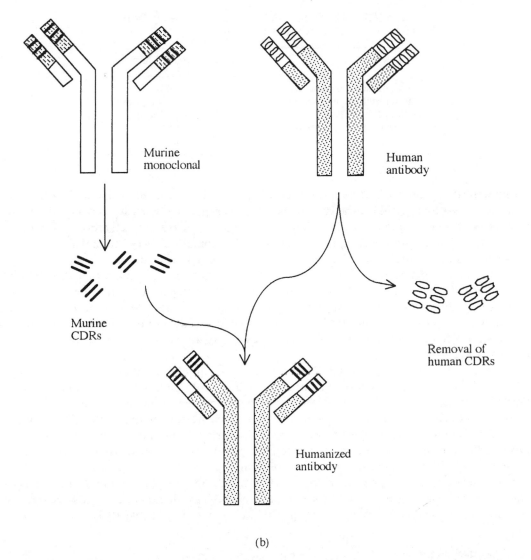

(b)

Figure 10.12b. Production of chimaeric (a) and humanized (b) antibodies (via recombinant DNA technology). Chimaeric antibodies consist of murine monoclonal V_H and V_L domains grafted onto the Fc region of a human antibody. Humanized antibody consists of murine CDR regions grafted into a human antibody

on the antibody's Fc domains. The variable region appears inherently less immunogenic. In practice, the expected reduced immunogenicity was observed. Early clinical trials with chimaerics have shown them to be safe and non-toxic. The rate of immune responses observed after single-dose administration dropped from almost 80% (murine) to ca. 5% (chimaeric). However, repeated administration of chimaerics did eventually raise an immune response in most recipients.

When compared to human monoclonals (half-life 14–21 days), murine monoclonals administered to humans display a relatively short half-life (30–40 h). Chimerization increased

Table 10.7.   The serum half-life values of some IgG antibody preparations when administered to humans

Antibody type	Serum half-life
Intact human monoclonal	14–21 days
Intact murine monoclonal	30–40 h
Chimaeric antibody	200–250 h
Murine F(ab)$_2$ fragment	20 h
Murine Fab fragment	2 h

serum half-life by five-fold, with typical values of 230 h being recorded (Table 10.7). A prolonged half-life is desirable if the antibody is to be used therapeutically, as it decreases the required frequency of product administration. Chimaeric antibodies also allow activation of Fc-mediated functions (e.g. activation of complement, etc.), as this domain displays human sequence.

While chimaeric antibodies contain an entire murine-derived variable region, it is only the complementarity-determining regions (CDRs) within this variable domain that actually dictate antigen specificity (Box 10.2). A method of reducing the antigenicity of murine antibodies still further is to 'humanize' them. This entails transferring the nucleotide sequences coding for the six CDR regions of the murine antibody of the desired specificity into a human antibody gene. The resulting hybrid antibody will, obviously, be entirely human in nature except for the CDRs (Figure 10.12).

Transfer of murine-derived CDR sequences into human antibody framework regions (Box 10.2) sometimes generates an antibody with greatly reduced antigen-binding affinity. Selected murine framework sequences are often also included in the humanized antibody. This process (known as 'reshaping' the human antibody) facilitates folding of the CDRs into their true native conformations. This, in turn, normally restores antibody–antigen binding affinity. Over 95% of such hybrid antibodies are human in sequence. Clinical trials indicate that such proteins do indeed behave similarly to native human antibodies.

Humanization has overcome many of the major factors that limited the therapeutic effectiveness of first-generation (murine) monoclonals as therapeutic agents. Several such humanized products have now gained marketing authorization (Table 10.4).

Antibody fragments

One limitation to antibody-mediated treatment of solid tumours relates to their poor penetration of tumour mass. Antibody-based tumour therapy (e.g. using radio-labelled murine monoclonals) have proved more effective in treating disseminated cancers (e.g. leukaemias and lymphomas) than solid tumours. The physical size of the intact antibody likely hinders tumour penetration. As a result, recent interest has focused upon using antibody fragments which retain their antigen-binding capabilities. Fragments, such as F(ab), F(ab)$_2$ and Fv (Box 10.2), can be easily generated, mainly via recombinant DNA technology. These have been labelled, e.g. with radio-active tags, with the intention of using them as diagnostic and therapeutic agents. While their lower molecular mass may aid more effective tumour penetration, whole chimaeric/humanized antibodies may be more effective, particularly if used for therapeutic purposes. Fragments generally display greatly reduced serum half-lives (Table 10.7) and cannot initiate effector functions. Radio-labelled fragments may be better suited to diagnostic imaging purposes.

Table 10.8. Some actual/potential medical applications of monoclonal antibodies (other than those relating to cancer). In many instances, these applications will entail use of chimaeric or humanized antibodies or antibody fragments

Imaging and/or therapy of cardiovascular diseases
Imaging of deep vein thrombosis
Imaging of sites of bacterial infection
Therapy associated with antigen transplantation
Therapy of septic shock
Treatment of autoimmune disorders

Additional therapeutic applications of monoclonal antibodies

Thus far, the discussion relating to the medical uses of monoclonals has focused exclusively upon cancer. Monoclonal antibodies (and their derivatives), however, have a far broader potential therapeutic application. Actual/potential additional uses include detection and treatment of cardiovascular disease, infectious agents, and various additional medical conditions. These are overviewed in Table 10.8. Specific examples of products already approved are provided in Table 10.4.

Cardiovascular and related disease

Various antibody preparations have been developed which facilitate imaging of vascular-related conditions, including myocardial infarction, deep vein thrombosis and artherosclerosis. Anti-myosin monoclonal antibody fragments (Fab) labelled with ^{111}In, for example, have been used for imaging purposes in conjunction with a planar γ-camera. The antibody displays specificity for intracellular cardiac myosin, which is exposed only upon death of heart muscle tissue induced by a myocardial infarction (heart attack). The product has proved non-toxic and capable of accurate detection of such infarctions.

Deep vein thrombosis refers to clot formation within the vascular system, usually in the lower extremities. It requires prompt medical attention, as it not only disrupts blood flow in the affected area but can also lead to the formation of emboli, with serious, often fatal, medical consequences (Chapter 9). Such thrombi may be pinpointed by immunoscintigraphy, utilizing a radio-labelled antibody directed against platelets or, more often, fibrin.

Atherosclerotic plaque also forms a target for imaging monoclonals. Most often, the antibodies employed display specificity for activated platelets, usually found in association with ruptured plaque.

Infectious diseases

Imaging monoclonals could be of use in visualizing the sites/extent of focused bacterial infections. This can be achieved by using radiolabelled antibodies displaying binding affinity for specific bacterial surface antigens. A related, but indirect, approach may entail use of imaging antibodies capable of detecting granulocytes and various other leukocytes that congregate at the sites of infection.

Various monoclonal preparations are also being assessed with regard to their ability to inhibit progression of various viral diseases. In most instances, the antibodies are capable of selectively binding to a viral surface epitope. Two viral agents receiving particular attention are hepatitis B virus and HIV. Both murine monoclonals as well as chimaeric and humanized antibody preparations raised against HIV surface antigens are currently being assessed with regard to their ability to alter the clinical course of AIDS.

One of the most serious consequences of (Gram-negative) bacterial infection is the possible development of septic shock. This is caused by the release of lipopolysaccharide (LPS; endotoxin) from the bacterial cell surface. Various anti-LPS monoclonals (mainly targeted at its lipid A component; Chapter 3) have been developed. It is hoped that administration of such monoclonals to affected individuals would effectively mop up free LPS, hence ameliorating the severity of the condition. Most trial results to date have proved disappointing in this regard.

Autoimmune disease

Autoimmunity describes any condition in which the body's immune system targets some elements of itself. This results from a failure of various immunological checking systems that are normally responsible for maintaining self-tolerance. It has been estimated that 1–2% of the US population suffer from autoimmune conditions, including rheumatoid arthritis, multiple sclerosis and some forms of diabetes. In many instances, an autoimmune response results from the inappropriate activation of a specific sub-set of B and/or T lymphocytes. The most common immunotherapeutic approach to potentially treat such diseases is to induce depletion of the individual's T and B cell populations. This could be achieved by administration of an antibody raised against a surface antigen present on such cells, e.g. initial trials have shown that injection of an (unconjugated) anti-CD 4 antibody (cell surface glycoprotein present on many T lymphocytes) over 7 days significantly reduced the clinical symptoms of rheumatoid arthritis for several months.

Selected adhesion molecules represent yet another antibody target. Adhesion molecules, such as LFA-1 (leukocyte function-associated antigen-1) and ICAM-1 (intercellular adhesion molecule 1), play central roles in promoting migration of inflammatory cells to the sites of damage. Such activities underlie many of the symptoms of conditions such as rheumatoid arthritis. Inhibition of adhesion molecule function by administration of antibodies raised against them may, therefore, demonstrate therapeutic potential in some instances.

Transplantation

Modern surgical techniques render the transplantation of various organs relatively straight-forward. Common examples include renal (kidney), cardiac (heart) and hepatic (liver) transplants. In general, cell-mediated immunological mechanisms are responsible for mediating rejection of transplanted organs. In many instances, transplant patients must be maintained on immunosuppressive drugs (e.g. some steroids and, often, the fungal metabolite cyclosporine). However, complications may arise if a rejection episode is encountered which proves unresponsive to standard immunosuppressive therapy. Orthoclone OKT-3 was the first monoclonal antibody-based product to find application in this regard. This antibody is raised against the protein-based CD3 antigen, present on the cell surface of most T lymphocytes. i.v. administration of (unconjugated) antibody appears to block normal functioning of such T cells and promote their clearance from the blood. However, upon cessation of antibody administration, CD3-positive cell numbers rapidly revert to normal values. Therefore, maintenance immunosuppression (e.g. with cyclosporine) must subsequently be restored.

OKT-3 was first approved for general medical use in the USA in 1986. Its indication was the treatment of acute kidney transplant rejection (Table 10.4). OKT-3 is produced via ascites grown in mice. The intact antibody is subsequently purified by a combination of ammonium sulphate fractionation and anion exchange chromatography. Despite its therapeutic effectiveness, the product does display some limitations. Its antigenicity in humans (the HAMA response) is one obvious factor which limits its prolonged use.

A number of additional antibody-based products aimed at preventing transplant rejection have now gained general marketing authorization. Simulect (chimaeric antibody) and Zenapax (humanized antibody) were approved in the late 1990s (Table 10.4). Their engineered nature has greatly reduced the HAMA response upon their administration to humans. Both products target the 1L-2 receptor and hence bind fairly selectively to activated immune system cells, especially activated T lymphocytes, monocytes and macrophages (Chapter 5). Binding prevents further cellular proliferation and hence dampens the immune system's attempts to destroy the transplanted tissue.

VACCINE TECHNOLOGY

The application of vaccine technology forms a core element of modern medicinal endeavour. It plays a central role, not only in human but also in veterinary medicine and represents the only commonly employed prophylactic (i.e. preventative) approach undertaken to control many infectious diseases. The current (annual) global vaccine market stands at in excess of $3 billion. Immunization programmes, particularly those undertaken on a multi-national scale, have served to reduce dramatically the incidence of many killer/disabling diseases, such as smallpox, polio and tuberculosis.

Continued/increased emphasis upon the implementation of such immunization programmes is likely. This is true not only of poorer world regions, but also amongst the most affluent nations. An estimated 500 000 adults die annually in the USA from conditions that could have been prevented by vaccination. These include pneumococcal pneumonia, influenza and hepatitis B.

Vaccination seeks to exploit the natural defence mechanisms conferred upon us by our immune systems. A vaccine contains a preparation of antigenic components consisting of, derived from or related to a pathogen. In most instances, upon vaccine administration, both the humoral and cell-mediated arms of the immune system are activated. The long-term immunological protection induced will normally prevent subsequent establishment of an infection by the same or antigenically-related pathogens. While some vaccines are active when administered orally, more are administered parenterally. Normally, an initial dose administration is followed by subsequent administration of one or more repeat doses over an appropriate time scale. Such booster doses serve to maximize the immunological response.

Traditional vaccine preparations have largely been targeted against viral and bacterial pathogens, as well as some bacterial toxins and, to a lesser extent, parasitic agents, such as malaria. However, an increased understanding of the molecular mechanisms underlying additional human diseases suggests several novel applications of vaccines to treat or prevent autoimmune conditions and cancer (Table 10.9). Such applications will be discussed later. Despite such potentially exciting future applications, recent scientific surveys indicate that the

436 BIOPHARMACEUTICALS

Table 10.9. Some important discoveries that chronicle the development of modern vaccine technology. Many of the initial landmark discoveries that underpinned our understanding of immunity and vaccination were made at the turn of the last century

A.D. 23	Romans investigate the possibility that liver extracts from rabid dogs could protect against rabies
1790s	Edward Genner uses Cowpox virus to successfully vaccinate against smallpox
1880s	Louis Pasteur develops first effective rabies vaccine
1890s	Emil von Behring and Kitasato Shibasaburo develop diphtheria and tetanus vaccines
1900s	Typhoid and cholera vaccines are first developed
1910s	Tetanus vaccine becomes widely available
1920s	Tuberculosis vaccine becomes available
1930s	Diphtheria and yellow fever vaccines come on stream
1940s	Influenza and pertussis vaccines are developed
1950s	Poliomyelitis vaccines (oral Sabin vaccine and injectable Salk vaccine) developed
1960s	Measles, mumps and rubella vaccines developed
1970s	Meningococcal vaccines developed
1980s	Initial subunit vaccines (e.g. hepatitis B) produced by recombinant DNA technology
1990s	Ongoing development of subunit vaccines and vaccines against autoimmune disease and cancer. Production of vaccines in recombinant viral vectors

most urgently required vaccines are those which protect against more mundane pathogens (Table 10.10). Although the needs of the developing world are somewhat different from those of developed regions, an effective AIDS vaccine is equally important to both. Approaches to development of such AIDS vaccines are discussed later in this chapter. Of particular consequence to developing world regions is the current lack of a truly effective malaria vaccine. With an estimated annual incidence of 300–500 million clinical cases (with up to 2.7 million resulting deaths), development of an effective vaccine in this instance is a priority.

Traditional vaccine preparations

For the purposes of this discussion, the term 'traditional' refers to those vaccines whose development predated the advent of recombinant DNA technology. Approximately 30 such vaccines remain in medical use (Table 10.11).

These can largely be categorized into one of several groups, including:

- Live, attenuated bacteria, e.g. Bacillus Calmette–Guérin (BCG) used to immunize against tuberculosis.
- Dead or inactivated bacteria, e.g. cholera and pertussis (whooping cough) vaccines.
- Live attenuated viruses, e.g. measles, mumps and yellow fever viral vaccines.

Table 10.10. Some diseases against which effective or more effective vaccines are urgently required. Diseases more prevalent in developing world regions differ from those that are most common in developed countries

Developing world regions	Developed world regions
AIDS	AIDS
Malaria	Respiratory syncytial virus
Tuberculosis	Pneumococcal disease

Table 10.11. Some traditional vaccine preparations which find medical application. In addition to being marketed individually, a number of such products are also marketed as combination vaccines. Examples include diphtheria, tetanus and pertussis vaccines and measles, mumps and rubella vaccines

Product	Description	Application
Anthrax vaccines	*Bacillus anthracis*-derived antigens found in a sterile filtrate of cultures of this microorganism	Active immunization against anthrax
BCG vaccine (Bacillus Calmette–Guérin vaccine)	Live attenuated strain of *Mycobacterium tuberculosis*	Active immunization against tuberculosis
Brucellosis vaccine	Antigenic extract of *Brucella abortus*	Active immunization against brucellosis
Cholera vaccine	Dead strain(s) of *Vibrio cholerae*	Active immunization against cholera
Cytomegalovirus vaccines	Live attenuated strain of human cytomegalovirus	Active immunization against cytomegalovirus
Diphtheria vaccine	Diphtheria toxoid formed by treating diphtheria toxin with formaldehyde	Active immunization against diphtheria
Japanese encephalitis vaccine	Inactivated Japanese encephalitis virus	Active immunization against viral agents causing Japanese encephalitis
Haemophilus influenzae vaccine	Purified capsular polysaccharide of *Haemophilus influenzae* type b (usually linked to a protein carrier, forming a conjugated vaccine)	Active immunization against *Haemophilus influenzae* type b infections (major causative agent of meningitis in young children)
Hepatitis A vaccine	(Formaldehyde)-inactivated hepatitis A virus	Active immunization against hepatitis A
Hepatitis B vaccine	Suspension of hepatitis B surface antigen (HBsAg) purified from the plasma of hepatitis B sufferers	Active immunization against hepatitis B (note: this preparation has largely been superseded by HBsAg preparations produced by genetic engineering)
Influenza vaccines	Mixture of inactivated strains of influenza virus	Active immunization against influenza
Leptospira vaccines	Killed strain of *Leptospira interogans*	Active immunization against leptospirosis icterohaemor-rhagica (Weil's disease)
Measles vaccines	Live attenuated strains of measles virus	Active immunization against measles
Meningococcal vaccines	Purified surface polysaccharide antigens of one or more strains of *Neisseria meningitidis*	Active immunization against *Neisseria meningitidis* (can cause meningitis and septicaemia)
Mumps vaccine	Live attenuated strain of the mumps virus (*Paramyxovirus parotitidus*)	Active immunization against mumps
Pertussis vaccines	Killed strain(s) of *Bordetella pertussis*	Active immunization against whooping cough
Plague vaccine	Formaldehyde-killed *Yersinia pestis*	Active immunization against plague
Pneumococcal vaccines	Mixture of purified surface polysaccharide antigens obtained from differing serotypes of *Streptococcus pneumoniae*	Active immunization against *Streptococcus pneumoniae*

(Continued)

Table 10.11 (*Continued*)

Product	Description	Application
Poliomyelitis vaccine (Sabin vaccine: oral)	Live attenutated strains of poliomyelitis virus	Active immunization against polio
Poliomyelitis vaccine (Salk vaccine: parenteral)	Inactivated poliomyelitis virus	Active immunization against polio
Rabies vaccines	Inactivated rabies virus	Active immunization against rabies
Rotavirus vaccines	Live attenuated strains of rotavirus	Active immunization against rotavirus (causes severe childhood diarrhoea)
Rubella vaccines	Live attenuated strain of rubella virus	Active immunization against rubella (German measles)
Tetanus vaccines	Toxoid formed by formaldehyde treatment of toxin produced by *Clostridium tetani*	Active immunization against tetanus
Typhoid vaccines	Killed *Salmonella typhi*	Active immunization against typhoid fever
Typhus vaccines	Killed epidemic *Rickettsia prowazekii*	Active immunization against louse-borne typhus
Varicella zoster vaccines	Live attenuated strain of herpes virus varicellae	Active immunization against chicken pox
Yellow fever vaccines	Live attenuated strain of yellow fever virus	Active immunization against yellow fever

- Inactivated viruses, e.g. hepatitis A and poliomyelitis (Salk) viral vaccines.
- Toxoids, e.g. diphtheria and tetanus vaccines.
- Pathogen-derived antigens, e.g. hepatitis B, meningococcal, pneumococcal and *Haemophilus influenzae* vaccines.

Attenuated, dead or inactivated bacteria

Attenuation (bacterial or viral) represents the process of elimination or greatly reducing the virulence of a pathogen. This is traditionally achieved by, for example, chemical treatment or heat, growing under adverse conditions or propagation in an unnatural host. The attenuated product should still immunologically cross-react with the wild-type pathogen. Although rarely occurring in practice, a theoretical danger exists in some cases that the attenuated pathogen might revert to its pathogenic state. An attenuated bacterial vaccine is represented by Bacillus Calmette–Guérin (BCG), which is a strain of tubercule bacillus (*Mycobacterium bovis*) that fails to cause tuberculosis but retains much of the antigenicity of the pathogen.

Killing or inactivation of pathogenic bacteria usually renders them suitable as vaccines. This is usually achieved by chemical or heat treatment, or both (Table 10.12). To be effective, the inactivated product must retain much of the immunological characteristics of the active pathogen. The killing or inactivation method must be consistently 100% effective in order to prevent accidental transmission of live pathogens. Cholera vaccines, for example, are sterile aqueous suspensions of killed *Vibrio cholerae*, selected for high antigenic efficiency. The preparation often consists of a mixture of smooth strains of the two main cholera serological

Table 10.12. Methods usually employed to inactivate bacteria or viruses subsequently used as dead/inactivated vaccine preparations

Heat treatment
Treatment with formaldehyde or acetone
Treatment with phenol or phenol and heat
Treatment with propiolactone

types: Inaba and Ogawa. A 1.0 ml typical dose usually contains not less than 8 billion *V. cholerae* particles and phenol (up to 0.5%) may be added as preservative. The vaccine can also be prepared in freeze-dried form. When stored refrigerated, the liquid vaccine displays a usual shelf-life of 18 months, while that of the dried product is 5 years.

Attenuated and inactivated viral vaccines

Viral particles destined for use as vaccines are generally propagated in a suitable animal cell culture system. While true cell culture systems are sometimes employed, many viral particles are grown in fertilized eggs, or cultures of chick embryo tissue (Table 10.13).

Many of the more prominent vaccine preparations in current medical use consist of attenuated viral particles (Table 10.11). Mumps vaccine consists of live attenuated strains of Paramyxovirus parotitidis. In many world regions, it is used to routinely vaccinate children, often a part of a combined measles, mumps and rubella (MMR) vaccine. Several attenuated strains have been developed for use in vaccine preparations. The most commonly used is the Jeryl Linn strain of the mumps vaccine, which is propagated in chick embryo cell culture. This vaccine has been administered to well over 50 million people worldwide and, typically, results in seroconversion rates of over 97%. The Sabin (oral poliomyelitis) vaccine consists of an aqueous suspension of poliomyelitis virus, usually grown in cultures of monkey kidney tissue. It contains approximately 1 million particles of poliomyelitis strains 1, 2 or 3 or a combination of all three strains.

Hepatitis A vaccine exemplifies vaccine preparations containing inactivated viral particles. It consists of a formaldehyde-inactivated preparation of the HM 175 strain of hepatitis A virus. Viral particles are normally propagated initially in human fibroblasts.

Table 10.13. Some cell culture systems in which viral particles destined for use as viral vaccines are propagated

Viral particle/vaccine	Typical cell culture system
Yellow fever virus	Chick egg embryos
Measles virus (attenuated)	Chick egg embryo cells
Mumps virus (attenuated)	Chick egg embryo cells
Polio virus (live, oral, i.e. Sabin and inactivated injectable, i.e. Salk)	Monkey kidney tissue culture
Rubella vaccine	Duck embryo tissue culture, human tissue culture
Hepatitis A viral vaccine	Human diploid fibroblasts
Varicella-zoster vaccines (chicken pox vaccine)	Human diploid cells

Table 10.14. Some vaccine preparations that consist not of intact attenuated/inactivated pathogens but of surface antigens derived from such pathogens

Vaccine	Specific antigen used
Anthrax vaccines	Antigen found in the sterile filtrate of *Bacillus anthracis*
Haemophilus influenzae vaccines	Purified capsular polysaccharide of *Haemophilus influenzae* type B
Hepatitis B vaccines	Hepatitis B surface antigen (HBsAg) purified from plasma of hepatitis B carriers
Meningococcal vaccines	Purified (surface) polysaccharides from *Neisseria meningitidis* (groups A or C)
Pneumococcal vaccine	Purified polysaccharide capsular antigen from up to 23 serotypes of *Streptococcus pneumoniae*

Toxoids, antigen-based and other vaccine preparations

Diphtheria and tetanus vaccine are two commonly used toxoid-based vaccine preparations. The initial stages of diphtheria vaccine production entails the growth of *Corynebacterium diphtheriae*. The toxoid is then prepared by treating the active toxin produced with formaldehyde. The product is normally sold as a sterile aqueous preparation. Tetanus vaccine production follows a similar approach; *Clostridium tetani* is cultured in appropriate media, the toxin is recovered and inactivated by formaldehyde treatment. Again, it is usually marketed as a sterile aqueous-based product.

Traditional antigen-based vaccine preparations consist of appropriate antigenic portions of the pathogen (usually surface-derived antigens; Table 10.14). In most cases, the antigenic substances are surface polysaccharides. Many carbohydrate-based substances are inherently less immunogenic than protein-based material. Poor immunological responses are thus often associated with administration of carbohydrate polymers to humans, particularly to infants. The antigenicity of these substances can be improved by chemically coupling (conjugating) them to a protein-based antigen. Several conjugated *Haemophilus influenzae* vaccine variants are available. In these cases, the *Haemophilus* capsular polysaccharide is conjugated variously to diphtheria toxoid, tetanus toxoid or an outer membrane protein of *Neisseria meningitidis* (group B).

All of the vaccine preparations discussed thus far are bacterial or viral-based. Typhus vaccine, on the other hand, targets a parasitic disease. Typhus (spotted fever) refers to a group of infections caused by *Rickettsia* (small, non-motile parasites). The disease is characterized by severe rash and headache, high fever and delirium. The most common form is that of epidemic typhus ('classical' or 'louse-borne' typhus). This is associated particularly with crowded, unsanitary conditions.

Without appropriate antibiotic treatment, fatality rates can approach 100%. The causative agent of epidemic typhus is *Rickettsia prowazekii*. Typhus vaccine consists of a sterile aqueous suspension of killed *R. prowazekii* which has been propagated in either yolk sacs of embryonated eggs, rodent lungs or the peritoneal cavity of gerbils.

To date, no effective vaccine has been developed for many parasites, notably the malaria-causing parasitic protozoa *Plasmodium*. One of the major difficulties in such instances is that parasites go through a complex life cycle, often spanning at least two different hosts.

The impact of genetic engineering on vaccine technology

The advent of recombinant DNA technology has rendered possible the large-scale production of polypeptides normally present on the surface of virtually any pathogen. These polypeptides, when purified from the producer organism (e.g. *Escherichia coli*, *Saccharomyces cerevisiae*) can then be used as 'sub-unit' vaccines. This method of vaccine production exhibits several advantages over conventional vaccine production methodologies. These include:

- Production of a clinically safe product; the pathogen-derived polypeptide now being expressed in a non-pathogenic recombinant host. This all but precludes the possibility that the final product could harbour undetected pathogen.
- Production of subunit vaccine in an unlimited supply. Previously, production of some vaccines was limited by supply of raw material (e.g. hepatitis B surface antigen; see below).
- Consistent production of a defined product which would thus be less likely to cause unexpected side effects.

A number of such recombinant (subunit) vaccines have now been approved for general medical use (Table 10.15). The first such product was that of hepatitis B surface antigen (rHBsAg), which gained marketing approval from the FDA in 1986. Prior to its approval, hepatitis B vaccines consisted of HBsAg purified directly from the blood of hepatitis B sufferers. When present in blood, HBsAg exists not in monomeric form, but in characteristic polymeric structures of 22 μm diameter. Production of hepatitis B vaccine by direct extraction from blood suffered from two major disadvantages:

- The supply of finished vaccine was restricted by the availability of infected human plasma.
- The starting material will likely be contaminated by intact, viable hepatitis B viral particles (and perhaps additional viruses, such as HIV). This necessitates introduction of stringent purification procedures to ensure complete removal of any intact viral particles from the product stream. A final product QC test to confirm this entails a 6 month safety test on chimpanzees.

The HBsAg gene has been cloned and expressed in a variety of expression systems, including *E. coli*, *S. cerevisiae* and a number of mammalian cell lines. The product used commercially is produced in *S. cerevisiae*. The yeast cells are not only capable of expressing the gene, but also assembling the resultant polypeptide product into particles quite similar to those found in the blood of infected individuals. This product proved safe and effective when administered to both animals and humans. An overview of its manufacturing process is presented in Figure 10.13.

Various other companies have also produced recombinant HBsAg-based vaccines. SmithKline Beecham secured FDA approval for such a product (trade name, Engerix-B) in 1989 (Figure 10.14). Subsequently, SmithKline Beecham have also generated various combination vaccines in which recombinant HBsAg is a component. 'Twinrix' (trade name), for example, contains a mixture of inactivated hepatitis A virus and recombinant HBsAg. Tritanrix, on the other hand, contains diphtheria and tetanus toxoids (produced by traditional means), along with recombinant HBsAg.

It seems likely that many such (recombinant) subunit vaccines will gain future regulatory approval. One such example is that of *B. pertussis* subunit vaccine. *B. pertussis* is a Gram-negative coccobacillus, transmitted by droplet infection, and is the causative agent of the upper respiratory tract infection commonly termed 'whooping cough'.

Table 10.15.   Recombinant subunit vaccines approved for human use

Product	Company	Indication
Recombivax (rHBsAg produced in *Saccharomyces cerevisiae*)	Merck	Hepatitis B prevention
Comvax (combination vaccine, containing rHBsAg produced in *S. cerevisiae*, as one component)	Merck	Vaccination of infants against *Haemophilus influenzae* type B and hepatitis B
Engerix B (rHBsAg produced in *S. cerevisiae*)	SmithKline Beecham	Vaccination against hepatitis B
Tritanrix-HB (combination vaccine, containing rHBsAg produced in *S. cerevisiae* as one component)	SmithKline Beecham	Vaccination against hepatitis B, diphtheria, tetanus and pertussis
Lymerix (rOspA, a lipoprotein found on the surface of *Borrelia burgdorferi*, the major causative agent of Lyme's disease. Produced in *E. coli*)	Smithkline Beecham	Lyme disease vaccine
Infanrix-Hep B (combination vaccine, containing rHBsAg produced in *S. cerevisiae* as one component)	SmithKline Beecham	Immunization against diphtheria, tetanus, pertussis and hepatitis B
Infanrix-Hexa (combination vaccine, containing rHBsAg produced in *S. cerevisiae* as one component)	SmithKline Beecham	Immunization against diphtheria, tetanus, pertussis, polio, *Haemophilus influenzae* b and hepatitis B
Infanrix-Penta (combination vaccine, containing rHBsAg produced in *S. cerevisiae* as one component)	SmithKline Beecham	Immunization against diphtheria, tetanus, pertussis, polio, and hepatitis B
Ambirix (combination vaccine, containing rHBsAg produced in *S. cerevisiae* as one component)	Glaxo SmithKline	Immunization against hepatitis A and B
Twinrix, Adult and pediatric forms in EU (combination vaccine containing rHBsAg produced in *S. cerevisiae* as one component)	SmithKline Beecham (EU), Glaxo SmithKline (USA)	Immunization against hepatitis A and B
Primavax (combination vaccine, containing rHBsAg produced in *S. cerevisiae* as one component)	Pasteur Merieux MSD	Immunization against diphtheria, tetanus and hepatitis B
Procomvax (combination vaccine, containing rHBsAg as one component)	Pasteur Merieux MSD	Immunization against *Haemophilus influenzae* type B and hepatitis B
Hexavac (combination vaccine, containing rHBsAg produced in *S. cerevisiae* as one component)	Aventis Pasteur	Immunization against diphtheria, tetanus, pertussis, hepatitis B, polio and *Haemophilus influenzae* type b
Triacelluvax (combination vaccine containing r(modified) pertussis toxin	Chiron SpA	Immunization against diphtheria, tetanus and pertussis
Hepacare (r S, pre-S and pre-S2 hepatitis B surface antigens, produced in a mammalian (murine) cell line	Medeva Pharma	Immunization against hepatitis B
HBVAXPRO (rHBsAg produced in *S. cerevisiae*)	Aventis Pharma	Immunization of children and adolescents against hepatitis B

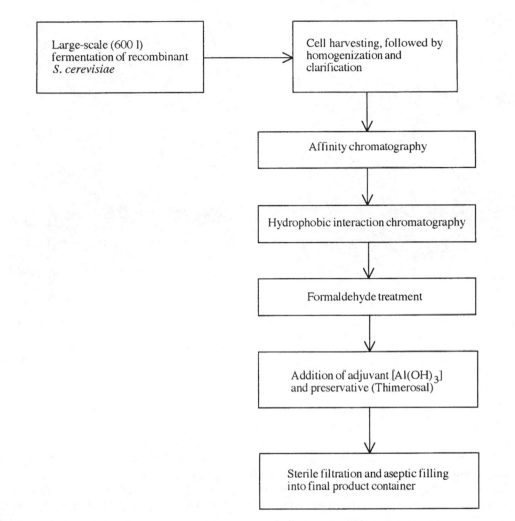

Figure 10.13. Overview of the production of recombinant HBsAg vaccine (Recombivax HB; Merck). A single dose of the product generally contains 10 μg of the antigen

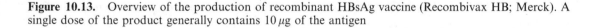

Whooping cough primarily affects children, with 90% of cases recorded in individuals under 5 years of age. Upon exposure, the bacteria adhere to the cilia of the upper respiratory tract, hence colonizing this area. They then synthesize and release several toxins which can induce both local and systemic damage.

Mass vaccination against whooping cough was introduced in the 1950s, using a killed *B. pertussis* suspension (i.e. a cellular vaccine). The incidence of whooping cough was subsequently reduced by up to 99% in countries where systematic vaccination was undertaken. Although clearly effective, some safety concerns accompany the use of this cellular vaccine. Severe side effects have been noted, albeit in an extremely low percentage of recipients.

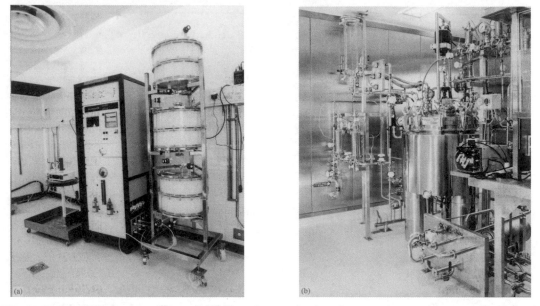

Figure 10.14. Photographs illustrating some clean room-based processing equipment utilized in the manufacture of SmithKline Beecham's hepatitis B surface antigen product. (a) represents a chromatographic fractionation system, consisting of (from left to right) fraction collector, control tower and chromatographic columns (stacked formation); (b) shows some of the equipment used to formulate the vaccine finished product. Photograph courtesy of SmithKline Beecham Biologicals s.a., Belgium

Complications have included anaphylaxis, brain damage and even death, typically occurring at an incidence of 3–9 cases per million doses administered.

Such safety concerns have, however, reduced the use of pertussis vaccination somewhat, particularly in several European countries. As a result, epidemics have once again been recorded in such jurisdictions. A safe pertussis vaccine is thus urgently required.

A number of *B. pertussis* (polypeptide) antigens have been expressed in *E. coli* and other recombinant systems. Several of these are being evaluated as potential subunit vaccines, including *B. pertussis* surface antigen, adhesion molecules and pertussis toxin. Pertussis toxin has been shown to protect mice from both aerosol and intracerebral challenge with virulent *B. pertussis*. The bacterial proteins that mediate surface adhesion protect mice from aerosol but not intracerebral challenge. Future pertussis subunit vaccines may well contain a combination of two or more pathogen-derived polypeptides.

Peptide vaccines

An alternative approach to the production of subunit vaccines entails their direct chemical synthesis. Peptides identical in sequence to short stretches of pathogen-derived polypeptide antigens can be easily and economically synthesized. The feasibility of this approach was first verified in the 1960s, when a hexapeptide purified from the enzymatic digest of tobacco mosaic virus was found to confer limited immunological protection against subsequent administration of the intact virus (the hexapeptide hapten was initially coupled to bovine serum albumin (BSA), used as a carrier to ensure an immunological response).

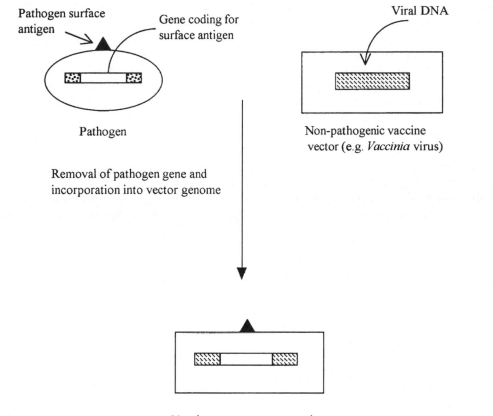

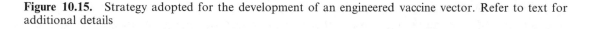

Figure 10.15. Strategy adopted for the development of an engineered vaccine vector. Refer to text for additional details

Similar synthetic vaccines have also been constructed which confer immunological protection against bacterial toxins, including diphtheria and cholera toxins. While coupling to a carrier is generally required to elicit an immunological response, some carriers are inappropriate due to their ability to elicit a hypersensitive reaction, particularly when repeat injections are undertaken. Such difficulties can be avoided by judicious choice of carrier. Often a carrier normally used for vaccination is itself used, e.g. tetanus toxoid has been used as a carrier for peptides derived from influenza haemagglutinin and *Plasmodium falciparum*.

Vaccine vectors

An alternative approach to the development of novel vaccine products entails the use of live vaccine vectors. The strategy followed involves incorporation of a gene/cDNA coding for a pathogen-derived antigen into a non-pathogenic species. If the resultant recombinant vector expresses the gene product on its surface, it may be used to immunize against the pathogen of interest (Figure 10.15).

Most vaccine vectors developed to date are viral-based, with poxviruses, picornaviruses and adenoviruses being used most. In general, such recombinant viral vectors elicit both strong humoral and cell-mediated immunity. The immunological response (particularly the cell-mediated response) to subunit vaccines is often less pronounced.

Poxviruses and, more specifically, the vaccinia virus, remain the most thoroughly characterized vector systems developed. These are large, enveloped double-stranded DNA viruses. They are the only DNA-containing viruses that replicate in the cytoplasm of infected cells. The most studied members of this family are variola and vaccinia. The former represents the causative agent of smallpox, while the latter — being antigenically related to variola but non-pathogenic — was used to immunize against smallpox. Vaccinia-based vaccination programmes led to the global eradication of smallpox, finally achieved by the early 1980s.

Poxvirus promoters are not recognized by eukaryotic transcription machinery. Transcription of poxviral genes is initiated only by virally encoded RNA polymerase, normally packaged alongside the DNA in the virion particles. Purified poxvirus DNA is, therefore, non-infectious.

A number of factors render vaccinia virus a particularly attractive vector system. These include:

- capacity to successfully assimilate large quantities of DNA in its genome;
- prior history of widespread and successful use as a vaccination agent;
- ability to elicit long-lasting immunity;
- ease of production and low production costs;
- stability of freeze-dried finished vaccine product.

The ability of vaccinia (and other poxviruses) to accommodate large sequences of heterologous DNA into its genome without adversely affecting its ability to replicate, remains one of its most attractive features. Integration of foreign genes must occur in regions of the viral genome not essential for viral replication. Two such sites are most often used. One is towards the left end of its genome, while the second is located within the thymidine kinase gene.

It is thought likely that up to 30 extra genes can be incorporated into vaccinia. The upper capacity has not been determined, but is likely to exceed 50 kb. This facilitates the development of a multivalent vaccine via expression of several pathogen-derived genes in the recombinant virus.

Early animal experiments have underlined the potential of vaccinia-based vector vaccines. Vaccinia virus-housing genes from HIV have clearly been found to elicit both humoral and cell-mediated immune responses in monkeys. Similar responses in other animals have been reported when surface polypeptides from a variety of additional pathogens have been expressed in recombinant vaccinia systems (Table 10.16). Human clinical trials are now in progress.

Adenoviruses also display potential as vaccine vectors. These double-stranded DNA viruses display a genome consisting of ca. 36 000 base pairs, encoding approximately 50 viral genes. Several antigenically distinct human adenovirus serotypes have been characterized and these viral species are endemic throughout the world. They can prompt respiratory tract infections and, to a lesser extent, gastrointestinal and genitourinary tract infections.

Live adenovirus strains have been isolated that cause asymptomatic infection and which have proved to be very safe and effective adenovirus vaccines. Unlike vaccinia, few sites exist in the adenoviral genome into which foreign DNA can be integrated without comprising viral function. Furthermore, packing limitations curb the quantity of foreign DNA that can be accommodated in the viral genome. However, a ca. 3000 base pair region can be removed from

Table 10.16. Some pathogens against which protective immunity was elicited by recombinant vaccinia vector systems. The virus invariably expressed a gene coding for a pathogen-derived surface polypeptide. The animal species in which the experiments were carried out is also listed

Pathogen	Protected species
Bovine leukaemia virus	Sheep
Bovine papilloma virus	Rats
Epstein–Barr virus	Cotton top tamarins
Equine herpes virus	Hamsters
Friend leukaemia virus	Mice
Hepatitis B virus	Chimpanzees
Herpes simplex virus	Mice
Human papilloma virus	Mice, rats
Human parainfluenza virus	Monkeys
Leishmania	Mice
Measles	Mice, rats, dogs
Polyoma virus	Rats
Pseudorabies virus	Mice, pigs
Rabies	Mice, foxes, raccoons, dogs
Respiratory syncytial virus	Rats, mice, monkeys
Yellow fever	Mice

a section of the genome, termed the E3 region. This facilitates incorporation of pathogen-derived or other DNA at this point.

Recombinant adenoviruses containing the hepatitis B surface antigen gene, the HIV P160 gene, the respiratory syncytial virus F gene, as well as the herpes simplex virus glycoprotein B gene, have all been generated using this approach. Many have been tested in animal models and have been found to elicit humoral and cell-mediated immunity against the pathogen of interest.

Picornaviruses are also being evaluated as potential vaccine vectors. Unlike the large pox- and adenoviruses discussed above, these are small viruses, incapable of carrying a gene coding for a complete foreign protein. However, such viral particles could easily house nucleotide sequences coding for short peptides representative of specific antigenic sites/epitopes present in pathogen-derived polypeptides. Studies continue in an effort to identify such putative short peptides.

The use of recombinant viral vectors as vaccination tools displays considerable clinical promise. One potential complicatory factor, however, centres around the possibility that previous recipient exposure to the virus being used as a vector would negate the therapeutic efficacy of the product. Such prior exposure would likely indicate the presence of circulating immune memory cells which could initiate an immediate immunological response upon re-entry of the virus into the host. Studies involving repeat administration of vaccinia virus have, to some extent, confirmed this possibility. However, the degree to which such an effect limits the applicability of this approach in a clinical setting remains to be elucidated.

Development of an AIDS vaccine

Acquired immune deficiency syndrome (AIDS) was initially described in the USA in 1981, although sporadic cases probably occurred for at least two decades prior to this. By 1983, the causative agent, now termed human immunodeficiency virus (HIV), was identified. HIV is a

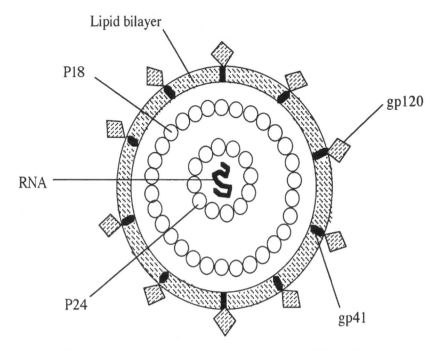

Figure 10.16. Simplified schematic representation of a cross-section of HIV. The central core contains the viral RNA, consisting of two identical single strand subunits (ca. 9.2 kb long). Associated with the RNA are two (RNA-binding) proteins, P7 and P9, as well as the viral reverse transcriptase complex (not shown above). Surrounding this is the protein P24, which forms the shell of the nuclear caspid. Covering this, in turn, is a lipid bilayer derived from the host cell, still carrying some host cell antigens. The viral protein, P18, is associated with the inner membrane leaflet. Viral gp41 represents a transmembrane protein, while viral gp120, residing on the outside of the lipid bilayer, is attached to gp41 via disulphide bonds

member of the lentivirus subfamily of retroviruses. It is a spherical, enveloped particle, 100–150 nm in diameter, and contains RNA as its genetic material (Figure 10.16).

The viral surface protein, gp120, is capable of binding to a specific site on the CD4 molecule, found on the surface of susceptible cells (Table 10.17). Some CD4-negative (CD4⁻) cells may (rarely) also become infected, indicating the existence of an entry mechanism independent of CD4.

Infection of CD4⁺ cells commences via interaction between gp120 and the CD4 glycoprotein, which effectively acts as the viral receptor. Entry of the virus into the cell, which appears to

Table 10.17. Some cell types whose susceptibility to infection by HIV is believed to be due to the presence of the CD4 antigen on their surface

T-helper lymphocytes
Blood monocytes
Tissue macrophages
Dendritic cells of skin and lymph nodes
Brain microglia

require some additional cellular components, occurs via endocytosis and/or fusion of the viral and cellular membranes. The gp41 transmembrane protein plays an essential role in this process.

Once released into the cell, the viral RNA is transcribed (by the associated viral reverse transcriptase) into double-stranded DNA. The retroviral DNA can then integrate into the host cell genome (or, in some instances, remain unintegrated). In resting cells, transcription of viral genes usually does not occur to any significant extent. However, commencement of active cellular growth/differentiation usually also triggers expression of proviral genes and, hence, synthesis of new viral particles. Aggressive expression of viral genes usually leads to cell death. Some cells, however (particularly macrophages), often permit chronic low-level viral synthesis and release without cell death.

Entry of the virus into the human subject is generally accompanied by initial viral replication, lasting a few weeks. High-level viraemia (presence of viral particles in the blood) is noted and p24 antigen can be detected in the blood. Clinical symptoms associated with the initial infection include an influenza-like illness, joint pains and general enlargement of the lymph nodes. This primary viraemia is brought under control within 3–4 weeks. This appears to be mediated largely by HIV-specific cytotoxic T lymphocytes, indicating the likely importance of cell-mediated immunity in bringing the initial infection under control. While HIV-specific antibodies are also produced at this stage, effective neutralizing antibodies are detected mainly after this initial stage of infection.

After this initial phase of infection subsides, the free viral load in the blood declines, often to almost undetectable levels. This latent phase may last for anything up to 10 years or more. During this phase, however, there does seem to be continuous synthesis and destruction of viral particles. This is accompanied by a high turnover rate of ($CD4^+$) T helper lymphocytes. The levels of these T lymphocytes decline with time, as do antibody levels specific for viral proteins. The circulating viral load often increases as a result and the depletion of T helper cells compromises general immune function. As the immune system fails, classical symptoms of AIDS-related complex (ARC) and, finally, full-blown AIDS begin to develop.

In excess of 40 million individuals are now thought to be infected by HIV. In 2001 alone it was estimated that 3 million people died from AIDS and a further 5 million became infected with the virus. Over 20 million people in total are now thought to have died from AIDS. The worst-affected geographical region is the southern half of Africa (Table 10.18). 90% of sufferers live in poorer world regions. So far, no effective therapy has been discovered and the main hope

Table 10.18. WHO-estimated numbers of individuals infected with HIV by the end of 2001. Almost 75% of these live in the southern half of Africa

World region	Numbers infected (millions)
Sub-Saharan Africa	28.5
South Asia	5.6
South America	1.5
North America	1.0
Eastern Europe and Central Asia	1.0
East Asia and Pacific	1.0
North Africa and Middle East	0.5
Western Europe	0.5
Caribbean	0.4
Australia and New Zealand	0.015

of eradicating this disease lies with the development of safe, effective vaccines. The first such putative vaccine entered clinical trials in 1987 but, thus far, no truly effective vaccine has been developed.

Difficulties associated with vaccine development

A number of attributes of HIV and its mode of infection conspire to render development of an effective vaccine less than straightforward. These factors include:

- HIV displays extensive genetic variation, often even within a single individual. Such genetic variation is particularly prominent in the viral *env* gene whose product, gp160, is subsequently proteolytically processed, yielding gp120 and gp41.
- HIV infects and destroys T helper lymphocytes, i.e. it directly attacks an essential component of the immune system itself.
- Although infected individuals display a wide range of anti-viral immunological responses, these ultimately fail to destroy the virus. A greater understanding of what elements of immunity are most effective in combating HIV infection is required.
- After initial virulence subsides, large numbers of cells harbour unexpressed proviral DNA. The immune system has no way of identifying such cells. An effective vaccine must thus induce the immune system to: (a) bring the viral infection under control before cellular infection occurs; or (b) destroy cells once they begin to produce viral particles and destroy the viral particles released.
- The infection may often be spread, not via transmission of free viral particles, but via direct transmission of infected cells harbouring the proviral DNA.

AIDS vaccines in clinical trials

A number of approaches are being assessed with regard to developing an effective AIDS vaccine. No safe attenuated form of the virus has been recognized to date or is likely to be developed in the foreseeable future. The high level of mutation associated with HIV would, in any case, heighten fears that spontaneous reversion of any such product to virulence would be possible.

The potential of inactivated viral particles as effective vaccines has gained some attention but again, fears of accidental transmission of disease if inactivation methods are not consistently 100% effective have dampened enthusiasm for such an approach. In addition, the stringent containment conditions required to produce large quantities of the virus renders such production processes expensive.

Despite such difficulties, at least one such inactivated product has reached clinical trials. The viral particles are initially propagated in cultured human T cells. They are then treated with formaldehyde to inactivate them—a process which also removes the viral envelope. The virion particles are then treated with γ-irradiation in order to ensure inactivation of the viral genome. The final product is administered along with an adjuvant in order to maximize the immunological response (see later).

Notwithstanding the possible value of such inactivated viral vaccines, the bulk of products developed to date are subunit vaccines. Live vector vaccines expressing HIV genes have also been developed (Table 10.19).

Table 10.19.   Some putative HIV vaccines that have made it to clinical trials

Vaccine preparation	Developing company
Inactivated viral particles	Immune response
rgp120 subunit vaccines	Genentech/Vaxgen
	Biocine
	Chiron/Ciba Geigy
rgp160 subunit vaccines	MicroGenes Sys. Inc.
	Immuno-Ag.
rp24 subunit vaccines	MicroGenes Sys. Inc.
Live vaccines based on viral vectors	Biocine
	Genentech
Octameric V3 peptide	UBI

Much of the pre-clinical data generated with regard to these vaccines entailed the use of one of two animal model systems: simian immunodeficiency virus (SIV) infection of macaque monkeys and HIV infection of chimpanzees. Most of the positive results observed in such systems have been in association with the chimp/HIV model. However, no such system can replace actual testing in humans.

Most of the recombinant subunit vaccines currently being tested employ gp120 or gp160 expressed in yeast, insect or mammalian (mainly CHO) cell lines. Eukaryotic systems facilitate glycosylation of the protein products. Like all subunit vaccines, these stimulate a humoral-based immune response while failing to elicit a strong T cell response. This approach thus presupposes that the production of neutralizing antibodies alone would be sufficient to defeat the viral infection. This may well not turn out to be the case. On the other hand, gp120/160-based subunit vaccines have been shown to protect chimps against HIV infection, albeit under very controlled laboratory conditions.

Much work has been invested into identification of which viral antigens are capable of producing the most effective anti-viral (i.e. neutralizing) antibodies. Such antibodies are mostly directed against gp120. Further studies have pinpointed the principal neutralizing domain of gp120. This short stretch of the polypeptide backbone is known as the V3 loop and it is located within one of the five hypervariable regions of gp120. Thus, while anti-V3 antibodies likely represent the most effective HIV-neutralizing species, these antibodies will also likely be strain-specific. Some protective vaccines based upon multimeric V3 loop peptide sequences have also been developed.

Some additional subunit vaccines are being developed, based upon internal viral polypeptides, particularly the p24 core protein. This was chosen as it is known to contain epitopes capable of eliciting a T cell response, and core proteins are generally less subject to antigenic drift than envelope proteins.

Several HIV vaccine systems based upon live vectors have also been developed, in an attempt to stimulate a significant T cell as well as B cell immune response. Both envelope and core antigens have been expressed in a number of recombinant viral systems, most notably in vaccinia. The clinical efficacy of these remain to be established.

Large-scale clinical trials are likely to be the only way by which any HIV vaccine may be properly assessed. In addition, a greater understanding of the molecular interplay between the viral and immune system may provide clues as to the development of novel vaccine and/or therapeutic products, e.g. a small proportion of infected individuals remain clinically asymptomatic for periods considerably greater than the average 10–15 years. An understanding of the immunological or other factors which delay onset of ARC/full-blown AIDS in these individuals may assist in the design of more effective vaccines. In addition, it has more recently been reported that a very small proportion of individuals exposed (often repeatedly) to the virus remain uninfected. The genetic/immunological mechanisms underlining such resistance may provide useful insights into the elements of immunity that an effective vaccine needs to trigger most.

Although the primary objective of any vaccine is its prophylactic use (i.e. prevention of future occurrence of a disease), AIDS vaccines may also be of therapeutic value. This supposition is based upon the fact that the immune system controls the viral infection for a time period. Hence, any agent capable of enhancing the anti-HIV immune response may prolong this effect.

Both industrial concerns and many government organizations continue to invest large capital sums in AIDS vaccine research. Although much progress has been made, the complexity of the disease has confounded the development of a truly effective vaccine thus far. By mid-2002 a preventitive AIDS vaccine 'AIDS VAX' (its trade name) had reached phase III clinical trials. The product, developed by a spin-off company of Genentech called Vaxgen is a recombinant gp120 glycoprotein produced in a CHO cell line.

Cancer vaccines

The identification of tumour-associated antigens could pave the way for the development of a range of cancer vaccines. A number of tumour-associated antigens have already been characterized, as previously described. Theoretically, administration of tumour-associated antigens may effectively immunize an individual against any cancer type characterized by expression of the tumour-associated antigen in question. Co-administration of a strong adjuvant (see later section) would be advantageous, as it would stimulate an enhanced immune response. This is important as many tumour-associated antigens appear to be weak immunogens. Administration of subunit-based tumor-associated antigen vaccines would primarily stimulate a humoral immune response. The use of viral vectors may ultimately prove more effective, as a T cell response appears to be central to the immunological destruction of cancer cells.

The latter approach has been adopted in experimental studies involving malignant melanoma. These transformed cells express significantly elevated levels of a surface glycoprotein, p97. p97 is also expressed — but at far lower levels — on the surface of many normal cell types. Initial animal studies have indicated that administration of a recombinant vaccinia vector expressing p97 has a protective effect against challenge with melanoma cells. However, protracted safety studies would be required in this, or similar, instances to prove that such vaccines would not, for example, induce an autoimmune response if the antigen was not wholly tumour-specific. The development of truly effective cancer vaccines probably requires a more comprehensive understanding of the transformed phenotype and how these cells normally evade immune surveillance in the first place. Notwithstanding this, limited clinical studies in this field have already begun.

Recombinant veterinary vaccines

Amongst the limited number of biopharmaceuticals approved for animal use (Chapter 1), recombinant vaccines represent the single largest sub-group. Several such products target pigs,

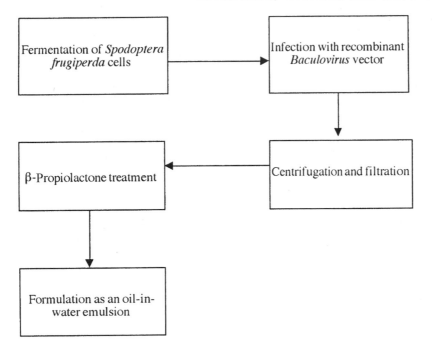

Figure 10.17. Overview of the manufacture of the veterinary vaccine Porcilis pesti. Refer to text for specific details

including Porcilis pesti and Bayovac CSF E2. *Porcilis pesti*, for example, contains a recombinant form of the classical swine fever virus E2 antigen, the immunodominant surface antigen associated with this viral pathogen. It is used to immunize young pigs. An overview of its manufacture is presented in Figure 10.17. The process is initiated by growth of *Spodoptera frugiperda* cells, typically in a 500 l fermenter. The cells are then infected with the recombinant baculovirus vector, resulting in high-level expression of the recombinant E2 antigen. The antigen is harvested from the production medium by low-speed centrifugation and membrane filtration steps, which serve to remove intact cells/cellular debris. The antigen-containing supernatant is then treated with β-propiolactone in order to inactivate any viral particles present. The antigen is not subjected to subsequent high-resolution chromatographic purification steps, and hence is not purified to homogeneity. The product is then formulated as an oil-in-water emulsion.

Adjuvant technology

Administration of many vaccines on their own stimulates a poor host immunological response. This is particularly true of the more recently developed subunit vaccines. An adjuvant is defined as any material that enhances the cellular and/or humoral immune response to an antigen. Adjuvants thus generally elicit an earlier, more potent and longer-lasting, immunological reaction against co-administered antigen. In addition, the use of adjuvants can often facilitate administration of reduced quantities of antigen to achieve an adequate immunological response.

Table 10.20. Overview of the adjuvant preparations that have been developed to date, or are under investigation. Of these, aluminium-based substances are the only adjuvants used to any significant degree in humans. Calcium phosphate and oil emulsions find very limited application in human medicine

Mineral compounds	Aluminium phosphate, $AlPO_4$
	Aluminium hydroxide, $Al(OH)_3$
	Alum, $AlK(SO_4)_2.12H_2O$
	Calcium phosphate, $CaPO_4$
Bacterial products	Mycobacterial species
	Mycobacterial components (e.g. trehalose dimycolate, muramyl dipeptide)
	Corynebacterium species
	Bordetella pertussis
	Lipopolysaccharide
Oil-based emulsions	Freund's complete/incomplete adjuvants (FCA/FIA)
	Starch oil
Saponins	Quil A
Liposomes	
Immunostimulatory complexes (ISCOMs)	
Some cytokines	Interleukins-1 and -2

This implies consequent economic savings, as vaccines (particularly subunit and vector vaccines) are far more expensive to produce than the adjuvant.

A number of different adjuvant preparations have been developed (Table 10.20). Most preparations also display some associated toxicity and, as a general rule, the greater the product's adjuvanticity, the more toxic it is likely to be. A few different adjuvants may be used in veterinary medicine; however, for safety reasons, aluminium-based products are the only adjuvants routinely used in human medicine. Application of many of the aggressive adjuvant materials is reserved for selected experimentation purposes in animals.

The concept of enhancing the immune response against an antigen by co-administration of an immunostimulatory substance dates back to the beginning of the 20th century. Oil-based emulsions were used from 1916 on, while in the mid-1920s, scientists discovered that the immunological response to administration of tetanus and diphtheria toxin was increased by co-administration of a range of (somewhat unlikely) substances, including agar, starch oil, saponin, tapioca and breadcrumbs.

Few of these substances remain in medical use, due to unacceptable side effects. An ideal adjuvant should display several specific characteristics. These include:

- safety (no unacceptable local/systemic responses);
- elicit protective immunity, even against weak immunogens;
- be non-pyrogenic;
- be chemically defined (facilitates consistent manufacture and quality control testing);
- be effective in infants/young children;
- yield stable formulation with antigen;
- be biodegradable;
- be non-immunogenic itself.

Adjuvant mode of action

Adjuvants are a heterogenous family of substances in terms of both their chemical structure and their mode of action. The observed adjuvanticity of any such substance may be due to one or more of the following factors:

- depot formation of antigen; this results in the subsequent slow release of the antigen from the site of injection which, in turn, ensures its prolonged exposure to the immune system;
- enhanced antigen presentation to the cells of the immune system;
- the direct induction of immunostimulatory substances, most notably interleukins and other cytokines.

In addition to the use of adjuvants *per se*, modification of the antigen may result in increasing its inherent immunogenicity. Such modifications can include:

- polymerization of protein antigens (e.g. by reaction with gluteraldehyde or other cross-linking agents); this approach has been successfully adopted with tetanus and diphtheria toxoids;
- conjugation of proteins to polysaccharides;
- cationization of protein antigens.

Mineral-based adjuvants

A number of mineral-based substances display an adjuvant effect. Although calcium phosphate, calcium chloride and salts of various metals (e.g. zinc sulphate and cerium nitrate) display some effect, aluminium-based substances are by far the most potent. Most commonly employed are aluminium hydroxide and aluminium phosphate (Table 10.20). Their adjuvanticity, coupled to their proven safety, renders them particularly valuable in the preparation of vaccines for young children. They have been incorporated into millions of doses of such vaccine products so far.

The principal method by which aluminium-adjuvanted vaccines are prepared entails mixing the antigen in solution with a pre-formed aluminium phosphate (or hydroxide) precipitate under chemically-defined conditions (e.g. of pH). Adsorption of the antigen to the aluminium-based gel ensues, with such preparations being generally termed 'aluminium-adsorbed vaccines'. 1 mg of aluminium hydroxide will usually adsorb ca. 50–200 μg of protein.

The major mode of action of such products appears to be depot formation at the site of injection. The antigen is only slowly released from the gel, ensuring its sustained exposure to immune surveillance. The aluminium compounds are also capable of activating complement. This can lead to a local inflammatory response, with consequent attraction of immunocompetent cells to the site of action.

Despite their popularity, aluminium-based adjuvants suffer from several drawbacks. They tend to effectively stimulate only the humoral arm of the immune response. They cannot be frozen or lyophylized, as either process promotes destruction of their gel-based structure. In addition, aluminium-based products display poor or no adjuvanticity when combined with some antigens (e.g. typhoid or *Haemophilus influenzae* type b capsular polysaccharides).

Oil-based emulsion adjuvants

The adjuvanticity of oil emulsions was first recognized in the early 1900s. However, the first such product to gain widespread attention was Freund's complete adjuvant (FCA), developed in 1937. This product essentially contained a mixture of paraffin (i.e. mineral) oil with dead

Table 10.21. Some toxic effects sometimes noted when Freund's complete adjuvant (FCA) is administered to experimental animals

Inflammation/abscess formation at the site of injection
Pyrogenic effect (fever)
Severe pain
Possible organ damage
Possible induction of autoimmune disease
Hypersensitization
Induction of cancer in some animals under some conditions

mycobacteria, formulated to form a water-in-oil emulsion. Arlacel A (mannide mono-oleate) is usually added as an emulsifier.

Freund's incomplete adjuvant (FIA) is a similar product. It differs from FCA in that it lacks the mycobacterial component and, consequently, displays somewhat lesser adjuvanticity. The mode of action of FIA is largely attributed to depot formation. The mycobacterial components in FCA have additional direct immunostimulatory activities.

Although it is one of the most potent adjuvant substances known, FCA is too toxic for human use. Some of its reported side effects are listed in Table 10.21. Its toxicity has also precluded its routine veterinary application, although it is sometimes used for experimental purposes. FIA is less toxic than its mycobacterial-containing counterpart. It has found used in the preparation of selected animal vaccines, and was even incorporated into some earlier human vaccines (Table 10.22). However, its use in humans (and to a large extent, animals) has been discontinued due to its reported toxic effects.

The presence in mineral oil of potential carcinogens also raised safety concerns relating to FCA/FIA. Mineral oil is composed of a complex mixture of both cyclic and non-cyclic hydrocarbons of varying chain length, some of which display carcinogenic potential. Arlacel A was also found to be capable of inducing cancer in mice.

Various additional oil-based adjuvants have subsequently been developed. Adjuvant 65, for example, consists of 86% peanut oil, 10% Arlacel A and 4% aluminium monostearate (as a stabilizer). Unlike mineral oil, peanut oil is composed largely of triglycerides, which are readily metabolized by the body. Although adjuvant 65 was initially proved safe and effective in humans, it displayed less adjuventicity than FIA. Its use was largely discontinued, mainly due to the presence in its formulation of Arlacel A.

Latterly, some oil-in-water adjuvants have been developed. Many are squalene-in-water emulsions. Emulsifiers most commonly used include polyalcohols, such as Tween and Span. In some cases, immunostimulatory molecules (including muramyl dipeptide and trehalose

Table 10.22. Some vaccine preparations in which Freund's incomplete adjuvant (FIA) was used as an adjuvant

Human vaccines	Influenza vaccines
	Dead poliomyelitis vaccines
Veterinary vaccines	Foot and mouth disease
	Newcastle disease
	Rabies
	Distemper
	Infectious canine hepatitis

dimycolate; see next section) have also been incorporated in order to enhance adjuvanticity. These continue to be carefully assessed and may well form a future family of useful adjuvant preparations.

Bacteria/bacterial products as adjuvants

Selected microorganisms have been identified which can trigger particularly potent immunological responses. The immunostimulatory properties of these cells has generated interest in their potential application as adjuvants. Examples include various Mycobacteria, *Corynebacterium parvum*, *C. granulosum* and *Bordetella pertussis*. Although some such microorganisms are used as antigens in vaccines, they are considered too toxic to be used solely in the role of adjuvant. Thus, researchers have sought to identify the specific microbial biomolecules responsible for the observed immunostimulatory activity. It was hoped that these substances, when purified, might display lesser/no toxic side effects, while retaining their immunostimulatory capacity.

Fractionation of mycobacteria resulted in the identification of two cellular immunostimulatory components, trehalose dimycolate (TDM) and muramyl dipeptides (MDP). Both are normally found in association with the mycobacterial cell wall. TDM is composed of a molecule of trehalose (a disaccharide consisting of two molecules of α-D-glucose linked via an α 1–1 glycosidic bond), linked to two molecules of mycolic acid (a long-chain aliphatic hydrocarbon-based acid) found almost exclusively in association with mycobacteria. TDM, while retaining its adjuvanticity, is relatively non-toxic.

The structure of the native immunostimulatory MDPs was found to be n-acetyl muramyl-L-alanyl-D-isoglutamine (N-acetyl muramic acid is a base component of bacterial peptidoglycan). Native TDM is a potent pyrogen and is too toxic for general use as an adjuvant. The molecular basis underlying MDP's adjuvanticity remains to be fully elucidated. Administration of MDP is, however, known to activate a number of cell types which play direct/indirect roles in immune function, and induces the secretion of various immunomodulatory cytokines (Table 10.23).

A number of derivatives were synthesized in the hope of identifying a modified form which retained its adjuvanticity but displayed lesser toxicity. Some such derivatives, most notably threonyl-MDP, muramyl tripeptide and murabutide, display some clinical promise in this regard.

Table 10.23. Some cell types activated upon administration of MDP. Activation induces synthesis of a range of immunomodulatory cytokines by these (and other) cells

Cell types activated	Macrophages
	Mast cells
	Polymorphonuclear leukocytes
	Endothelial cells
	Fibroblasts
	Platelets
Cytokines and other molecules induced	Interleukin-1
	Colony stimulating factors
	Fibroblast activating factor
	B cell growth factor
	Prostaglandins

Table 10.24. Some characteristic biological effects induced by lipopolysacharide

---

Pyrogenicity
Generalized and severe toxicity
Adjuvanticity
Activation of macrophages and granulocytes
B lymphocyte mitogen
Activation of complement
Induction of synthesis of TNF, CSF, IL-1, IFN
Some anti-tumour activity

Threonyl-MDP, for example, has been included in the formulation known as Syntex adjuvant formulation-1 (SAF-1). Animal studies suggest that this adjuvant is non-toxic and elicits a good B and T cell response.

An additional bacterial component displaying appreciable adjuvanticity is the *Corynebacterium granulosum*-derived p40 particulate fraction. p40 is composed of fragments of cell wall peptidoglycan and associated glycoproteins. Its administration to animals results in activation of various elements of immune function while displaying little or no toxic effects. In addition to activation of macrophages, p40 induces synthesis of a variety of cytokines, most notably IL-2, TNF, IFN-α and IFN-γ. Not surprisingly, p40 was found to enhance both specific and non-specific resistance to a wide range of pathogens and was also shown to display anti-tumour activity. Clinical trials in humans appear to confirm many of these observations. p40, or derivatives thereof, may therefore yet play a role in human or veterinary immunization programmes.

The observed adjuvanticity of *Bordetella pertussis* is largely attributable to the presence of pertussis toxin and lipopolysaccharide (LPS). LPS, a constituent of the cell envelope of Gram-negative bacteria (Chapter 3), essentially consists of polysaccharide moieties to which lipid (lipid A) is covalently attached.

While purified LPS displays potent immunostimulatory properties, it also induces various toxic side effects (Table 10.24), the most prominent of which is pyrogenicity. These effects render application of LPS as an adjuvant unacceptable. Both its immunostimulatory and toxic properties are mainly associated with the lipid A portion of the molecule. Attempts have been made to chemically or otherwise alter the lipid A portion in order to ameliorate the observed toxicity.

Succinylated or phthalylinated LPS displays significant reduction in toxicity (up to 100 000-fold) while retaining its adjuvanticity. Acid treatment (0.1 M HCl) of LPS obtained from various *Salmonella* species resulted in the production of an LPS-derivative termed monophosphoryl lipid A (MPL). This also displays adjuvanticity, with little associated pyrogenicity or toxicity. This alteration of biological activity can also be achieved by removal of some of the fatty acids found in the LPS lipid A region. As LPS is effective in activating both cellular and humoral immune responses, research in this area continues to be pursued.

Additional adjuvants

In addition to the immunostimulatory substances discussed above, the adjuvanticity of a variety of other substances is also being appraised. These include saponins, liposomes and immuno-stimulatory complexes (ISCOMS).

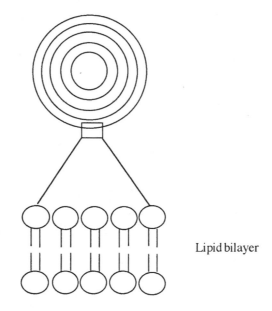

Figure 10.18.   Generalized liposome structure. Refer to text for details

Saponins are a family of glycosides (sugar derivatives) widely distributed in plants. Each saponin consists of a sugar moiety bound to a 'sapogenin'–either a steroid or a triterpene. The immunostimulatory properties of the saponin fraction isolated from the bark of *Quillaja* (a tree) has been long recognized; Quil A (which consists of a mixture of related saponins) is used as an adjuvant in selected veterinary vaccines. However, its haemolytic potential precludes its use in human vaccines. Research efforts continue in an attempt to identify individual saponins (or derivatives thereof) that would make safe and effective adjuvants for use in human medicine.

Liposomes are membrane-based supramolecular particles which consist of a number of concentric lipid membrane bilayers separated by aqueous compartments (Figure 10.18). They were developed initially as carriers for therapeutic drugs. Initially, the bilayers were almost exclusively phospholipid-based. More recently, non-phospholipid-based liposomes have been developed.

The adjuvanticity of liposomes depends upon their composition, number of layers and charge characteristics. They act as effective adjuvants for both protein and carbohydrate-based antigen and help stimulate both B and T cell responses. Their likely mode of action includes depot formation, but they also possibly increase/enhance antigen presentation to macrophages. The exact molecular mechanism(s) by which they stimulate a T cell response remains to be elucidated, but it appears to be associated with their hydrophobicity. Liposomes are likely to gain more widespread use as adjuvants when technical difficulties associated with their stability and consistent/reproducible production are resolved.

ISCOMs are stable (non-covalent) complexes composed of a mixture of Quil A, cholesterol and (an amphipathic) antigen. ISCOMs stimulate both humoral and cellular immune responses and have been used in the production of some veterinary vaccines. Their use in humans, however, has not been licensed so far, mainly due to safety concerns relating to the Quil A component.

In summary, therefore, a whole range of adjuvants have thus far been identified/developed. Problems of toxicity have precluded use of many of these adjuvants (particularly in humans). However, research efforts continue in an attempt to develop the next generation of safe and, hopefully, even more effective vaccine adjuvants.

FURTHER READING

Books

Amyes, S. (2002). *Tumour immunology*. Taylor & Francis, London.
Grossbard, M. (1998). *Monoclonal Antibody-based Therapy of Cancer*. Marcel Dekker, New York.
Harris, W. (1997). *Antibody Therapeutics*. CRC Press, Boca Raton, FL.
Kontermann, R. (2001). *Antibody Engineering*. Springer-Verlag, Berlin.
Liddell, J. (1995). *Antibody Technology*. BIOS Scientific, Oxford.
Plotkin, S. (1999). *Vaccines*. W.B. Saunders, London.
Powell, M. (1995). *Vaccine Design: The Subunit and Adjuvant Approach*. Plenum, New York.
Stern, P. (2000). *Cancer Vaccines and Immunotherapy*. Cambridge University Press, Cambridge.
Talwar, G. (1994). *Synthetic Vaccines*. Springer-Verlag, Berlin.
Woodrow, G. (1997). *New Generation Vaccines*. Marcel Dekker, New York.

Articles

Antibody technology

Benhar, I. (2001). Biotechnological applications of phage and cell display. *Biotechnol. Adv.* **19**, 1–33.
Berger, M. *et al.* (2002). Therapeutic applications of monoclonal antibodies. *Am. J. Med. Sci.* **324**(1), 14–30.
Breedveld, F. (2000). Therapeutic monoclonal antibodies. *Lancet* **355**, 735–740.
Chapman, P. (2002). PEGylated antibodies and antibody fragments for improved therapy: a review. *Adv. Drug Deliv. Rev.* **54**(4), 531–545.
Chester, K. & Hawkins, R. (1995). Clinical issues in antibody design. *Trends Biotechnol.* **13**, 294–300.
Funaro, A. *et al.* (2000). Monoclonal antibodies and the therapy of human cancers. *Biotechnol. Adv.* **18**(5), 385–401.
Goldenberg, D. *et al.* (2002). Targeted therapy of cancer with radiolabeled antibodies. *J. Nuclear Med.* **43**(5), 693–713.
Hoogenboom, H. *et al.* (1998). Antibody phage display technology and its applications. *Immunotechnology* **4**, 1–20.
Huennekens, F. (1994). Tumor targeting: activation of prodrugs by enzyme-monoclonal antibody conjugates. *Trends Biotechnol.* **12**, 234–239.
Keating, G. & Perry, C. (2002). Infliximab—an updated review of its use in Crohn's disease and rheumatoid arthritis. *Biodrugs* **16**(2), 111–148.
Kohler, G. & Milstein, C. (1975). Continuous culture of fused cells secreting antibody of pre-defined specificity. *Nature* **256**, 495–497.
Murry, J. (2000). Monoclonal antibody treatment of solid tumors: a coming of age. *Semin. Oncol.* **27**(6), 64–70.
Senter, P. & Springer, C. (2001). Selective activation of anticancer prodrugs by monoclonal antibody–enzyme conjugates. *Adv. Drug Deliv. Rev.* **53**(3), 247–264.
Trail, P. & Bianchi, A. (1999). Monoclonal antibody drug conjugates in the treatment of cancer. *Curr. Opin. Immunol.* **11**(5), 584–588.
Umemura, S. *et al.* (2002). Pathological evaluation of HER2 overexpression for the treatment of metastatic breast cancers by humanized anti-HER2 monoclonal antibody (Trastuzumab). *Acta Biochim. Cytochim.* **35**(2), 77–81.
Wang, R. (1999). Human tumor antigens: implications for cancer vaccine development. *J. Mol. Med.* **77**(9), 640–655.
Wang, R. & Rosenberg, S. (1999). Human tumor antigens for cancer vaccine development. *Immunol. Rev.* **170**, 85–100.
Winter, G. & Milstein, C. (1991). Man-made antibodies. *Nature* **349**, 293–299.

Vaccine technology

Andino, R. *et al.* (1994). Engineering poliovirus as a vaccine vector for the expression of diverse antigens. *Science* **265**, 1448–1451.
Chauhan, V. (1996). Progress towards malaria vaccine. *Curr. Sci.* **71**(12), 967–975.
Cox, J. & Coutter, A. (1997). Adjuvants—a classification and review of their modes of action. *Vaccine* **15**(3), 248–256.
Doolan, D. & Hoffman, S. (1997). Multigene vaccination against malaria—a multistage, multi-immune response approach. *Parasitol. Today* **13**(5), 171–178.

Edelman, R. (2002). The development and use of vaccine adjuvants. *Mol. Biotechnol.* **21**(2), 129–148.

Esparza, J. *et al.* (1995). HIV-preventive vaccines, progress to date. *Drugs* **50**(5), 792–804.

Frontiers in Medicine: Vaccines (1994). *Science* **265** (Special Issue, September 2).

Gaschen, B. *et al.* (2002). AIDS — diversity considerations in HIV-1 vaccine selection. *Science* **296**(5577), 2354–2360.

Gupta, R. & Siber, G. (1995). Adjuvants for human vaccines — current status, problems and future prospects. *Vaccine* **13**(14), 1263–1274.

Hilton, L. *et al.* (2002). The emerging role of avian cytokines as immunotherapeutics and vaccine adjuvants. *Vet. Immunol. Immunopathol.* **85**(3–4), 119–128.

Lachman, L. *et al.* (1996). Cytokine-containing liposomes as vaccine adjuvants. *Eur. Cytokine Network* **7**(4), 693–698.

Lemon, S. & Thomas, D. (1997). Drug therapy — vaccines to prevent viral hepatitis. *N. Engl. J. Med.* **336**(3), 196–204.

Mason, H. *et al.* (2002). Edible plant vaccines: applications for prophylactic and therapeutic molecular medicine. *Trends Mol. Med.* **8**(7), 324–329.

Ohagan, D. *et al.* (1997). Recent advances in vaccine adjuvants — the development of Mf59 emulsion and polymeric microparticles. *Mol. Med. Today* **3**(2), 69–75.

Perkus, M. *et al.* (1995). Poxvirus-based vaccine candidates for cancer, AIDS and other infectious diseases. *J. Leukocyte Biol.* **58**, 1–10.

Plotkin, S. (2002). Vaccines in the twenty-first century. *Hybridoma Hybridom.* **21**(2), 135–145.

Poland, G. *et al.* (2002). Science, medicine and the future — new vaccine development. *Br. Med. J.* **324**(7349), 1315–1319.

Russo, S. *et al.* (1997). What's going on in vaccine technology? *Med. Res. Rev.* **17**(3), 277–301.

Sandhu, J. (1994). Engineered human vaccines. *Crit. Rev. Biotechnol.* **14**(1), 1–27.

Sela, M. *et al.* (2002). Therapeutic vaccines: realities of today and hopes for the future. *Drug Discovery Today* **7**(12), 664–673.

Singh, M. & O'Hagan, D. (2002). Recent advances in vaccine adjuvants. *Pharmaceut. Res.* **19**(6), 715–728.

Strominger, J. (1995). Peptide vaccination against cancer? *Nature Med.* **1**(11), 1140.

Wang, R. & Rosenberg, S. (1999). Human tumor antigens for cancer vaccine development. *Immun. Rev.* **170**, 85–100.

Yokoyama, N. *et al.* (1997). Recombinant viral vector vaccines for veterinary use. *J. Vet. Med. Sci.* **59**(5), 311–322.

Chapter 11
Nucleic acid therapeutics

Throughout the 1980s and early 1990s, the term 'biopharmaceutical' had become virtually synonymous with 'proteins of therapeutic use' (Chapter 1). Nucleic acid-based biopharmaceuticals, however, harbour great potential — a potential which is likely to become a medical reality within this decade. Current developments in nucleic acid based-therapeutics centre around gene therapy and antisense technology. These technologies have the potential to revolutionize medical practice. Their full benefit, however, will accrue only after the satisfactory resolution of several technical difficulties currently impeding their routine medical application.

Despite all the hype, it is important to note that, by mid-2002 at least, only a single nucleic acid-based product has been approved for medical use (an antisense-based product, discussed later). No gene therapy-based product had been approved for general medical use by that time.

GENE THERAPY

The fundamental principle underpinning gene therapy is theoretically straightforward, but difficult to satisfactorily achieve in practice. The principle entails the stable introduction of a gene into the genetic complement of a cell, such that subsequent expression of the gene achieves a therapeutic goal. The potential of gene therapy as a curative approach for inborn errors of metabolism and other conditions induced by the presence of a defective copy of a specific gene (or genes) is obvious.

An increased understanding of the molecular basis of various other diseases, including cancer, some infectious diseases (e.g. AIDS) and some neurological conditions, also suggest a role for gene therapy in combating these. Indeed, well over half of all gene therapy trials conducted to date aim to treat cancer. Table 11.1 lists the major disease types for which a gene therapy treatment is currently being assessed in clinical trials. The first such trial was initiated in the USA in 1990. Thus far, over 400 different clinical studies have been or are being undertaken, involving ca. 6000 patients worldwide. Despite initial enthusiasm, only a handful of such studies have revealed any therapeutic benefit to the patient and, thus far, no complete, permanent cures have been recorded.

Moreover, gene therapy — like all other medical interventions — is not without associated risk. A US patient died in 1999 as a result of participating in a gene therapy-based trial. Even more disturbingly, the ensuing FDA investigation unearthed allegations that at least six other

Biopharmaceuticals: Biochemistry and Biotechnology, Second Edition by Gary Walsh
John Wiley & Sons Ltd: ISBN 0 470 84326 8 (ppc), ISBN 0 470 84327 6 (pbk)

Table 11.1.   Some diseases for which gene-based therapeutic approaches are currently being appraised in clinical trials. Many of these examples are discussed in more detail later in this chapter

Cancer — various forms	AIDS
Cystic fibrosis	Haemophilia
Familial hypercholesterolemia	Severe combined immunodeficiency diseases
Gaucher's disease	(SCID)
Purine nucleoside phosphorylase	α_1-Antitrypsin deficiency
deficiency	Chronic granulomatous disease
Rheumatoid arthritis	Peripheral vascular disease

deaths attributed to clinical trial treatments had gone unreported to the regulatory agency and, further, that only a fraction of serious adverse effects had been reported. As a result, regulatory regulation and monitoring of gene therapy-based trials has been increased.

Such disappointing results do not reflect any flaw in the concept of gene therapy. Instead, they reflect the need to develop more effective technical means of accomplishing gene therapy in practice. Such initial studies have highlighted the technical innovations required to achieve successful gene transfer and expression. These, in turn, should render future ('second-generation') gene therapy protocols more successful.

Basic approach to gene therapy

The basic approach to gene therapy is outlined in Figure 11.1. The desired gene must usually be packaged into a vector system capable of delivering it safely inside the intended recipient cells. A variety of vectors can be used to effect gene transfer. These include both viruses (particularly retroviruses) and non-viral carriers, such as plasmid-containing liposomes/lipoplexes (Table 11.2). Each such vector has its own unique set of advantages and disadvantages, as discussed subsequently in this chapter.

Once assimilated by the cell, the exogenous nucleic acid must now travel or be delivered to the nucleus. In some cases, the mechanism by which this transfer occurs is understood, at least in part (e.g. in the case of retroviral vectors). In other cases (e.g. use of liposome vectors, or naked DNA), this process is less well understood. At a practical level, gene therapy protocols may entail one of three different strategies (Figure 11.2).

The *in vitro* approach entails initial removal of the target cells from the body. These are then cultured *in vitro* and incubated with a vector containing the nucleic acid to be delivered. The genetically altered cells are then re-introduced into the patient's body. This approach represents the most commonly adopted protocol to date. In order to be successful, however, the target cells must be relatively easy to remove from the body and reintroduce into the body. Such *in vitro* approaches have successfully been undertaken, utilizing various body cell types, including blood cells, stem cells, epithelial cells, muscle cells and hepatocytes.

A second approach involves direct injection/administration of the nucleic acid-containing vector to the target cell, *in situ* in the body. Examples of this approach have included the direct injection of vectors into a tumour mass, as well as aerosol administration of vectors (e.g. containing the cystic fibrosis gene) to respiratory tract epithelial cells.

While less complicated than the *in vitro* approach, direct *in situ* injection of vector into the immediate vicinity of target cells is not always feasible. This would be true, for example, if the

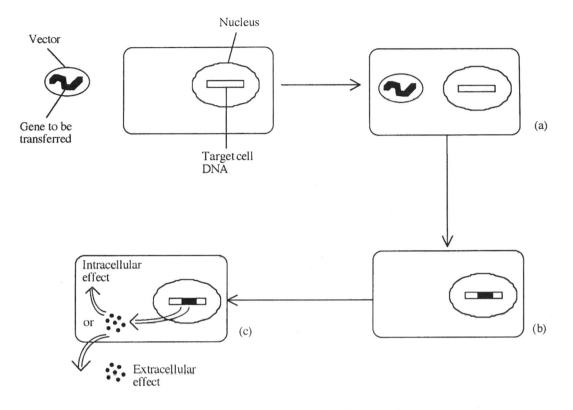

Figure 11.1. Simplified schematic representation of the basis of gene therapy. The genetic material to be transferred is firstly usually packaged into some form of vector, which serves to deliver the nucleic acid to the target cell. (a) Entry of the therapeutic nucleic acid — often still associated with its vector — into the cell cytoplasm. (b) Transfer of the nucleic acid into the nucleus of the recipient cell. This is often, although not always, followed by integration of the foreign genetic material into the cellular DNA. (c) The foreign gene (whether integrated or not) is expressed, resulting in the synthesis of the desired protein product. Regulatory elements of the nucleic acid transferred may be designed to ensure that the protein product is retained within the cell, or is exported from the cell, as necessary. Refer to the text for further details

Table 11.2. Vector systems used to deliver genes into mammalian cells. To date, the majority of clinical trials undertaken have utilized retroviral vector systems. Non-viral systems have generally been employed least often, although some, e.g. nucleic acid-containing liposomes, may be used more extensively in the future. Some of the methods tested, e.g. calcium phosphate precipitation, electroporation and particle acceleration, are unlikely to be employed to any great extent in gene therapy protocols

Viral-based vector systems	Non-viral-based vector systems
Retroviruses	Nucleic acid containing liposomes
Adenoviruses	Molecular conjugates
Adeno-associated virus	Direct injection of naked DNA
Herpes virus	$CaPO_4$ precipitation
Polio virus	Electroporation
Vaccinia virus	Particle acceleration

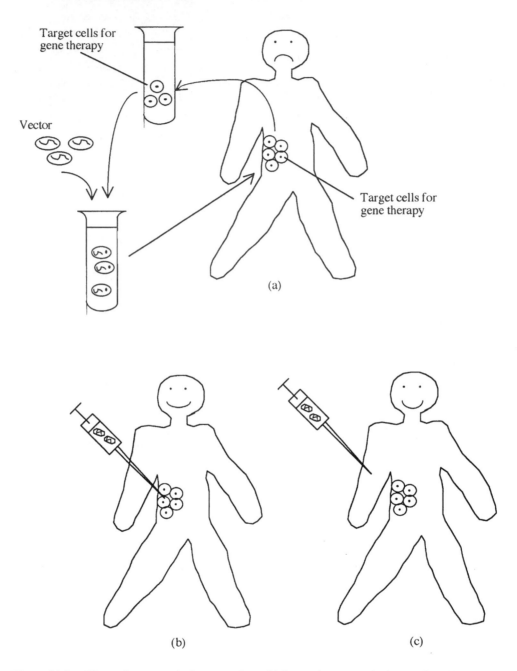

Figure 11.2. The various practical approaches which may be pursued when undertaking gene therapy. *In vitro* gene therapy (a) entails removal of target cells from the body, followed by their incubation with nucleic acid-containing vector. After the vector delivers the nucleic acid into the human cells, they are placed back in the body. *In situ* gene therapy (b) entails direct injection of the vector immediately adjacent to the body target cells. *In vivo* gene therapy involves intravenous administration of the vector (c) The vector has been designed such that it will only recognize and bind the intended target cells. In this way, the nucleic acid is delivered exclusively to those cells. Refer to text for further details

target cells are not localized to one specific area of the body (e.g. blood cells). An alternative (*in vivo*) approach entails the development of vectors capable of recognizing and binding only to specific, pre-defined cell types. Such vectors could then be administered easily, e.g. by intravenous injection. Through appropriate bio-specific interactions, they would only deliver their nucleic acid payload to the specified target cells. The simplicity and specificity of this approach renders it the method of choice. However, thus far, no such vector systems have been developed for routine therapeutic use. Intensive efforts to develop these are under way and a number of different strategies are being pursued. For example, the inclusion of an antibody on the vector surface, which specifically binds a surface antigen uniquely associated with the target cell, would allow selective delivery. Another approach entails engineering the vector to display a specific hormone which would bind only to cells displaying the hormone receptor. The feasibility of this approach has been demonstrated using retroviral vectors engineered to display erythropoietin on their surface.

Some additional questions

The choice of vector, target cell and protocol used will depend upon a number of considerations. The major consideration is obviously what the ultimate goal of the gene therapy treatment is in any given case, e.g. in some instances it may be to correct an inherited genetic defect, whereas in other instances it may be to confer a novel function upon the recipient cell. An example of the former would be the introduction of the cystic fibrosis transmembrane conductance regulator (CFTR) gene (the cystic fibrosis gene) into the airway epithelial cells of CF sufferers. An example of the latter would be the introduction of a novel gene into white blood cells whose protein product is capable of in some way interfering with HIV replication; such an approach might prove an effective therapeutic strategy for the treatment of AIDS.

An additional consideration that may influence the protocol used is the desired duration of subsequent expression of the gene product. In most cases of genetic disease, long-term expression of the inserted gene would be required. In other instances (e.g. some forms of cancer therapy, or the use of gene therapy to deliver a DNA-based vaccine), short-term expression of the gene introduced would be sufficient/desirable.

For most applications of gene therapy, straightforward expression of the gene product itself will suffice. However, in some instances, regulation of expression of the transferred gene would be required, e.g. if gene therapy combating insulin-dependent diabetes mellitus was to be considered. Achieving such expressional control over transferred genes is a pursuit that is only in the early stages of development.

The choice of target cells is another point worthy of discussion. In some instances, this choice is pre-determined, e.g. treatment of the genetic condition familial hypercholesterolemia would require insertion of the gene coding for the low-density lipoprotein receptor specifically in hepatocytes.

In other cases, however, some scope may be available to choose a target cell population. Even in the case of redressing some genetic diseases, it may not be necessary to genetically correct the exact population of cells affected, e.g. a hallmark of several of the best-characterized genetic diseases is the exceedingly low production of a circulatory gene product; examples include clotting factors VIII and IX, a lack of which leads to haemophilia. It may be possible to correct such defects by introducing the appropriate gene into any recipient cell capable of exporting the gene product into the blood. In such cases, choosing a target cell could be made upon practical considerations, such as their ease of isolation and culture, their capacity to express (and excrete) the protein product, and their half-lives *in vivo*.

Several cell types, including keratinocytes, myoblasts and fibroblasts, have been studied in this regard. It has been shown, for example, that myoblasts into which the factor IX gene and the growth hormone gene have been introduced could express their protein products and secrete them into the circulation.

Vectors used in gene therapy

A list of the various vectors capable of introducing genes into recipient cells has been provided in Table 11.2. These vectors are conveniently categorized as being viral-based or non-viral-based systems. The main vector systems developed thus far are discussed in somewhat more detail below.

Retroviral vectors

In the region of 80% of gene therapy clinical trials undertaken to date have employed retroviral vectors as gene delivery systems. Retroviruses are enveloped viruses. Their genome consists of single-stranded RNA (ssRNA) of approximately 5–8 kb. Upon entry into sensitive cells, the viral RNA is reverse-transcribed and eventually yields double-stranded DNA. This subsequently integrates into the host cell genome (Box 11.1). The basic retroviral genome contains a minimum of three structural genes; *gag* (codes for core viral protein), *pol* (codes for reverse transcriptase) and *env* (codes for the viral envelope proteins). At either end of the viral genome are the long terminal repeats (LTRs), which harbour powerful promoter and enhancer regions and sequences required to promote integration into the host DNA. Also present, immediately adjacent to the 5′ LTR, is the packing sequence (ψ). This is required to promote viral RNA packaging.

The ability of such retroviruses to (a) effectively enter various cell types and (b) integrate their genome into the host cell genome in a stable, long-term fashion, made them obvious potential vectors for gene therapy.

The construction of retroviruses to function as gene vectors entails replacing the endogenous viral genes, required for normal viral replication, with the exogenous gene of interest (Figure 11.3a). Removal of the viral structural genes means that the resulting vector cannot itself replicate. In order to generate mature virion particles harbouring the vector nucleic acid (Figure 11.3b), this genetic material must be introduced into a 'packing cell'. These are recombinant cells that have previously been engineered to contain the *gag*, *pol* and *env* structural genes (Figure 11.4). In this way, packing cells are capable of producing mature but replication-deficient viral particles, harbouring the gene to be transferred (see later section on Manufacture of viral vectors). These viral particles function as so-called 'one-time, single-hit' gene transfer systems.

More recently, various modifications have been introduced to this basic retroviral system. The inclusion of the 5′ end of the gag gene is shown to enhance levels of vector production by up to 200-fold. Additionally, specific promoters have been introduced in order to attempt to control expression of the inserted gene. Most work has focused upon the use of tissue-specific promoters in an effort to limit expression of the desired gene to a specific tissue type. The most commonly employed (recombinant-deficient) retrovirus used in this regard has been derived from the Maloney murine leukaemia virus (MoMuLV).

Box 11.1.   The retroviral life cycle

The retroviral life cycle begins with the entry of the enveloped virus into the cell. The viral reverse transcriptase enzyme then copies the viral RNA genome into a single (minus) DNA strand and, using this as a template, generates double-stranded (ds) DNA. The dsDNA is then randomly integrated into the host cell genome (the proviral DNA). Transcription of the proviral genes host cell's transcription machinery yields mRNA that directs synthesis of mature virion particles. The viral particles bud out from the cell's plasma membrane, picking up a membrane-derived outer coat as they do so.

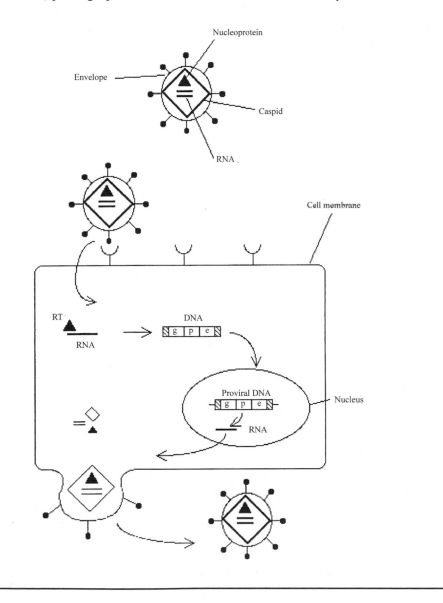

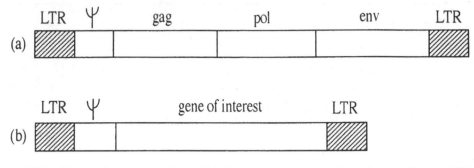

Figure 11.3. Schematic representation of (a) the proviral genome of a basic retrovirus and (b) the genome of a basic engineered retroviral vector carrying the gene of interest. Refer to text for further details

Retroviruses display a number of properties/characteristics that influences their potential as vectors in gene therapy protocols. These may be summarized as follows:

- Retroviruses as a group have been studied in detail and their biochemistry and molecular biology is well understood.
- Most retroviruses can integrate their proviral DNA only into actively replicating cells.
- The efficiency of gene transfer to most sensitive cell types is very high, often approaching 100%.
- Integrated DNA can be subject to long-term, relatively high-level expression.
- Proviral DNA integrates randomly into the host chromosomes.
- Retroviruses are promiscuous in that they infect a variety of dividing cell types.
- Complete copies of the proviral DNA are passed on to daughter cells if the original recipient cell divides.
- Good, high-level titre stocks of replication-incompetent retroviral particles can be produced.
- Safety studies using retroviral vectors have already been carried out on various animal species.

The fact that they have been well studied, display almost 100% transduction efficacy in sensitive cells and that the transferred genes are usually subject to long-term, fairly high-level expression renders retroviruses powerful potential vectors. These advantages form the basis of their widespread use in this regard.

However, many of the other characteristics listed serve to curtail the application of retroviruses as gene therapy vectors. In most instances, their ability to infect only dividing cells clearly restricts their use. Their lack of selectivity in terms of the dividing cell types they infect is also a disadvantage. They will not infect all dividing cell types—the entry of any specific retrovirus being dependent upon the existence of an appropriate viral receptor on the surface of a target cell. As the identity of most retroviral receptors is still unknown, it remains difficult to predict the entire range of cell types any retrovirus is likely to infect during a gene therapy protocol. Integration and expression of the exogenous gene in cells other than target cells could result in physiological complications.

An additional drawback with regard to retroviral-based vectors is the propensity of the transferred gene to integrate randomly into the chromosomes of the recipient cells. Integration of the transferred DNA in the middle of a gene whose product plays a critical role in the cell

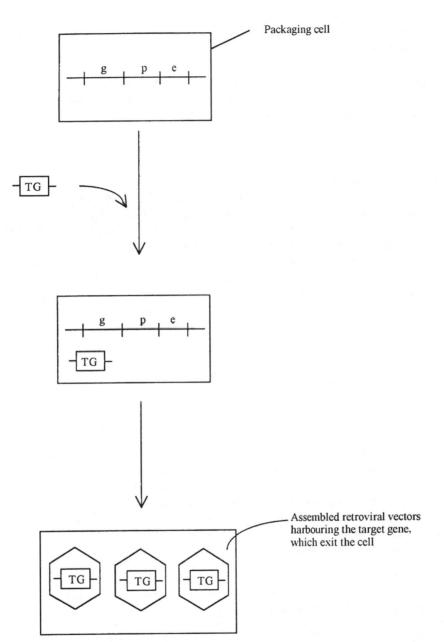

Figure 11.4. The use of packaging cells to generate replication-deficient retroviral vectors. The packaging cell is an engineered animal cell into which the retroviral *gag* (g), *pol* (p) and *env* (e) genes have been introduced. The cell line chosen must be one which the (replication deficient) virus can infect. The engineered retroviral vector genome (which is carrying the target gene; TG) is then incubated with the packaging cell. This results in the generation and assembly of mature replication-deficient retroviral vector particles. These exit the cell and will replicate by entering other packaging cells. By completing a number of such replication cycles, large quantities of the desired retroviral vectors are produced

could irrevocably damage cellular function, e.g. disruption of a central metabolic enzyme could cause cell death, while disruption of a tumour suppresser gene could give rise to cellular transformation; in addition, integration of the proviral nucleic acid to sites adjacent to quiescent cellular proto-oncogenes could result in their activation. Another impediment to routine use of retroviral vectors is the relatively labile nature of these particles. Thus, while retroviruses are relatively easy to propagate, they are often damaged by subsequent purification and concentration — steps essential for their clinical use.

Additional viral-based vectors

A number of additional viral types may also prove useful as vectors in the practice of gene therapy. Chief amongst these are the adenoviruses. Adeno-associated virus, the herpes virus and a number of other viruses are also being considered (Table 11.2).

Adenoviruses are relatively large, non-enveloped structures, housing double-stranded DNA as their genetic material. Their genome is much larger (approximately 35 kb), and more complex than those of retroviruses. In most instances, only a small fraction of this genome is removed when constructing an adenovirus-based vector. Upon cellular infection, adenoviral DNA becomes localized in the nucleus, but does not integrate into the host cell DNA. Usually, infection by wild-type adenoviruses is associated with, at most, mild clinical symptoms in humans.

As potential vectors for gene therapy, adenoviruses display a number of both advantages and disadvantages (Table 11.3). Their major advantage relates to their ability to efficiently infect non-dividing cells and the usually observed expression of large quantities of the desired gene products. However, the failure of the adenoviral-based DNA to integrate into the host cell generally means that its survival, and hence the duration of gene expression, is limited. Adenovirus-based vectors carrying various marker genes (i.e. a gene whose expression product is easily detected) have been administered to animals. Marker gene expression has been subsequently noted in various tissues, including heart, liver, muscle, bone marrow, CNS and endothelial cells. Duration of marker gene expression ranged from 2–3 weeks to several months.

While short-term, high-level gene expression may be appropriate for some gene therapy applications, it would be of less use for the treatment of, for example, genetic diseases, where long-term gene expression would be required. This could be achieved in theory by repeat administration of the adenoviral vector. However, adenoviruses prompt a strong immune response, which limits the efficacy of repeat administration.

Table 11.3. Some characteristic advantages and disadvantages of adenoviruses as potential vectors for gene therapy. Refer to text for further details

Advantages	Disadvantages
Adenoviruses are capable of gene transfer to non-dividing cells	Adenoviruses are highly immunogenic in man
They are easy to propagate in large quantities	The duration of expression of transferred genes can vary, and is usually transient
High levels of gene expression are usually recorded	Infection of permissive cells with wild-type adenovirus usually results in cell lysis
They are relatively stable viruses	Adenoviruses display a broad selectivity in the cell types they can infect

Additional viruses that may prove of some use as future viral vectors include adeno-associated virus and herpes virus. Adeno-associated virus is a very small, single-stranded DNA (ssDNA) virus — its genome consists of only two genes. It does not have the ability to replicate autonomously and can do so only in the presence of a co-infecting adenovirus (or other selected viruses).

Although it is found in the human population, it does not appear to be associated with any known diseases. Not surprisingly, only relatively small genes can be introduced into adeno-associated viral vector systems. Such systems, however, do provide a mechanism of gene transfer into non-dividing cells. It also seems to facilitate long-term expression of the transferred genetic material. In contrast to adenoviruses, nucleic acid transferred by adeno-associated viruses appears to be integrated into the recipient cell genome.

The herpes simplex virus (HSV) represents another potential vector system which is receiving increased attention. Because HSV is a neurotrophic virus, it may prove to be particularly useful in delivering genes to neurons of the peripheral and central nervous system. Upon infection, HSV usually remains latent in non-dividing neurons — with its genome remaining in an unintegrated form. Thus far, it has proved difficult to generate a replication-incompetent, but yet viable, herpes simplex particle. Moreover, some of the replication-incompetent viruses generated still retain an ability to damage/destroy the cells they infect. While herpes-based vector systems may one day prove useful in gene therapy, suitable and safe vector variants of HSV must first be generated and tested.

An additional virus, which has more recently gained some attention as a possible vector, is that of the sindbis virus. A member of the alphavirus family, this ssRNA virus can infect a broad range of both insect and vertebrate cells. The mature virion particles consist of the RNA genome complexed with a capsid protein C. This, in turn, is enveloped by a lipid bilayer in which two additional viral proteins, E1 and E2, are embedded. The E2 polypeptide appears to mediate viral binding to the surface receptors of susceptible cells (the major mammalian cell surface receptor it targets appears to be the highly conserved, widely distributed laminin receptor).

The sindbis virus is simple, robust, capable of infecting non-dividing cells and generally supports high levels of gene expression. However, it does display a broad host range and, hence, lacks the inherent targeting specificity characteristic of an idealized viral vector.

Recently a novel recombinant sindbis virus displaying altered host cell specificity has been generated. Scientists inserted a nucleotide sequence coding for the IgG-binding domain of *Staphyloccus aureus* into the E2 viral gene. Disruption of the E2 gene renders its protein product incapable of binding laminin (hence destroying the natural viral tropism). However, the protein A domain allows the chimeric E2 product to bind monoclonal antibodies. This altered virus may prove to be a useful generic or 'null' vector, potentially capable of being specifically targeted to any desired cell type. This would simply necessitate pre-incubation of the virus with monoclonal antibodies raised against a surface antigen unique to the proposed target cell population (Figure 11.5). Binding of the monoclonal antibody to the protein A domain would ensue and the immobilized monoclonal antibody would dictate the cell type targeted.

Initial studies using this system have proved encouraging. The altered virus (without associated monoclonal antibody) failed to infect a wide variety of human cell lines. By initially incubating with monoclonal antibody of the appropriate specificity, however, the viral particles were capable of efficiently transducing cells expressing surface receptors such as CD4, CD33 and human leukocyte antigen (HLA).

A number of other issues must now be addressed, including determining whether the IgG–protein A affinity is sufficiently high to keep the antibody associated with the virus *in vivo*. The

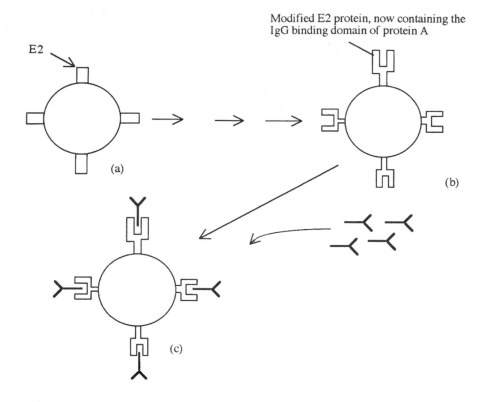

Figure 11.5.   Generation of engineered sindbis virus capable of being targeted to bind specific cell types. (a) Simplified depiction of the virus, displaying the surface E2 protein. Genetic engineering facilitates disruption of the E2 gene by incorporation of the IgG-binding domain of protein A (b). Incubation of such engineered viral particles with most monoclonal antibody types results in effective immobilization of the antibody on the viral surface (c). Thus, the engineered viral vector should be targetable to any specific cell type, simply by its pre-incubation with monoclonal antibodies, which selectively bind a surface antigen uniquely associated with the target cell

full potential of this approach will also require more detailed characterization of surface markers uniquely associated with different cell types. However, the approach exemplifies the types of technical innovations now being introduced, which will make second-generation vectors more suited to their role in gene therapy.

Manufacture of viral vectors

Literature reports describing the large-scale manufacture of viral vectors for gene therapy application are few and far between. Development of manufacturing protocols has largely been undertaken by companies engaged in gene therapy product development and, consequently, protocol details remain confidential. The overall approach likely taken is not too dissimilar to that of therapeutic protein manufacture (Chapter 3). It involves synthesis in cells, recovery, concentration, purification and formulation steps. A likely generalized manufacturing scenario for retroviral-based vectors is outlined in Figure 11.6. The manufacture of alternative viral

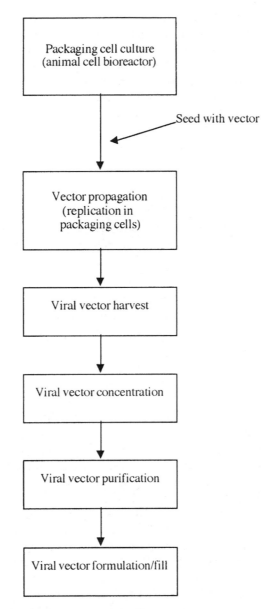

Figure 11.6. Large-scale manufacture of retroviral vectors for use for gene therapy-based clinical protocols. Refer to text for details

vectors likely follow a similar approach. The process is initiated by the culture of packing cells in suitable animal cell bioreactors. The principles and practice of animal cell culture have been overviewed in Chapter 3. To date, bioreactor size of 100 l or less have been used, which are sufficient to satisfy clinical trial demand. The packing cells are then seeded with the replication-deficient virus, allowing vector propagation (see also Figure 11.4). Viral harvest may then be undertaken by methods of microfiltration, which separates intact packing cells/cell debris from the vector-containing product stream. Viral vector concentration can then be undertaken by ultrafiltration (Chapter 3). Subsequent vector purification strategies employed include chromatographic approaches similar to those used to purify proteins. Ion exchange and various forms of affinity chromatography have received most attention. A detailed under-standing of the interactions between chromatographic media and viral surface molecules is currently lacking and hence is the subject of ongoing research. A comprehensive understanding of such interactions would be required to optimize chromatographic purification protocols. After purification, final product analysis and formulation is undertaken. Again, few details of these steps have been openly published.

Non-viral vectors

Although viral-mediated gene delivery systems currently predominate, some 20–25% of current clinical trials use non-viral-based methods of gene delivery. General advantages quoted with respect to non-viral delivery systems include:

- their low/non-immunogenicity;
- non-occurrence of integration of the therapeutic gene into the host chromosome (this eliminates the potential to disrupt essential host genes or to activate host oncogenes.

The initial approach adopted entailed administration of 'naked' plasmid DNA housing the gene of interest. This avenue of research was first opened in 1990, when it was shown that naked plasmid DNA was expressed in mice muscle cells subsequent to its i.m. injection. The plasmid DNA concerned housed the β-galactosidase gene as a reporter. Subsequent expression of β-galactosidase activity could persist for anything from a few months to the remainder of the animal's life. The transfection rate recorded was low (1–2% of muscle fibres assimilated the DNA) and the DNA was not integrated into the host cell's chromosomes.

Up until this point, it was assumed that naked DNA injected into animals would not be spontaneously taken up and expressed in host cells. This finding vindicated the cautious approach taken by the FDA and other regulatory authorities with regard to the presence of free DNA in biopharmaceutical products (Chapter 3).

Scientists have also since demonstrated that DNA (coated on microscopic gold beads) propelled into the epidermis of test animals with a 'gene gun' is expressed in the animal's skin cells. Furthermore, the introduction in this fashion of DNA coding for human influenza viral antigens resulted in effective immunization of the animal against influenza. Similar results, using other pathogen models, have also now been generated. It is assumed that expressed antigen is secreted by the cell and, in this way, is exposed to immune surveillance. Further research has illustrated that systematic administration via i.v. injection rarely achieves meaningful cell transfection. This is most likely due to the high nuclease levels present in serum. In contrast, free nuclease activity in muscle tissue is extremely low.

Modern non-viral-based systems generally entail complexing/packaging the gene of interest (present, along with appropriate promoters, etc., in a circular plasmid) with additional molecules, particularly various lipids or some polypeptides. These generally display a positive charge and hence interact with the negatively-charged DNA molecules. The function of such carrier molecules is to stabilize the DNA, protect it, e.g. from serum nucleases, and ideally to modulate interaction with the biological system, e.g. help target the DNA to particular cell types — or away from other cell types.

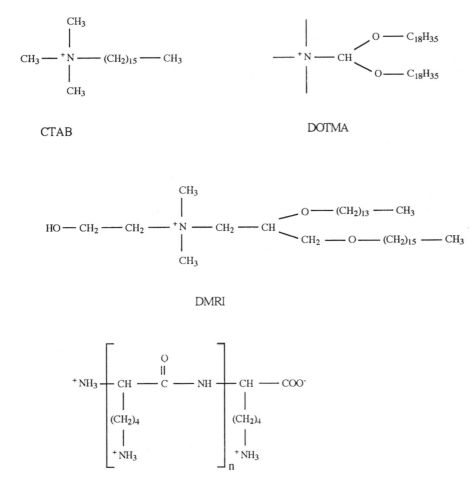

Figure 11.7. Structure of some cationic lipids and polylysine

The most commonly used polymers are the cationic lipids and polylysine chains (Figure 11.7). Cationic lipids can aggregate in aqueous-based systems to form vesicles/liposomes, which in turn will interact spontaneously with DNA (Figure 11.8). Initially, the negatively-charged plasmid DNA probably acts as a bridge between adjacent vesicles. Further DNA–vesicle interactions quickly generate a complex 3-D lattice-like system composed of flattened vesicles (some of which probably rupture) interspersed with plasmid DNA. The lipid component of such 'lipoplexes' should therefore provide a measure of physical protection to the therapeutic gene.

Gene therapy results to date using this approach have been mixed. The process of lipoplex formation is not easily controlled and hence different batches made under seemingly identical conditions may not be structurally identical. Furthermore, *in vitro* test results using such lipoplexes can correlate very poorly with subsequent *in vivo* performance. Clearly, more research is required to underpin the rational use of lipoplexes for gene therapy purposes. The same is true

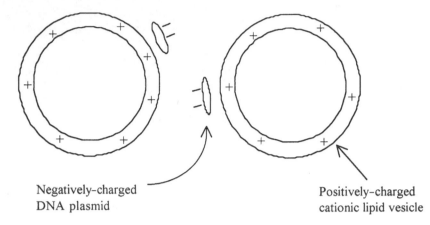

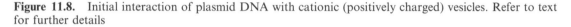

Negatively-charged   Positively-charged
DNA plasmid   cationic lipid vesicle

Figure 11.8.   Initial interaction of plasmid DNA with cationic (positively charged) vesicles. Refer to text for further details

for other polymer-based synthetic gene delivery systems, the most significant of which is the polylysine-based system. Polylysine molecules, due to their positive charge (Figure 11.7) can also form electrostatic complexes with DNA. However, the stability of such 'polyplexes' in biological fluids can be problematic. Furthermore, polyplexes tend to be rapidly removed from the circulation, prompting a low plasma half-life. These difficulties can be alleviated in part by the attachment of polyethylene glycol (PEG) molecules. PEG attachment is also used to increase the serum half-life of various therapeutic proteins, such as some interferons (Chapter 4).

No matter what their composition, such synthetic gene delivery systems also meet various biological barriers to efficient cellular gene delivery. Viral vector-based systems are far less prone to such problems, as the viral carrier has evolved in nature to overcome such obstacles. Obstacles relate to:

- blood-related issues;
- biodistribution profile;
- cellular targeting;
- cellular entry and nuclear delivery.

While lipoplexes/polyplexes generally protect the plasmid from serum nucleases, the overall positive charge characteristic of these structures leads to their non-specific interactions with cells (both blood cells and vascular endothelial cells) and serum proteins. Also, following i.v. injection, such DNA complexes tend in practice to accumulate in the lung and liver. Targeting of DNA complexes to specific cell types also poses a considerable (largely unmet) technical challenge. Approaches such as the incorporation of antibodies directed against specific cell surface antigens may provide a future avenue of achieving such cell-selective targeting. However, it is currently believed that ionic interactions constitute a predominant binding force between the positively-charged lipoplexes/polyplexes and the negatively charged eukaryotic cell surface. Such electrostatic interactions may even override more biospecific interactions characteristic of antibody- or receptor-based systems. Currently, probably the most effective means of delivering such vectors to target tissue/cells is to inject them into or beside the target area.

However targeted to the appropriate cell surface, if it is to be clinically effective, the therapeutic plasmid must enter the cell and reach the nucleus intact. Cellular entry is generally achieved via endocytosis (Figure 11.9). A proportion of endocytosed plasmid DNA escapes from the endosome by entering the cytoplasm (thereby escaping liposomal destruction (Figure 11.9). The molecular mechanism by which escape is accomplished is, at best, only partially understood. Anionic lipid constituents of lipoplexes, for example, may fuse directly with the endosomal membranes, facilitating direct expulsion of at least a portion of the plasmid DNA into the cytoplasm. Generally, the DNA is released in free form (i.e. uncomplexed to any lipid).

Some attempts have been made to rationally increase the efficiency of endosomal escape. One such avenue entails the incorporation of selected hydrophobic (viral) peptides into the gene delivery systems. Many viruses naturally enter animal cells via receptor-mediated endocytosis. These viruses have evolved efficient means of endosomal escape, usually relying upon membrane-disrupting peptides derived from the viral coat proteins.

Once in the cytoplasm, a proportion of plasmid molecules are probably degraded by cytoplasmic nucleases, effectively further reducing transfection efficiencies. There are two potential routes by which plasmid DNA could reach the nucleus:

- direct nuclear entry as a consequence of nuclear membrane breakdown associated with mitosis;
- transport through nuclear pores, which may occur via passive diffusion or specific energy-requiring transport processes.

Overall, it is estimated that only one in 10^4–10^5 plasmids taken up by endocytosis will enter the nucleus intact and be successfully expressed.

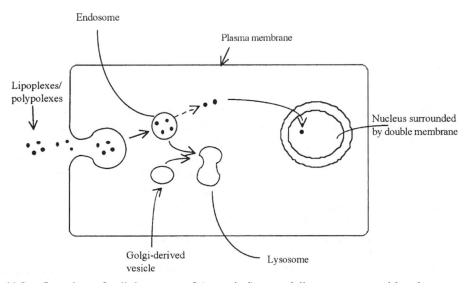

Figure 11.9. Overview of cellular entry of (non-viral) gene delivery systems, with subsequent plasmid relocation to the nucleus. The delivery systems (e.g. lipoplexes and polyplexes) initially enter the cell via endocytosis (the invagination of a small section of plasma membrane to form small membrane-bound vesicles termed endosomes). Endosomes subsequently fuse with Golgi-derived vesicles forming lysosomes. Golgi derived hydrolytic lysosomal enzymes then degrade the lysosomal contents. A proportion of the plasmid DNA must escape lysosomal destruction via entry into the cytoplasm. Some plasmids subsequently enter the nucleus. Refer to text for further details

Manufacture of plasmid DNA

Plasmid DNA is routinely extracted and purified from various microbial cells at the research level. However, industrial-scale manufacture to the exacting standards of purity demanded of pharmaceutical products is a pursuit still in its infancy, and little has been published on the subject. The overall generalized approach used to produce plasmid DNA for the purposes of gene therapy trials is presented in Figure 11.10. Prior to its manufacture, researchers would have constructed an appropriate vector housing the therapeutic gene and introduced it into a producer microorganism, such as *E. coli*. Routine large-scale plasmid manufacture then entails culture of a batch of producer microorganisms by fermentation, followed by plasmid extraction and purification. In this regard, the overall approach used resembles the approaches taken in the large-scale manufacture of recombinant therapeutic proteins, as described in Chapter 3.

Industrial-scale microbial fermentation (upstream processing) has also been described in Chapter 3, to which the reader is referred. Fermentation promotes microbial cell replication and thus the biosynthesis of large quantities of plasmid. Subsequent to fermentation, the microbial cells are harvested (collected) by either centrifugation or microfiltration. Following resuspension in a low volume of buffer, the cells must be disrupted in order to release the plasmids therein. This appears to be most commonly achieved by the addition of a lysis reagent, consisting of NaOH and SDS (sodium dodecyl sulphate). The combination of high pH and detergent action disrupts the microbial cell wall and membranes, with consequent release of the intracellular contents. In addition to the desired plasmid DNA, this crude mixture will also contain various impurities that must be removed by subsequent downstream processing steps. Notable impurities include:

- cell wall debris and some intact cells;
- proteins;
- genomic DNA;
- RNA;
- low molecular mass metabolites;
- endotoxin.

After lysis is complete, the next step can entail the addition of a high-salt neutralization solution, such as potassium acetate. This promotes formation of aggregates of genomic DNA (gDNA) and SDS–protein complexes, which can subsequently be removed by centrifugation or filtration. The plasmids can then be themselves precipitated from the resultant solution by the addition of appropriate solvent (usually either isoproponal or ethanol). Upon resuspension, the plasmid preparation can then be subjected to chromatographic purification. The major contaminants likely still present include RNA, gDNA fragments, nicked or other plasmid variants and endotoxins. Gel filtration chromatography can effectively remove contaminants that differ substantially in shape/size from the desired plasmid. These can include most gDNA fragments, RNA and (most) endotoxins. It can also achieve partial removal of plasmid variants, such as open circular plasmids, from the main (supercoiled) plasmid preparation. Ion exchange can remove many protein contaminants, as well as RNA. However, gDNA and endotoxins generally co-purify with the plasmid DNA. Additional chromatographic approaches based upon reverse-phase and affinity systems have been developed at laboratory scale at least.

A significant feature of plasmid purification employing capture chromatography (i.e. involves plasmids binding to the chromatographic beads) is the low plasmid-binding capacities observed.

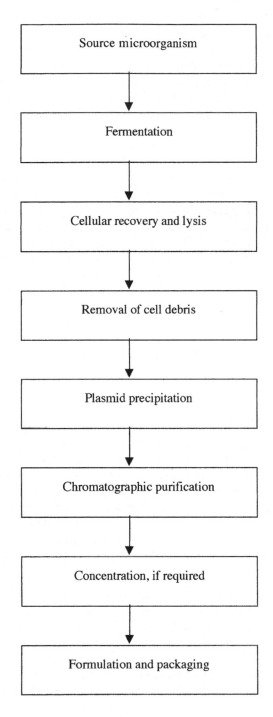

Figure 11.10. Overview of the manufacturing process for the large-scale production of plasmid DNA. Refer to the text for further details

The pore size of commercially-available capture chromatographic media is insufficiently large to allow entry of plasmids, restricting binding to the bead surface. Binding capacities can, therefore, be 100-fold or more lower than those observed when the same medium is used to purify (much smaller) therapeutic proteins (Chapter 3).

Purified plasmids may then be analysed using various analytical techniques. Freedom from contaminating nucleic acid and/or proteins can be assessed electrophoretically. Endotoxin and sterility tests would also be routinely undertaken. The purified plasmid DNA must next be formulated to yield the final non-viral delivery system. Formulation studies relating to such systems remain an area requiring further investigation. Most work reported to date relates to formulating and stabilizing lipoplex-based gene delivery systems. Aqueous suspensions of these (and other) non-viral based systems tend to quickly aggregate (in a matter of minutes to hours). In order to circumvent this problem, the final delivery systems were often actually formulated at the patient's bedside in earlier clinical trials.

Research aimed at identifying appropriate stabilizing excipients and formulation formats is ongoing. Simple freezing is an option, particularly as frozen formulations would be immune to agitation-induced aggregation. However, the process of freezing, particularly slow freezing, in itself induces aggregation. This can be minimized by flash freezing (e.g. by immersion in liquid nitrogen), although this approach may not prove practicable at an industrial scale. The addition of cryoprotectants may help minimize this problem and initial studies indicate that various sugars (e.g. glucose, sucrose and trehalose) show some potential in this regard. Another avenue under investigation relates to the generation of a final freeze-dried product. Again issues, such as the (relatively) slow freezing process characteristic of industrial-scale freeze-driers, complicate attaining this goal in practice.

Gene therapy and genetic disease

Well over 4000 genetic diseases have been characterized to date. Many of these are caused by lack of production of a single gene product or are due to the production of a mutated gene product incapable of carrying out its natural function. Gene therapy represents a seemingly straightforward therapeutic option which could correct such genetic-based diseases. This would be achieved simply by facilitating insertion of a 'healthy' copy of the gene in question into appropriate cells of the sufferer.

Although simple in concept, the application of gene therapy to treat or cure genetic diseases has, thus far, made little impact in practice. The slow progress in this regard is likely due to a number of factors. These include:

- The number of genetic diseases for which the actual gene responsible has been identified and studied is relatively modest, although completion of the human genome project should rapidly accelerate identification of such genes.
- As discussed previously, none of the first-generation gene-delivering vectors have proved fully satisfactory.
- Some genetic diseases are quite complex, with several organs/cell types being affected. In most instances, it has proved difficult in practice to introduce the required gene into all the affected cell types.
- Regulation of expression levels of the genes transferred has proved problematic.
- Drug companies often display greater interest in applying gene therapy to more prevalent diseases, such as cancer. The patient population suffering from many genetic diseases is

Table 11.4. Some examples of genetic diseases for which the defective gene responsible has been identified

Disease	Defective genes protein product
Haemophilia A	Factor VIII
Haemophilia B	Factor IX
Thalassemia	β-Globin
Sickle cell anaemia	β-Globin
Familial hypercholesterolemia	Low-density protein receptor
Severe combined immunodeficiency	Adenosine deaminase, purine nucleoside phosphorylase
Niemann–Pick disease	Sphingomylinase
Gaucher's disease	Glucocerebrosidase
Cystic fibrosis	Cystic fibrosis transmembrane regulator
Emphysema	α_1-Antitrypsin
Leukocyte adhesion deficiency	CD18
Hyperammonemia	Ornithine transcarbamylase
Citrullinemia	Arginosuccinate synthetase
Phenylketonuria	Phenylalanine hydroxylase
Maple syrup disease	Branched chain α-ketoacid dehydrogenase
Tyrosinemia type 1	Fumarylacetoacetate hydrolase
Glycogen storage deficiency type 1A	Glucose-6-phosphatase
Fucosidosis	α-L-Fucosidase
Mucopolysaccharidosis type VII	β-Glucuronidase
Mucopolysaccharidosis type I	α-L-Iduronidase
Galactosemia	Galactose-1-phosphate uridyl transferase

relatively modest. In some instances, a limited patient population may not be sufficient to allow the developing company to recoup the cost of drug development.

Some of the genetic conditions for which the defective gene has been pinpointed are summarized in Table 11.4. Many of the initial attempts to utilize gene therapy in practice focused upon haemoglobinopathies (e.g. sickle cell anaemia and thalassemias). These conditions were amongst the first genetic disorders to be characterized at a molecular level, with the defect centring around the haemoglobin α- or β-chain genes. Furthermore, the target cells in the bone marrow could be removed and subsequently replaced with relative ease. However, these conditions proved to be a difficult initial choice for the gene therapist. The production of the appropriate quantities of functional haemoglobin is dependent not only upon the presence of α- and β-globin genes of the correct sequence, but also upon detailed regulation of gene expression. Such tight regulation of expression of transferred genes is beyond the capability of gene therapy technology as it currently stands.

Another early genetic disease for correction by gene therapy was severe combined immunodeficiency (SCID). This disease is caused by a lack of adenosine deaminase (ADA) activity. ADA is an enzyme that plays a central role in the degradation of purine nucleosides (it catalyzes the removal of ammonia from adenosine, forming inosine which, in turn, is usually eventually converted to uric acid). This leads to T and B lymphocyte dysfunction. Lack of an effective immune system means that SCID sufferers must be kept in an essentially sterile environment.

When compared to treating diseases such as thalassemia, regulation of the level of expression of a corrected ADA gene was believed to be less important for a successful therapeutic outcome (in most — although not all — metabolic diseases caused by an enzyme deficiency, it appears that expression of even a fraction of normal enzyme levels is sufficient to ameliorate the disease symptoms).

Gene therapy trials aimed at counteracting ADA deficiency were initiated in 1990. The first recipient was a 4 year-old SCID sufferer. The protocol used entailed the isolation of the child's peripheral lymphocytes, followed by the *in vitro* introduction of the human ADA gene into these cells, using a retroviral vector. After a period of expansion (by culture *in vitro*), these treated cells were re-injected into the patient. As the lymphocytes (and by extension, the corrective gene) had a finite life span, the therapy was repeated every 6–8 weeks. This approach appeared successful in that it has resulted in a marked and sustained improvement in the recipient's immune function. Critically, however, interpetration of this outcome was made more difficult, owing to the later revelation that the patient also initiated more conventional SCID therapy just prior to the gene therapy treatment.

Stem cells are attractive potential recipients cells, as they are immortal. Successful introduction of the target gene into these cells should facilitate ongoing production of the gene product in mature blood cells, which are continually derived from the stem cell population. This would likely remove the requirement for repeat gene transfers to the affected individual.

The routine transduction of stem cells has, thus far, proved technically difficult. They are found only in low quantities in the bone marrow, and there is a lack of a suitable assay for stem cells. However, recent progress has been made in this regard and routine transduction of such cells will likely be achievable within the next few years.

Additional genetic diseases for which a gene therapy approach is currently being evaluated include familial hypercholesterolaemia and cystic fibrosis. Familial hypercholesterolaemia is caused by the absence (or presence of a defective form of) low-density lipoprotein receptors on the surface of liver cells. This results in highly elevated serum cholesterol levels, normally accompanied by early onset of serious vascular disease. Gene therapy approaches that have been attempted thus far to counteract this condition have entailed the initial removal of a relatively large portion of the liver. Hepatocytes derived from the liver are then cultured *in vitro*, with gene transfer being undertaken using retroviral vectors. The corrected hepatocytes are then usually infused back into the liver via a catheter. Although studies in animals have been partially successful, transduction of only a small proportion of the hepatocytes is normally observed. Subsequent expression of the corrective gene can also be variable. *In vivo* approaches to hepatic gene correction, using both viral and non-viral approaches, are also currently being assessed.

The cystic fibrosis (*cf*) gene was first identified in 1989. It codes for a 170 kDa protein, the cystic fibrosis transmembrane conductance regulator (CFTR), which serves as a chloride channel in epithelial cells. Inheritance of a mutant *cftr* gene from both parents results in the CF phenotype. While various organs are affected, the most severely affected are the respiratory epithelial cells, which have, unsurprisingly, become the focus of attempts at corrective gene therapy.

Several vectors have been used in an attempt to deliver the *cf* gene to the airway epithelial cells of sufferers. The most notable systems include adenoviruses and cationic liposomes. Vector delivery to the target cells can be achieved directly by aerosol technology. Delivery of *cftr* cDNA to airway epithelial cells (and subsequent gene expression) has been demonstrated with the use of both vector types. However, in order to be of therapeutic benefit, it is essential that 5–10% of the target cell population receive and express the *cftr* gene. This level of integration has not been

Table 11.5. Some therapeutic strategies being pursued in an attempt to treat cancer using a gene therapy approach. Refer to text for details

---

Modifying lymphocytes in order to enhance their anti-tumour activity
Modifying tumour cells to enhance their immunogenicity
Inserting tumour suppressor genes into tumour cells
Inserting toxin genes in tumour cells in order to promote tumour cell destruction
Inserting suicide genes into tumour cells
Inserting genes, such as a multiple drug resistance (*mrd*) gene, into stem cells to protect
  them from chemotherapy-induced damaged
Counteracting the expression of oncogenes in tumour cells by inserting an appropriate
  antisense gene

---

achieved so far and, furthermore, gene expression has often been transient. However, it is considered likely that ongoing developments in this field will render gene therapy a useful treatment for CF within the earlier part of the twenty-first century.

Gene therapy and cancer

To date, the majority of gene therapy trials undertaken aim to cure not inherited genetic defects, but cancer. The average annual incidence of cancer reported in the USA alone stands at ca. 1.4 million cases. Survival rates attained by pursuit of conventional therapeutic strategies (surgery, chemo-therapy, radio-therapy) stands at about 50%. Gene therapy will likely provide the medical community with an additional therapeutic tool with which to combat cancer within the next 10–15 years.

Initial gene therapy trials aimed at treating/curing cancer began in 1991. Various strategic approaches have since been developed in this regard (Table 11.5). Numerous trials aimed at assessing the application of gene therapy for the treatment of a wide variety of cancer types are now under way (Table 11.6).

While many of the results generated to date provide hope for the future, thus far gene therapy has failed to provide a definitive cure for any cancer type. The lack of success is likely due to a number of factors, including:

- a requirement for improved, more target-specific vector systems;
- a requirement for a better understanding of how cancer cells evade the normal immune response;
- for ethical reasons, most patients treated to date were suffering from advanced and widespread terminal cancer (i.e. little/no hope of survival if treated using conventional

Table 11.6. Some specific cancer types for which human gene therapy trials have been initiated. Although several of the strategies listed in Table 11.5 are being employed in these trials, many focus upon the introduction of various cytokines into the tumour cells themselves in order to attract and enhance a tumour-specific immune response

---

Breast cancer	Colorectal cancer
Malignant melanoma	Tumours of the CNS
Ovarian cancer	Renal cell carcinoma
Small-cell lung cancer	Non-small-cell lung cancer

---

therapies); cancers at earlier stages of development will probably prove to be more responsive to gene therapy.

One of the earliest cancer gene therapy trials attempted involved the introduction of the TNF gene into tumour-infiltrating lymphocytes (TILs). The rationale was that if, as expected, TIL cells reintroduced into the body could infiltrate the tumour, TNF synthesis would occur at the tumour site, where it is required. This approach has since been broadened, by introducing genes coding for a range of immunostimulatory cytokines (e.g. IL-2, IL-4, IFN-γ and GM-CSF) into TILs. A variation of this approach involves the introduction of such cytokine genes directly into tumour cells themselves. It is hoped that reintroduction of such cytokine-producing cells into the body will result in a swift and effective immune response — killing the tumour cells and vaccinating the patient against recurrent episodes. In most instances so far, this strategy has been carried out in practice by removal of the target cells from the body, culture *in vitro*, introduction of the desired gene (mainly using retroviral vectors), followed by reintroduction of the altered cells into the body.

An alternative anti-cancer strategy entails insertion of a copy of a tumour suppresser gene into cancer cells. For example, a deficiency in one such gene product, p53, has been directly implicated in the development of various human cancers. It has been shown *in vitro* that insertion of a p53 gene into p53-deficient tumour cells induces the death of such cells. A weakness of such an approach, however, is that 100% of the transformed cells would have to be successfully treated to fully cure the cancer.

Yet another strategy that may prove useful is the introduction into tumour cells of a 'sensitivity' gene. This concept dictates that the gene product should harbour the ability to convert a non-toxic pro-drug into a toxic substance within the cells — thus leading to their selective destruction. The model system most used to appraise such an approach entails the use of the thymidine kinase gene of the herpes simplex virus (Figure 11.11).

A different gene therapy-based approach to cancer entails introduction of a gene into haemopoietic stem cells in order to protect these cells from the toxic effects of chemotherapy. Most cancer drugs display toxic side effects, which usually limits the upper dosage levels that can be safely administered. One common toxic side effect is the destruction of stem cells. If these cells could be protected or made resistant to the chemotherapeutic agent, it might be possible to administer higher concentrations of the drug to the patient. In practice, such a protective effect could be conferred by the multiple drug resistance (type 1; MDR-1) gene product. This is often expressed by cancer cells resistant to chemotherapy. It functions to pump a range of chemotherapeutic drugs (e.g. daunorubicin, taxol, vinblastine, vincristine, etc.) out of the cell. Animal studies have confirmed that introduction of the MDR-1 gene into stem cells subsequently protects these cells from large doses of taxol. This approach is now being appraised in patients receiving high-dose chemotherapy for a range of cancer types, including breast and ovarian cancer and brain tumours.

Gene therapy and AIDS

It is likely that gene therapy will prove useful in treating a far broader range of medical conditions than simply those of inherited genetic disease and cancer. Prominent additional disease targets are those caused by infectious agents, particularly intracellular pathogens such as HIV. The main strategic approach adopted entails introducing a gene into pathogen-susceptible

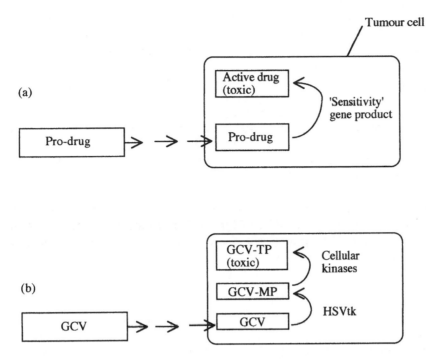

Figure 11.11. Schematic representation of the therapeutic rationale underpinning the introduction of a 'sensitivity' gene into tumour cells in order to promote their selective destruction. As depicted in (a), the gene product should be capable of converting an inactive pro-drug into a toxic drug, capable of killing the cell. A specific example of this approach is presented in (b): introduction of the herpes simplex thymidine kinase (HSVtk) gene confers sensitivity to the anti-herpes drug, Ganciclovir (GCV) on the cell. GCV is converted by HSVtk into a monophosphorylated form (GCV-MP). This, in turn, is phosphorylated by endogenous kinases, yielding ganciclovir triphosphate (GCV-TP). GCV-TP induces cell death by inhibiting DNA polymerase. A potential advantage of this system is that some adjacent tumour cells (which themselves lack the HSVtk gene) are also destroyed. This is most likely due to diffusion of the GCV-MP or GCV-TP (perhaps via gap junctions) into such adjacent cells. This so-called 'bystander effect' means that all the transformed cells in a tumour would not necessarily need to be transduced for the therapy to be successful

cells whose product will interfere with pathogen survival/replication within that cell. Such a strategy is sometimes termed 'intracellular immunization'.

One such anti-AIDS strategy being pursued is the introduction into virus-sensitive cells of a gene coding for an altered (dysfunctional) HIV protein, such as *gag*, *tat* or *env*. The presence of such mutant forms of *gag*, in particular, was shown to be capable of inhibiting viral replication. This is probably due to interference by the mutated *gag* product with correct assembly of the viral core. An additional approach entails the transfer to sensitive cells of a gene coding for antibody fragments capable of binding to the HIV envelope proteins. This may also interfere with viral assembly in infected cells.

Scientists have also generated recombinant cells capable of synthesizing and secreting soluble forms of the HIV cell surface receptor, the CD4 antigen. It was suggested that release of such soluble viral receptors into the blood would bind circulating virions, hence blocking their ability to 'dock' at sensitive cells. Although this proved to be the case *in vitro*, early *in vivo* studies have not proved as encouraging.

Yet additional therapeutic approaches to AIDS, based upon antisense technology, will be discussed later in this chapter. The use of gene therapy to combat this disease has now become firmly established as an approach worthy of significant future research.

Gene-based vaccines

Conventional vaccine technology, including the generation of modern recombinant 'subunit' vaccines, has been discussed in Chapter 10. An additional gene therapy-based approach to vaccination is also now under investigation. The approach entails the administration of a DNA vector housing the gene coding for a surface antigen protein from the target pathogen. In this way, the body itself would produce the pathogen-associated protein. Theoretically, virtually any body cell could be targeted, the only requirement being that target cells export the resultant antigenic protein such that it is encountered by the immune system. Additionally, gene expression need only be transient; sufficiently long to facilitate the induction of an immune response. Target conditions for gene-based vaccines that have entered clinical trials thus far include malaria, hepatitis B and AIDS.

Gene therapy: some additional considerations

The importance of gene therapy to the future practice of medicine is no longer being seriously questioned. However, in addition to technical difficulties, a number of non-technical issues must be satisfactorily addressed before its practice becomes widespread. Chief amongst these issues are the questions of public perception, ethics and costs.

Gene therapy is not, and will not be, an inexpensive therapeutic tool. The cost of such treatments will likely be broadly similar to the cost of present-day biopharmaceuticals. However, if proved successful in treating many currently incurable conditions, the cost:benefit ratio will greatly favour its medical use.

Public perception and ethical considerations are, in many ways, inter-linked. The ability to so readily modify our genetic complement holds great therapeutic promise. However, strict regulations overseeing the use of this technology are required (and are being enforced). Without proper controls, the danger exists that gene therapy could eventually be used to 'improve' human characteristics. The technical know-how to underpin a new era of eugenics is now almost a reality. The most important safeguard aimed at preventing eugenic-type developments is already in place. Currently, gene therapy is restricted to somatic cells—the genetic manipulation of human germ cells is banned. Any genetic alterations achieved thus will not be transmitted to future generations. Like nuclear technology, there is no 'going back' in relation to gene therapy. The challenge is to ensure that human genetic manipulation is used only for purposes that clearly represent the 'common good'.

ANTI-SENSE TECHNOLOGY

Various disease states are associated with the inappropriate production or overproduction of gene products. Examples include:

- the expression of oncogenes, leading to the transformed state;
- the overexpression of cytokines during some disease states, with associated worsening of disease symptoms;
- the overproduction of angiotensinogen, which ultimately results in hypertension.

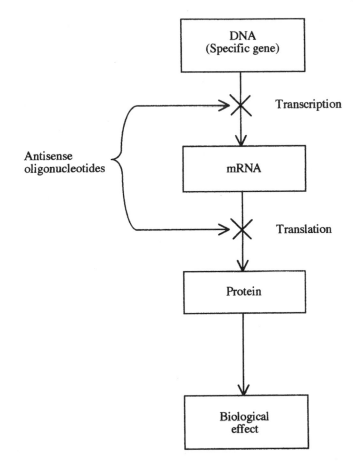

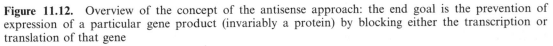

Figure 11.12. Overview of the concept of the antisense approach: the end goal is the prevention of expression of a particular gene product (invariably a protein) by blocking either the transcription or translation of that gene

An additional example includes the intracellular transcription and translation of virally-encoded genes during intracellular viral replication. In all such instances, the medical consequences of such inappropriate gene (over)expression could be ameliorated or prevented if this expression could be downregulated. A nucleic acid-based approach to achieve just this is termed 'antisense technology'.

The antisense approach is based upon the generation of short, single-stranded stretches of nucleic acids (which can be DNA- or RNA-based) displaying a specific nucleotide sequence. These are generally termed 'antisense oligonucleotides'. These oligonucleotides are capable of binding to DNA (at specific gene sites) or, more commonly, to mRNA derived from specific genes. This binding, in most cases, occurs via Watson and Crick-based nucleotide base pair complementarity. Binding prevents expression of the gene product by preventing either the transcription or the translation process (Figure 11.12). There are three major classes of antisense agents: antisense oligonucleotides, antigene sequences and ribozymes. Antisense oligonucleotides represent the family of antisense agents that have, thus far, received most attention by

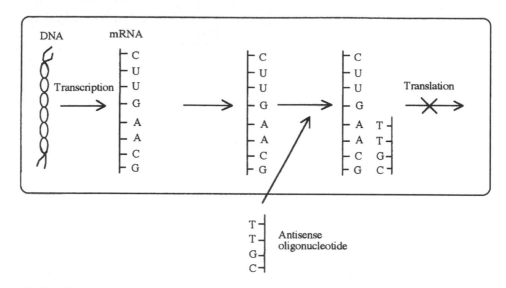

Figure 11.13. Outline of how an antisense oligonucleotide can prevent synthesis of a gene product by blocking translation. In practice, antisense oligos are 12–18 nucleotides in length. In many instances antisense binding is believed to occur in the nucleus

medical researchers. These are discussed below. Antigene sequences and ribozymes are briefly overviewed towards the end of this chapter.

Anti-sense oligonucleotides

The nucleotide sequence of a mRNA molecule contains the encoded blueprint which dictates the amino acid sequence of a protein. Because of this, the mRNA sequence is said to make 'sense' (this mRNA is therefore complementary to an 'antisense' DNA strand, i.e. it is the antisense strand of DNA in a given gene that serves as template for the mRNA synthesis). As long as at least part of the nucleotide sequences of any mRNA is known, it becomes potentially possible to chemically synthesize an oligonucleotide, either a ribo- or deoxyribo-nucleotide, whose base sequence is complementary to at least a section of the mRNA sequence. As long as such an 'antisense' oligonucleotide can enter the cell, the complementarity of sequences can promote hybridization between the mRNA and the antisense oligonucleotide (Figure 11.13).

Successful binding, however, does not depend alone upon Watson and Crick base complementarity. It is also influenced by higher-order secondary and tertiary structures adopted by the RNA. Intramolecular complementary base pairing can occur (particularly within transfer and ribosomal RNA, but also within messenger RNA), resulting in the formation of short duplex sequences, separated by stems and loops. Such higher-order structure seems to be functionally important, conferring recognition motifs for proteins and additional nucleic acids, as well as helping to stabilize the RNA. Regions engaged in intramolecular base pairing are obviously poor targets for antisense oligos. It is thus desirable to synthesize a nucleotide whose sequence is complementary to an accessible sequence along the mRNA backbone. Various approaches are taken to identify such suitable sequences (remember, the entire sequence of the mRNA will be known). The 'blind' or 'shotgun' approach entails synthesizing large numbers of oligos targeted to various (often overlapping) regions of the mRNA. The ability of each oligo to block translation of the mRNA is then directly assessed in an *in vitro* assay system using cell-free extracts. The second design approach entails the use of various computer programmes to interrogate the mRNA sequence in an attempt to predict its higher-order structure (and hence identify accessible sequences). This approach remains to be optimized. The translation initiation site of mRNAs are often popular targets because they are essential to translation and they are generally free from secondary structure. However, sequence homologies can exist within these sequences in unrelated genes. This reduces the specificity of the blocking effect and could lead to clinically significant side effects.

Binding results in the blocking of translation of the mRNA, and hence prevents synthesis of, the mature gene's protein product. Indeed, certain microorganisms appear to synthesize antisense molecules naturally as a means of regulating gene expression.

The prevention of mRNA translation by duplex formation with antisense oligonucleotides appears to be underpinned by twin mechanisms. First, the oligonucleotides act as steric blockers, i.e. prevent proteins involved in translation, or other aspects of mRNA processing, from binding to appropriate sequences in the mRNA. The generation of duplexes also likely allows targeting by intracellular RNases such as RNase H. This enzyme is capable of binding to RNA–DNA duplexes and degrading the RNA portion of the duplex (most synthetic antisense oligonucleotides are DNA-based).

Uses, advantages and disadvantages of 'oligos'

Antisense oligonucleotides ('oligos') are being assessed in pre-clinical and clinical studies as therapeutic agents in the treatment of cancer, as well as a variety of viral diseases (e.g. HIV, hepatitis B, herpes virus and papillomavirus infections). They also have potential application in treating other disease states for which blocking of gene expression would likely have a beneficial effect. Such medical conditions include restenosis, rheumatoid arthritis and allergic disorders. As potential drugs, antisense oligos display a number of desirable characteristics, the most significant of which is extreme specificity. Statistical analysis reveals that any specific base sequence of 17 or more bases is extremely unlikely to occur more than once in a human cell's nucleic acid complement. It thus follows that an oligonucleotide of 17 or more nucleotide units in length, which is designed to successfully duplex with a specific mRNA species, is unlikely to form a duplex with any other (unintended) mRNA species. Most synthetic oligos are therefore in the region of 17 nucleotides units long. These will display virtually an absolute specificity for the target sequence. Additional advantages of the oligonucleotide antisense approach include:

- minimal toxicity: thus far, most trials report few or no side effects. This is likely due to the highly specific nature of oligo duplexing, and the fact that they are 'natural' biomolecules;
- the requirement for only low levels of the oligo to be present inside the cell, as target mRNA is, itself, usually present only in nanomolar (nM) concentrations;
- the ability to manufacture oligos of specified nucleotide sequence is relatively straightforward using automated synthesizers.

However, native antisense oligonucleotides also suffer from a number of disadvantages, which include:

- sensitivity to nucleases;
- very low serum half-lives;

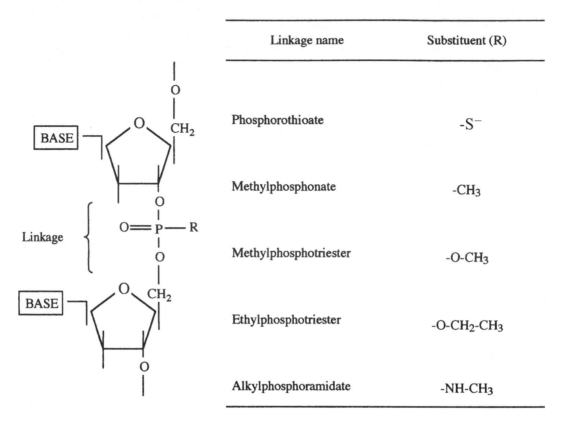

Linkage name	Substituent (R)
Phosphorothioate	$-S^-$
Methylphosphonate	$-CH_3$
Methylphosphotriester	$-O-CH_3$
Ethylphosphotriester	$-O-CH_2-CH_3$
Alkylphosphoramidate	$-NH-CH_3$

Figure 11.14.   Major types of modification potentially made to an oligo's phosphodiester linkage in order to increase its stability or enhance some other functional characteristic

- poor rate of cellular uptake;
- orally inactive.

Some progress has been made in overcoming such difficulties, and continued progress in the area is expected to render the next generation of oligos more therapeutically effective.

Native oligonucleotides display a 3′–5′ phosphodiester linkage in their backbone (Figure 11.14). These are sensitive to a range of nucleases naturally present in most extracellular fluids and intracellular compartments. The half-life of native oligonucleotides in serum is only ca. 15 min, and oligoribonucleotides are less stable than oligodeoxynucleotides. Selective modification of the native phosphodiester bond can render the product resistant to nuclease degradation.

Modification usually entails replacement of one of the free (non-bridging) oxygens of the phosphodiester linkage with an alternative atom or chemical group (Figure 11.14). Most commonly, the oxygen has been replaced with a sulphur atom and the resultant phosphoro-thioates display greatest clinical promise. Phosphorothioate-based oligos ('S'-oligos), display increased resistance to nuclease attack, while remaining water-soluble. They are also easy to synthesize chemically and display a biological half-life of up to 24 h. Most antisense oligos currently being assessed in clinical trials are S-oligos.

Delivery and cellular uptake of oligonucleotides

Oligo administration during many clinical trials entails direct i.v. infusion, often over a course of several hours. Although relatively stable in serum, the commonly employed phosphorothioate oligos (and indeed most other oligo types) encounter several barriers to reaching their final destinations. They bind various serum proteins, including serum albumin, as well as a range of heparin-binding and other proteins, which commonly occur on many cell surfaces. Targeting of naked oligos to specific cell types is therefore not possible. Following administration, these oligos tend to be distributed to many tissues, with the highest proportion accumulating in the liver and kidney.

The precise mechanism(s) by which oligos enter cells are not fully understood. Most are charged molecules, sometimes displaying a molecular mass of up to 10–12 kDa. Receptor-mediated endocytosis appears to be the most common mechanism by which charged oligos, such as phosphorothioates, enter most cells. One putative phosphorothioate receptor appears to consist of an 80 kDa surface protein, associated with a smaller 34 kDa membrane protein. However, this in itself seems to be an inefficient process, with only a small proportion of the administered drug eventually being transferred across the plasma membrane.

Uncharged oligos appear to enter the cell by passive diffusion, as well as possibly by endocytosis. However, elimination of the charges renders the resultant oligos relatively hydrophobic, thus generating additional difficulties with their synthesis and delivery.

Attempts to increase delivery of oligos into the cell centre mainly on the use of suitable carrier systems. Liposomes, as well as polymeric carriers (e.g. polylysine-based carriers), are gaining most attention in this regard. Details of such carriers have already been discussed earlier in this chapter.

An alternative system, which effectively results in the introduction of antisense oligonucleotides into the cell, entails the application of gene therapy. In this case, a gene which, when transcribed, yields (antisense) mRNA of appropriate nucleotide sequence, is introduced into the cell by a retroviral or other appropriate vector. This approach, as applied to the treatment of cancer and AIDS, is being appraised in a number of trials.

Oligos, including modified oligos, appear to be ultimately metabolized within the cell by the action of nucleases, particularly 3'-exonucleases. Breakdown metabolic products are then mainly excreted via the urinary route.

Manufacture of oligonucleotides

In contrast to the biopharmaceuticals thus far discussed (recombinant proteins and gene therapy plasmids), antisense oligonucleotides are manufactured by direct chemical synthesis. Organic synthetic pathways have been developed, optimized and commercialized for some time, as oligonucleotides are widely used reagents in molecular biology. They are required as primers, probes and for the purposes of site-directed mutagenesis. The basic synthetic strategy is very similar in concept to the means by which peptides are synthesized via the Merrifield method, as described in Chapter 2 (Box 2.1). The nucleotides required (themselves either modified or unmodified, as desired) are first reacted with a protecting chemical group. Each protected nucleotide is then coupled in turn to the growing end of the nucleotide chain, itself attached to a solid phase. After coupling, the original protecting group is removed and, when chain synthesis is complete, the bond anchoring the chemical to the solid phase is hydrolysed, releasing the free oligo. This may then be purified by HPLC. The most common synthetic method used is known as the phosphoramidite method, which uses a dimethoxytrityl (DMTr) protecting group and tetrazole as the coupling agent. Automated synthesizers are commercially available which can quickly and inexpensively synthesize oligos of over 100 nucleotides.

Vitravene, an approved antisense agent

On 26 August 1998, Vitravene became the first (and thus far apparently the only) antisense product to be approved for general medical use by the FDA. It gained approval within the European Union the following year, although it has since been withdrawn from the EU market for commercial rather than technical reasons. Vitravene is the trade name given to a 21-nucleotide phosphorothioate based product of the following base sequence:

5'-G–C–G–T–T–T–G–C–T–C–T–T–C–T–T–C–T–T–G–C–G-3'

Developed by the US company Isis, Vitravene is used to treat cytomegalovirus (CMV) retinitis in AIDS patients. It is formulated as a sterile solution in WFI (Chapter 3) using a bicarbonate buffer to maintain a final product pH of 8.7. Administration is by direct injection into the eye (intravitreal injection) and each ml of product contains 6.6 mg of active ingredient.

The product inhibits replication of human cytomegalovirus (HCMV) via an antisense mechanism. Its nucleotide sequence is complementary to a sequence in mRNA transcripts of the major immediate early region (IE2 region) of HCMV. These mRNAs code for several essential viral proteins and blocking their synthesis effectively inhibits viral replication.

Antigene sequences and ribozymes

Antigene sequences and ribozymes form two additional classes of antisense agents. However, the therapeutic potential of these agents is only now beginning to be appraised. Certain RNA sequences can function as catalysts. These so-called 'ribozymes' function to catalyse cleavage at specific sequences in a specific mRNA substrate. Many ribozymes will cleave their target mRNA where there exists a particular triplet nucleotide sequence G–U–C. Statistically, it is likely that this triplet will occur at least once in most mRNAs.

Ribozymes can be directed to a specific mRNA by introducing short-flanking oligonucleotides, which are complementary to the target mRNA (Figure 11.15). The resultant cleavage of the target obviously prevents translation. One potential advantage of ribozymes is that, as catalytic agents, a single molecule could likely destroy thousands of copies of the target mRNA. Such a drug should, therefore, be very potent.

'Antigene' (oligonucleotide) sequences function to inhibit transcription of a specific gene (as opposed to inhibition of translation of a mRNA species). These oligonucleotides achieve this by hybridizing with appropriate stretches of double-stranded DNA, forming a triple helix. This inhibits initiation of transcription of the genes in this region.

The binding of antigene sequences occurs only in the so-called 'major groove' of DNA. The incoming oligonucleotide does not disrupt the double-stranded DNA. It binds to it, forming what are termed 'Hoogsteen base pairs' — each base in the antigene sequence forming two new

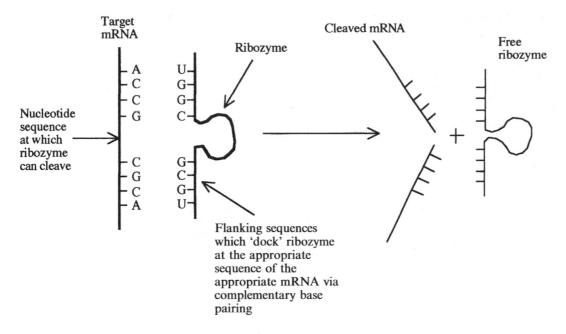

Figure 11.15. Outline of how ribozyme technology could prevent translation of specific mRNA, thus preventing synthesis of a specific target protein

hydrogen bonds with a purine base in the targeted region of the double helix. Much research, however, must be undertaken before it will become clear whether such antigene sequences will be of therapeutic use.

CONCLUSION

Every few decades, a medical innovation is perfected that profoundly influences the practice of medicine. Widespread vaccination against common infectious agents and the discovery of antibiotics serve as two such examples. Many scientists now believe that the potential of gene therapy and antisense technology rivals even the most significant medical advances achieved to date.

It is now just over a decade since the first nucleic acid-based drugs began initial tests. Several such drugs will likely be in routine medical use in less than one decade more. The application of gene technology could also change utterly the profile of biopharmaceutical drugs currently on the market. Virtually all such products are proteins, currently administered to patients for short or prolonged periods, as appropriate. Gene therapy offers the possibility of equipping the patient's own body with the ability to synthesize these drugs itself, and over whatever time scale is appropriate. Taken to its logical conclusion, gene therapy thus offers the potential to render obsolete most of the biopharmaceutical products currently on the market. Of all the biopharmaceuticals discussed throughout this text, nucleic acid-based drugs may well turn out to have the most profound influence on the future practice of molecular medicine.

FURTHER READING

Books

Blankenstein, T. (Ed.) (1999). *Gene Therapy: Principles and Applications*. Birkhauser-Verlag.
Crooke, S. (Ed.) (2001). *Antisense Drug Technology*. Marcel Dekker, New York.
Kresina, T. (Ed.) (2001). *An Introduction to Molecular Medicine and Gene Therapy*, Parts I and II. Wiley-Liss, New York.
Lowrie, D. (1999). *DNA Vaccines*. Humana, New York.
Phillips, M. (2000). *Antisense Technology (Methods in Enzymology*, Vol. 313). Academic Press, New York.
Stein, C. & Krieg, A. (1998). *Applied Antisense Oligonucleotide Technology*. Wiley, Chichester.

Articles

Gene therapy

Buchschacher, G. & Wong-Staal, F. (2001). Approaches to gene therapy for human immunodeficiency virus infection. *Human Gene Ther.* **12**(9), 1013–1019.
Davies, J. *et al.* (2001). Gene therapy for cystic fibrosis. *J. Gene Med.* **3**(5), 409–417.
Demeterco, C. & Levine, F. (2001). Gene therapy for diabetes. *Frontiers Biosci.* **6**, D175–D191.
Demoly, P. *et al.* (1997). Gene therapy strategies for asthma. *Gene Therapy* **4**(6), 507–516.
Docherty, K. (1997). Gene therapy for diabetes mellitus. *Clin. Sci.* **92**(4), 321–330.
Donnelly, J. (1997). DNA vaccines. *Ann. Rev. Immunol.* **15**, 617–648.
Felgner, P. (1997). Nonviral strategies for gene therapy. *Sci. Am.* **June**, 86–90.
Ferreira, G. *et al.* (2000). Downstream processing of plasmid DNA for gene therapy and DNA vaccine applications. *Trends Biotechnol.* 18(9), 380–388.
Lewin, A. & Hauswirth, W. (2001). Ribozyme gene therapy: applications for molecular medicine. *Trends Mol. Med.* **7**(5), 221–228.
Liras, A. (2001). Gene therapy for haemophilia: the end of a 'royal pathology' in the third millennium? *Haemophilia* **7**(5), 441–445.
Mhashilkar, A. *et al.* (2001). Gene therapy—therapeutic approaches and implications. *Biotechnol. Adv.* **19**(4), 279–297.
Moller, P. & Schadendorf, D. (1997). Somatic gene therapy and its implications in melanoma treatment. *Arch. Dermatol. Res.* **289**(2), 71–77.
Mulligan, R. (1993). The basic science of gene therapy. *Science* **260**, 926–931.
Pfeifer, A. & Verma, I. (2001). Gene therapy: promises and problems. *Ann. Rev. Genom. Hum. Genet.* **2**, 177–211.
Phillips, A. (2001). The challenge of gene therapy and DNA delivery. *J. Pharm. Pharmacol.* **53**(9), 1169–1174.
Robertson, J. & Griffiths, E. (2001). Assuring the quality, safety and efficacy of DNA vaccines. *Mol. Biotechnol.* **17**(2), 143–149.
Rosenberg, S. (1997). Cancer vaccines based on the identification of genes encoding cancer regression antigens. *Immunol. Today* **18**(4), 175–182.
Schatzlein, A. (2001). Non-viral vectors in cancer gene therapy: principles and progress. *Anti-cancer Drugs* **12**(4), 275–304.
Scott-Taylor, T. & Dalgeish, A. (2000). DNA vaccines. *Expert Opin. Invest. Drugs* **9**(3), 471–480.
Smith, A. (1995). Viral vectors in gene therapy. *Ann. Rev. Microbiol.* **49**, 807–838.
Smith, H. & Klinman, D. (2001). The regulation of DNA vaccines. *Curr. Opin. Biotechnol.* **12**(3), 299–303.
Wu, N. & Ataai, M. (2000). Production of viral vectors for gene therapy applications. *Curr. Opin. Biotechnol.* **11**(2), 205–208.

Antisense technology

Adah, S. *et al.* (2001). Chemistry and biochemistry of 2′-5′ oligoadenylate-based antisense strategy. *Cur. Med. Chem.* **8**(10), 1189–1212.
Akhtar, S. *et al.* (2000). The delivery of antisense therapeutics. *Adv. Drug Delivery Rev.* **44**(1), 3–21.
Askari, F. (1996). Molecular medicine: antisense-oligonucleotide therapy. *N. Engl. J. Med.* **334**(5), 316–318.
Galderisi, U. *et al.* (2001). Antisense oligonucleotides as drugs for HIV treatment. *Expert Opin. Therapeut. Patents* **11**(10), 1605–1611.
Hughes, M. *et al.* (2001). The cellular delivery of antisense oligonucleotides and ribozymes. *Drug Discovery Today* **6**(6), 303–315.
Lebedeva, I. & Stein, C. (2001). Antisense oligonucleotides: promise and reality. *Ann. Rev. Pharmacol. Toxicol.* **41**, 403–419.
Pawlak, W. *et al.* (2000). Antisense therapy in cancer. *Cancer Treatment Rev.* **26**(5), 333–350.

Reddy, D. (1996). Antisense oligonucleotides: a new class of potential anti-AIDS and anti-cancer drugs. *Drugs Today* **32**(2), 113–137.

Taylor, M. (2001). Emerging antisense technologies for gene functionalization and drug discovery. *Drug Discovery Today* **6**(15), S97–S101.

Wagner, R. & Flanagan, W. (1997). Antisense technology and prospects for therapy of viral infections and cancer. *Mol. Med. Today* **3**(1), 31–38.

Wickstrom, E. (1992). Strategies for administering targeted therapeutic oligodeoxynucleotides. *Trends Biotechnol.* **10**, 281–286.

Appendix 1

Biopharmaceuticals thus far approved in the USA or European Union

Notes: (a) Several products have been approved for multiple indications. Only the first indication for which each was approved is listed. (b) 'Vet' listing in therapeutic indication column indicates an animal application. All other products are used in human medicine.

Abbreviations: r=recombinant, rh=recombinant human, CHO=Chinese hamster ovary, BHK=baby hamster kidney, Mab=monoclonal antibody, tPA=tissue plasminogen activator, hGH=human growth hormone, FSH=follicle stimulating hormone, TSH=thyroid stimulating hormone, EPO=erythropoietin, GM-CSF=granulocyte-macrophage colony stimulating factor, IFN=interferon, IL=interleukin, HBsAg=hepatitis B surface antigen, PDGF=platelet-derived growth factor, TNFR=tumour necrosis factor receptor, *E. coli*=*Escherichia coli*, *S. cerevisiae*=*Saccharomyces cerevisiae*.

Product	Company	Therapeutic indication	Date approved
Recombinant blood factors			
Bioclate (rhFactor VIII produced in CHO cells)	Centeon	Haemophilia A	1993 (USA)
Benefix (rhFactor IX produced in CHO cells)	Genetics Institute	Haemophilia B	1997 (USA, EU)
Kogenate (rhFactor VIII produced in BHK cells. Also sold as **Helixate** by Centeon via a license agreement)	Bayer	Haemophilia A	1993 (USA), 2000 (EU)
Helixate NexGen (octocog-α; rhFactor VIII produced in BHK cells)	Bayer	Haemophilia A	2000 (EU)
NovoSeven (rhFactor VIIa produced in BHK cells)	Novo Nordisk	Some forms of haemophilia	1995 (EU), 1999 (USA)

(Continued)

Biopharmaceuticals: Biochemistry and Biotechnology, Second Edition by Gary Walsh
John Wiley & Sons Ltd: ISBN 0 470 84326 8 (ppc), ISBN 0 470 84327 6 (pbk)

Product	Company	Therapeutic-indication	Date approved
Recombinate (rhFactor VIII produced in an animal cell line)	Baxter Healthcare/ Genetics Institute	Haemophilia A	1992 (USA)
ReFacto (Moroctocog-α, i.e. B-domain-deleted rhFactor VIII produced in CHO cells)	Genetics Institute	Haemophilia A	1999 (EU), 2000 (USA)

Recombinant tissue plasminogen activator-based products

Activase (Alteplase, rh-tPA produced in CHO cells)	Genentech	Acute myocardial infarction	1987 (USA)
Ecokinase (Reteplase, rtPA; differs from human tPA in that three of its five domains have been deleted. Produced in *E. coli*)	Galenus Mannheim	Acute myocardial infarction	1996 (EU)
Retavase (Reteplase, rtPA; see Ecokinase)	Boehringer-Mannheim/ Centocor	Acute myocardial infarction	1996 (USA)
Rapilysin (Reteplase, rtPA; see Ecokinase)	Boehringer-Mannheim	Acute myocardial infarction	1996 (EU)
Tenecteplase (also marketed as Metalyse) (TNK-tPA, modified rtPA produced in CHO cells)	Boehringer-Ingelheim	Myocardial infarction	2001 (EU)
TNKase (Tenecteplase; modified rtPA produced in CHO cells; see Tenecteplase)	Genentech	Myocardial infarction	2000 (USA)

Recombinant hormones

Humulin (rhInsulin produced in *E. coli*)	Eli Lilly	Diabetes mellitus	1982 (USA)
Novolin (rhInsulin)	Novo Nordisk	Diabetes mellitus	1991 (USA)
Humalog (Insulin Lispro, an insulin analogue produced in *E. coli*)	Eli Lilly	Diabetes mellitus	1996 (USA, EU)
Insuman (rhInsulin produced in *E. coli*)	Hoechst AG	Diabetes mellitus	1997 (EU)
Liprolog (Bio Lysprol, a short-acting insulin analogue produced in *E. coli*)	Eli Lilly	Diabetes mellitus	1997 (EU)
NovoRapid (Insulin Aspart, short-acting rhInsulin analogue)	Novo Nordisk	Diabetes mellitus	1999 (EU)
Novomix 30 (contains Insulin Aspart, short acting rhInsulin analogue — see NovoRapid — as one ingredient)	Novo Nordisk	Diabetes mellitus	2000 (EU)
Novolog (Insulin Aspart, short-acting rhInsulin analogue produced in *S. cerevisiae*. See also Novorapid)	Novo Nordisk	Diabetes mellitus	2001 (USA)
Novolog mix 70/30 (contains Insulin Aspart, short-acting rhInsulin analogue, as one ingredient. See also Novomix 30)	Novo Nordisk	Diabetes mellitus	2001 (USA)

Product	Company	Therapeutic indication	Date approved
Actrapid/Velosulin/Monotard/ Insulatard/Protaphane/Mixtard/ Actraphane/Ultratard (All contain rhInsulin produced in *S. cerevisiae*, formulated as short–intermediate– long-acting products)	Novo Nordisk	Diabetes mellitus	2002 (EU)
Lantus (Insulin glargine, long- acting rhInsulin analogue produced in *E. coli*)	Aventis Pharmaceuticals	Diabetes mellitus	2000 (USA, EU)
Optisulin (Insulin glargine, long-acting rhInsulin analogue produced in *E. coli*. See Lantus)	Aventis Pharmaceuticals	Diabetes mellitus	2000 (EU)
Protropin (rhGH, differs from human hormone only by containing an additional N-terminal methionine residue. Produced in *E. coli*)	Genentech	hGH deficiency in children	1985 (USA)
Glucagen (rhGlucagon. produced in *S. cerevisiae*)	Novo Nordisk	Hypoglycaemia	1998 (USA)
Thyrogen (Thyrotrophin-α, rhTSH produced in CHO cells)	Genzyme	Detection/treatment of thyroid cancer	1998 (USA), 2000 (EU)
Humatrope (rhGH, produced in *E. coli*)	Eli Lilly	hGH deficiency in children	1987 (USA)
Nutropin (rhGH, produced in *E. coli*)	Genentech	hGH deficiency in children	1994 (USA)
Nutropin AQ (rhGH, produced in *E. coli*)	Schwartz Pharma AG	Growth failure, Turner's syndrome	2001 (EU)
BioTropin (rhGH)	Biotechnology General	hGH deficiency in children	1995 (USA)
Genotropin (rhGH, produced in *E. coli*)	Pharmacia and Upjohn	hGH deficiency in children	1995 (USA)
Saizen (rhGH)	Serono Laboratories	hGH deficiency in children	1996 (USA)
Serostim (rhGH)	Serono Laboratories	Treatment of AIDS- associated catabolism/ wasting	1996 (USA)
Norditropin (rhGH)	Novo Nordisk	Treatment of growth failure in children due to inadequate growth hormone secretion	1995 (USA)
Gonal F (rhFSH, produced in CHO cells)	Serono	Anovulation and superovulation	1995 (EU), 1997 (USA)
Puregon (rhFSH, produced in CHO cells)	N.V. Organon	Anovulation and superovulation	1996 (EU)
Follistim (follitropin-β, rhFSH produced in CHO cells)	Organon	Some forms of infertility	1997 (USA)
Luveris (lutropin-α; rhLH produced in CHO cells)	Ares-Serono	Some forms of infertility	2000 (EU)
Ovitrelle also termed **Ovidrelle**; (rhCG, produced in CHO cells)	Serono	Used in selected assisted reproductive techniques	2001 (EU), 2000 (USA)

Continued

Product	Company	Therapeutic indication	Date approved
Forcaltonin (r salmon calcitonin, produced in *E. coli*)	Unigene	Paget's disease	1999 (EU)

Haemopoietic growth factors

Product	Company	Therapeutic indication	Date approved
Epogen (rhEPO, produced in a mammalian cell line)	Amgen	Treatment of anaemia	1989 (USA)
Procrit (rhEPO, produced in a mammalian cell line)	Ortho Biotech	Treatment of anaemia	1990 (USA)
Neorecormon (rhEPO, produced in CHO cells)	Boehringer-Mannheim	Treatment of anaemia	1997 (EU)
Aranesp (darbepoetin-α; long-acting rEPO analogue produced in CHO cells)	Amgen	Treatment of anaemia	2001 (EU, USA)
Nespo (darbepoetin-α; see also Aranesp; long-acting rEPO analogue produced in CHO cells)	Dompe Biotec	Treatment of anaemia	2001 (EU)
Leukine (rGM-CSF, differs from the native human protein by one amino acid, Leu 23. Produced in *S. cerevisiae*)	Immunex	Autologous bone marrow transplantation	1991 (USA)
Neupogen (Filgrastim, rG-CSF; differs from human protein by containing an additional N-terminal methionine. Produced in *E. coli*)	Amgen	Chemotherapy-induced neutropenia	1991 (USA)
Neulasta (PEGfilgrastim, rPEGylated filgrastim—see Neupogen). Also marketed in EU as **Neupopeg**	Amgen	Neutropenia	2002 (USA, EU)

Recombinant interferons and interleukins

Product	Company	Therapeutic indication	Date approved
Intron A (rIFN-α-2b, produced in *E. coli*)	Schering Plough	Cancer, genital warts, hepatitis	1986 (USA), 2000 (EU)
PegIntron A (PEGylated rIFN-α-2b, produced in *E. coli*)	Schering Plough	Chronic hepatitis C	2000 (EU), 2001 (USA)
Viraferon (rIFN-α-2b, produced in *E. coli*)	Schering Plough	Chronic hepatitis B and C	2000 (EU)
ViraferonPeg (PEGylated rIFN-α-2b, produced in *E. coli*)	Schering Plough	Chronic hepatitis C	2000 (EU)
Roferon A (rhIFN-α-2a, produced in *E. coli*)	Hoffman-La Roche	Hairy cell leukaemia	1986 (USA)
Actimmune (rhIFN-γ-1b, produced in *E. coli*)	Genentech	Chronic granulomatous disease	1990 (USA)
Betaferon (rIFN-β-1b, differs from human protein in that Cys 17 is replaced by Ser. Produced in *E. coli*)	Schering AG	Multiple sclerosis	1995 (EU)
Betaseron (rIFN-β-1b, differs from human protein in that Cys 17 is replaced by Ser. Produced in *E. coli*)	Berlex Laboratories and Chiron	Relapsing, remitting multiple sclerosis	1993 (USA)

Product	Company	Therapeutic indication	Date approved
Avonex (rhIFN-β-1a, produced in CHO cells)	Biogen	Relapsing multiple sclerosis	1997 (EU), 1996 (USA)
Infergen (rIFN-α, synthetic type 1 interferon produced in *E. coli*)	Amgen (USA), Yamanouchi Europe (EU)	Chronic hepatitis C	1997 (USA), 1999 (EU)
Rebif (rh IFN-β-1a, produced in CHO cells)	Ares-Serono	Relapsing/remitting multiple sclerosis	1998 (EU), 2002 (USA)
Rebetron (combination of ribavirin and rhIFN-α-2b produced in *E. coli*)	Schering Plough	Chronic hepatitis C	(1999 USA)
Alfatronol (rhIFN-α-2b, produced in *E. coli*)	Schering Plough	Hepatitis B, C, and various cancers	2000 (EU)
Virtron (rhIFN-α-2b, produced in *E. coli*)	Schering Plough	Hepatitis B and C	2000 (EU)
Pegasys (PEGinterferon α-2a, produced in *E. coli*)	Hoffman-La Roche	Hepatitis C	2002 (EU, USA)
Vibragen Omega (rFeline interferon ω)	Virbac	Vet. (reduce mortality/ clinical signs of canine parvovirus)	2001 (EU)
Proleukin (rIL-2, differs from human molecule in that it is devoid of an N-terminal alanine and Cys 125 has been replaced by a Ser. Produced in *E. coli*)	Chiron	Renal cell carcinoma	1992 (USA)
Neumega (rIL-11, lacks N-terminal proline of native human molecule. Produced in *E. coli*)	Genetics Institute	Prevention of chemotherapy-induced thrombocytopenia	1997 (USA)
Kineret (anakinra; rIL-1 receptor antagonist produced in *E. coli*)	Amgen	Rheumatoid arthritis	2001 (USA)

Vaccines

Product	Company	Therapeutic indication	Date approved
Recombivax (rHBsAg produced in *S. cerevisiae*)	Merck	Hepatitis B prevention	1986 (USA)
Comvax (Combination vaccine, containing rHBsAg produced in *S. cerevisiae* as one component)	Merck	Vaccination of infants against *Haemophilus influenzae* type B and hepatitis B	1996 (USA)
Engerix B (rHBsAg, produced in *S. cerevisiae*)	SmithKline Beecham	Vaccination against hepatitis B	1998 (USA)
Tritanrix-HB (Combination vaccine, containing rHBsAg, produced in *S. cerevisiae* as one component)	SmithKline Beecham	Vaccination against hepatitis B, diphtheria, tetanus and pertussis	1996 (EU)
Lymerix (rOspA, a lipoprotein found on the surface of *Borrelia burgdorferi*, the major causative agent of Lyme's disease. Produced in *E. coli*)	SmithKline Beecham	Lyme disease vaccine	1998 (USA)
Infanrix-Hep B (Combination vaccine, containing rHBsAg produced in *S. cerevisiae* as one component)	SmithKline Beecham	Immunization against diphtheria, tetanus, pertussis and hepatitis B	1997 (EU)

Continued

Product	Company	Therapeutic indication	Date approved
Infanrix-Hexa (Combination vaccine, containing rHBsAg produced in *S. cerevisiae* as one component)	SmithKline Beecham	Immunization against diphtheria, tetanus, pertussis, polio, *H. influenzae* b and hepatitis B	2000 (EU)
Infanrix-Penta (Combination vaccine, containing rHBsAg produced in *S. cerevisiae* as one component)	SmithKline Beecham	Immunization against diphtheria, tetanus, pertussis, polio and hepatitis B	2000 (EU)
Ambirix (Combination vaccine, containing rHBsAg produced in *S. cerevisiae* as one component)	Glaxo SmithKline	Immunization against hepatitis A and B	2002 (EU)
Twinrix (Adult and paediatric forms in EU. Combination vaccine containing rHBsAg produced in *S. cerevisiae* as one component)	SmithKline Beecham (EU), Glaxo SmithKline (USA)	Immunization against hepatitis A and B	1996 (EU) (adult), 1997 (EU) (paediatric), 2001 (USA)
Primavax (Combination vaccine, containing rHBsAg produced in *S. cerevisiae* as one component)	Pasteur Mérieux MSD	Immunization against diphtheria, tetanus and hepatitis B	1998 (EU)
Procomvax (Combination vaccine, containing rHBsAg as one component)	Pasteur Mérieux MSD	Immunization against *H. influenzae* type B and hepatitis B	1999 (EU)
Hexavac (Combination vaccine, containing rHBsAg produced in *S. cerevisiae* as one component)	Aventis Pasteur	Immunization against diphtheria, tetanus, pertussis, hepatitis B, polio and *H. influenzae* type b	2000 (EU)
Triacelluvax (Combination vaccine containing r(modified) pertussis toxin)	Chiron SpA	Immunization against diphtheria, tetanus and pertussis	1999 (EU)
Hepacare (r S, pre-S and pre-S2 hepatitis B surface antigens, produced in a murine cell line)	Medeva Pharma	Immunization against hepatitis B	2000 (EU)
HBVAXPRO (rHBsAg produced in *S. cerevisiae*)	Aventis Pharma	Immunization of children and adolescents against hepatitis B	2001 (EU)
Porcilis Porcoli (combination vaccine containing r *E. coli* adhesins)	Intervet	Vet (active immunization of sows)	1996 (EU)
Fevaxyn Pentofel (Combination vaccine containing r feline leukaemia viral antigen as one component)	Fort Dodge Laboratories	Vet. (immunization of cats against various feline pathogens)	1997 (EU)
Porcilis AR-T DF (Combination vaccine containing a modified toxin from *Pasteurella multocida* expressed in *E. coli*)	Intervet	Vet. (reduction in clinical signs of progressive atrophic rhinitis in piglets: oral administration)	2000 (EU)

Product	Company	Therapeutic indication	Date approved
Porcilis pesti (vaccine containing r classical swine fever virus E_2 subunit antigen, produced in an insect cell baculovirus expression system)	Intervet	Vet. (immunization of pigs against classical swine fever virus)	2000 (EU)
Bayovac CSF E2 (vaccine consisting of r classical swine fever virus E_2 subunit antigen, produced using a baculovirus vector system)	Bayer	Vet. (immunization of pigs against classical swine fever virus)	2001 (EU)

Monoclonal antibody-based products

Product	Company	Therapeutic indication	Date approved
CEA-scan (Arcitumomab, murine Mab fragment (Fab), directed against human carcinoembryonic antigen, CEA)	Immunomedics	Detection of recurrent/ metastatic colorectal cancer	1996 (USA, and EU)
MyoScint (Imiciromab-Pentetate, murine Mab fragment directed against human cardiac myosin)	Centocor	Myocardial infarction imaging agent	1996 (USA)
OncoScint CR/OV (Satumomab Pendetide, murine Mab directed against TAG-72, a high molecular weight tumour-associated glycoprotein)	Cytogen	Detection/staging/ follow-up of colorectal and ovarian cancers	1992 (USA)
Orthoclone OKT3 (Muromomab CD3, murine Mab directed against the T lymphocyte surface antigen CD3)	Ortho Biotech	Reversal of acute kidney transplant rejection	1986 (USA)
ProstaScint (Capromab Pentetate, murine Mab directed against the tumour surface antigen PSMA)	Cytogen	Detection/staging/ follow-up of prostate adenocarcinoma	1996 (USA)
ReoPro (Abciximab, Fab fragments derived from a chimaeric Mab, directed against the platelet surface receptor $GPII_b/III_a$)	Centocor	Prevention of blood clots	1994 (USA)
Rituxan (Rituximab chimaeric Mab directed against CD20 antigen found on the surface of B lymphocytes)	Genentech/IDEC Pharmaceuticals	Non-Hodgkin's lymphoma	1997 (USA)
Verluma (Nofetumomab murine Mab fragments (Fab) directed against carcinoma-associated antigen)	Boehringer Ingelheim/NeoRx	Detection of small cell lung cancer	1996 (USA)
Zenapax (Daclizumab, humanized Mab directed against the α-chain of the IL-2 receptor)	Hoffman-La Roche	Prevention of acute kidney transplant rejection	1997 (USA), 1999 (EU)
Simulect (Basiliximab, chimaeric Mab directed against the α-chain of the IL-2 receptor)	Novartis	Prophylaxis of acute organ rejection in allogeneic renal transplantation	1998 (EU, USA)

Continued

Product	Company	Therapeutic indication	Date approved
Remicade (Infliximab, chimaeric Mab directed against TNF-α)	Centocor	Treatment of Crohn's disease	1998 (USA), 1999 (EU)
Synagis (Palivizumab, humanized Mab directed against an epitope on the surface of respiratory syncytial virus)	MedImmune (USA), Abbott (EU)	Prophylaxis of lower respiratory tract disease caused by respiratory syncytial virus in paediatric patients	1998 (USA), 1999 (EU)
Herceptin (Trastuzumab, humanized antibody directed against HER2, i.e. human epidermal growth factor receptor 2)	Genentech (USA), Roche Registration (EU)	Treatment of metastatic breast cancer if tumour overexpresses HER2 protein	1998 (USA), 2000 (EU)
Indimacis 125 (Igovomab, murine Mab fragment (Fab$_2$) directed against the tumour-associated antigen CA 125)	CIS Bio	Diagnosis of ovarian adenocarcinoma	1996 (EU)
Tecnemab KI (murine Mab fragments (Fab/Fab$_2$ mix) directed against HMW-MAA, i.e. high molecular weight melanoma-associated antigen)	Sorin	Diagnosis of cutaneous melanoma lesions	1996 (EU)
LeukoScan (Sulesomab, murine Mab fragment (Fab) directed against NCA 90, a surface granulocyte non-specific cross-reacting antigen)	Immunomedics	Diagnostic imaging for infection/inflammation in bone of patients with osteomyelitis	1997 (EU)
Humaspect (Votumumab, human Mab directed against cytokeratin tumour-associated antigen)	Organon Teknika	Detection of carcinoma of the colon or rectum	1998 (EU)
Mabthera (Rituximab, chimaeric Mab directed against CD20 surface antigen of B lymphocytes. See also Rituxan)	Hoffmann-La Roche	Non-Hodgkin's lymphoma	1998 (EU)
Mabcampath (EU) or **Campath** (USA) (Alemtuzumab; a humanized monoclonal antibody directed against CD52 surface antigen of B lymphocytes)	Millennium & ILEX (EU); Berlex, ILEX Oncology and Millennium Pharmaceuticals (USA)	Chronic lymphocytic leukaemia	2001 (EU, and USA)
Mylotarg (Gemtuzumab zogamicin; a humanized antibody–toxic antibiotic conjugate targeted against CD33 antigen, found on leukaemic blast cells)	Wyeth Ayerst	Acute myeloid leukaemia	2000 (USA)
Zevalin (Ibritumomab Tiuxetan, murine monoclonal antibody, produced in a CHO cell line, targeted against the CD20 antigen)	IDEC pharma-ceuticals	Non-Hodgkin's lymphoma	2002 (USA)

Product	Company	Therapeutic indication	Date approved
Additional products			
Beromun (rhTNF-α, produced in *E. coli*)	Boehringer-Ingelheim	Adjunct to surgery for subsequent tumour removal, to prevent or delay amputation	1999 (EU)
Revasc (Anticoagulant; hirudin produced in *S. cerevisiae*)	Ciba Novartis, Europharm	Prevention of venous thrombosis	1997 (EU)
Refludan (Anticoagulant; hirudin produced in *S. cerevisiae*)	Hoechst Marion Roussel (in USA), Behringwerke AG (in EU)	Anticoagulation therapy for heparin-associated thrombocytopenia	1998 (USA), 1997 (EU)
Cerezyme (rβ-Glucocerebrosidase, produced *in E. coli*. Differs from native human enzyme by one amino acid; Arg 495 is substituted with a His, also has modified oligosaccharide component)	Genzyme	Treatment of Gaucher's disease	1994 (USA), 1997 (EU)
Pulmozyme (dornase-α, rDNase produced in CHO cells)	Genentech	Cystic fibrosis	1993 (USA)
Fabrazyme (rhα-Galactosidase, produced in CHO cells)	Genzyme	Fabry's disease (α-galactosidase A deficiency)	2001 (EU)
Replagal (rhα-Galactosidase produced in a continuous human cell line)	TKT Europe	Fabry's disease (α-galactosidase A deficiency)	2001 (EU)
Fasturtec (Elitex in USA) (rasburicase; rUrate oxidase, produced in *S. cerevisiae*)	Sanofi-Synthelabo	Hyperuricaemia	2001 (EU), 2002 (USA)
Regranex (rhPDGF, produced in *S. cerevisiae*)	Ortho-McNeil Pharmaceuticals (USA), Janssen-Cilag (EU)	Lower extremity diabetic neuropathic ulcers	1997 (USA), 1999 (EU)
Vitravene (Fomivirsen, an antisense oligonucleotide)	ISIS Pharmaceuticals	Treatment of cytomegalovirus (CMV) retinitis in AIDS patients	1998 (USA)
Ontak (rIL-2–diphtheria toxin fusion protein, which targets cells displaying a surface IL-2 receptor)	Seragen inc/Ligand Pharmaceuticals	Cutaneous T cell lymphoma	1999 (USA)
Enbrel (rTNFR–IgG fragment fusion protein, produced in CHO cells)	Immunex (USA) Wyeth Europa (EU)	Rheumatoid arthritis	1998 (USA), 2000 (EU)
Osteogenic protein 1 (rhOsteogenic protein-1–BMP-7, produced in CHO cells)	Howmedica (EU), Stryker (USA)	Treatment of non-union of tibia	2001 (EU, and USA)
Inductos (Dibotermin-α; rBone morphogenic protein-2, produced in CHO cells)	Genetics Institute BV	Treatment of acute tibia fractures	2002 (EU)
Xigris (Drotrecogin-α; rh activated protein C, produced in a mammalian (human) cell line)	Eli Lilly	Severe sepsis	2001 (USA), 2002 (EU)

Appendix 2

Some Internet addresses relevant to the biopharmaceutical sector

Note: most home pages listed themselves contain relevant and extensive Internet site links

SOME BIOTECHNOLOGY/PHARMACEUTICAL/ MEDICAL ORGANIZATIONS

BIO home page

Site address: http://www.bio.org
Home page of the biotechnology industry organization. Also contains many excellent links.

Pharmaceutical researchers and manufacturers of America

Site address: http//phrma.org
Excellent site, providing information on a wide range of pharmaceutical issues, including reports such as the annual 'Biotechnology Medicines in Development' series.

Drug Information Association (DIA)

Site address: http://www.diahome.org
Home page of the DIA, contains information on various facets of the pharmaceutical industry, including pharmaceutical biotechnology.

European Association of Pharma Biotechnology (EAPB)

Site address: http://www.eapb.org
Home page of the EAPB, containing selected pharmaceutical biotechnology information.

Biopharmaceuticals: Biochemistry and Biotechnology, Second Edition by Gary Walsh
John Wiley & Sons Ltd: ISBN 0 470 84326 8 (ppc), ISBN 0 470 84327 6 (pbk)

European Federation of Biotechnology (EFB)

Site address: http://www.efbweb.org
Home page of the EFB, containing information on various facets of biotechnology, including pharmaceutical biotechnology.

World Health Organization (WHO)

Site address: http//www.who.int/en/
Excellent although general site. Contains information regarding e.g. global disease incidence, vaccination/immunization, etc.

REGULATORY AND ASSOCIATED SITES

Food and Drug Administration (FDA) home page

Site address: http://www.fda.gov
FDA home page. A key reference for regulatory issues (United States) for (bio)pharmaceutical development and production. Also contains information on approved products.

European Medicines Evaluation Agency (EMEA) home page

Site address: http://www.emea.eu.int
EMEA home page. A key reference for regulatory issues (European) for biopharmaceutical development and production. Also contains information on approved products.

International Conference on Harmonization (ICH)

Site address: http://www.ich.org
ICH home page. The International Conference on Harmonization of Technical Requirements for Registration of Pharmaceuticals for Human Use (ICH), a unique project that brings together the regulatory authorities of Europe, Japan and the USA, and experts from the pharmaceutical industry.

Pharmacos (European Commission)

Site address: http://pharmacos.eudra.org
Pharmaceuticals home page of the EC. Contains documents relating to various aspects of the European pharmaceutical industry, including the text of *The Rules Governing Medicinal Products in the EU* and a register of all approved pharmaceutical products.

US Patent Office

Site address: http://www.uspto.gov
This site from the US government contains a wealth of information on patenting of materials and has a searchable database of patents.

European Directorate for the Quality of Medicines

Site address: http//www.pheur.org
Houses information relating to various quality aspects of pharmaceuticals, including details of the *European Pharmacopoeia*.

United States Pharmacopoeia (USP)

Site address: http//www.usp.org
Houses information detailing the USP.

SOME BIOPHARMACEUTICAL COMPANIES

Amgen

Site address: http//www.amgen.com

Genentech

Site address: http//www.genentech.com

Biogen

Site address: http://www.biogen.com

Genzyme

Site address: http://www.genzyme.com

Wyeth

Site address: http://wyeth.com

Eli Lilly

Site address: http://www.lilly.com

Novo

Site address: http://www.novonordisk.com

Schering Plough

Site address: http//www.sch-plough.com/

PROTEINS AND GENES

The genome database

Site address: http//gdbwww.gdb.org
A focal database for human gene mapping that attempts to integrate physical and genetic maps.

The Institute for Genomics Research

Site address: http//www.tigr.org/tdb/
Excellent source of information regarding various completed/ongoing genome sequencing projects.

Databases at the European Bioinformatics Institute (EBI)

Site address: http//www.ebi.ac.uk/dbases/topdata.html
Databases at the EBI for nucleotide/protein searches (data largely overlap that at National Center for Biotechnology Information (NCBI)).

Protein Databank (PDB)

Site address: http//www.rcsb.org/pdb
Searchable repository of 3-D protein structure.

ExPASy

Site address: http//www.expasy.org/
Proteomics server of the Swiss institute of bioinformatics. Dedicated to analysis of protein sequences and structure, as well as 2-D SDS–PAGE.

PredictProtein

Site address: http//www.embl-heidelberg.de/Services/sander/predictprotein/
Submit a protein sequence and you will receive secondary structure prediction via e-mail.

Principles of Protein Structure

Site address: http//www.cryst.bbk.ac.uk/pps2
Provides information relating to protein structure, including some basic course material.

3D searching with receptor-based queries

Site address: http//www.ch.ic.ac.uk:80/ectoc/papers/guner/
This is an interesting site presenting information on the ability to search for molecules with similar chemical structures.

The Immunology Link

Site address: http://www.immunologylink.com
Site provides links to additional immunology-related sites.

American Society for Gene Therapy

Site address: http//www.asgt.org

European Society for Gene Therapy

Site address: http://www.esgt.org

Appendix 3

Two selected monographs reproduced from the *European Pharmacopoeia*, with permission from the European Commission*

I. RECOMBINANT DNA TECHNOLOGY, PRODUCTS OF

Producta ab ADN recombinante

This monograph provides general requirements for the development and manufacture of products of recombinant DNA technology. These requirements are not necessarily comprehensive in a given case and requirements complementary or additional to those prescribed in this monograph may be imposed in an individual monograph or by the competent authority.

The monograph is not applicable to modified live organisms that are intended to be used directly in man and animals, for example as live vaccines.

Definition

Products of rDNA technology are produced by genetic modification in which DNA coding for the required product is introduced, usually by means of a plasmid or a viral vector, into a suitable microorganism or cell line, in which that DNA is expressed and translated into protein. The desired product is then recovered by extraction and purification.

The cell or microorganism before harbouring the vector is referred to as the host cell, and the stable association of the two used in the manufacturing process is referred to as the host–vector system.

*Copyright holder: European Directorate for the Quality of Medicines

Biopharmaceuticals: Biochemistry and Biotechnology, Second Edition by Gary Walsh
John Wiley & Sons Ltd: ISBN 0 470 84326 8 (ppc), ISBN 0 470 84327 6 (pbk)

Production

Production is based on a validated seed-lot system using a host–vector combination that has been shown to be suitable to the satisfaction of the competent authority. The seed-lot system uses a master cell bank and a working cell bank derived from the master seed lot of the host–vector combination. A detailed description of cultivation, extraction and purification steps and a definition of the production batch shall be established.

The determination of the suitability of the host–vector combination and the validation of the seed-lot system include the following elements.

Cloning and expression

The suitability of the host–vector system, particularly as regards microbiological purity, is demonstrated by:

- *Characterization of the host cell, including source, phenotype and genotype, and of the cell-culture media. Documentation of the strategy for the cloning of the gene and characterization of the recombinant vector, including*:
  i.   the origin and characterization of the gene;
  ii. nucleotide-sequence analysis of the cloned gene and the flanking control regions of the expression vector. The cloned sequences are kept to a minimum and all relevant expressed sequences are clearly identified and confirmed at the RNA level. The DNA sequence of the cloned gene is normally confirmed at the seed-lot stage, up to and beyond the normal level of population doubling for full-scale fermentation. In certain systems, for example, where multiple copies of the gene are inserted into the genome of a continuous cell line, it may be inappropriate to sequence the cloned gene at the production level. Under these circumstances, Southern blot analysis of total cellular DNA or sequence analysis of the messenger RNA (mRNA) may be helpful, particular attention being paid to characterization of the expressed protein;
  iii. the construction, genetics and structure of the complete expression vector.
- *Characterization of the host–vector system, including:*
  i.   mechanism of transfer of the vector into the host cells;
  ii. copy number, physical state and stability of the vector inside the host cell;
  iii. measures used to promote and control the expression.

Cell banking system

The master cell bank is a homogeneous suspension of the original cells already transformed by the expression vector containing the desired gene, distributed in equal volumes into individual containers for storage (e.g. in liquid nitrogen). In some cases it may be necessary to establish separate master cell banks for the expression vector and the host cells.

The working cell bank is a homogeneous suspension of the cell material derived from the master cell bank(s) at a finite passage level, distributed in equal volumes into individual containers for storage (e.g. in liquid nitrogen).

In both cell banks, all containers are treated identically during storage and, once removed from storage, the containers are not returned to the cell stock.

The cell bank may be used for the production at a finite passage level or for continuous-culture production.

Production at a finite passage level

This cultivation method is defined by a limited number of passages or population doublings which must not be exceeded during production. The maximum number of cell doublings, or passage levels, during which the manufacturing process routinely meets the criteria described below, must be stated.

Continuous-culture production

By this cultivation method the number of passages or population doublings is not restricted from the beginning of production. Criteria for the harvesting as well as for the termination of production have to be defined by the manufacturer. Monitoring is necessary throughout the life of the culture: the required frequency and type of monitoring will depend on the nature of the production system and the product.

Information is required on the molecular integrity of the gene being expressed and on the phenotypic and genotypic characteristics of the host cell after long-term cultivation. The acceptance of harvests for further processing must be clearly linked to the schedule of monitoring applied and a clear definition of a 'batch' of product for further processing is required.

Validation of the cell banks

Validation of the cell banks includes:
i. stability, by measuring viability and the retention of the vector;
ii. identity of the cells by phenotypic features;
iii. where appropriate, evidence that the cell banks are free from potentially oncogenic or infective adventitious agents (viral, bacterial, fungal or mycoplasmal). Special attention has to be given to viruses that can commonly contaminate the species from which the cell line has been derived. Certain cell lines contain endogenous viruses, e.g. retroviruses, which may not readily be eliminated. The expression of these organisms, under a variety of condition known to cause their induction, shall be tested:
iv. for mammalian cells, details of the tumorigenic potential of the cell bank shall be obtained.

Control of the cells

The origin, form, storage, use and stability at the anticipated rate of use must be documented in full for all cell banks under conditions of storage and recovery. New cell banks must be fully validated.

Validation of the production process

Extraction and purification

The capacity of each step of the extraction and purification procedure to remove and/or inactivate contaminating substances derived from the host cell or culture medium, including, in particular, virus particles, proteins, nucleic acids and added substances, must be validated.

Validation studies are carried out to demonstrate that the production process routinely meets the following criteria:

- Exclusion of extraneous agents from the product. Studies including, for example, viruses with relevant physico-chemical features are undertaken, and a reduction capacity for such contaminants at each relevant stage of purification is established.
- Adequate removal of vector, host cell culture medium and reagent-derived contaminants from the product. The reduction capacity for DNA is established by spiking. The reduction of proteins of animal origin can be determined by immunochemical methods.
- Maintenance within stated limits of the yield of product from the culture.
- Adequate stability of any intermediate of production and/or manufacturing when it is intended to use intermediate storage during the process.

Characterization of the substance

The identity, purity, potency and stability of the final bulk product are established initially by carrying out a wide range of chemical, physical, immunochemical and biological tests. Prior to release, each batch of the product is tested by the by the manufacturer for identity and purity and an appropriate assay is carried out.

Production consistency

Suitable tests for demonstrating the consistency of the production and purification are performed. The tests include, especially, characterization tests, in-process controls and final-product tests, for example.

Amino acid composition

Partial amino acid sequence analysis.   The sequence data permit confirmation of the correct N-terminal processing and detection of the loss of the C-terminal amino acids.

Peptide mapping.   Peptide mapping using chemical and/or enzymatic cleavage of the protein product and analysis by a suitable method such as two-dimensional gel electrophoresis, capillary electrophoresis or liquid chromatography must show no significant difference between the test protein and the reference preparation. Peptide mapping can also be used to demonstrate correct disulphide bonding.

Determination of molecular mass

Cloned-gene retention.   The minimum amount in percentage of the cells containing the vector or the cloned gene after cultivation is approved by the relevant authority.

Total protein.   The yield of protein is determined.

Chemical purity.   The purity of the protein product is analysed in comparison with a reference preparation by a suitable method, such as liquid chromatography, capillary electrophoresis or sodium dodecyl sulphate polyacrylamide gel electrophoresis (SDS–PAGE).

Host-cell-derived proteins. Host-cell-derived proteins are detected by immunochemical methods, using, for example, polyclonal antisera raised against protein components of the host–vector system used to manufacture the product, unless otherwise prescribed. The following types of procedure may be used: liquid-phase displacement assays (e.g. radio-immunoassay), liquid-phase direct-binding assays and direct-binding assays using antigens immobilized on nitrocellulose (or similar) membranes (e.g. dot-immunoblot assays, Western blots). General requirements for the validation of immunoassay procedures are given under 2.7.1, *Immunochemical Methods*. In addition, immunoassay methods for host–cell contaminants meet the following criteria:

- *Antigen preparations.* Antisera are raised against a preparation of antigens derived from the host organism, into which has been inserted the vector used in the manufacturing process that lacks the specific gene coding for the product. This host cell is cultured, and proteins are extracted, using conditions identical to those used for culture and extraction in the manufacturing process. Partly purified preparations of antigens, using some of the purification steps in the manufacturing process, may also be used for the preparation of antisera.
- *Calibration and standardization.* Quantitative data are obtained by comparison with dose–response curves obtained using standard preparations of host-derived protein antigens. Since these preparations are mixtures of poorly defined proteins, a standard preparation is prepared and calibrated by a suitable protein determination method. This preparation is stored in a stable state suitable for use over an extended period of time.
- *Antisera.* Antisera contain high-avidity antibodies recognizing as many different proteins in the antigen mixture as possible, and do not cross react with the product.

Host-cell and vector-derived DNA.   Residual DNA is detected by hybridization analysis, using suitably sensitive sequence-independent analytical techniques or other suitably sensitive analytical techniques.

Hybridization analysis

DNA in the test sample is denatured to give single-stranded DNA, immobilized on a nitrocellulose or other suitable filter and hybridized with labelled DNA prepared from the host–vector manufacturing system (DNA probes). Although a wide variety of experimental approaches is available, hybridization methods for measurement of host–vector DNA meet the following criteria:

- *DNA probes.* Purified DNA is obtained from the host–vector system grown under the same conditions as those used in the manufacturing process. Host chromosomal DNA and vector DNA may be separately prepared and used as probes.
- *Calibration and standardization.* Quantitative data are obtained by comparison with responses obtained using standard preparations. Chromosomal DNA probes and vector DNA probes are used with chromosomal DNA and vector DNA standards, respectively. Standard preparations are calibrated by spectroscopic measurements and stored in a state suitable for use over an extended period of time.

- *Hybridization conditions.* The stringency of hybridization conditions is such as to ensure specific hybridization between probes and standard DNA preparations and the drug substances must not interfere with hybridization at the concentrations used.

Sequence-independent techniques

Suitable procedures include: detection of sulphonated cytosine residues in single-stranded DNA (where DNA is immobilized on a filter and cytosines are derivatized *in situ*, before detection and quantitation using an antibody directed against the sulphonated group); detection of single-stranded DNA using a fragment of single-stranded DNA bound to a protein and an antibody of this protein. Neither procedure requires the use of specific host or vector DNA as an assay standard. However, the method used must be validated to ensure parallelism with the DNA standard used, linearity of response and non-interference of either the drug substance or excipients of the formulation at the dilutions used in the assay.

Identification, tests and assay

The requirements with which the final product (bulk material or dose form) must comply throughout its period of validity, as well as specific test methods, are stated in the individual monograph.

Storage

See the individual monographs.

Labelling

See the individual monographs.

II. INTERFERON-α2 CONCENTRATED SOLUTION

(Interferoni-α2 solutio concentrata)

CDLPQTHSLG   SRRTLMLLAQ   MRX$_1$ISLFSCL   KDRHDFGFPQ
EEFGNQFQKA   ETIPVLHEMI   QQIFNLFSTK   DSSAAWDETL
LDKFYTELYQ   QLDNLEACVI   QGVGVTETPL   MKEDSILAVR
KYFQRITLYL   KEKKYSPCAW   EVVRAEIMRS   FSLTSNLQES
LRSKE

Definition

Interferon-α2 concentrated solution is a solution of a protein that is produced according to the information coded by the α2 sub-species of interferon-α gene and that exerts non-specific antiviral activity, at least in homologous cells, through cellular metabolic processes involving synthesis of both ribonucleic acid and protein. Interferon-α2 concentrated solution also exerts antiproliferative activity. Different types of interferon α2, varying in the amino acid residue at position 23, are designated by a letter in lower case.

Designation	Residue at position 23 (X_1)
α2a	Lys
α2b	Arg

This monograph applies to interferon-α2a and α2b concentrated solutions. The potency of interferon-α2 concentrated solution is not less than 1.4×10^8 IU per milligram of protein. Interferon-α2 concentrated solution contains not less than 2×10^8 IU of interferon-α2 per millilitre.

Production

Interferon-α2 concentrated solution is produced by a method based on recombinant DNA (rDNA) technology using bacteria as host cells. It is produced under conditions designed to minimize microbial contamination of the product. Interferon-α2 concentrated solution complies with the following additional requirements:

- *Host cell-derived proteins.*   The limit is approved by the competent authority.
- *Host cell- or vector-derived DNA.*   The limit is approved by the competent authority.

Characteristics

A clear, colourless or slightly yellowish liquid.

Identification

(A) It shows the expected biological activity (see Assay)
(B) Examine by isoelectric focusing

Test solution. Dilute the preparation to be examined with *water R* to a protein concentration of 1 mg/ml.

Reference solution. Prepare a 1 mg/ml solution of the appropriate *interferon-α2 CRS* in *water R*

Isoelectric point calibration solution, pI range 3.0–10.0. Prepare and use according to the manufacturer's instructions.
   Use a suitable apparatus connected with a recirculating temperature-controlled water bath set at 10°C and gels for isoelectric focusing with a pH gradient of 3.5–9.5. Operate the apparatus in accordance with the manufacturer's instructions. Use as the anode solution *phosphoric acid R* (98 g/l H_3PO_4) and as the cathode solution 1 *M sodium hydroxide*. Samples are applied to the gel by filter papers. Place sample application filters on the gel close to the cathode.
   Apply 15 μl of the test solution and 15 μl of the reference solution. Start the isoelectric focusing at 1500 V and 50 mA. Turn off the power after 30 min, remove the application filters and reconnect the power supply for 1 h. Keep the power constant during the focusing process. After focusing, immerse the gel in a suitable volume of a solution containing 115 g/l of

trichloroacetic acid R and 34.5 g/l of *sulphosalicylic acid R* in *water R* and agitate the container gently for 60 minutes. Transfer the gel to a mixture of 32 volumes of *glacial acetic acid R*, 100 volumes of *ethanol R* and 268 volumes of *water R*, and soak for 5 minutes. Immerse the gel for 10 minutes in a staining solution pre-warmed to 60°C in which 1.2 g/l of *acid blue 83 R* has been added to the previous mixture of glacial acetic acid, ethanol and water. Wash the gel in several containers with the previous mixture of glacial acetic acid, ethanol and water and keep the gel in this mixture until the background is clear (12 h to 24 h). After adequate destaining, soak the gel for 1 h in a 10% (V/V) solution of *glycerol R* in the previous mixture of glacial acetic acid, ethanol and water.

The principal bands of the electropherogram obtained with the test solution correspond in position to the principal bands of the electropherogram obtained with the reference solution. Plot the migration distances of the isoelectric point markers versus their isoelectric points and determine the isoelectric points of the principal components of the test solution and the reference solution. They do not differ by more than 0.2 pI units. The test is not valid unless the isoelectric point markers are distributed along the entire length of the gel and the isoelectric points of the of the principal bands in the electrogram obtained with the reference solution are between 5.8 and 6.3.

(C) Examine the electropherograms obtained under reducing conditions in the test for impurities of molecular masses differing from that of interferon-α2. The principal band in the electropherogram obtained with test solution (a) corresponds in position to the principal band in the electropherogram obtained with reference solution (a).

(D) Examine by peptide mapping

Test solution. Dilute the preparation to be examined in *water R* to a protein concentration of 1.5 mg/ml. Transfer 25 μl to a polypropylene or glass tube of 1.5 ml capacity. Add 1.6 μl of 1 *M phosphate buffer solution pH 8.0 R*, 2.8 μl of a freshly prepared 1.0 mg/ml solution of *trypsin for peptide mapping R* in *water R* and 3.6 μl of *water R* and mix vigorously. Cap the tube and place it in a waterbath at 37°C for 18 h, then add 100 μl of a 573 g/l solution of *guanidine hydrochloride R* and mix well. Add 7 μl of 154.2 g/l solution of *dithiothreitol R* and mix well. Place the capped tube in boiling water for 1 min. Cool to room temperature.

Reference solution. Prepare at the same time and in the same manner as for the test solution but use a 1.5 mg/ml solution of the appropriate *interferon-α2 CRS* in *water R*.

Examine by liquid chromatography (2.2.29). The chromatographic procedure may be carried out using:

- a stainless steel column 0.10 m long and 4.6 mm in internal diameter packed with *octadecylsilyl silica gel for chromatography R* (5 μm) with a pore size of 30 nm;
- as mobile phase at a flow rate of 1.0 ml/min. *Mobile phase A*; dilute 1 ml of *trifluoroacetic acid* to 1000 ml with *water R*; *Mobile phase B*; to 100 ml of *water R* add 1 ml of *trifluoroacetic acid R* and dilute to 1000 ml with *cetonitrile for chromatography R*;
- as detector a spectrophotometer set at 214 nm, maintaining the temperature of the column at 30°C.

Time (min)	Mobile phase A (% V/V)	Mobile phase B (% V/V)	Comment
0–8	100	0	Isocratic
8–68	100 → 40	0 → 60	Linear gradient
68–72	40	60	Isocratic
72–75	40 → 100	60 → 0	Linear gradient
75–80	100	0	Re-equilibration

Equilibrate the column with mobile phase A for at least 15 min. Inject 100 μl of the reference solution. The test is not valid unless the chromatogram obtained with each solution is qualitatively similar to the appropriate *Ph. Eur. Reference chromatogram of interferon-α2 digest.* The profile of the chromatogram obtained with the test solution corresponds to that of the chromatogram obtained with the reference solution.

Tests

Impurities of molecular mass differing from that of interferon-α2

Examine by SDS–PAGE (2.2.31). The test is performed under both reducing and non-reducing conditions, using resolving gels of 14% acrylamide and silver staining as the detection method.

- Sample buffer (non-reducing conditions). Mix equal volumes of *water R* and *concentrated SDS–PAGE sample buffer R.*
- *Sample buffer (reducing conditions).* Mix equal volumes of *water R* and *concentrated SDS–PAGE sample buffer for reducing conditions R* containing *2-mercaptoethanol* as the reducing agent.
- *Test solution (a).* Dilute the preparation to be examined in sample buffer to a protein concentration of 0.5 mg/ml.
- *Test solution (b).* Dilute 0.20 ml of test solution (a) to 1 ml with sample buffer.
- *Reference solution (a).* Prepare a 0.625 mg/ml solution of the appropriate *interferon-α2 CRS* in sample buffer.
- *Reference solution (b).* Dilute 0.20 ml of reference solution (a) to 1 ml with sample buffer.
- *Reference solution (c).* Dilute 0.20 ml of reference solution (b) to 1 ml with sample buffer.
- *Reference solution (d).* Dilute 0.20 ml of reference solution (c) to 1 ml with sample buffer.
- *Reference solution (e).* Dilute 0.20 ml of reference solution (d) to 1 ml with sample buffer.
- *Reference solution (f).* Use a solution of molecular mass standards suitable for calibrating SDS–PAGE gels in the range 15–67 kDa.

Place test and reference solutions, contained in covered test-tubes, in a waterbath for 2 min.

Apply 10 μl of reference solution (f) and 50 μl of each of the other solutions to the stacking gel wells. Perform the electrophoresis under the conditions recommended by the manufacturer of the equipment. Detect proteins in the gel by silver staining.

The test is not valid unless: the validation criteria are met (2.2.31); a band is seen in the electropherogram obtained with reference solution (e); and a gradation of intensity of staining is seen in the electropherograms obtained, respectively, with test solution (a) and test solution (b) and with reference solutions (a) to (e).

The electropherogram obtained with test solution (a) under reducing conditions may show, in addition to the principal band, less intense bands with molecular masses lower than the principal band. No such band is more intense than the principal band in the electropherogram with the reference solution (d) (1%) and not more than three such bands are more intense than the principal band in the electropherogram obtained with reference solution (e) (0.2%).

The electropherogram obtained with test solution (a) under non-reducing conditions may show, in addition to the principal band, less intense bands with molecular masses higher than the principal band. No such band is more intense than the principal band in the electropherogram obtained with reference solution (d). (1%) and not more than 3 such bands are more intense than the principal band in the electropherogram obtained with reference solution (e) (0.2%).

Related proteins

Examine by liquid chromatography (2.2.29).

- *Test solution*. Dilute the preparation to be examined with *water R* to a protein concentration of 1 mg/ml.
- *0.25% V/V hydrogen peroxide solution*. Dilute *dilute hydrogen peroxide solution R* in *water R* in order to obtain a 0.25% V/V solution.
- *Reference solution*. To a volume of the test solution, add a suitable volume of 0.25% V/V hydrogen peroxide solution to give a final hydrogen peroxide concentration of *0.005 % V/V*, and allow to stand at room temperature for 1 h, or for the length of time that will generate about 5% oxidized interferon. Add 12.5 mg of *L-methionine R* per millilitre of solution. Allow to stand at room temperature for 1 h. Store the solutions for not longer than 24 h at a temperature of 2–8°C. The chromatographic procedure may be carried out using:

    a stainless steel column 0.25 m long and 4.6 mm in internal diameter packed with *octadecylsilyl silica chromatography R* (5 μm) with a pore size of 30 nm,

    as mobile phase at a flow rate of 1.0 ml/min: *Mobile phase A*. To 700 ml of *water R* add 2 ml *of trifluoroacetic acid* R and 300 ml of *acetonitrile for chromatography R*; *Mobile phase B*. To 200 ml of *water R* add 2 ml *of trifluoroacetic acid* R and 800 ml of *acetonitrile for chromatography R*;

    as detector a spectrophotometer set at 210 nm.

Time (min)	Mobile phase A (%V/V)	Mobile phase B (% V/V)	Comment
0–1	72	28	Isocratic
1–5	72 $\longrightarrow$ 67	28 $\longrightarrow$ 33	Linear gradient
5–20	67 $\longrightarrow$ 63	33 $\longrightarrow$ 37	Linear gradient
20–30	63 $\longrightarrow$ 57	37 $\longrightarrow$ 43	Linear gradient
30–40	57 $\longrightarrow$ 40	43 $\longrightarrow$ 60	Linear gradient
40–42	40	60	Isocratic
42–50	40 $\longrightarrow$ 72	60 $\longrightarrow$ 28	Linear gradient
50–60	72	28	Re-equilibration

Equilibrate the column with the mobile phases in the initial gradient ratio for at least 15 min. Inject $50\,\mu l$ of each solution.

In the chromatograms obtained, interferon-α2 elutes at a retention time of about 20 min. In the chromatogram obtained with the reference solution a peak related to oxidized interferon appears at a retention time of about 0.9 relative to the principal peak. The test is not valid unless the resolution between the peaks corresponding to oxidized interferon and interferon is at least 1.0. Consider only the peak whose retention time is 0.7 and 1.4 relative to that of the principal peak. In the chromatogram obtained with the test solution, the area of any peak, apart from the principal peak, is not greater than 3.0% of the total area of all of the peaks. The sum of the areas of any peaks other than the principal peak is not greater than 5.0% of the total area of all the peaks.

Bacterial endotoxins (2.6.14)

Less than 100 IU in the volume that contains 1.0 mg of protein.

Assay

Protein

- *Test solution.* Dilute the preparation to be examined with water R to obtain a concentration of about 0.5 mg/ml of interferon-α2.
- *Reference solutions.* Prepare a stock solution of 0.5 mg/ml of *bovine albumin R*. Prepare 8 dilutions of the stock solution containing between $3\,\mu g/ml$ and $30\,\mu g/ml$ of bovine albumin R.

Prepare 30-fold and 50-fold dilutions of the test solution. Add 1.25 ml of a mixture prepared the same day by combining 2.0 ml of a 20 g/l solution of *copper sulphate R* in water R, 2.0 ml of a 40 g/l solution of *sodium tartrate R* in *water R* and 96.0 ml of a 40 g/l solution of *sodium carbonate R* in 0.2 M sodium hydroxide to test tubes containing 1.5 ml of *water R* (blank), 1.5 ml of the different dilutions of the test solution or 1.5 ml of the reference solutions. Mix after each addition. After approximately 10 min, add to each test-tube 0.25 ml of a mixture of equal volumes of *water R* and *phosphomolybdotungstic reagent R*. Mix each addition. After approximately 30 min, measure the absorbance (2.2.25) of each solution at 750 nm using blank as the compensation liquid. Draw a calibration curve (from the absorbances of the eight reference solutions; the corresponding protein contents and read from the curve the content of protein in the test solution.

Potency

The potency of interferon-α2 is estimated by comparing its effect to protect cells against a viral cytopathic effect with the same effect of the appropriate International Standard of human recombinant interferon-α2 or of a reference standard calibrated in International Units.

The International Unit is the activity contained in a stated amount of the appropriate International Standard. The equivalence in International Units of the International Standard is stated by the World Health Organization.

Carry out the assay by a suitable method, based on the following design.

Use, in standard culture conditions, an established cell line sensitive to the cytopathic effect of a suitable virus (a human diploid fibroblast cell line, free of microbial contamination, responsive to interferon and sensitive to encephalomyocarditis virus, is suitable).

The following cell cultures and virus have shown to be suitable: MDBK cells (ATCC No. CCL22), or Mouse L cells (NCTC clone 929; ATCC No. CCL I) as the cell culture and vesicular stomatitis virus VSV:Indiana strain (ATCC No. VR-158) as the infective agent; or human diploid fibroblast FS-71 cells responsive to interferon as the cell culture, and encephalomyocarditis virus (ATCC No. VR-129B) as the infective agent.

Incubate at least four series, cells with three or more different concentrations of the preparation to be examined and the reference preparation in a microtitre plate and include in each series appropriate controls of untreated cells. Choose the concentrations of the preparations such that the lowest concentration produces some protection and the largest concentration produces less than maximal protection against the viral cytopathic effect. At a suitable time add the cytopathic virus to the wells with the exception of a sufficient number of wells in all series, which are left with uninfected control cells. Determine the cytopathic effect of virus quantitatively with a suitable method. Calculate the potency of the preparation to be examined by the usual statistical methods for a parallel line assay.

The estimated potency is not less than 80% and not more than 125% of the stated potency. The fiducial limits of error of the estimated potency ($p = 0.95$) are not less than 64% and not more than 156% of the stated potency.

Storage

Store in an airtight container, protected from light, at or below $-20°C$.

Labelling

The label states:

- the type of interferon (α2a or α2b);
- the type of production.

Appendix 4

Annex 2 'Manufacture of biological medicinal products for human use'[1]

SCOPE

The methods employed in the manufacture of biological medicinal products are a critical factor in shaping the appropriate regulatory control. Biological medicinal products can be defined therefore largely by reference to their method of manufacture. Biological medicinal products prepared by the following methods of manufacture will fall under the scope of this annex[2]:

(a) Microbial cultures, excluding those resulting from rDNA techniques;
(b) Microbial and cell cultures, including those resulting from recombinant DNA or hybridoma techniques;
(c) Extraction from biological tissues;
(d) Propagation of live agents in embryos or animals.

Not all of the aspects of this annex may necessarily apply to products in category (a).

Note: In drawing up this guidance, due consideration has been given to the general requirements for manufacturing establishments and control laboratories proposed by the WHO.

The present guidance does not lay down detailed requirements for specific classes of biological products, and attention is therefore directed to other guidelines issued by the Committee for Proprietary Medicinal Products (CPMP), e.g. the note for guidance on monoclonal antibodies and the note for guidance on products of recombinant DNA technology (*The Rules Governing Medicinal Products in the European Community*, Volume III).

[1]From *The Rules Governing Medicinal Products in the European Community. Vol. 4, Good Manufacturing Practice for Medicinal Products*. Reproduced by permission of the European Union Publications Office, Luxembourg
[2]Biological medicinal products manufactured by these methods include: vaccines, immunosera, antigens, hormones, cytokines, enzymes and other products of fermentation (including monoclonal antibodies and products derived from rDNA).

Biopharmaceuticals: Biochemistry and Biotechnology, Second Edition by Gary Walsh
John Wiley & Sons Ltd: ISBN 0 470 84326 8 (ppc), ISBN 0 470 84327 6 (pbk)

PRINCIPLE

The manufacture of biological medicinal products involves certain specific considerations arising from the nature of the products and the processes. The way in which biological medicinal products are produced, controlled and administered make some particular precautions necessary.

Unlike conventional medicinal products, which are produced using chemical and physical techniques capable of a high degree of consistency, the production of biological medicinal products involves biological processes and materials, such as cultivation of cells or extraction of material from living organisms. These biological processes may display inherent variability, so that the range and nature of by-products are variable. Moreover, the materials used in these cultivation processes provide good substrates for growth of microbial contaminants.

Control of biological medicinal products usually involves biological analytical techniques which have a greater variability than physico-chemical determinations. In-process controls, therefore, take on a great importance in the manufacture of biological medicinal products.

PERSONNEL

1. All personnel (including those concerned with cleaning, maintenance or quality control) employed in areas where biological medicinal products are manufactured should receive additional training specific to the products manufactured and to their work. Personnel should be given relevant information and training in hygiene and microbiology.

2. Persons responsible for production and quality control should have an adequate background in a relevant scientific discipline, such as bacteriology, biology, biometry, chemistry, medicine, pharmacy, pharmacology, virology, immunology and veterinary medicine, together with sufficient practical experience to enable them to exercise their management function for the process concerned.

3. The immunological status of personnel may have to be taken into consideration for product safety. All personnel engaged in production, maintenance, testing and animal care (and inspectors) should be vaccinated, where necessary, with appropriate specific vaccines and have regular health checks. Apart from the obvious problem of exposure of staff to infectious agents, potent toxins or allergens, it is necessary to avoid the risk of contamination of a production batch with infectious agents. Visitors should generally be excluded from production areas.

4. Any changes in the immunological status of personnel, which could adversely affect the quality of the product, should preclude work in the production area. Production of BCG vaccine and tuberculin products should be restricted to staff who are carefully monitored by regular checks or immunological status or chest X-ray.

5. In the course of a working day, personnel should not pass from areas where exposure to live organisms or animals is possible to areas where other products or different organisms are handled. If such passage is unavoidable, clearly defined decontamination measures, including change of clothing and shoes and, where necessary, showering, should be followed by staff involved in any such production.

PREMISES AND EQUIPMENT

6. The degree of environmental control of particulate and microbial contamination of the production premises should be adapted to the product and the production step, bearing in mind the level of contamination of the starting materials and the risk to the finished product.

7. The risk of cross-contamination between biological medicinal products, especially during those stages of the manufacturing process in which live organisms are used, may require additional precautions with respect to facilities and equipment, such as the use of dedicated facilities and equipment, production on a campaign basis and the use of closed systems. The nature of the product, as well as the equipment used, will determine the level of segregation needed to avoid cross-contamination.

8. In principle, dedicated facilities should be used for the production of BCG vaccine and for the handling of live organisms used in production of tuberculin products.

9. Dedicated facilities should be used for the handling of *Bacillus anthracis*, of *Clostridium botulinum* and of *Clostridium tetani* until the inactivation process is accomplished.

10. Production on a campaign basis may be acceptable for other spore-forming organisms provided that the facilities are dedicated to this group of products and not more than one product is processed at any one time.

11. Simultaneous production in the same area, using closed systems of biofermenters, may be acceptable for products such as monoclonal antibodies and products prepared by rDNA techniques.

12. Processing steps after harvesting may be carried out simultaneously in the same production area provided that adequate precautions are taken to prevent cross-contamination. For killed vaccines and toxoids, such parallel processing should only be performed after inactivation of the culture or after detoxification.

13. Positive-pressure areas should be used to process sterile products but negative pressure in specific areas at point of exposure of pathogens is acceptable for containment reasons.

    Where negative-pressure areas or safety cabinets are used for aseptic processing of pathogens, they should be surrounded by a positive-pressure sterile zone.

14. Air filtration units should be specific to the processing area concerned and recirculation of air should not occur from areas handling live pathogenic organisms.

15. The layout and design of production areas and equipment should permit effective cleaning and decontamination (e.g. by fumigation). The adequacy of cleaning and decontamination procedures should be validated.

16. Equipment used during handling of live organisms should be designed to maintain cultures in a pure state and uncontaminated by external sources during processing.

17. Pipework systems, valves and vent filters should be properly designed to facilitate cleaning and sterilization. The use of 'clean in place' and 'sterilize in place' systems should be encouraged. Valves on fermentation vessels should be completely steam sterilizable. Air vent filters should be hydrophobic and validated for their scheduled lifespan.

18. Primary containment should be designed and tested to demonstrate freedom from leakage risk.

19. Effluents which may contain pathogenic microorganisms should be effectively decontaminated.

20. Due to the variability of biological products or processes, some additives or ingredients have to be measured or weighed during the production process (e.g. buffers). In these cases, small stocks of these substances may be kept in the production area.

ANIMAL QUARTERS AND CARE

21. Animals are used for the manufacture of a number of biological products, e.g. polio vaccine (monkeys), snake antivenoms (horses and goats), rabies vaccine (rabbits, mice and

hamsters) and serum gonadotropin (horses). In addition, animals may also be used in the quality control of most sera and vaccines, e.g. pertussis vaccine (mice), pyrogenicity (rabbits), BCG vaccine (guinea-pigs).

22. General requirements for animal quarters, care and quarantine are laid down in Directive 86/609/EEC. Quarters for animals used in production and control of biological products should be separated from production and control areas. The health status of animals from which some starting materials are derived, and of those used for quality control and safety testing, should be monitored and recorded. Staff employed in such areas must be provided with special clothing and changing facilities. Where monkeys are used for the production or quality control of biological medicinal products, special consideration is required as laid down in the current WHO Requirements for Biological Substances No. 7.

DOCUMENTATION

23. Specifications for biological starting materials may need additional documentation on the source, origin, method of manufacture and controls applied, particularly microbiological controls.

24. Specifications are routinely required for intermediate and bulk biological medicinal products.

PRODUCTION

Starting materials

25. The source, origin and suitability of starting materials should be clearly defined. Where the necessary tests take a long time, it may be permissible to process starting materials before the results of the tests are available. In such cases, release of a finished product is conditional on satisfactory results of these tests.

26. Where sterilization of starting materials is required, it should be carried out, where possible, by heat. Where necessary, other appropriate methods may also be used for inactivation of biological materials (e.g. irradiation).

Seed lot and cell bank system

27. In order to prevent the unwanted drift of properties which might ensue from repeated subcultures or multiple generations, the production of biological medicinal products obtained by microbial culture, cell culture or propagation in embryos and animals should be based on a system of master and working seed lots and/or cell banks.

28. The number of generations (doublings, passages) between the seed lot or cell bank and the finished product should be consistent with the marketing authorization dossier. Scaling up of the process should not change this fundamental relationship.

29. Seed lots and cell banks should be adequately characterized and tested for contaminants. Their suitability for use should be further demonstrated by the consistency of the characteristics and quality of the successive batches of product. Seed lots and cell banks should be established, stored and used in such a way as to minimize the risks of contamination or alteration.

30. Establishment of the seed lot and cell bank should be performed in a suitably controlled environment to protect the seed lot and the cell bank and, if applicable, the personnel handling it. During the establishment of the seed lot and cell bank, no other living or infectious material (e.g. virus, cell lines or cell strains) should be handled simultaneously in the same area or by the same persons.

31. Evidence of the stability and recovery of the seeds and banks should be documented. Storage containers should be hermetically sealed, clearly labelled and kept at an appropriate temperature. An inventory should be meticulously kept. Storage temperature should be recorded continuously for freezers and properly monitored for liquid nitrogen. Any deviation from set limits and any corrective action taken should be recorded.

32. Only authorized personnel should be allowed to handle the material and this handling should be done under the supervision of a responsible person. Access to stored material should be controlled. Different seed lots or cell banks should be stored in such a way to avoid confusion or cross-contamination. It is desirable to split the seed lots and cell banks and to store the parts at different locations so as to minimize the risks of total loss.

33. All containers of master or working cell banks and seed lots should be treated identically during storage. Once removed from storage, the containers should not be returned to the stock.

Operating principles

34. The growth-promoting properties of culture media should be demonstrated.

35. Addition of materials or cultures to fermenters and other vessels, and the taking of samples, should be carried out under carefully controlled conditions to ensure that absence of contamination is maintained. Care should be taken to ensure that vessels are correctly connected when addition or sampling take place.

36. Centrifugation and blending of products can lead to aerosol formation and containment of such activities to prevent transfer of live microorganisms is necessary.

37. If possible, media should be sterilized *in situ*. In-line sterilizing filters for routine addition of gases, media, acids or alkalis, defoaming agents, etc., to fermenters should be used where possible.

38. Careful consideration should be given to the validation of any necessary virus removal or inactivation undertaken (see CPMP notes for guidelines).

39. In cases where a virus inactivation or removal process is performed during manufacture, measures should be taken to avoid the risk of recontamination of treated products by non-treated products.

40. A wide variety of equipment is used for chromatography and, in general, such equipment should be dedicated to the purification of one product and should be sterilized or sanitized between batches. The use of the same equipment at different stages of processing should be discouraged. Acceptance criteria, lifespan and sanitation or sterilization method of columns should be defined.

QUALITY CONTROL

41. In-process controls play a specially important role in ensuring the consistency of the quality of biological medicinal products. Those controls which are crucial for quality (e.g. virus

removal) but which cannot be carried out on the finished product, should be performed at an appropriate stage of production.

42. It may be necessary to retain samples of intermediate products in sufficient quantities, and under appropriate storage conditions, to allow the repetition or confirmation of a batch control.

43. Continuous monitoring of certain production processes is necessary, e.g. fermentation. Such data should form part of the batch record.

44. Where continuous culture is used, special consideration should be given to the quality control requirements arising from this type of production method.

Index

Page numbers in *italic* indicate figures or tables.

Biopharmaceuticals: Biochemistry and Biotechnology, Second Edition by Gary Walsh
John Wiley & Sons Ltd: ISBN 0 470 84326 8 (ppc), ISBN 0 470 84327 6 (pbk)

sex hormones *13*, 14–19
Shc 290
sheep
    defleecing 287
    milk 118
Shope fibroma virus 196
short stature 283, 327, 328–30
shotgun approach 490–1
sickle cell anaemia 353, 483
Sicor 10
silkworms 123, 124, 219
silver-binding method *163*, 164
Simulect *416*, 435, *505*
sindbis virus 473
single nucleotide polymorphisms (SNPs) 52
single peak insulins 310
sissomicin *38*
site-directed mutagenesis 5, 7
size exclusion HPLC 168
Smad proteins 293
smallpox 446
SmithKline Beecham 441, *442, 503, 504*
snake venom 5
    antisera *406*, 408–9
SNT-1 290
SOCS/Jab/Cis family 202
sodium caprylate 356
sodium dodecyl sulphate polyacrylamide gel elec-
    trophoresis (SDS–PAGE) 164, *165*
sodium hydroxide 104
soft tissue sarcoma 252
somatomedins 279
somatorelin 324
somatostatin 325
somatotrophin 9, 324
sorbitol *152*
Sorin *416, 506*
Span 456
specifications 110
sperm cell production 334
spider antivenins *406*, 408–9
split synthesis 56–7, *60*
Spodoptera frugiperda 123
Src 290
stabilizing agents 143, 150–2
standard operating procedures (SOPs) 110
stanozolol *15, 16*
staphylokinase *381*, 386–8
starvation 283
STATs 200
steam 178
stem cells 255, 484, 486
sterility testing 180
steroid (sex) hormones *13*, 14–19
stilboesterol 15, *17, 18*
stomach acid 66

stomach ulcers 29
streptokinase *381*, 385
streptomycin 35, 38
Streptozon *7*
stress response 330
stroke 372, 381
structural genomics 50
structure-based drug design 54
Stryker *507*
Stuart factor *359*
study population 75
subfertility 339, 341–2, 344
subunit vaccines 441–4, 451
succinylation 390
sufficiency of disclosure 62
sulpha drugs 4, *6, 7*
sulphanilamide *6, 7*
superovulation 339, 344–5
superoxide dismutase 397
superoxide radical 397
surfactant
    lungs 67, 260
    stabilizers 152
SV40 427
swine fever vaccine 124
Synagis *416, 506*
synapse 295
Syntex adjuvant formulation-1 (SAF-1) 458
synthetic immune libraries 414
syphilis 3

T-bag synthesis 56
T cell growth factor 225
T cytotoxic cells 191
T helper cells 191
T helper type 1 lymphocytes 244
T lymphocytes 191, 417
T suppressor cells 191
tamoxifen 16, *18*
targeted screening 53
tat 487
taxol *4, 28, 31*, 32–3
^{99m}TC (technetium) 420–1
Tecnemab-K-1 421–2
Tecnemab KI *416, 506*
Tenecteplase *381*, 385, *500*
teratogenicity 71
terpenoids 30–3
tertiary structure analysis 173
testosterone 14, *15, 16*, 335, 336, 337
testosterone–oestradiol binding globulin (TEBG)
    14
tetanus
    antitoxin *406*
    immunoglobulin *406*, 408
    vaccine *438*, 440